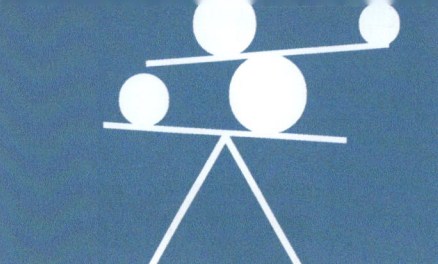

HEALTH SERVICES MANAGEMENT

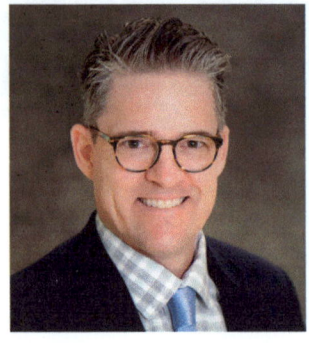

ZACHARY PRUITT, PhD, MHA, FACHE, is an associate professor at the University of South Florida College of Public Health. Dr. Pruitt teaches health services management, quality management, strategic planning, and topics related to the U.S. healthcare delivery system. Dr. Pruitt cowrote *Healthcare Quality Management: A Case Study Approach*, also from Springer Publishing Company, LLC, and has written a variety of book chapters, including the health care management chapter in *Jonas and Kovner's Health Care Delivery in the United States*. His health services research scholarship relates to the integration of medical and social care services. Dr. Pruitt is a Fellow of the American College of Healthcare Executives and of the Commission on Accreditation of Healthcare Management Education. He serves on the board of directors for the Association of University Programs in Health Administration. He earned his bachelor's degree from the University of Texas at Austin and his Master of Health Administration and doctorate in health services research from the University of South Florida.

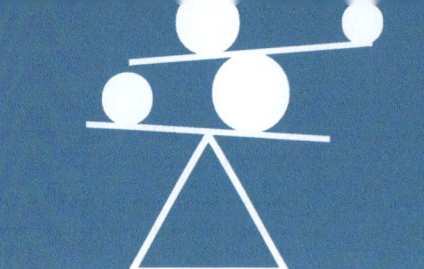

HEALTH SERVICES MANAGEMENT

COMPETENCIES AND CAREERS

Zachary Pruitt, PhD, MHA, FACHE

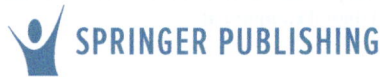

Copyright © 2025 Springer Publishing Company, LLC
All rights reserved.

No part of this publication may be reproduced, stored in a retrieval system, or transmitted in any form or by any means, electronic, mechanical, photocopying, recording, or otherwise, without the prior permission of Springer Publishing Company, LLC, or authorization through payment of the appropriate fees to the Copyright Clearance Center, Inc., 222 Rosewood Drive, Danvers, MA 01923, 978-750-8400, fax 978-646-8600, info@copyright.com or at www.copyright.com.

Springer Publishing Company, LLC
902 Carnegie Center, Suite 140, Princeton, NJ 08540
www.springerpub.com
connect.springerpub.com

Acquisitions Editor: David D'Addona
Compositor: Amnet
Production Editor: Joseph Stubenrauch

ISBN: 978-0-8261-4806-3
ebook ISBN: 978-0-8261-4807-0
DOI: 10.1891/9780826148070

SUPPLEMENTS:

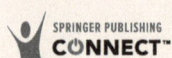

A robust set of instructor resources designed to supplement this text is located at http://connect.springerpub.com/content/book/978-0-8261-4807-0.
Qualifying instructors may request access by emailing textbook@springerpub.com.

Instructor Materials:
LMS Common Cartridge–With All Instructor Resources ISBN: 978-0-8261-7989-0
Instructor Manual ISBN: 978-0-8261-4808-7
Instructor Test Bank ISBN: 978-0-8261-4805-6
Instructor PowerPoint Presentations ISBN: 978-0-8261-4809-4
Instructor Sample Syllabus ISBN: 978-0-8261-5726-3

Student Materials:
Informational Interviews Transcripts ISBN: 978-0-8261-4817-9

24 25 26 27 / 5 4 3 2 1

The author and the publisher of this Work have made every effort to use sources believed to be reliable to provide information that is accurate and compatible with the standards generally accepted at the time of publication. The author and publisher shall not be liable for any special, consequential, or exemplary damages resulting, in whole or in part, from the readers' use of, or reliance on, the information contained in this book. The publisher has no responsibility for the persistence or accuracy of URLs for external or third-party Internet websites referred to in this publication and does not guarantee that any content on such websites is, or will remain, accurate or appropriate.

Library of Congress Cataloging-in-Publication Data
Names: Pruitt, Zachary, author.
Title: Health services management : competencies and careers / Zachary Pruitt.
Description: First Springer Publishing edition. | New York : Springer Publishing Company, 2024. | Includes bibliographical references and index.
Identifiers: LCCN 2024024572 (print) | LCCN 2024024573 (ebook) | ISBN 9780826148063 | ISBN 9780826148070 (ebook)
Subjects: MESH: Health Services Administration | Administrators | United States
Classification: LCC RA425 (print) | LCC RA425 (ebook) | NLM W 84 AA1 | DDC 362.1--dc23/eng/20240723
LC record available at https://lccn.loc.gov/2024024572
LC ebook record available at https://lccn.loc.gov/2024024573

Contact sales@springerpub.com to receive discount rates on bulk purchases.

Publisher's Note: **New and used products purchased from third-party sellers are not guaranteed for quality, authenticity, or access to any included digital components.**

Printed in the United States of America.

CONTENTS

Informational Interviews xix
Preface xxiii
Resources xxvii

1. ROLE OF THE HEALTH SERVICES MANAGER 1

Competencies 1
Chapter Outline 1
Introduction 1
Management Practices 2
    Fayol's Management Functions 2
    Drucker's Five Basic Functions of the Manager 3
    Mintzberg's Management Roles 4
    Definitions of Management 5
    Management and Systems Theory 7
Health Services Management 8
    Evolution of the Health Services Manager 8
    Responsibilities of Health Services Managers 9
    Managing in the Continuum of Care 10
    Inpatient Settings 11
    Outpatient Settings 12
    Long-Term Care Settings 14
    Ancillary Services 15
    Operations Support Services 15
Competencies of Health Services Management 17
    Fundamental Domains of Competencies 17
    Management Challenges Unique to the Healthcare Sector 18
    Contributing to the Interprofessional Team 18
    Diversity, Equity, and Inclusion 21
Health Services Management Careers 22
    Managing Oneself 22
    Managing Careers 23
Future Directions 24
Summary 24
Key Terms 24
Learning Activities 25
    Professional Development and Reflection 25
    Discussion Questions 25
Recommended Reading and Media 26
References 26

2. PROBLEM-SOLVING AND EVIDENCE-BASED MANAGEMENT 31

Competencies 31
Chapter Outline 31
Introduction 31
Evidence-Based Management 32
    Critical Thinking and Bias 32
    Evidence-Based Problem-Solving 34
    Systematic Approaches to Problem-Solving 34
Define Problems 36
    Stakeholder Analysis 36
    Problem Analysis 37
    Framing and Reframing Problems 40
Identify Potential Solutions and Generate Hypotheses 42
    Hypothesis-Driven Thinking 43
    Set Decision Criteria 43
Analyze Alternative Solutions 45
    Analytical Plan 45
    Analysis of Alternative Solutions 46
    Sources of Data 47
    Synthesize Findings, Conclusions, and Recommendations 48
    Transform Decisions Into Action 50
Future Directions 50
Summary 50
Key Terms 51
Learning Activities 51
    Professional Development and Reflection 51
    Discussion Questions 52
Recommended Reading and Media 52
References 52

3. MANAGING INTERPERSONAL COMMUNICATIONS 57

Competencies 57
Chapter Outline 57
Introduction 57
Interpersonal Communications 58
    Managing Interpersonal Relationships 58
    Creating Psychological Safety 59
    Managing Conflict 61
    Negotiating and Contracting 62
Professional Reputation 64
    Executive Presence 64
    Personal Brand 65
    Networking 66
Communicating in Meetings 67

  Participating in Meetings *67*
  Planning, Coordinating, and Facilitating Meetings *67*
  Types of Meetings *68*
 Presentation Skills *70*
  Verbal Presentation Competency *70*
  Presentation Delivery *71*
  Presentation Content *72*
  Presentation Materials *76*
 Written Communications *76*
  Business Writing Style *76*
  Business Reports *76*
  Emails and Collaboration Tools *78*
 Future Directions *78*
 Summary *79*
 Key Terms *79*
 Learning Activities *80*
  Professional Development and Reflection *80*
  Discussion Questions *80*
 Recommended Reading and Media *80*
 References *81*

4. LEADERSHIP AND CHANGE MANAGEMENT *87*

 Competencies *87*
 Chapter Outline *87*
 Introduction *87*
 Vision Setting *88*
  Management and Leadership *88*
  Imagining the Future *89*
  Gaining Commitment to a Shared Vision *89*
  Planning Future Action *90*
 Leadership and Organizational Culture *90*
  Role Modeling *90*
  Teamwork and Collaborative Leadership *91*
  Positive Theories of Leadership *93*
  Leadership Styles *94*
 Emotional and Social Intelligence *96*
  Emotional Intelligence Model *96*
  Self-Awareness *96*
  Self-Management *97*
  Social Awareness *98*
  Relationship Management *99*
 Power and Influence *99*
  Dark-Side Leaders *99*
  Self-Protective Behaviors *100*
  Sources of Power *101*
  Political Skill *102*
  Checks on Power and Abusive Behaviors *102*

Change Management   *103*
   A Leadership Process   *103*
   Kotter's 8 Steps of Change   *104*
Future Directions   *107*
Summary   *108*
Key Terms   *108*
Learning Activities   *109*
   Professional Development and Reflection   *109*
   Discussion Questions   *109*
Recommended Reading and Media   *109*
References   *110*

5. PROFESSIONALISM AND ETHICS   117

Competencies   *117*
Chapter Outline   *117*
Introduction   *117*
Professionalism   *118*
   Trusting Relationships   *118*
   Education   *118*
   Credentials   *119*
   Adapting to Organizational Norms   *120*
   Work Ethic   *121*
   Self-Management   *123*
   Lifelong Learning   *123*
   Contribute to the Community   *123*
   Build Professional Connections   *124*
   Valuing Diversity, Equity, and Inclusion   *126*
   Integrity   *126*
Professional Ethics   *127*
   Ethics for Health Services Managers   *127*
   Ethical Analysis and Decision-Making   *129*
   Ethical Dilemmas in Business of Healthcare   *129*
Organizational Ethics   *131*
   Creating Ethical Cultures   *131*
   Compliance Programs   *132*
Clinical and Research Ethics   *134*
   Clinical Ethics   *134*
   Research Ethics   *135*
Future Directions   *136*
Summary   *136*
Key Terms   *137*
Learning Activities   *138*
   Professional Development and Reflection   *138*
   Discussion Questions   *138*
Recommended Reading and Media   *138*
References   *139*

6. POPULATION HEALTH AND COMMUNITY COLLABORATION   *145*

Competencies   145
Chapter Outline   145
Introduction   145
Population Health Assessment   146
   Community Health Needs Assessments   146
   Community Stakeholders   146
   Geographic and Demographic Characteristics   147
   Community Assets   148
   Health Status   148
   Health Behaviors   149
   Physical Environment   151
   Social and Economic Factors   151
Population Health Management   153
   Management Functions in Population Health   153
   Population Health Financial Management   153
   Value-Based Health Care Organizational Design   155
   Health Information Technology   157
   Program Planning and Evaluation   157
   Cost-Efficient Care   158
   Health Promotion   159
   Integrating Medical and Social Care   159
Community Collaboration   160
   Community Engagement   160
   Health Policy Advocacy   160
   Anchor Institutions   161
   Emergency Preparedness and Response   162
   Community Volunteerism   163
Future Directions   163
Summary   163
Key Terms   164
Learning Activities   165
   Professional Development and Reflection   165
   Discussion Questions   165
Recommended Reading and Media   165
References   166

7. HEALTHCARE GOVERNANCE   *171*

Competencies   171
Chapter Outline   171
Introduction   171
Role of Management in Governance   172
   Relationship Between the Board and the CEO   172
   Support the Board of Directors   174

Engage Medical Staff in Governance   174
Include Nurses and Other Clinicians in Governance   175
Role of Boards of Directors in Governance   175
  Set the Strategic Direction   175
  Oversee Management and Clinicians   176
  Recruit New Board Members   177
  Ethical Principles of Board Practice   178
  Representation of External Stakeholders   179
Role of Clinicians in Governance   179
  Medical Staff Governance   179
  Shared Governance Councils   180
  Medical Practice and Other Governance Structures   181
Role of Patients in Governance   183
  Patient-Centered Governance   183
  Patient and Family Advisory Councils   183
  Community Representation   184
Governance Structures and Processes   184
  Charters and Bylaws   184
  Committee Membership and Structures   185
  Governance Policies and Procedures   186
  Multi-Organization Governance   186
Future Directions   189
Summary   189
Key Terms   189
Learning Activities   190
  Professional Development and Reflection   190
  Discussion Questions   190
Recommended Reading and Media   190
References   191

8. HEALTHCARE STRATEGY AND MARKETING   *195*

Competencies   195
Chapter Outline   195
Introduction   195
Strategic Analysis   196
  Internal Environment Assessment   196
  External Environmental Assessment   199
  Competitive Advantage   202
Three Levels of Strategy   203
  Corporate Strategy   203
  Business Unit Strategy   207
  Functional Level Strategy   208
Marketing Health Services   209
  Trust and Ethics in Health Services Marketing   209
  Market Segmentation and Targeting   210
  Marketing Mix (Four Ps of Marketing)   212

Promotional Mix   *214*
    Branding, Advertising, and Public Relations   *214*
    Internal Marketing   *215*
    Marketing to Clinicians   *216*
Future Directions   *216*
Summary   *217*
Key Terms   *217*
Learning Activities   *218*
    Professional Development and Reflection   *218*
    Discussion Questions   *218*
Recommended Reading and Media   *219*
References   *219*

9. HUMAN RESOURCE MANAGEMENT   *225*

Competencies   *225*
Chapter Outline   *225*
Introduction   *225*
Human Resources and Early Careerists   *226*
    Administrative Functions of Human Resources   *226*
    Job Analysis   *226*
    Job Applications   *227*
    Recruiting   *227*
    Interviewing   *229*
    Selection   *230*
    Compensation and Benefits   *230*
    Onboarding   *232*
Human Resources Business Partners and Health Services Managers   *232*
    Human Resources Business Partners   *232*
    Employee Relations   *233*
    Human Resources Laws and Regulations   *233*
    Staffing   *235*
    Workload Forecasting   *235*
    Performance Evaluations   *237*
    Training and Organizational Development   *237*
    Employee Safety and Well-Being   *239*
Strategic Human Resources and Healthcare Executives   *239*
    Strategic Human Resources Management   *239*
    Workforce Planning   *240*
    Unions and Collective Bargaining   *240*
    Physician Recruitment and Retention   *241*
    Succession Planning   *241*
    Organizational Culture   *241*
Future Directions   *242*
Summary   *243*
Key Terms   *243*
Learning Activities   *244*

Professional Development and Reflection   244
Discussion Questions   244
Recommended Reading and Media   244
References   245

10. ORGANIZATIONAL DESIGN   249

Competencies   249
Chapter Outline   249
Introduction   249
Defining the Work   250
   Standardized Work   250
   Standard Operating Procedures   250
   Clinical Protocols   251
Assigning the Work   252
   Division of Labor   252
   Authority and Responsibility   252
   The Professional Bureaucracy   255
   Dyad Models of Authority and Responsibility   257
   Alternatives to the Functional Structure   258
Coordinating the Work   259
   Coordinating Health Services   259
   Clarifying Health Services Roles   259
   Coordinating Processes and Structures   260
Expanding the Organization   261
   Divisionalized Organizations   261
   Centralized and Decentralized Organizations   261
   Service Line Structures   262
   Coordinated Divisional Structures   264
Extending the Organization   265
   Organizational Affiliations and Alliances   265
   Outsourcing to Suppliers   266
   Cooperation Among Competitors   267
Future Directions   267
Summary   267
Key Terms   268
Learning Activities   268
   Professional Development and Reflection   268
   Discussion Questions   269
Recommended Reading and Media   269
References   269

11. PERFORMANCE MANAGEMENT   273

Competencies   273
Chapter Outline   273
Introduction   273

Accountability to Stakeholders   274
   Stakeholder View of Performance   274
   Boards of Directors   274
   Regulators   275
   Payers   275
   Accreditors   276
   Awards and Recognitions   276
   Ranking Organizations   276
Strategic Performance   277
   Benchmarking   277
   Strategic Scorecard   277
   Healthcare Perspectives   278
Performance Management Process   278
   Strategic Scorecard   278
   Set Strategic Objectives   280
   Communicate Strategic Objectives   281
Goal Setting   281
   Link Strategic Objectives to Goals   281
   Common Healthcare Goals   282
   Define Targets   286
Executing, Monitoring, and Learning   286
   Creating Short-Term Initiatives   286
   Monitor Performance   290
   Feedback and Learning in the Health Care Organization   291
Individual Performance   293
   Performance Evaluations   293
   Delivering Performance Evaluations   294
   Performance Incentives   295
Future Directions   296
Summary   296
Key Terms   297
Learning Activities   297
   Professional Development and Reflection   297
   Discussion Questions   298
Recommended Reading and Media   298
References   298

12. HEALTHCARE QUALITY MANAGEMENT   303

Competencies   303
Chapter Outline   303
Introduction   303
Healthcare Quality Organization   304
   Health Services Managers   304
   Board of Directors   305
   Clinicians   305
   Quality Improvement Teams   305

Risk Management Professionals   306
Administrative and Clinical Support Services   307
Patient and Family Involvement in Quality   307
External Quality and Safety Stakeholders   307
Quality and Safety Culture   308
Promoting Quality and Safety Culture   308
Empowering Self-Reliance and Responsibility   309
A Just Culture   310
Quality Measurement and Improvement   311
Quality Measurement   311
Patient Safety   311
Workplace Safety   313
Access to Care   314
Patient Experience   314
Quality Management Methodologies   317
Methodologies and Philosophies   317
Lean   317
Six Sigma   321
High-Reliability Health Care Organizations   322
Future Directions   324
Summary   324
Key Terms   325
Learning Activities   325
Professional Development and Reflection   325
Discussion Questions   326
Recommended Reading and Media   326
References   326

13. PROJECT MANAGEMENT   335

Competencies   335
Chapter Outline   335
Introduction   335
Project Constraints   336
Temporary Work Under Tight Deadlines   336
Project Constraints   337
Project Initiation   338
Project Authorization   338
Initial Project Scoping   339
Project Procurement   340
Project Planning   341
Project Plan   341
Responsibility Matrix   342
Project Schedule   343
Activity Sequencing   345
Visualizing Project Timelines   346
Budget Estimation   347

Project Execution, Monitoring, and Control   *350*
   Project Risk Management   *350*
   Change Control   *351*
   Project Monitoring and Communication   *351*
Project Closure   *353*
   Project Sign Off   *353*
   Project Transition to Operations   *353*
   Celebrating Successes   *354*
Future Directions   *354*
Summary   *354*
Key Terms   *355*
Learning Activities   *355*
   Professional Development and Reflection   *355*
   Discussion Questions   *356*
Recommended Reading and Media   *356*
References   *356*

14. HEALTHCARE FINANCIAL MANAGEMENT   *359*

Competencies   *359*
Chapter Outline   *359*
Introduction   *359*
Healthcare Finance Organization   *360*
   Chief Financial Officer   *360*
   Controller   *360*
   Treasurer   *361*
   Board of Directors   *362*
Healthcare Revenue   *363*
   Seeking Revenue Growth   *363*
   Third-Party Payers   *363*
   Payments to Health Care Organizations   *365*
   Revenue Cycle Management   *367*
   Philanthropy   *369*
Expenses and Costing Methods   *369*
   Controlling Costs   *369*
   Types of Expenses   *371*
   Traditional Costing   *372*
   Activity-Based Costing   *373*
Financial Statements   *375*
   Importance of Financial Statements   *375*
   Income Statement   *375*
   Balance Sheet   *378*
   Cash Flow Statement   *379*
Financial Ratios and Metrics   *380*
   Analyzing and Interpreting Financial Reports   *380*
   Profitability Ratios   *380*
   Liquidity Ratios   *381*

Capital Structure Ratios　　382
　　　Asset Efficiency Ratios　　382
　　　Labor Cost Ratios and Metrics　　383
　Budgeting and Planning　　383
　　　Budgeting as a Management Competency　　383
　　　Operational Budgeting　　383
　　　Budget Variance　　384
　　　Capital Budgeting　　384
　　　Analysis of Capital Allocation Options　　386
　Future Directions　　388
　Summary　　388
　Key Terms　　389
　Learning Activities　　390
　　　Professional Development and Reflection　　390
　　　Discussion Questions　　390
　Recommended Reading and Media　　390
　References　　391

15. HEALTH SERVICES MANAGEMENT SCENARIOS AND PROJECTS　　*397*

　Case Scenarios and Projects Outline　　397
　Case Scenarios and Projects　　397
　1. Conflict on the Interprofessional Team　　397
　　　Competencies　　397
　　　Introduction　　397
　　　Scenario　　398
　　　Project Assignments　　398
　　　References　　399
　2. The Diversity, Equity, and Inclusion Initiative at the Health Care Organization　　399
　　　Competencies　　399
　　　Introduction　　400
　　　Scenario　　400
　　　Project Assignments　　400
　　　References　　402
　3. Triple Bottom Line: People, Planet, and Profit　　402
　　　Competencies　　402
　　　Introduction　　402
　　　Scenario　　402
　　　Project Assignments　　403
　　　References　　405
　4. The Dark-Side Leader　　405
　　　Competencies　　405
　　　Introduction　　405
　　　Scenario　　406
　　　Project Assignments　　406
　　　Reference　　407

5. Resisting Private Equity Investors   *407*
   Competencies   *407*
   Introduction   *407*
   Scenario   *408*
   Project Assignments   *409*
   References   *409*
6. Medical Model Versus Population Health Model   *410*
   Competencies   *410*
   Introduction   *410*
   Scenario   *410*
   Project Assignments   *411*
   Reference   *412*
7. Assessing Community Health Needs   *412*
   Competencies   *412*
   Introduction   *412*
   Scenario   *413*
   Project Assignments   *414*
   References   *415*
8. Design an Accountable Care Organization   *415*
   Competencies   *415*
   Introduction   *415*
   Scenario   *415*
   Project Assignments   *416*
   Reference   *417*
9. Home Health Business Plan   *417*
   Competencies   *417*
   Introduction   *418*
   Scenario   *418*
   Project Assignments   *420*
   References   *421*
10. Performance Review Gone Wrong   *421*
    Competencies   *421*
    Introduction   *421*
    Scenario   *422*
    Project Assignments   *422*
    References   *423*

Appendix 1. Examples of Health Services Management Problems   *425*
Appendix 2. Chapter to Case Scenarios and Projects Crosswalk   *431*
Appendix 3. Chapter to the American College of Healthcare Executives Knowledge Crosswalk   *433*
Appendix 4. Career Content at a Glance   *439*
Index   *441*

Glossary is available online by accessing Springer Connect™ at http://connect.springerpub.com/content/book/978-0-8261-4807-0.

INFORMATIONAL INTERVIEWS

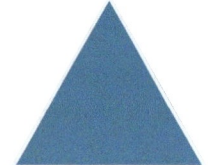

CHAPTER 1

Informational Interview 1.1: Career Advice from an Administrator in Training, Long-Term Care
Santiago Vera, MHA

Informational Interview 1.2: Career Advice from a Director, Hospital-Based Physician Services
Kathryn McGonegal, MHSA

Informational Interview 1.3: Career Advice from a Chief Operating Officer
Kory Thomas, MPH

CHAPTER 2

Informational Interview 2.1: Career Advice from a Human Capital Consultant
Fernando Chero, MHA

Informational Interview 2.2: Career Advice from a Clinic Administrator
Natalie Leone, MHA

CHAPTER 3

Informational Interview 3.1: Career Advice from a CEO and Brand Strategist
Mary E. Maloney, FACHE

Informational Interview 3.2: Career Advice from a Founder and CEO
Paul Grossman, BA, BS

CHAPTER 4

Informational Interview 4.1: Career Advice from a Director of Programming/Operations
Sydney Grant, MHA

Informational Interview 4.2: Career Advice from a Chief Development Officer
Bland Eng, MBA, MHS, FACHE

CHAPTER 5

Informational Interview 5.1: Career Advice from a System Leader, Supplier Diversity
Stacy Crouther, MPH, CPH

Informational Interview 5.2: Career Advice from a Market Director of Oncology
Frantz M. Berthaud, MPH

CHAPTER 6

Informational Interview 6.1: Career Advice from a Manager of Population Health
Ella Elizee, APRN, FNP-C, CCDS

Informational Interview 6.2: Career Advice from a Chief Executive Officer, Community Health Center
Bradley Herremans, MBA, FACHE

CHAPTER 7

Informational Interview 7.1: Career Advice from a Board of Directors Member, Community Health Center
Krystal Lockhart, BA

Informational Interview 7.2: Career Advice from a Manager, Corporate Governance
Paula Zieben, MHA

CHAPTER 8

Informational Interview 8.1: Career Advice from a Senior Marketing Coordinator
Taylor Howard, MAMC

Informational Interview 8.2: Career Advice from a Director, Business Development and Physician Relations
Ashley Abbondandolo, MHA

Informational Interview 8.3: Career Advice from an Executive Director, Strategic Planning
Dustin S. Zabokrtsky, MA, MBA

CHAPTER 9

Informational Interview 9.1: Career Advice from a Human Resources Coordinator
Lily Goodman, MHA

Informational Interview 9.2: Career Advice from a Senior Human Resources Business Partner
Kimberly Steadman, BS in Human Resources Management

Informational Interview 9.3: Career Advice from a Vice President, Human Resources
Nicki Hancock, MBA, FACHE, SPHR

CHAPTER 10

Informational Interview 10.1: Career Advice from an Integration Project Manager
Reem Yousif, MHA

Informational Interview 10.2: Career Advice from a Vice President, Service Lines
Steven Chew, MHA, CPC

Informational Interview 10.3: Career Advice from a Chief Transformation and Service Line Officer
Emily Allinder Scott, MHA, FACHE

CHAPTER 11

Informational Interview 11.1: Career Advice from a Manager, Patient Experience
Sabrina Rice, MHA, MPH, CPXP

Informational Interview 11.2: Career Advice from a Chief Executive Officer, Academic Medical Center Physician Practice
Mark G. Moseley, MD, MHA, CPE, FACEP

CHAPTER 12

Informational Interview 12.1: Career Advice from a Performance Improvement Coordinator
Lauren Kiskunes, MPH

Informational Interview 12.2: Career Advice from a Performance Program Manager
Jennifer Ammerman, MHA, CPHQ

Informational Interview 12.3: Career Advice from a Chief Executive Officer, The Quality Coaching Co.
Jarvis T. Gray, MHA, MPM

CHAPTER 13

Informational Interview 13.1: Career Advice from a Project Coordinator
Erika Domenech, MHA, CAPM

Informational Interview 13.2: Career Advice from a Program Manager, Informatics
Ibrahim Akorede, MHA, PMP

Informational Interview 13.3: Career Advice from a Vice President, Operations
Tyler Hillis, MHA

CHAPTER 14

Informational Interview 14.1: Career Advice from a Financial Analyst
Dominic Patete, MHS

Informational Interview 14.2: Career Advice from a Revenue Cycle Support Manager
Ariela Sancho, MHA

Informational Interview 14.3: Career Advice from a Senior Vice President, Patient Financial Services
Anthony Escobio, MPH

PREFACE

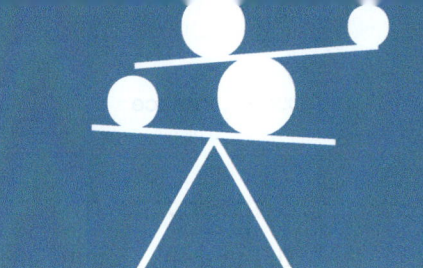

TEXTBOOK THEMES

The health services management profession—mysterious to students and misconstrued by clinicians—deserves a clear explanation, free of jargon and overly complicated conceptual models. Confusion about the role of the health services manager is understandable. Arcane knowledge and highly specialized skills can be intimidating, and the health services management profession seems to be full of contradictory motivations. However, as this textbook explains, technical management skills can be learned, and the contradictions actually make the profession worth pursuing.

The textbook is written for undergraduate or graduate students who seek an introduction to the health services management role and related careers. The main goals of the textbook are to (a) provide knowledge on the fundamental competencies needed to succeed in the health services management profession and (b) expose students to different health services management career options. The 15 chapters of the textbook address the knowledge, skills, and abilities commonly taught in undergraduate and graduate health services management courses.

In addition, this textbook is useful for mid- and late-career health services managers who seek to prepare for the American College of Healthcare Executives (ACHE) Board of Governor's Exam. Earning a Fellow of the American College of Healthcare Executives (FACHE) designation is an important career step. The rigorous exam is based on the competencies necessary to perform the role of health services manager (Bowen & Hahn, 2012). Health services managers can take the board exam once they earn a graduate degree, attain a certain level of professional responsibility, and complete ACHE continuing education requirements. This textbook, along with other educational materials offered by ACHE and local ACHE chapters' professional development programming, is designed to assist FACHE candidates with passing the exam.

Competencies

True professional competence in health services management is demonstrated through action, not just the recall of facts. As such, contemporary academic health administration programs focus less on theoretical and research-oriented curricula in favor of what is called competency-based education (Broom et al., 2016). Programs teaching under this philosophy often look to professional authorities, such as the ACHE, the National Center for Healthcare Leadership, and the Association of University Programs of Health Administration, to develop their competency models. Health administration education programs use competency models to assess student readiness to practice the health services management profession.

This textbook covers a wide range of competencies, incorporating different conceptions of health services management practice. Because there are dozens of different health services management competencies, a person does not need to be expert in all of them. Graduates of health administration education programs are expected to be a novice in numerous competencies, proficient in others, and experts in a few that will make them valuable to health services organizations. Acquiring expertise normally takes decades of practice. If a person achieves excellence in health services management by 30 years old, then they are considered a prodigy (Griffith, 2007). Mastery of the health services management profession requires years of hard work and a deep commitment to the profession (Garman & Lemak, 2011).

Careers

This textbook supports integration of professional development content into undergraduate or graduate health services management courses. Most academic health administration programs teach professionalism (Agris et al., 2018). While stand-alone professional development courses are common, the majority of programs choose to incorporate content related to careers into other courses (Meacham et al., 2017). To advance professional development, this textbook covers a variety of topics identified by Meacham and colleagues (2017) as fundamental to professional development courses, such as interview skills, professional networking, and personal career planning. Other professional development topics include professional codes of conduct, emotional and social intelligence, job search guidance, executive presence, and service to one's community.

In addition to plenty of real-world examples in the core content of each chapter, the textbook includes a variety of features the support career and professional development, including the following:

- *Informational interviews:* Hosted by the author, each chapter features multiple conversations with health services managers. These 15- to 20-minute edited audio discussions model informal discussions called informational interviews and serve as examples to early careerists regarding how they should engage with experienced professionals to increase their understanding of career possibilities.
- *Career boxes:* Each chapter contains career development advice related to the chapter content, including building a strong work ethic, exploring career options in health services management, engaging a career board of directors, and more. See Appendix 4 for a full list of Career Box content by chapter.
- *Professional development and reflections:* Knowing oneself requires reflection. Each chapter presents students with chapter-specific management concepts to consider for their own professional development.
- *Recommended reading and media:* In addition to the numerous scholarly references, each chapter lists additional readings and other media for students to learn more about the relevant health services management topics.

Management and Administration Terms

There are hundreds of thousands of health services managers and administrative staff who work in organizations that directly care for patients, such as hospitals, clinics, nursing homes, pharmacies, and other care delivery settings (BLS, 2024). Multiple terms are used in popular and scholarly literature to describe this role, including healthcare managers, health administrators, and healthcare leaders. This textbook treats these terms as synonymous and uses the term health services manager. The use of the term administration, instead of management, stems from the mid-20th-century distaste for profit in public institutions, such as hospitals. Administration implied running large public institutions, whereas management implied a profit motive (Drucker & Maciariello, 2008). This distinction has disappeared over the decades, and today, the healthcare sector uses the terms management and administration interchangeably, as does this textbook. Most graduate programs in this field are known as Master of Health Administration, Master of Health Services Administration, or Master of Business Administration with a healthcare concentration.

Healthcare Systems and Roles of Health Services Managers

While other texts focus on the complexities of the U.S. healthcare system, this textbook addresses the role of the health services manager within that system. Learning about the healthcare settings, roles, financing, and policy becomes more manageable to students when focusing on the roles of health services managers. Awash in too much information, students prefer textbooks to be concise and easy to read with practical instruction and plenty of relevant examples. This textbook provides many examples to illustrate the roles of health services managers and, in doing so, explains many of the intricacies of the healthcare system.

TEXTBOOK STRUCTURE

Chapters 1 through 5 address the fundamentals of health services management.
- Chapter 1, "Role of the Health Services Manager," shares how the unique professional role of health services management contributes to the interprofessional healthcare team.
- Chapter 2, "Problem-Solving and Evidence-Based Management," explains how managers solve problems using the best available evidence and critical thinking skills.
- Chapter 3, "Managing Interpersonal Communications," covers how health services managers express self-confidence, listen to others, and excel at many types of oral and written communication.
- Chapter 4, "Leadership and Change Management," reviews key concepts associated with leading health care organizations (HCOs), such as leadership theory, organizational culture, emotional intelligence, change management, and power and influence.
- Chapter 5, "Professionalism and Ethics," describes how professional and ethical conduct of health services managers models behaviors for strong organizational cultures, earn the trust of clinicians, and serves patients, employees, clinicians, the profession, the HCO, and society.

Chapters 6 through 14 cover the specialized skills, knowledge, and functions of the health services management profession.
- Chapter 6, "Population Health and Community Collaboration," illustrates the latest management approaches for keeping communities healthy and prosperous.
- Chapter 7, "Healthcare Governance," reviews how health services managers, boards of directors, clinicians, and patients work together to achieve common goals.
- Chapter 8, "Healthcare Strategy and Marketing," explains the strategic planning process, including how health services managers align strategy with the operational functions of the HCO, including marketing.
- Chapter 9, "Human Resource Management," highlights how the human resources function supports health services managers throughout their career.
- Chapter 10, "Organizational Design," reviews how health services managers divide, organize, and coordinate work across complex HCOs.
- Chapter 11, "Performance Management," describes the competencies associated with performance measurement, monitoring, and evaluation of individuals and business operations.
- Chapter 12, "Healthcare Quality Management," explains the various tools and approaches used to improve medical care processes, reduce safety issues, enhance patient experience, and optimize clinical and operational performance.
- Chapter 13, "Project Management," examines the skills health services managers need to effectively and efficiently initiate and coordinate team projects.
- Chapter 14, "Healthcare Financial Management," summarizes the finance competencies required to succeed throughout health services management careers, including knowledge of financial statements, revenue cycle, budgeting, and more.

TEACHING AND LEARNING SUPPORT

The textbook supports teaching and learning with a variety of features:
- *Competencies:* Each chapter features a list of competencies and sub-competencies necessary to succeed in the health services management role.
- *Discussion questions:* Each chapter provides content-related discussion questions designed to promote active engagement, critical thinking, and a deeper understanding of the content.

- *Instructor's manual:* Accessible to instructors only, this document provides course syllabi examples, chapter activities, multiple choice and essay questions with answer keys, and guidance on accommodating diverse learning styles and teaching modalities.
- *Online content:* Instructors and health services managers studying for the ACHE Board of Governors Exam can access additional online content on Springer CONNECT or request access by emailing textbook@springerpub.com.

Finally, Chapter 15, "Health Services Management Scenarios and Projects," includes a series of integrated health services management case scenarios and project assignments. Scenarios are brief descriptions (i.e., short case studies) of current challenges in health services management. These integrative case scenarios and project assignments can be used to assess student competency attainment.

ACKNOWLEDGMENTS

A special thanks to my wife, Becky, and children, Cole and Mia, for their unwavering support and unconditional love. I am also grateful to the best leaders I know, Susy Sportsman and Kate Chapin, for their emotional support and excellent advice. Thank you to all my students, especially Stephanie Hersman and William Steed, for their reviews and feedback; I wrote this textbook for you. To Sandra J. Potthoff, thank you for teaching me how to teach problem-solving and for co-writing your excellent textbook (Potthoff, Mishek, & Hart, 2020). I deeply appreciate the support and expertise of my friends Natalie Leone, Nicki Hancock, and Victor D. Weeden for their subject matter expertise and input on early drafts of the textbook. Also, thanks to the dozens of informational interview guests who gave their time to help students learn about the important health services management role. Finally, thank you to my mentor Anthony R. Kovner for his encouragement and discerning point of view.

Zachary Pruitt, PhD, MHA, FACHE

REFERENCES

Agris, J., Brichto, E., Meacham, M., & Louis, C. (2018). Developing professionalism in healthcare management programs: An examination of accreditation outcomes. *Journal of Health Administration Education, 35*(2), 187–203.

Bowen, D. J., & Hahn, C. A. (2012). Credentialing for health care leaders: an overview of ACHE's FACHE credential and its contributions to the health care management field. *World Hospitals and Health Services: The Official Journal of the International Hospital Federation, 48*(3), 30–32.

Broom, K., Turner, J., & Brichto, E. (2016). How well do programs fulfill their role in management development? An analysis of competency assessments using CAHME accreditation outcomes. *Journal of Health Administration Education, 33*(4), 559–579.

Bureau of Labor Statistics [BLS]. (2024). U.S. Department of Labor, Occupational Outlook Handbook, Medical and Health Services Managers. https://www.bls.gov/ooh/management/medical-and-health-services-managers.htm

Drucker, P. F., & Maciariello, J. A. (2008). *Management* (rev. ed.). HarperCollins.

Meacham, M. R., Thompson, J. M., & Hall, R. S. (2017). Professional development of healthcare management students: A survey of programs. *Journal of Health Administration Education, 34*(1), 49–61.

Potthoff, S. J., Mishek, J. H., & Hart, G. W. (2020). *Applied problem-solving in healthcare management.* Springer Publishing, Inc.

RESOURCES

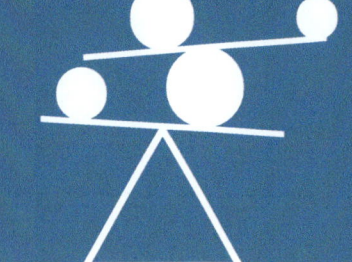

All purchasers have access to the following resources:

STUDENT RESOURCES

- **Informational Interviews (Audio)**
- **Informational Interviews Transcripts**
- **Online Glossary featuring 750+ Key Terms**

These resources are available at http://connect.springerpub.com/content/book/978-0-8261-4807-0

INSTRUCTOR RESOURCES

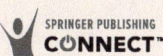 A robust set of instructor resources designed to supplement this text is located at http://connect.springerpub.com/content/book/978-0-8261-4807-0. Qualifying instructors may request access by emailing textbook@springerpub.com.

- **LMS Common Cartridge**–With All Instructor Resources
- **Instructor Manual**
  - Group Activities
  - Discussion and Essay Questions
- **Instructor Test Bank** With Multiple-Choice Questions and Detailed Rationales
- **Instructor PowerPoint Presentations**
- **Instructor Sample Syllabus**

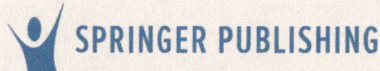

Visit http://connect.springerpub.com/content/book/978-0-8261-4807-0 and look for the "**Show Supplementary**" button on the **book homepage**.

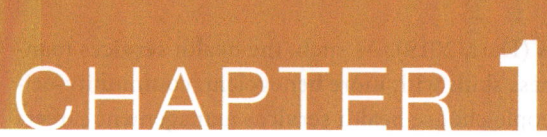
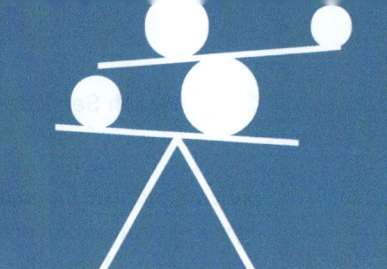

CHAPTER 1

ROLE OF THE HEALTH SERVICES MANAGER

Health services management is a goal-directed, action-oriented, and people-focused role that contributes to the interprofessional health care team by planning, organizing, directing, coordinating, and controlling information, physical, financial, and human resources.

COMPETENCIES

- Perform management functions including planning, organizing, directing, coordinating, and controlling.
- Apply management practices to health care organizations.
- Maintain or enhance operations of health care organizations.
- Promote systems thinking in healthcare.
- Contribute to the interprofessional healthcare team.
- Balance the concerns of health care access, quality, and cost.
- Accept professional and social responsibility for diversity, equity, and inclusion.
- Manage career and professional self-development.

CHAPTER OUTLINE

- Management Practices
- Health Services Management
- Competencies of Health Services Management
- Health Services Management Careers

INTRODUCTION

Health services management often goes unrecognized for its career potential and contribution to health care organizations (HCOs). Few children dream of becoming health services managers, instead aspiring to become physicians, nurses, or other clinicians acclaimed for their lifesaving skills. However, after learning more about the day-to-day duties of clinical professions, some people opt to pursue other meaningful careers. In this search, some people discover a talent for management, recognizing that they are planners and organizers, goal oriented, and strategically minded. Because they enjoy working in teams and solving difficult problems, organizations value them for their management potential.

However, some high-potential future health services managers resist management careers due to suspicions of typical business goals (Drucker, 1990). After all, they respect the clinical professions because they help patients, not because they are motivated by profits. They may not know that the primary ethical responsibility of the health services management profession is to patients, not the financial needs of their HCOs (Darr, 2019). As such, the health services management profession combines traditional business skills with more benevolent, community-oriented values (White & Griffith, 2019). Most people choose health services management careers to empower clinicians, build community connections, and serve society (Schuller et al., 2018). Health services managers concentrate on the financial, human resources, and operational functions of HCOs so that physicians, nurses, and other clinicians can focus their energies on caring for patients.

Health services managers, also known as healthcare administrators, ensure efficient and effective operational, financial, and administrative functions of HCOs. For the purposes of this textbook, health services managers are those who work in organizations that directly care for patients, such as hospitals, clinics, nursing homes, pharmacies, and other care delivery settings. Over 350,000 health services managers and administrative staff work for these organizations, ranging from small physician practices to very large multistate health systems (U.S. Bureau of Labor Statistics [BLS], 2022a). Employment in these positions is projected to grow several times faster than the average for all occupations and the management positions of other industries (U.S. BLS, 2022b).

There are also thousands of managers who work in pharmaceutical companies, durable medical equipment, health information technology, consulting, health insurance, research laboratories, professional associations, and more. Like HCOs that directly care for patients, these healthcare businesses require professional managers with extensive business training and experience. However, one could argue that management roles in these types of organizations have more in common with non-healthcare business managers than with health services managers. For one, managers in these other healthcare businesses are physically removed from direct patient care delivery settings. Also, there are relatively fewer clinicians than in direct care settings, where clinicians dominate the social and political power structures. Finally, direct care HCOs are mostly not-for-profit, publicly owned, or physician owned, whereas the other healthcare businesses are generally for profit, whose investors prioritize efficiency over community commitment (Franz et al., 2021; Pruitt & Pracht, 2013).

On the other hand, the healthcare sector is rapidly privatizing and consolidating, which is erasing the boundaries between direct service HCOs and other healthcare businesses (Southwick, 2022). Large insurance companies are purchasing physician practices and pharmacies. Hospitals are buying physician practices to form integrated health systems. Health systems are merging with other health systems to compete with the insurance companies. Despite the developments of these large-scale healthcare enterprises, some industry dynamics—sick patients, highly trained clinicians, complex operations, and expensive care—are unlikely to disappear, which makes managers who understand health services delivery business even more valuable.

MANAGEMENT PRACTICES

Fayol's Management Functions

Management as a distinct professional practice emerged from Henri Fayol's (1916) experiences as an executive manager at a large mining company in the 19th century. Its industrial origins have led some to misinterpret the term management as synonymous with business (Drucker, 1990). In reality, the management profession exists in all sectors of the economy and all types of organizations. One can manage a charity just as one can manage a corporation.

⚠ KEY IDEA

The management profession exists in all sectors of the economy and all types of organizations. One can manage a charity just as one can manage a corporation.

Some jobs may have the title of a manager but do not perform management functions. For example, some companies use the term manager to indicate administrative responsibilities, such as an office manager. Such roles do not necessarily perform the functions of a manager. Moreover, high performers are sometimes promoted to top positions in an organization to reflect their accomplishments and value to the organization. However, these executive titles do not necessarily mean that they practice management. Some people are individual contributors, even if they have titles that imply that they are managers.

In fact, management involves practices or functions that distinguish it from other occupations. Fayol's (1916) classical conception of management provides the foundation for today's management definitions:

1. *Planning:* Evaluate alternative courses of action, decide in advance what needs to be done, explain desired outcomes, and develop objectives.
2. *Organizing:* Arrange people and activities to complete the work. Managers create the organizational structure, which includes division of labor (who does what), chain of command (who reports to whom), and spans of control (who is responsible for what).
3. *Commanding:* Set expectations for performance and give clear instructions. Today's management theory has relabeled commanding as **directing** or leading.
4. *Coordinating:* Through instilling discipline within teams, ensure that people are working toward the same goals. Synchronize people with resources, such as material and information.
5. *Controlling:* Monitor and evaluate performance. If goals are not met, then implement initiatives to improve results. Managers regularly track performance against plans through systems and processes, such as budgeting and performance evaluations.

Fayol's five functions assumed high levels of control over workers enforced with strict discipline. Early managers commanded their subordinates, imposed objectives, and delivered negative consequences for failing to perform. While some managers still behave this way, most management experts reject the authoritarian management style (Pizzolitto et al., 2022). By the mid-20th century, the nature of work—and the workers themselves—had changed, and managers responded accordingly.

Drucker's Five Basic Functions of the Manager

By the 1950s, management scholar Peter Drucker realized that a large portion of the workforce had transformed from unskilled labor to highly educated professionals. Drucker coined the term *knowledge workers* to describe people who analyze information, solve problems, generate ideas, and make decisions (1954). Because knowledge workers are capable of deciding how to perform their work to achieve the best results, managers do not command or control their subordinates. Instead, managers collaborate with knowledge workers, form effective teams, motivate them to achieve goals, and measure and communicate results. In this new conception of management, Drucker (1954) argued that managers perform five basic functions, illustrated in Figure 1.1.

FIGURE 1.1 Drucker's management functions.

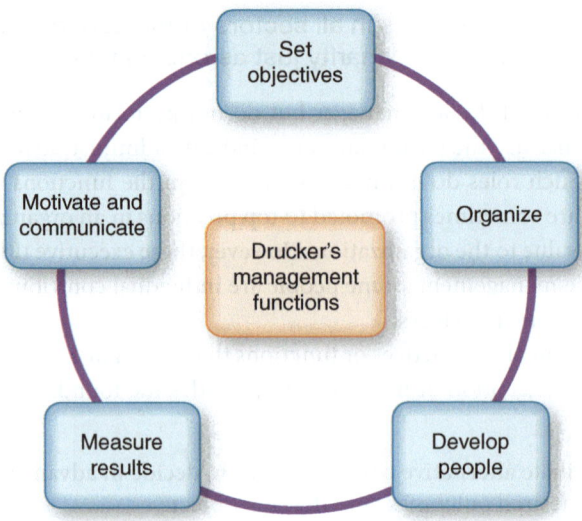

1. *Set objectives:* Create mutual understanding among teams about what is important to achieve. Individual goals should be connected to personal motivations and aligned with the organizational strategy. Drucker used the term *management by objectives* to describe how managers set shared objectives.
2. *Organize:* Evaluate the work that needs to be accomplished, divide it into manageable parts, organize it by common types, and assign people to perform it. Managers integrate people into teams.
3. *Develop people:* Add people to the team, help them grow professionally and personally, and reward them when they meet or exceed expectations. An effective manager maximizes peoples' strengths and minimizes their weaknesses.
4. *Measure results:* Evaluate performance, identify shortfalls, and implement improvements. Effective managers continuously seek ways to improve.
5. *Motivate and communicate:* Motivate team members to accomplish goals. Resolve any conflicts and keep team focused on performance. Communicate information throughout the organization.

Drucker emphasized that competent managers create organizations in which people can develop new skills so that their organizations can improve performance and respond to emerging opportunities. In other words, when workers thrive, organizations succeed.

Mintzberg's Management Roles

Henry Mintzberg was another well-regarded management theorist of the 20th century who identified roles common to all managers. His management concepts, illustrated in Figure 1.2, remain popular in management education and research (Korica et al., 2017). Mintzberg (1973) categorized 10 different managerial roles, in parentheses, into three groups:

1. Interpersonal roles require the manager to serve as a figure of authority (figurehead), act as the person responsible and accountable for the performance of the organization (leader), and function as the facilitator of internal and external communications (liaison).

FIGURE 1.2 Mintzberg's 10 management roles.

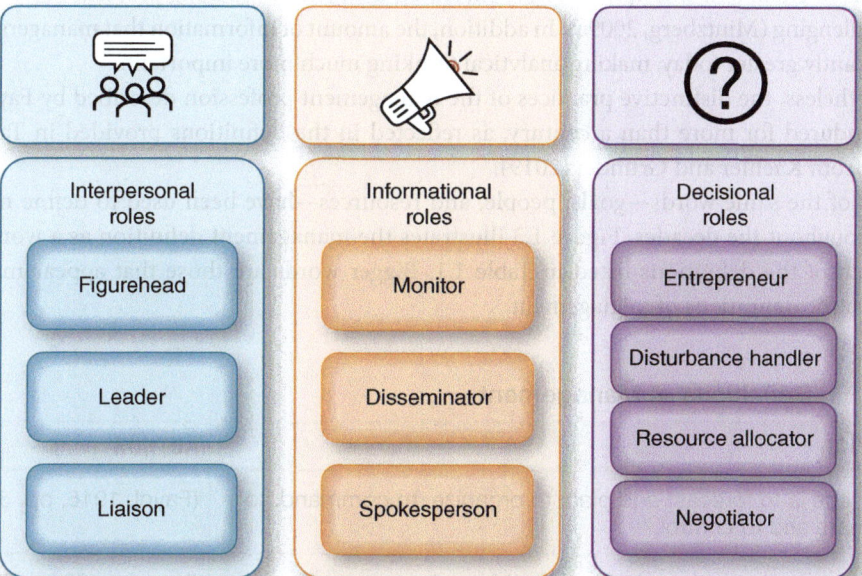

2. Informational roles involve seeking information about industry changes, assessing the current operations of the organization, identifying potential opportunities for improvement (monitoring), sharing important information with team members to help them perform their jobs (disseminator), and representing the organization to external stakeholders (spokesperson).
3. Decisional roles require the manager to solve problems and develop new strategies (entrepreneur), direct corrective action when the organization faces unexpected crises (disturbance handler), decide where organizational resources are best applied (resource allocator), and represent the organization in decisions about committing resources (negotiator).

Mintzberg (1994) cautioned against breaking apart management into too many small functional pieces because it can obscure the comprehensive nature of the role. Responsible for integrating many different parts into a whole, managers meld people into teams, teams into organizations, and organizations into society.

Definitions of Management

Management is goal directed, action oriented, and people focused. Managers do not perform the work themselves; they plan, organize, direct, coordinate, and control the work of others. However, it is not enough to simply be in charge or to tell people what to do. Managers must also contribute to the organization's goals using profession-specific practices, knowledge, skills, and abilities.

In many respects, managers perform the same core functions today as they did 50 years ago (Korica et al., 2017). On the other hand, some substantial changes have occurred since then. Managers spend far less time confined to their offices, instead interacting with colleagues in all sorts of short information exchanges. Managers also attend many types of scheduled meetings, including one-on-one interactions and large group collaborations. Meanwhile, other aspects of the management profession have intensified. While constant interruptions have always been a part of the job, the inventions of email and smartphones have increased distractions, making problem-solving much more challenging (Mintzberg, 2009a). In addition, the amount of information that managers receive is significantly greater today, making analytical thinking much more important.

Nevertheless, the distinctive practices of the management profession described by Fayol have largely endured for more than a century, as reflected in the definitions provided in Table 1.1, adapted from Kaehler and Grundei (2019).

Many of the same words—goals, people, and resources—have been used to define management throughout the decades. Figure 1.3 illustrates the management definition as a word cloud using each of the definitions listed in Table 1.1. Bigger words are those that appear more frequently in the definitions of management.

TABLE 1.1 Definitions of Management

DEFINITION	AUTHOR
"To manage is to forecast and plan, to organize, to command, to co-ordinate and to control."	(Fayol, 1916, pp. 5–6)
"[. . .] management is the art of getting things done through and with people in formally organized groups, the art of creating an environment in such an organized group where people can perform as individuals and yet cooperate toward attainment of group goals, the art of removing blocks to such performance, the art of optimizing efficiency in effectively reaching goals."	(Koontz, 1961, p. 186)
"[. . .] management can be defined as the process of achieving organizational goals through planning, organizing, leading, and controlling the human, physical, financial, and information resources of the organization in an effective and efficient manner."	(Bovée et al., 1993, p. 5)
"Management is the process of achieving organisational objectives, within a changing environment, by balancing efficiency, effectiveness and equity, obtaining the most from limited resources, and working with and through other people."	(Naylor, 2004, p. 6)
"Management, to repeat, means getting things done through other people—Whether that be on the people plane (leading and linking) or on the information plane (controlling and communicating)."	(Mintzberg, 2009b, p. 168)
"Management: A set of activities (including planning and decision making, organizing, leading, and controlling) directed at an organization's resources (human, financial, physical, and information), with the aim of achieving organizational goals in an efficient and effective manner."	(Griffin, 2013, p. 5)
"Management is the process of working with people and resources to accomplish organizational goals. Good managers do those things both effectively and efficiently."	(Bateman et al., 2017, p. 13)
"[. . .] management is defined as (1) the pursuit of organizational goals efficiently and effectively by (2) integrating the work of people through (3) planning, organizing, leading, and controlling the organization's resources."	(Kinicki & Williams, 2018, p. 5)

Source: Kaehler, B., & Grundei, J. (2019). The concept of management: In search of a new definition. *HR Governance: A Theoretical Introduction*, 3–26. https://doi.org/10.1007/978-3-319-94526-2_2

FIGURE 1.3 Word cloud of management definitions.

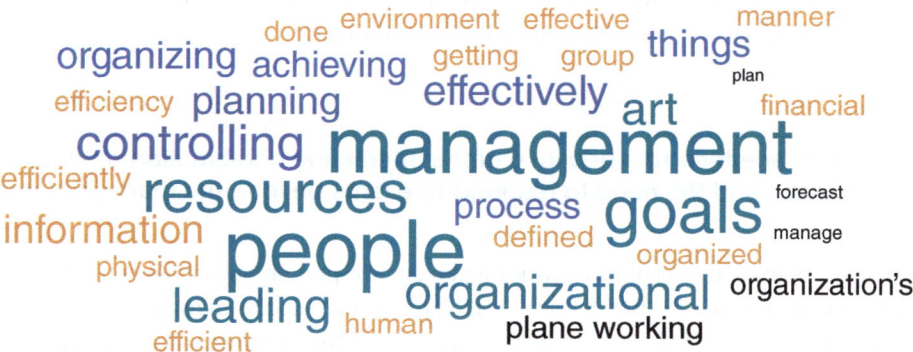

Management and Systems Theory

Systems thinking is a mental model that recognizes that all the parts of an organization connect, interact, and contribute to outcomes (Daellenbach et al., 2017). According to **systems theory**, no element of a system is independent of one another, and all can affect how the system operates. As illustrated in Figure 1.4, the simple system includes input, processes, and outputs. Inputs are people and material resources; outputs are the products created by the system; and processes are the steps taken to transform an input into an output. Managers use feedback to adjust inputs or processes, as necessary, in order to maintain the overall equilibrium (i.e., balance) of the system. Within the system, managers make sure that the inputs, processes, and feedback loops are monitored, maintained, repaired, or enhanced so that the system can produce predictable outputs.

When the organization is considered a **closed system** (i.e., not subject to any external force), then creating equilibrium in the system is relatively straightforward, as long as the feedback loops are monitored. In reality, however, all managers contend with complex **open systems** that are influenced by changes in the external environment. To track disruptions in the system, effective managers conduct **boundary spanning** activities that require them to engage with the environments outside the organization to build relationships of all types. In this way, managers monitor

FIGURE 1.4 Systems theory of management.

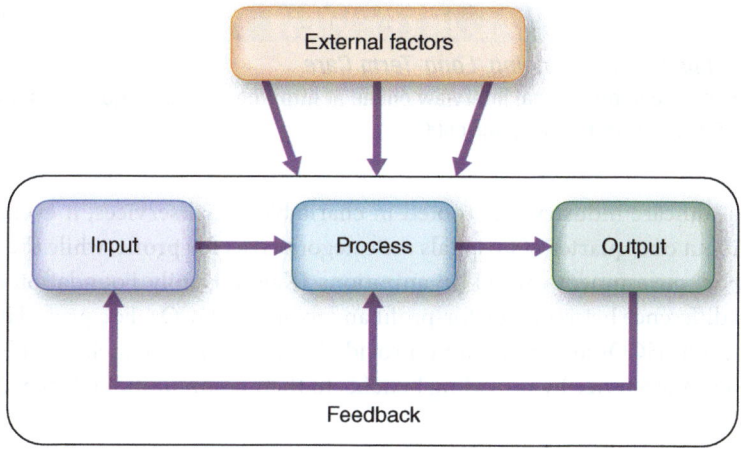

the external environment for potential disruptions, industry trends, competitive challenges, policy changes, and customer preferences. Successful managers anticipate troubles and act as a catalyst to improvement when faced with a changing environment.

> ⚠ **KEY IDEA**
>
> **Managers embrace their role because of the interesting combination of stability-seeking activities and the need to respond to events beyond the manager's control.**

Balancing systems within chaotic environments can be especially stressful when the challenges occur at an unrelenting pace (Mintzberg, 1973). Nevertheless, successful managers embrace their role because of the interesting combination of stability-seeking activities and creating change in the organization.

HEALTH SERVICES MANAGEMENT

Evolution of the Health Services Manager

Management emerged as a separate discipline in the early 20th century, when healthcare institutions were still mostly run by charitable and religious organizations, such as the Catholic church (Starr, 1982). At that time, hospitals were more social care organizations than businesses. Physician practices were usually solo practitioners or small partnerships and pharmacies still sold more soda than prescriptions (Urick & Meggs, 2019).

By the mid-20th century, most hospital boards in the United States split responsibilities among hospital management and clinicians. Management was put in charge of buildings, equipment, employees, and finances, and clinicians were responsible for patients at the bedside, patient safety, and clinical performance. Due to population growth, medical advances, and technological innovations, the federal government invested billions of dollars to building new hospitals by passing the **Hill-Burton Act** in 1946. More complex hospitals gave rise to the health services managers, who were the financial and operational experts who could allocate resources and coordinate the work between the various functions. Health services managers became a specialty within the management profession who sought to balance their business acumen with a social mission, community relationships, and respect for the clinical professions (Davis, 1929; Stevens, 1989).

 INFORMATIONAL INTERVIEW 1.1
Administrator in Training, Long-Term Care
Access the informational interview online at http://connect.springerpub.com/content/book/978-0-8261-4807-0/chapter/ch00.

While the healthcare industry was rooted in charitable social services, it eventually became big business. About one-quarter of hospitals are categorized as **for profit**, while the rest are either **not-for-profit** or government-owned organizations (Kaiser Family Foundation [KFF], 2019). There is a legal difference between not-for-profit and for-profit HCOs. For-profit HCOs must pay taxes. Not-for-profit HCOs are tax-exempt, provided that they justify their tax advantage to the U.S. Internal Revenue Service by providing benefits to their communities (Rozier, 2020). Still, all

HCOs seek to make more money than they spend (i.e., profits) so that they can support research, acquire new technologies, recruit leading clinicians, and fund charity care programs. This means that all HCOs must consider revenue and expenses in their decision-making processes, even if not necessarily motivated by profits.

> ⚠ **KEY IDEA**
> All health care organizations must consider revenue and expenses, even if not necessarily motivated by profits.

Responsibilities of Health Services Managers

According to Haddock et al. (2002), health services managers accept three main responsibilities. First, health services managers are responsible for business aspects of HCOs, including making business decisions about where to allocate resources, often for clinical matters about which they have little expertise. This is especially challenging because clinicians and patients often demand the latest new technologies which may provide marginal improvement in the quality of care but are often too costly to justify the expense (Balak et al., 2020; Burns, 2012). When declining to make these investments, health services managers can become the target of blame and disappointment from clinicians who fail to consider the needs of the entire HCO.

Second, health services managers are responsible for HCOs that care for people in their most vulnerable state (Haddock et al., 2002). Because they are ultimately responsible for patient care delivered at the HCO, ethical managers prioritize the health outcomes over financial interests (Darr, 2019). In some instances, health services managers may choose to invest in unprofitable services in an effort to ensure access to needed health care. The balance between patient care and profits is the responsibility of the health services manager.

> **CAREER BOX 1.1: Early Career Health Services Management**
>
> Health services managers rarely start their careers in management positions. Instead, aspiring managers start in entry-level, nonmanagement administrative positions and work their way up. Early careerists usually perform basic administrative tasks associated with the business of healthcare, such as processing, documenting, tracking, retrieving, and assisting. The following terms are common position titles for early career management jobs:
> - *Representatives:* Handle customer service issues, such as assisting with patient flow in a clinic, scheduling patient visits with physicians, or handling patient billing questions.
> - *Specialists:* Work in functional areas, such as finance or human resources, and perform administrative tasks, such as processing authorizations for inpatient admissions, reviewing credential applications, or maintaining a database of contracts.
> - *Coordinators:* Act as an operational resource for the HCO, such as patient experience, marketing, or continuing medical education.
> - *Analysts:* Work with clinical, financial, or administrative data to produce internal reports that managers use to make decisions.
>
> Despite the abundance administrative tasks these early career positions entail, those who apply themselves, accept responsibility for results, and build specialized skills can expect to earn promotions into management roles.

Finally, health services managers are responsible for the employees of the organization. Britt Berrett and Paul Spiegelman (2013), in their book, *Patients Come Second*, provocatively declared that health services managers should prioritize employees over patients. To create better patient health outcomes, they argued, managers must create a happy workplace, invest in the development of employees, and reward excellent performance. Health services managers also defend their teams and keep the peace when conflict arises, especially among patients and clinicians (Haddock et al., 2002). Sometimes, putting employees first means purposefully removing negative patients or employees from the work environment lest they contaminate the culture.

> ⚠ **KEY IDEA**
> Sometimes, putting employees first means purposefully removing negative patients or employees from the work environment lest they contaminate the culture.

Managing in the Continuum of Care

Health services managers perform their professional roles in every health care setting. The **continuum of care** is the phrase used to define the full range of health and medical services across multiple settings, providers, and institutions. There are several ways to frame the continuum of care, including the life span (i.e., birth, health maintenance, sickness, and dying) or stages of disease (i.e., screening, diagnosis, treatment, and recovery). Figure 1.5 illustrates the continuum of care based on the severity of patient condition (i.e., acuity of care).

HCOs are progressively consolidating the care continuum under single ownership structures to better negotiate prices with health insurance and suppliers. Over two thirds of all hospitals are a part of a system, and more consolidation is expected in the near future (American Hospital Association [AHA], 2021a; Southwick, 2022). A **health system**, sometimes called an **integrated delivery network**, is a phrase used to define a collection of HCOs, including at least one hospital and a group of physicians, who are connected through common ownership or joint management (Agency for Healthcare Research and Quality [AHRQ], 2023). Combined, the 10 largest health systems comprise about 15% of the approximately 6,100 nonfederal hospitals in the country, as shown in Table 1.2 (Falvey, 2023). The federal government operates the **Veterans Health Administration** (VHA) hospital system, which includes 171 different facilities, and the Military Health System, a part of the U.S. Department of Defense, which includes another 45 facilities (Defense Health Agency [DHA], 2022; VHA, 2023).

FIGURE 1.5 Continuum of care by severity of illness.

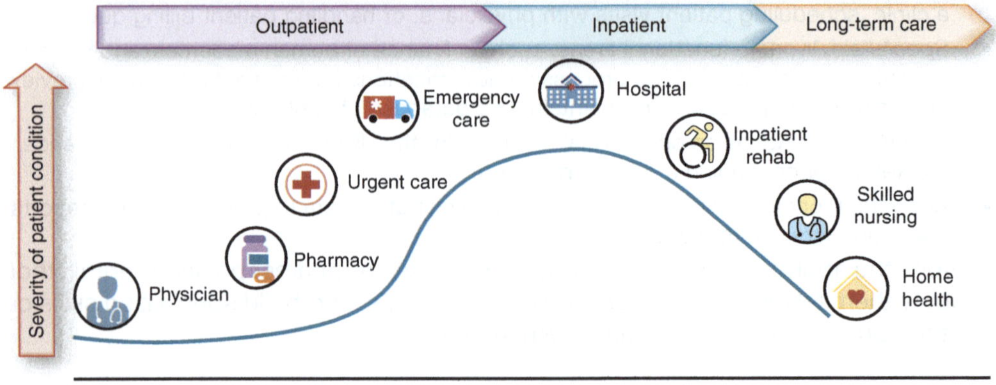

TABLE 1.2 Top 10 Health Systems in the United States by Number of Hospitals

HEALTH SYSTEM	TYPE	NUMBER OF HOSPITALS
HCA Healthcare	For-profit	182
CommonSpirit Health	Not-for-profit, Catholic	140
Ascension Health	Not-for-profit, Catholic	139
Trinity Health	Not-for-profit, Catholic	88
LifePoint Health	For-profit	84
Community Health Systems	For-profit	79
Advocate Health (NC)	Not-for-profit	67
Tenet Healthcare	For-profit	61
Christus Health	Not-for-profit, Catholic	60
Providence (WA)	Not-for-profit, Catholic	52

HCA, Hospital Corporation of America; NC, North Carolina; WA, Washington.

Consolidated organizations are also known by other names in healthcare. A **clinically integrated network** is a legal collaboration between hospitals and a wide range of physician specialties that is created to aggressively negotiate better rates with insurance companies, share information about their patients, enhance care quality, and reduce costs. An **accountable care organization** (ACO) is also a type of collaboration among hospitals, physicians, and other health care providers designed to improve care and decrease spending (Huang et al., 2023). ACOs contract with Centers for Medicare & Medicaid Services to accept a set amount of money to care for a group of Medicare patients. If the ACO decreases costs while achieving certain quality targets, then the ACO is eligible for a performance bonus.

Inpatient Settings

Over 100,000 health services managers and administrative staff work in hospitals, also called **inpatient** settings, in which patients are admitted to the hospital for an overnight stay, either for emergency situations or for scheduled surgeries (BLS, 2022b). Inpatient facilities provide **acute care**, which involves treatment for brief but severe episodes of illness as the result of disease or trauma. Among more than 48,000 health services managers who belong to the American College of Healthcare Executives (ACHE), over 60% of them work in hospitals and health systems (ACHE, 2023).

The nature of work in hospital management jobs depends on the size of the facility. Smaller hospitals with less than 150 staffed beds provide managers with broad experiences in many different departments, giving the sense of closeness to the patient and the confidence to get things done (Aldrich, 2015). Large hospitals, on the other hand, allow health services managers to specialize in certain functions, such as strategic planning or supply chain management, or to gain broad experience by holding different types of positions within the same HCO. However, large hospitals are incredibly complex and bureaucratic, which can make it difficult for managers to feel like they are making a difference in the overall organization. Table 1.3 defines the various inpatient settings and types (AHA, 2021a, 2021b).

TABLE 1.3 Inpatient Care Settings and Types

SETTING	DEFINITION
Academic medical center	A hospital, sometimes called a teaching hospital, that is integrated with a medical school and that serves as the main location for the education of medical students and trainees
Community hospitals	A technical term for all nonfederal, short-term general, and other special hospitals, including academic medical centers if they are nonfederal, short-term hospitals
Critical access hospitals	Rural hospitals with no more than 25 acute care beds and located more than 35 miles from the nearest hospital (or 15 miles if by mountainous terrain or secondary roads)
Disproportionate share hospitals	Hospitals that care for a disproportionate number of low-income patients and receive payments from the federal government to care for uninsured patients
Intensive care units	Units of hospitals with specialized staff and equipment that care for acutely ill and injured patients. May also be called critical care units or intensive therapy units
Inpatient rehabilitation facilities	Freestanding rehabilitation hospitals or rehabilitation units within acute care hospitals. Most patients are treated at an acute care hospital before admission to an inpatient rehabilitation facility.
Medical-surgical	Units of hospitals dedicated to general medical and surgical services, usually called "med-surg"
Rural hospital	Hospitals not located within a metropolitan area, almost half of which have fewer than 25 staffed beds
Safety-net hospital	Hospitals that treat the highest number of patients insured by Medicaid (state-funded health insurance) or uninsured
Specialty hospitals	Hospitals that offer specialized services through a particular subset of skills and technology, including children's, psychiatric, rehabilitation, and cancer hospitals
Trauma center	Capable of providing emergency medical services to patients suffering from the most serious injuries. The different levels of trauma centers (Level I, II, III, IV, or V) refer to the resources available and the annual number of patients admitted yearly. Level I is the highest level of trauma center.

Outpatient Settings

Medical services that do not require overnight stays are called **outpatient** care. Outpatient care is also called **ambulatory care**, meaning that patients are able to walk in and out of the care settings. When clinically appropriate, outpatient care is the preferred setting for insurance companies and government payers because these services are less expensive than inpatient care. Growth in outpatient care has led to substantial growth in health services management career opportunities. Physician practices are increasingly owned by health systems or corporate entities, such as health insurers or private equity groups, and more physicians are joining large physician groups each year (American Medical Association [AMA], 2021; Physicians Advocacy Institute [PAI], 2021). Whereas smaller practices can operate effectively with health services management generalists with less training, large physician groups require managers with specialized business skills to help run the practices.

Health services managers who are experts in physician practice management can also run **independent practice associations** (IPAs), which are businesses that provide services to smaller physician groups, such as negotiating insurance company contracts. **Management services organizations** are similar support businesses that provide independent physician practices with administrative services, such as technology support, staff education and training, coding compliance, and patient billing and collection services.

The professional association for physician practices is Medical Group Management Association (MGMA), which serves over 60,000 medical practice management professionals and certifies qualified managers with the Certified Medical Practice Executive (CMPE) board certification (MGMA, 2023). Health services managers specialize in operating a variety of outpatient settings, as described in Table 1.4 (Aliber, 2016; AMA, 2021).

TABLE 1.4 Outpatient Care Settings and Types

SETTING	DEFINITION
Ambulatory surgery centers	A facility not part of a hospital with the primary purpose of providing elective, same-day, minimally invasive surgical care. Orthopedic care, such as muscle, tendon, and cartilage repairs, is commonly performed in the outpatient setting.
Community health centers	Community-based clinics that provide primary care to patients, regardless of their ability to pay and charge for services on a sliding fee scale. Health centers that receive federal grant funding are called federally qualified health centers.
Convenient care and retail clinics	Typically located in existing pharmacies, grocery stores, and large retailers, these clinics treat a limited number of conditions and are staffed by physician assistants or nurse practitioners who see patients on a first come, first seen basis.
Dialysis centers	Provide care for patients with kidney disease or kidney failure. During dialysis, blood is filtered to remove waste and excess fluid.
Emergency departments	An emergency facility that is open 24 hours per day, 7 days a week and is connected to an inpatient facility that provides treatment of acute life- or limb-threatening medical and potentially surgical needs
Freestanding emergency departments	Emergency facilities that are not physically connected to inpatient services and typically do not include the full range of diagnostic capabilities. Capabilities generally fall between those of urgent care clinics and hospital-based emergency departments.
Hospital outpatient centers	A general term for the outpatient service settings owned and operated by hospitals, including primary care, secondary care, pain management, chemotherapy, wound care, and physical therapies

(Continued)

TABLE 1.4 Outpatient Care Settings and Types (*continued*)

SETTING	DEFINITION
Physician practice	A private or independent practice owned by physicians who also provide the care. Fewer than half of physicians work in physician-owned practices (American Medical Association, 2021).
Primary care clinics	Primary care is preventive care and treatment for common illnesses provided by specialists in family medicine, general internal medicine, general pediatrics, and nurse practitioners.
Urgent care clinics	Clinics open for extended hours that provide care for people who need care right away (no appointment needed) but not so severe enough for emergency department care

Long-Term Care Settings

Long-term care or post-acute care occurs in facilities or at home and is primarily intended for improving functional abilities associated with daily tasks or for those who have dementia. Long-term care is a growing and essential service for older adults, who are more likely to have various illnesses and disabilities that make recovery from acute illness take longer. Health services managers in nursing homes are required to become licensed nursing home administrators, which necessitates hundreds of hours of supervised training and a passing score on a qualifying exam (National Association of Long-Term Care Administrator Boards [NAB], 2022). The NAB administers a national licensing exam for the state boards and agencies that license long-term care administrators. Table 1.5 describes the various post-acute care settings and types (Sanford et al., 2015; Wang et al., 2019).

INFORMATIONAL INTERVIEW 1.2
Director, Hospital-Based Physician Services
Access the informational interview online at http://connect.springerpub.com/content/book/978-0-8261-4807-0/chapter/ch00.

TABLE 1.5 Post-Acute Care Settings and Types

SETTING	DEFINITION
Assisted living facilities	Provides room and board along with management of medical conditions and other support for patients who are physically and/or cognitively impaired
Comprehensive outpatient rehabilitation facilities	A medical facility that provides outpatient diagnostic and therapeutic care, including physical, occupational, and/or speech therapy with the goal of improving functional status after acute illness or hospitalization. Also called outpatient rehabilitation care
Home health	Care delivered to patients in their own homes through regular visits by caregivers, aides, nurses, and physical or occupational therapists. Home health can be augmented by specialized remote monitoring to provide hospital-at-home services through specialized monitoring equipment, hospital beds, and constant remote medical supervision.

TABLE 1.5 Post-Acute Care Settings and Types (*continued*)

SETTING	DEFINITION
Hospice homes	Offers patients who are near the end of life and their families a variety of physical, emotional, social, and spiritual support
Inpatient rehabilitation facilities	For patients who require hospital-level care directed by a physician in conjunction with daily intensive rehabilitation delivered. Care can be provided in a freestanding building or a department within a hospital. Patients are typically recovering from burns, complex trauma, strokes, and other neurological and orthopedic conditions.
Long-term acute care facilities	Facilities that specialize in caring for patients with serious medical conditions that require care on an ongoing basis. Patients are typically discharged from intensive care units and require more care than other long-term care facilities.
Nursing homes	Long-term residential care facility for people with chronic disease or disability, particularly elderly people who require supportive and a safe environment to maintain functional abilities for as long as possible
Palliative care	Specialized medical care for anyone living with a serious illness that is designed to improve quality of life and help with symptoms. Appropriate at any age and at any stage in a serious illness, palliative care can be provided along with curative treatment.
Skilled nursing facilities	Established within nursing homes, provide rehabilitation, nutrition care, and skilled nursing care, such as drug treatment, wound treatment, and ventilator care under physician supervision

Ancillary Services

Health services managers also run the business operations of **ancillary services**, which include a wide range of supportive therapies and specialized diagnostic services. These services can be located in a variety of settings, such as hospitals, outpatient care centers, medical laboratories, urgent care facilities, or medical practices. Managers over these areas tend to have professional clinical training in the specialization, although not always. For example, the manager of radiology services may need the knowledge and skills of a radiologic technologist. Ancillary services managers oversee staff, maintain equipment, track budgets, and optimize patient throughput (Green, 2022). Table 1.6 describes the various ancillary service types.

Operations Support Services

HCOs provide dozens of nonclinical operations **support services** that complement patient care services. Health services managers can specialize in the support services operational functions. In some HCOs, executives with experience managing nonclinical operations can hold the title of chief operating officer. Table 1.7 describes various support services in HCOs (Aucamp, 2016; Nugent & Emmerich, 2014).

TABLE 1.6 Ancillary Service Types and Professions

TYPES	DEFINITION
Clinical laboratories	Provide a wide range of diagnostic tests performed on samples of biological specimens from patients
Pharmacies	The manufacturing, procurement, storage, compounding, dispensing, and testing of pharmaceuticals. Pharmacy settings include hospitals, clinics, retail stores, and nursing homes.
Imaging and radiology services	Radiology uses imaging technology and may be divided into two different areas: diagnostic radiology and interventional radiology. Diagnostic radiology exams include CT scan, MRI, mammography, and X-rays. Interventional radiology uses imaging to guide procedures, such as cardiac catheterization that removes blockages in the arteries and veins.
Physical therapy, occupational therapy, and speech-language pathology	Often collectively called the rehabilitation therapy team, these professions offer evaluations, interventions, and treatments that help patients move, speak, eat, walk, and dress themselves.
Medical social work	Helps patients understand their illness or condition and attends to the psychosocial needs of patients and families to promote overall well-being

TABLE 1.7 Operations Support Service Functional Departments

TYPE	DEFINITION
Environmental services	Sometimes referred to as housekeeping; prioritizes infection prevention through disinfection and cleaning of patient rooms, nursing units, equipment, offices, and clinical areas
Facilities management	Manages building maintenance and repair, heating and air conditioning, energy, plumbing, construction, and servicing clinical equipment
Food services	In inpatient settings, provides clinical nutrition menus, develops service style and systems for meal ordering, and delivery; manages cafeteria for hospital employees, patients, and family members
Health information management	Manage health information systems, including telehealth, electronic health records, clinical decision support systems, and business analytics, according to legal and regulatory standards
Laundry and linens services	Responsible for washing, sanitizing, and distributing clothes, bed linen, and surgical linen; ensure that workers are protected from harm associated with physical, chemical, and biological exposures to waste
Patient services	Serve as the point of contact for patients and families, including telephone inquiries, problem resolution, appointment scheduling, and insurance verification

TABLE 1.7 Operations Support Service Functional Departments (*continued*)

TYPE	DEFINITION
Patient transportation services	Manage processes related to requesting, scheduling, and moving patients between inpatient units safely, timely, and efficiently
Safety and security	Manage security personnel, communications, monitoring, and responding to security-related events
Supply chain	Manages supply inventory and relationships with suppliers. Responsible for purchasing, storing, and delivering material resources to providers and patients

COMPETENCIES OF HEALTH SERVICES MANAGEMENT

Fundamental Domains of Competencies

Competency-based education means that students are trained to perform discipline-specific actions. For at least 2 decades, academic health administration programs have moved away from theoretical and research-oriented curricula to competency-based education (Bradley et al., 2008). By specifying the behaviors that students must perform, educators are able assess readiness to practice the health services management profession. Upon graduation, employers expect a minimum level of competency from graduates of health administration education programs.

The competency-based education approach has also been adopted by clinical education fields (Edgar et al., 2020). For example, medical training programs recognize that patients want to know that their physician is competent to practice medicine. When a patient arrives to the emergency department with severe chest pain, they expect the physician to be able to effective care for them. This means, of course, that an emergency medicine physician must have knowledge of how the heart works. But knowledge is not enough. Physicians need to also have the skills to effectively diagnose whether the patient is having a heart attack. But diagnosis is not enough. The physician

---

CAREER BOX 1.2: Specialist Versus Generalist Health Services Management

Hospitals and large outpatient organizations employ most of the mid-career health services managers. Because large HCOs are very complex, health services managers sometimes need to specialize in certain functional areas, such as operations, quality, marketing, strategy, information technology, finance, compliance, and human resources. The management positions that support the core operations of the organization are called staff roles. Alternatively, some mid-career professionals gain expertise in the general management of the various HCO businesses or departments, usually called line management roles. Line management in HCOs means overseeing the businesses that directly care for patients, such as the emergency department or surgical services. Promotions to executive roles can happen through line or staff roles, although health services managers in staff positions are more likely to be promoted if they have experience in a number of functional areas. Some line managers gain experience in smaller HCOs before moving into positions in larger organizations. Line managers generally specialize in managing particular settings of HCOs, such as community health centers or physician practices.

must also remain calm, think analytically, and communicate with the patient. All of these skills in isolation are insufficient. Competency requires applying all knowledge, experience, judgment, and skills to complicated, ill-defined, and unexpected circumstances. Competency in medicine means being able to save a patient's life.

Therefore, competence in the practice of health services management does not just mean the recall of facts. True competence means the effective application of discipline-specific knowledge, skills, and abilities to complex situations. Just like other professions in healthcare, there is an expectation that health services managers demonstrate essential discipline-specific behaviors or actions. Because there can be dozens of different health services management competencies, a person does not need to be an expert in each and every one. Graduates of health administration education programs are expected to be a novice in numerous competencies, proficient in others, and experts in areas that will make them valuable to the HCO.

△ **KEY IDEA**
True competence means the effective application of discipline-specific knowledge, skills, and abilities to complex situations.

Competency models are collections of statements defining the performance expectations of a particular job or profession. Each academic program or professional association develops their own competency model consistent with their mission, vision, and values (Standish, 2018). Because of this flexibility, there are dozens of health management competency models, each of which reflect slightly different conceptions of health services management practice. Two of the more prominent competency models are the Healthcare Leadership Alliance model (Stefl, 2008) and the National Center for Healthcare Leadership model (Garman et al., 2020). The ACHE and the MGMA use the Healthcare Leadership Alliance competency model to develop their healthcare management certification programs.

Management Challenges Unique to the Healthcare Sector

Some health services management competencies, such as interpersonal skills and leadership, are common to management in all fields. However, the health care industry is special in many ways, so managers need to develop certain industry-specific competencies. Table 1.8 lists some unique health services management competencies that are addressed in chapters of this textbook.

Contributing to the Interprofessional Team

Collaboration with other kinds of professions is not particularly unique to health services managers. Like healthcare, other industries require managers to coordinate and integrate specialists into cohesive teams (Drucker & Maciariello, 2008). For example, the gaming, sports, and film and television industries involve professionals who perform the work (e.g., game designers, athletes, actors) and managers who manage the work. Like these other industries, managers either contribute to the work or risk losing the respect of the other professionals. However, health services managers typically lack clinical practice knowledge. As such, clinicians may view health services managers as their "support staff" who supplement the important work of providing patient care and underestimate the contribution of the health services manager to the healthcare interprofessional team (Pruitt et al., 2020).

TABLE 1.8 Examples of Management Competencies Unique to Health Services

COMPETENCY AREA	KEY ISSUES
Professionalism and ethics (Chapter 5)	Professionalism and ethics are key competencies of managers in other industries, but health services managers embrace special professional motivations, such as helping patients, empowering clinicians, building community ties, and serving society. Health services managers also accept responsibilities uncommon in most other industries, such as intense regulatory oversight, nonstop demands for services, and life-and-death consequences of business decisions.
Population health and community collaboration (Chapter 6)	While HCOs primarily provide medical care, health services managers need to be well versed in the broader health and wellness needs of their communities. The government and insurance companies are moving toward paying for keeping patients healthy, not just paying for each service delivered.
Healthcare governance (Chapter 7)	Health services managers do not usually have direct authority over physicians and other clinicians. Medical staffs and other shared governance structures require that health services managers develop competency in using institutional governance to enhance the overall performance of the HCOs.
Healthcare quality management (Chapter 12)	Health services managers are responsible for clinical care quality even though they do not have authority over clinicians. Successful managers learn to influence clinician behaviors to improve patient care outcomes.
Healthcare financial management (Chapter 14)	All managers must be competent in the general financial functions of business, such as accounting, budgeting, and finance. However, because patients rely on third-party payers, such as health insurance companies and Medicare, to pay most of the costs, health services managers need to contend with payers by negotiating and managing contracts, navigating benefit and payment rules, and tracking paid and denied payment claims.

INFORMATIONAL INTERVIEW 1.3
Chief Operating Officer
Access the informational interview online at http://connect.springerpub.com/content/book/978-0-8261-4807-0/chapter/ch00.

Even without detailed clinical knowledge, health services managers uniquely contribute to patient care. Interprofessionalism occurs when individuals from multiple healthcare disciplines collaborate to care for patients. Health services managers play an important role on the interprofessional healthcare team, including the following (Begun, White, & Mosser, 2011):

- Allocate resources to interprofessional practice, including clinician training and staffing of teams.
- Apply management practices, such as planning, organizing, and coordinating to improve clinical processes.
- Develop interprofessional governance committees.
- Strengthen ties among the professions.
- Define processes for escalation of concerns among the team.

- Establish and monitor goals for the interprofessional team.
- Hold teams accountable for clinical quality.
- Evaluate teams and individuals and reward achievement.
- Resolve power struggles and conflict among clinical professions.
- Gain consensus among clinicians regarding profession-specific roles and patient care task assignments.

Table 1.9 identifies example competencies (knowledge, technical skills, and interpersonal skills) for five different roles of the interprofessional team.

Health services managers impact patient health outcomes without directly delivering medical care (Chandra et al., 2016; McConnell et al., 2013). For example, management practices are related to decreased mortality rates for heart attacks, including actions leading to improved patient flow efficiencies (Jain et al., 2019). However, health services managers should remain humble, recognizing the sharp divide between clinical and nonclinical professional competencies. Managers do not provide care to patients. Gaining the respect from the interprofessional team requires

TABLE 1.9 Select Competencies From the Interprofessional Team

	KNOWLEDGE	TECHNICAL SKILLS	INTERPERSONAL SKILLS
Health services manager[a]	Demonstrate understanding of health system operations and financing systems.	Measure and monitor clinical and organizational performance.	Lead teams toward shared visions and goals.
Physician[b]	Apply anatomy and physiology knowledge to clinical situations.	Make informed diagnostic and therapeutic decisions.	Maintain an open dialogue and flow of information with patients.
Nurse practitioner[c]	Interpret diagnostic information.	Analyze and prioritize patient problems.	Demonstrate strong patient interviewing skills.
Physical therapist[d]	Demonstrate understanding of the human movement system.	Apply current knowledge, theory, and evidence to make effective clinical decisions.	Interact with patients in a manner congruent with situational and cultural needs.
Social worker[e]	Demonstrate understanding of social and medical service resources.	Manage patients' transitions from hospital discharge to care at their homes.	Communicate with family members to evaluate patients in their social contexts.

[a]National Center for Healthcare Leadership. (2018). *Healthcare leadership competency model 3.0*. https://nchl.member365.org/publicFr/store/item/19
[b]Edgar, L., McLean, S., Hogan, S. O., Hamstra, S., & Holmboe, E. S. (2020). *The milestones guidebook*. Accreditation Council for Graduate Medical Education. https://www.acgme.org/globalassets/milestones guidebook.pdf
[c]D'Aoust, R. F., Brown, K. M., McIltrot, K., Adamji, J. M. D., Johnson, H., Seibert, D. C., & Ling, C. G. (2022). A competency roadmap for advanced practice nursing education using PRIME-NP. *Nursing Outlook, 70*(2), 337–346. https://doi.org/10.1016/j.outlook.2021.10.009
[d]Grignon, T. P., Henley, E., Lee, K. M., Abentroth, M. J., & Jette, D. U. (2014). Expected graduate outcomes in US physical therapist education programs: A qualitative study. *Journal of Physical Therapy Education, 28*(1), 48–57. https://doi.org/10.1097/00001416-201410000-00010
[e]Kangasniemi, M., Karki, S., Voutilainen, A., Saarnio, R., Viinamäki, L., & Häggman-Laitila, A. (2022). The value that social workers' competencies add to health care: An integrative review. *Health & Social Care in the Community, 30*(2), 403–414. https://doi.org/10.1111/hsc.13266

that managers understand the roles of clinicians and how they contribute to the patient health outcomes. When managers bring value to the team, they enhance the stature of the management profession. This means acting with integrity, treating people fairly, admitting mistakes, and continuously seeking ways to improve as a professional. When health services managers behave contrary to these values, they diminish the authority of the profession and weaken their effectiveness within the organization (Griffith, 1993).

Diversity, Equity, and Inclusion

Health disparities continue to be pervasive and persistent among ethnic and racial minorities in the United States (Lavizzo-Mourey et al., 2021). Because health services managers hold a special role in healthcare, they have the professional responsibility to reduce health disparities among patients and the communities served by the HCO (Brooks-Williams, 2022). However, some health services managers who claim to want greater health equity may not be willing to invest the time, effort, resources, and commitment necessary to make it happen. The extent to which HCOs succeed in reducing health disparities depends on how much responsibility managers accept and whether they hold themselves and others accountable. Good intentions are no substitute for good management.

> ⚠ **KEY IDEA**
>
> The extent to which HCOs succeed in reducing health disparities depends on how much managers accept the responsibility and hold themselves and others accountable. Good intentions are no substitute for good management.

One way to achieve **health equity**—where everyone, especially individuals who have the greatest need, can achieve optimal health—is to maximize diversity and inclusion in the workplace (Institute for Diversity and Health Equity [IFDHE], 2020). This means HCOs that create workplaces that reflect the communities they serve are able to more effectively reduce health disparities (Gomez & Bernet, 2019). **Diversity** is the variation in characteristics within a group of people that makes people unique, including race, age, gender, religion, sexual orientation, experiences, talents, skills, opinions, and personalities. **Inclusion** in the workplace entails recognizing, appreciating, and utilizing employees of diverse backgrounds, talents, and skills. Diversity and inclusion help to create organizational understanding about the best ways to care for populations of people who most need it. Health services managers—if prepared—can use classical management practices to improve diversity and inclusion and impact health equity in their communities.

1. *Planning:* Evaluate best approaches and allocate funding for diversity and inclusion initiatives.
2. *Organizing:* Appoint chief diversity officer with responsibility and authority for achieving health equity through workplace diversity and inclusion.
3. *Directing:* Set performance expectations for diversity, equity, and inclusion.
4. *Coordinating:* Connect executives from clinical and social care departments in order to address social risks, such as poverty, food insecurity, and domestic violence.
5. *Controlling:* Allocate budgets and evaluate performance based on the results of diversity, equity, and inclusion improvement initiatives.

In addition, creating health equity requires a shift from caring for individual patients to addressing the health of populations, which requires an additional set of management skills, such as epidemiology, social marketing, and community collaboration. Knowledge of population health fundamentals facilitates better decisions in the efforts to improve diversity, equity, and inclusion.

HEALTH SERVICES MANAGEMENT CAREERS

Managing Oneself

Successful health services managers ascend to the executive ranks because they can effectively manage themselves. Self-management involves applying management competencies to one's career and professional development. Of course, this is not easy, and for many people, this is the greatest challenge of their careers. This textbook will address the practices associated with managing HCOs, but the competencies can be applied to professional development as well. Table 1.10 lists professional development questions related to each chapter of the textbook that health services managers can ask.

Answering these questions requires deliberate examination of one's values, strengths, development needs, learning style, and time management tactics. Managing oneself effectively requires initiative, self-awareness, reflection, discipline, and purposeful self-directed learning.

TABLE 1.10 Professional Development Questions Related to Chapter Content

CHAPTER	CHAPTER TITLE	PROFESSIONAL DEVELOPMENT QUESTIONS
1	Role of the Health Services Manager	How can I contribute to HCO goals? What is my role on the team?
2	Problem-Solving and Evidence-Based Management	What are the most effective ways to overcome my weaknesses? What evidence supports my professional advancement?
3	Managing Interpersonal Communications	How do others perceive my competence? Can I advocate for my professional advancement?
4	Leadership and Change Management	How does my ability to control my emotions impact my ability to manage my organization? How can I develop myself professionally?
5	Professionalism and Ethics	What is the right thing to do?
6	Population Health and Community Collaboration	How should I spend my time? Who are my allies in my professional development effort?
7	Healthcare Governance	Who can advise me on my career?
8	Healthcare Strategy and Marketing	What am I good at? Which of my strengths do employers most value?
9	Human Resource Management	What job would be the best fit for me? What HCO would be the best fit for me?

TABLE 1.10 Professional Development Questions Related to Chapter Content (*continued*)

CHAPTER	CHAPTER TITLE	PROFESSIONAL DEVELOPMENT QUESTIONS
10	Organizational Design	What style of boss suits me best? How much responsibility do I desire in my work?
11	Performance Management	What are my goals? How can I get feedback to accelerate my personal growth?
12	Healthcare Quality Management	How do I learn new knowledge, skills, and abilities to improve my work quality?
13	Project Management	What is the action plan that will advance my career?
14	Healthcare Financial Management	How much money do I need to leave a job without serious financial repercussions?

> **CAREER BOX 1.3:** Late-Career Health Services Management
>
> Late-career health care management success can be defined in many different ways. Although the idea of being the top boss is appealing, not every manager wants to become the chief executive officer (CEO). The CEO position is a distinct role within HCOs that requires a specific set of responsibilities, including attending board meetings, strategic retreats, community social events, and news conferences with politicians. Sometimes, late-career managers would prefer the role of the chief operating officer, an executive who specializes in day-to-day operations of the HCO, or dozens of other late-career positions.

Managing Careers

As a person progresses in their health services management career, each promotion provides new opportunities for professional development. To earn promotions, however, a person needs to accept additional responsibility and accountability for performance, which requires them to take on more work than they are paid to do. Working hard may sound obvious, but people rarely ask for more responsibility without expecting to be compensated. Instead, successful careers are built on asking the bosses, "What can I do to help you?" and then performing well, not because of expectations for a raise but with the intention of being useful (Drucker & Maciariello, 2008). Health services managers who are most effective will be given additional responsibilities and financial rewards. Minimally effective managers do not advance in their careers. Ineffective managers will change occupations—voluntarily or involuntarily.

△ KEY IDEA

To earn promotions, however, a person needs to accept additional responsibility and accountability for performance, which requires them to take on more work than they are paid to do.

FUTURE DIRECTIONS

Health services management job opportunities will grow much faster in the next decade than the average for all occupations (U.S. BLS, 2021). However, there will be significant challenges for the profession. In addition to the aforementioned consolidation of the healthcare sector, health services managers will have to deal with workforce shortages; supply chain issues; environmental impacts of HCOs; transforming care delivery models; and growth of advanced technologies, such as telemedicine, artificial intelligence, and gene editing. Health services managers will face demands from patients, governments, and insurance companies to improve care quality, patient experience, and health equity, all while reducing costs of medical care. Meeting these challenges will require management competence gained through academic training, hard work, and years of experience.

SUMMARY

- Management does not necessarily mean business management. Managers exist in all sectors of the economy and all types of organizations.
- Management involves practices that distinguish it from other occupations, including planning, organizing, directing, coordinating, and controlling.
- Most health services managers work in inpatient settings, although the most substantial growth in employment will be in outpatient and long-term care settings. Thousands of managers also work in healthcare businesses that do provide direct health care services.
- Health services management competence means the effective application of discipline-specific knowledge, skills, and abilities to complex situations.
- Health services management requires certain competencies that are unique to management practice that must be performed under circumstances uncommon to most industries, such as lack of authority over physicians and other clinicians, third-party payers, intense regulatory oversight, nonstop demands for services, and life-and-death consequences of business decisions.
- Health services managers make business choices that consider clinical investments of uncertain marginal value, requiring them to negotiate the trade-offs between profits and patient care.
- Even without detailed clinical knowledge, health services managers uniquely contribute to the interprofessional team, including allocating resources and holding teams accountable for outcomes.
- Health services managers have the professional obligation to reduce health disparities and increase diversity and inclusion in the workplace.

END-OF-CHAPTER RESOURCES

KEY TERMS*

*For the full list of key terms, please see the online glossary at **http://connect.springerpub.com/content/book/978-0-8261-4807-0.**

academic medical center
accountable care organization
acute care
ambulatory care
ancillary services
boundary spanning

community health centers
community hospitals
commanding
controlling
coordinating
clinically integrated network
critical access hospital
directing
disproportionate share hospital
diversity
for-profit
health disparities
health equity
health services managers
health systems
Hill-Burton Act
hospice
inclusion
independent practice association
inpatient
integrated delivery network
line position
long-term care
management
management by objectives
management services organizations
not-for-profit
organizing
outpatient
palliative care
planning
pharmacies
physician practices
safety-net provider
staff position
staffing
support services
systems thinking
systems theory
urgent care
Veterans Health Administration

LEARNING ACTIVITIES

Professional Development and Reflection

1. Reflect on career options along the continuum of care. Using Figure 1.5 that illustrates the continuum of care, identify at least five health services management positions that most interest you. Write your reflection on what interests you about the positions; work settings; and the skills, education, and experience level required to obtain those jobs.
2. Each chapter features "Informational Interviews" conducted with related health services management practitioners. An informational interview is a question-and-answer discussion with a more experience professional to learn about career paths and build future relationships. Conduct an informational interview with a health services manager working in a healthcare setting or type that interests you. When complete, describe the most important piece of advice that you were given.

Discussion Questions

1. Discuss the significance of the legal distinction between for-profit and not-for-profit HCOs. How does this difference, particularly in tax obligations, influence the operations and decision-making of each type of organization?
2. Which of the roles, functions, practices, or responsibilities of the health services manager described in the chapter make diversity, equity, and inclusion a professional obligation?
3. In what ways can the competencies associated with managing health care organizations be translated and applied to an individual's professional development?

RECOMMENDED READING AND MEDIA

Berrett, B., & Spiegelman, P. (2013). *Patients come second: Leading change by changing the way you lead.* An Inc. Original.

Clear, J. (2018). *Atomic habits: Tiny changes, remarkable results.* Avery.

Covey, S. R. (2020). *The 7 habits of highly effective people: Powerful lessons in personal change.* Simon & Schuster.

Zhuo, J. (2019). *The making of a manager: What to do when everyone looks to you.* Portfolio/Penguin.

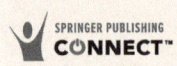

A robust set of instructor resources designed to supplement this text is located at http://connect.springerpub.com/content/book/978-0-8261-4807-0. Qualifying instructors may request access by emailing textbook@springerpub.com.

REFERENCES

Agency for Healthcare Research and Quality. (2023). *Defining health systems.* https://www.ahrq.gov/chsp/defining-health-systems/index.html

Aldrich, J. (2015). *Climbing the healthcare management ladder: Career advice from the top on how to succeed.* Health Professions Press.

Aliber, J. (2016, February 8). *The 8 types of ambulatory care settings.* AHA Trustee Services. https://trustees.aha.org/articles/1046-the-8-types-of-ambulatory-care-settings

American College of Healthcare Executives. (2023). *Members and fellows profile.* https://www.ache.org/learning-center/research/members-and-fellows-profile

American Hospital Association. (2021a). *Fast facts: U.S. health systems infographic.* https://www.aha.org/infographics/2021-01-15-fast-facts-us-health-systems-infographic

American Hospital Association. (2021b). *Fast facts: U.S. rural hospitals infographic.* https://www.aha.org/infographics/2021-05-24-fast-facts-us-rural-hospitals-infographic

American Medical Association. (2021). *AMA analysis shows most physicians work outside of private practice.* https://www.ama-assn.org/press-center/press-releases/ama-analysis-shows-most-physicians-work-outside-private-practice

Aucamp, M. (2016). Housekeeping and linen management. In C. Friedman (Ed.), *Basic concepts of infection control* (3rd ed.). International Federation of Infection Control.

Balak, N., Tisell, M., & Honeybul, S. (2020). Healthcare economics. In S. Honeybul (Ed.), *Ethics in neurosurgical practice* (pp. 73–84). Cambridge University Press.

Bateman, T. S., Snell, S., & Konopaske, R. (2017). *Management:Leading & collaborating in a competitive world* (12th ed.). McGraw-Hill Education.

Begun, J. W., White, K. R., & Mosser, G. (2011). Interprofessional care teams: The role of the healthcare administrator. *Journal of Interprofessional Care, 25*(2), 119–123. https://doi.org/10.3109/13561820.2010.504135

Berrett, B., & Spiegelman, P. (2013). *Patients come second: Leading change by changing the way you lead.* An Inc. Original.

Bovée, C. L., Thill, J. V., Wood, M. B., & Dovel, G. P. (1993). *Management.* McGraw-Hill.

Bradley, E. H., Cherlin, E., Busch, S. H., Epstein, A., Helfand, B., & White, W. D. (2008). Adopting a competency-based model: Mapping curricula and assessing student progress. *Journal of Health Administration Education, 25*(1), 37–51.

Brooks-Williams, D. (2022). An effective response to healthcare disparities begins with a strategic plan. *Frontiers of Health Services Management, 39*(2), 27–31. https://doi.org/10.1097/hap.0000000000000153

Burns, L. R. (Ed.). (2012). *The business of healthcare innovation* (2nd ed.). Cambridge University Press.

Chandra, A., Finkelstein, A., Sacarny, A., & Syverson, C. (2016). Health care exceptionalism? Performance and allocation in the US health care sector. *American Economic Review, 106*(8), 2110–2144. https://doi.org/10.1257%2Faer.20151080

Daellenbach, H. G., McNickle, D. C., & Dye, S. (2017). *Management science: Decision making through systems thinking*. Palgrave Macmillan.

Darr, K. (2019). *Ethics in health services management* (6th ed.). Health Professions Press.

D'Aoust, R. F., Brown, K. M., McIltrot, K., Adamji, J. M. D., Johnson, H., Seibert, D. C., & Ling, C. G. (2022). A competency roadmap for advanced practice nursing education using PRIME-NP. *Nursing Outlook, 70*(2), 337–346. https://doi.org/10.1016/j.outlook.2021.10.009

Davis, M. M. (1929). *Hospital administration: A career*. Rockefeller Foundation.

Defense Health Agency. (2022). *MHS health facilities*. https://www.health.mil/Military-Health-Topics/MHS-Toolkits/Media-Resources/Media-Center/MHS-Health-Facilities

Drucker, P. F. (1954). *The practice of management*. Harper & Row, Publishers, Inc.

Drucker, P. F. (1990). *Managing the nonprofit organization: Practices and principles*. HarperCollins.

Drucker, P. F., & Maciariello, J. A. (2008). Management (rev. ed.). New York: HarperCollins.

Edgar, L., McLean, S., Hogan, S. O., Hamstra, S., & Holmboe, E. S. (2020). *The milestones guidebook*. Accreditation Council for Graduate Medical Education. https://www.acgme.org/globalassets/milestonesguidebook.pdf

Falvey, A. (2023, February 28). 100 of the largest hospitals and health systems in America. *Becker's Hospital Review*. https://www.beckershospitalreview.com/lists/100-of-the-largest-hospitals-and-health-systems-in-america-2023.html

Fayol, H. (1916). General principles of management. *Classics of Organization Theory, 2*(15), 57–69.

Franz, B., Cronin, C. E., Rodriguez, V., Choyke, K., Simon, J. E., & Hall, M. T. (2021). For-profit hospitals as anchor institutions in the United States: A study of organizational stability. *BMC Health Services Research, 21*(1), 1–9. https://doi.org/10.1186/s12913-021-07307-1

Garman, A. N., Boren, S., Masuda, D., & Shah, S. C. (2020). Mapping national center for healthcare leadership competencies to the CAHME accreditation competency domains. *The Journal of Health Administration Education, 37*(1), 349–354.

Gomez, L. E., & Bernet, P. (2019). Diversity improves performance and outcomes. *Journal of the National Medical Association, 111*(4), 383–392. https://doi.org/10.1016/j.jnma.2019.01.006

Green, C. (2022). *Being intentional when adding ancillary services*. Medical Group Management Association. https://www.mgma.com/mgma-stats/being-intentional-when-adding-ancillary-services

Griffin, R. W. (2013). *Management: Principles and practices* (11th ed.). Cengage Learning South-Western.

Griffith, J. R. (1993). *The moral challenges of health care management*. Health Administration Press.

Grignon, T. P., Henley, E., Lee, K. M., Abentroth, M. J., & Jette, D. U. (2014). Expected graduate outcomes in US physical therapist education programs: A qualitative study. *Journal of Physical Therapy Education, 28*(1), 48–57. https://doi.org/10.1097/00001416-201410000-00010

Haddock, C. C., McLean, R. A., & Chapman, R. C. (2002). *Careers in healthcare management: How to find your path and follow it*. Health Administration Press.

Huang, H., Zhu, X., Ullrich, F., MacKinney, A. C., & Mueller, K. (2023). The impact of Medicare shared savings program participation on hospital financial performance: An event-study analysis. *Health Services Research, 58*(1), 116–127. https://doi.org/10.1111/1475-6773.14085

Institute for Diversity and Health Equity. (2020). *Health equity, diversity & inclusion measures for hospitals and health system dashboards*. American Hospital Association. https://ifdhe.aha.org/system/files/media/file/2020/12/ifdhe_inclusion_dashboard.pdf

Jain, S., Thorpe, K. E., Hockenberry, J. M., & Saltman, R. B. (2019). Strategies for delivering value-based care: Do care management practices improve hospital performance? *Journal of Healthcare Management, 64*(6), 430–444. https://doi.org/10.1097/jhm-d-18-00049

Kaehler, B., & Grundei, J. (2019). The concept of management: In search of a new definition. *HR Governance: A Theoretical Introduction*, 3–26. https://doi.org/10.1007/978-3-319-94526-2_2

Kaiser Family Foundation. (2019). *Hospitals by ownership type*. State Health Facts. https://www.kff.org/other/state-indicator/hospitals-by-ownership

Kangasniemi, M., Karki, S., Voutilainen, A., Saarnio, R., Viinamäki, L., & Häggman-Laitila, A. (2022). The value that social workers' competencies add to health care: An integrative review. *Health & Social Care in the Community, 30*(2), 403–414. https://doi.org/10.1111/hsc.13266

Kinicki, A., & Williams, B. K. (2018). *Management: A practical introduction* (8th ed.). McGraw-Hill.

Koontz, H. (1961). The management theory jungle. *Academy of Management Journal, 4*(3), 174–188. https://doi.org/10.5465/254541

Korica, M., Nicolini, D., & Johnson, B. (2017). In search of 'managerial work': Past, present and future of an analytical category. *International Journal of Management Reviews, 19*(2), 151–174. https://doi.org/10.1111/ijmr.12090

Lavizzo-Mourey, R. J., Besser, R. E., & Williams, D. R. (2021). Understanding and mitigating health inequities—Past, current, and future directions. *New England Journal of Medicine, 384*(18), 1681–1684. https://doi.org/10.1056/nejmp2008628

McConnell, K. J., Lindrooth, R. C., Wholey, D. R., Maddox, T. M., & Bloom, N. (2013). Management practices and the quality of care in cardiac units. *JAMA Internal Medicine, 173*(8), 684–692. https://doi.org/10.1001/jamainternmed.2013.3577

Medical Group Management Association. (2023). *MGMA home*. https://www.mgma.com

Mintzberg, H. (1973). *The nature of managerial work*. Harper & Row.

Mintzberg, H. (1994). Rounding out the manager's job. *Sloan Management Review, 36*(1), 11–26.

Mintzberg, H. (2009a). *Managing*. Berret-Koehler Publishers.

Mintzberg, H. (2009b, August 17). What managers really do. *Wall Street Journal*. http://www.mintzberg.org/sites/default/files/article/download/mgrsreallydo.pdf

National Association of Long Term Care Administrator Boards. [NAB]. (2022). *Who we are*. https://www.nabweb.org/about-nab/who-we-are

National Center for Healthcare Leadership. (2018). *Healthcare leadership competency model 3.0*. https://nchl.member365.org/publicFr/store/item/19

Naylor, J. (2004). *Management* (2nd ed.). Pearson Education/Prentice Hall.

Nugent, B., & Emmerich, C. (2014). Top 4 sources of savings in support services. *Healthcare Financial Management, 68*(12), 74–78.

Physician's Advocacy Institute. (2021, June). *COVID-19's impact on acquisitions of physician practices and physician employment 2019–2020*. http://www.physiciansadvocacyinstitute.org/Portals/0/assets/docs/Revised-6-8-21_PAI-Physician-Employment-Study-2021-FINAL.pdf

Pizzolitto, E., Verna, I., & Venditti, M. (2022). Authoritarian leadership styles and performance: A systematic literature review and research agenda. *Management Review Quarterly, 73*(2), 841–871. https://doi.org/10.1007/s11301-022-00263-y

Pruitt, Z., Mhaskar, R., & Greenberg, M. R. (2020). Interprofessional collaboration between medical and health administration students. *The Journal of Health Admin Education, 36*(4), 317–334.

Pruitt, Z., & Pracht, E. (2013). Emergency admissions for non-life-threatening injuries to children. *American Journal of Managed Care, 19*(11), 917–924.

Rozier, M. D. (2020). Nonprofit hospital community benefit in the US: A scoping review from 2010 to 2019. *Frontiers in Public Health, 8*, 72. https://doi.org/10.3389/fpubh.2020.00072

Sanford, A. M., Orrell, M., Tolson, D., Abbatecola, A. M., Arai, H., Bauer, J. M., Cruz-Jentoft, A. J., Dong, B., Ga, H., Goel, A., Hajjar, R., Holmerova, I., Katz, P. R., Koopmans, R. T., Rolland, Y., Visvanathan, R., Woo, J., Morley, J. E., & Vellas, B. (2015). An international definition for "nursing home". *Journal of the American Medical Directors Association, 16*(3), 181–184. https://doi.org/10.1016/j.jamda.2014.12.013

Schuller, K. A., Cronin, C. E., & Buchman, S. A. (2018). Measuring motivational differences for selecting a nursing or health services administration major and examining opportunities for shared learning. *The Journal of Health Administration Education, 35*(4), 439.

Southwick, R. (2022, December 5). *Atrium Health, Advocate Aurora Health complete merger, and more hospital deals could follow*. Chief Healthcare Executive. https://www.chiefhealthcareexecutive.com/view/atrium-health-advocate-aurora-health-complete-merger-and-more-hospital-deals-could-follow

Standish, M. P. (2018). Competency models in graduate healthcare management education: Analysis of current practices and recommendations for getting to best practices. *The Journal of Health Administration Education, 35*(2), 269.

Starr, P. (1982). *The social transformation of American medicine: The rise of a sovereign profession and the making of a vast industry*. Basic Books.

Stefl, M. E. (2008). Common competencies for all healthcare managers: The healthcare leadership alliance model. *Journal of Healthcare Management, 53*(6), 360–374. https://doi.org/10.1097/00115514-200811000-00004

Stevens, R. (1989). *In sickness and in wealth: American hospitals in the twentieth century*. Johns Hopkins University Press.

U.S. Bureau of Labor Statistics. (2021). *Employment projections, 2021–2031*. https://data.bls.gov/projections/nationalMatrix?queryParams=11-9111

U.S. Bureau of Labor Statistics. (2022a). *Health care and social assistance: NAICS 62*. https://www.bls.gov/iag/tgs/iag62.htm

U.S. Bureau of Labor Statistics. (2022b). *Healthcare occupations*. https://www.bls.gov/ooh/healthcare/home.htm

Urick, B. Y., & Meggs, E. V. (2019). Towards a greater professional standing: Evolution of pharmacy practice and education, 1920–2020. *Pharmacy, 7*(3), 98. https://doi.org/10.3390/pharmacy7030098

Veteran Health Administration. (2023, May 9). *Health home page*. https://www.va.gov/health

Wang, Y. C., Chou, M. Y., Liang, C. K., Peng, L. N., Chen, L. K., & Loh, C. H. (2019). Post-acute care as a key component in a healthcare system for older adults. *Annals of Geriatric Medicine and Research, 23*(2), 54–62. https://doi.org/10.4235/agmr.19.0009

White, K. R., & Griffith, J. R. (2019). Foundations of well-managed healthcare organizations. In *The well-managed healthcare organization* (9th ed., pp. 3–33). Chicago: Health Administration Press.

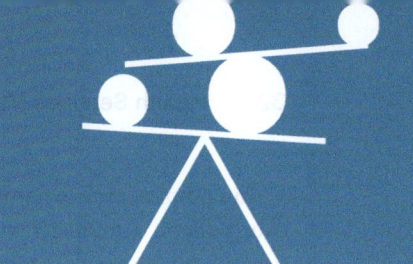

CHAPTER 2

PROBLEM-SOLVING AND EVIDENCE-BASED MANAGEMENT

Problem-solving involves investigating and analyzing problems, generating and evaluating alternative solutions, and developing and communicating recommendations for action. Evidence-based management combines critical thinking with the best available evidence to improve decision-making.

COMPETENCIES

- Solve problems through critical thinking and analysis of the best available evidence.
- Apply evidence-based management skills to health services management challenges.
- Proactively identify current and future problems.
- Define problems, challenges, or opportunities thoroughly and succinctly.
- Formulate alternative solutions using a variety of credible sources.
- Analyze quantitative and qualitative evidence to evaluate alternative solutions.
- Generate conclusions based on findings.
- Connect recommendations to supportable conclusions.

CHAPTER OUTLINE

- Evidence-Based Management
- Define Problems
- Identify Potential Solutions and Generate Hypotheses
- Analyze Alternative Solutions
- Types of Health Services Management Problems

INTRODUCTION

With foresight and planning, health services managers create stability and reliability in health care organizations (HCOs). Despite their best efforts, however, constant disruptions require health services managers to solve problems. A **problem** is simply a gap between how things are and how they should be (Potthoff, Mishek, & Hart, 2020). In other words, problems are issues that get in the way of achieving organizational objectives. Problems can be obstacles to achievement or unpleasant predicaments but can also present opportunities for improvement. When performance is below expectations or when something presents a threat to future success, health services managers take the initiative to address the issue (Drucker, 1954).

In complex and dynamic HCOs, problems are everywhere. When a project threatens to go over budget, a manager intervenes to prevent escalating costs. If a medical supplier increases prices, a health services manager finds more cost-effective alternatives. If a formidable competitor enters the market, a health services manager responds with strategic moves of their own. When two proposals seem equally attractive, a health services manager analyzes the alternatives. When too many patients wait in the emergency department, a manager redesigns the processes, fine-tunes the staffing, or expands the facilities. Effective health services managers constantly solve these kinds of problems and more. Appendix 1 provides examples of health services management problems.

Unfortunately, many health services managers do not solve problems effectively (London, Conn, & Sarrazin, 2019). Without a deliberate approach, managers resort to solving problems by using management fads, uninspired fixes, or even just the whims of powerful people. Clouded by overconfidence or simply overwhelmed, some managers jump to solutions without defining the problem. Other managers avoid difficult issues by solving easier problems, often unaware of time being wasted solving the wrong problems (Kahneman, 2011). Some managers fail to generate new ideas or ask others for input, thereby missing out on better solutions and ruining any chance for innovation (Chevallier & Enders, 2022).

This chapter will explain how health services managers can apply established problem-solving methodologies to make better decisions. The fundamental steps of problem-solving—rooted in the scientific method and common to most approaches—will be defined, described, and clarified with health services management examples.

EVIDENCE-BASED MANAGEMENT

Critical Thinking and Bias

Successful problem-solving requires sound reasoning based on facts. **Critical thinking** is the term used to describe purposeful reflection and logical analysis of information to generate supportable conclusions (Ennis, 2015; Moon, 2007). The opposite of critical thinking is indiscriminately accepting information, ideas, or opinions without analysis or evaluation. This type of thinking can be called intuition, instinct, or gut feelings. Advocating for something that feels true despite any evidence, referred to as **truthiness**, is a mistake in thinking driven by egotism and intellectual self-satisfaction (Payette & Barnes, 2017). Without critical thinking, health services managers are bound to create further problems or worsen existing ones.

> △ **KEY IDEA**
>
> **Advocating for something that feels true despite any evidence, referred to as *truthiness*, is a mistake in thinking driven by egotism and intellectual self-satisfaction. Without critical thinking, health services managers are bound to blunder.**

But arrogance cannot always be blamed for errors in thinking. Frustration, fear, fatigue, ignorance, and distraction also undercut critical thinking (Erwin, 2019). Under duress and without discipline, health services managers resort to mental shortcuts, also known as **heuristic** decision-making. While intuitive thinking can improve creativity and save time, the assumptions that accompany heuristics can lead to poor decision-making (Rasiel & Friga, 2001). Erroneous assumptions, attitudes, and behaviors that cause errors in thinking are known as **cognitive biases**

(Tversky & Kahneman, 1974). Cognitive bias means not just bad thinking but systematically bad thinking. Unfortunately, no one escapes biased thinking; all human judgment suffers from cognitive limitations and irrationality of various kinds (Simon, 1955). Effective problem solvers are aware of the human tendencies to commit these mental errors and use critical thinking to negate irrationality. Table 2.1 presents some of the common cognitive biases that negatively impact problem-solving (Hardman, 2009; Kahneman, 2011; Rynes et al., 2017).

TABLE 2.1 Common Cognitive Biases That Negatively Impact Problem-Solving

BIAS	DEFINITION	EXAMPLE THINKING
Affect heuristic	Occurs when emotions and mood heavily influence thinking	"Maybe I was having a bad day, but I just don't think that candidate fits our organizational culture."
Anchoring bias	Relying too heavily on the first piece of information when making subsequent judgments or decisions	"After reviewing the proposal of $1 million, the $100,000 proposal seems much more reasonable."
Confirmation bias	Confirming existing beliefs or rejecting evidence that contradicts beliefs	"I found evidence to support the solution that I prefer."
Law of the instrument	Exaggerated enthusiasm for a preferred method of analysis or type of solution; also known as Maslow's hammer	"Let's fix the problem by hiring more staff."
Groupthink	Making decisions based on the collective opinion of the group rather than individual thought	"We've already discussed this, so let's not waste any more time on discussion. I think we should make the investment. Who agrees?"
Representativeness bias	Estimating the probability of an event based on how similar it is to a known situation	"He looks just like our CEO, so he must be the best candidate."
Self-serving bias	To claim more responsibility for successes than failures in order to maintain self-esteem	"I never supported that bad decision."
Solution bias	Defining a problem with the solution in mind instead of defining the problem thoroughly	"I have an idea for a solution that I've wanted to try. Let's solve this problem with my idea."
Sunk-cost fallacy	Continuing something because of previously invested resources; often described by the idiom "throwing good money after bad"	"Since so much money has been spent on the project so far, we should keep trying to make it a success."

CEO, chief executive officer.

> **CAREER BOX 2.1: Cognitive Bias in Career Decision-Making**
>
> When planning careers, cognitive bias can create barriers to success. For example, availability bias can cause you to think too narrowly about career options (Whittlestone, 2013). Early-career health services managers tend to set their sights on becoming the chief executive officer of a hospital. However, many excellent health services management careers are found in other positions and health care settings. To expand career options and increase chances for success, widen your perspective by investigating many career options. By investigating many potential alternative career options, you can improve your chances to identify opportunities that are more likely to develop into a high-impact career (and for which you are better suited).

Evidence-Based Problem-Solving

Medical knowledge has advanced at an unparalleled pace. While beneficial to patient care, the vast number of research studies take too much time to review for even the most diligent physicians (Subbiah, 2023). In response to the information explosion, the **evidence-based medicine** movement has sought to make it easier for physicians to integrate research-derived evidence into clinical decision-making (Guyatt & Rennie, 1993; Sackett et al., 1996). Scholars and clinicians critically appraise thousands of research articles published each year and summarize them into a small number of systematic reviews and clinical practice guidelines (Djulbegovic & Guyatt, 2017). Evidence-based medicine enables physicians to efficiently adopt medical practices that are consistent with evidence, but also consider clinical judgment and patient preferences.

> **INFORMATIONAL INTERVIEW 2.1**
>
> *Human Capital Consultant*
> Access the informational interview online at http://connect.springerpub.com/content/book/978-0-8261-4807-0/chapter/ch00.

The **evidence-based management** movement also seeks to enable better decisions through critical thinking and the systematic application of the best available evidence. However, integration of evidence into practice has been less successful for managers than for physicians due to several reasons (Rynes & Bartunek, 2017). First, health services managers often lack skills necessary to assess and utilize evidence in decision-making (Guo et al., 2016). Managers also discount the usefulness of scholarly literature, erroneously claiming that science is not applicable to them because their problems are unique (Kovner & D'Aunno, 2016; Pfeffer & Sutton, 2006). Also, management research often produces weaker evidence than medicine because management scholars rarely conduct rigorous randomized controlled trials on the business of healthcare. Finally, a disconnect exists between health services management practitioners and scholars about what is important to research. Regrettably, this leads to irrelevant research generated by the academic community (Begun et al., 2018). While these challenges stifle the practice of evidence-based management, these approaches can still be a valuable part of effective problem-solving.

Systematic Approaches to Problem-Solving

To avoid bias and more intentionally incorporate evidence, various professions have developed systematic problem-solving methods based on the **scientific method**. The scientific method refers to the objective, systematic process of investigating natural phenomena, answering questions, and solving problems. This means that science-based problem-solving is deliberative, rational, and logical. Like the scientific method, these problem-solving methods attempt to avoid cognitive biases through structured thinking.

> ⚠ **KEY IDEA**
>
> **To avoid bias and more intentionally incorporate evidence, various professions have developed systematic problem-solving methods based on the scientific method.**

The scientific approach to problem-solving has existed for thousands of years, dating back at least to the time of the ancient Greek philosopher Aristotle (Quarantotto, 2020). There are at least 150 problem-solving strategies used by professional disciplines, each using slightly different terminologies (Woods, 2000). However, each approach follows a similar pattern: define the problem, generate potential solutions, test alternatives through structured analysis, and repeat. The following are examples from medicine, engineering, and aviation:

- *Physicians:* In the **differential diagnosis**, physicians identify a problem (patient complaint), gather diagnostic data (e.g., X-rays), generate a list of possible diagnoses, prioritize the diagnoses by severity and likelihood, and systematically test the validity of each potential diagnosis until one cannot be ruled out (Stern et al., 2020).
- *Engineers:* When solving design problems, engineers first recognize and define the problem, then prepare, analyze, synthesize, evaluate, and present their findings (Woods, 2000).
- *Airplane pilots:* The FOR-DEC method stands for **F**acts, **O**ptions, **R**isks and benefits, **D**ecision, **E**xecution, and **C**heck and asks flight crews to assess the facts of the situation, identify the possible ways to solve the problem, weight the risks and benefits, make a decision, assign responsibilities, and check that the plan is working (Orasanu-Engel & Mosier, 2019).

In the management profession, a multitude of structured problem-solving approaches have emerged, each rooted in scientific thinking. In his classic management book, *The Practice of Management*, Peter F. Drucker (1954) described the five phases of decision-making, which are representative of most management problem-solving methods. The steps Drucker proposed include the following:

1. *Define the problem:* Spend substantial time investigating the underlying causes of the problem.
2. *Analyze the problem:* Scrutinize the facts to understand the problem. It is not necessary to have all of the information but just enough to reduce the risk of making a bad decision.
3. *Develop alternative solutions:* Train the imagination to search for multiple alternative solutions to a problem. Taking no action is always a viable solution.
4. *Decide upon the best solution:* Create criteria for objectively judging the best solution. Choose a solution that has the best chance of working in practice.
5. *Convert decision into effective action:* Communicate the decision clearly, precisely, and unambiguously. Describe what needs to change within the organization in order to solve the problem.

Throughout the 20th century, other management problem-solving methods evolved to fit the times and circumstances. This chapter will focus on three different types of management problem-solving methods, listed in Figure 2.1. First, health management teacher and scholar James A. Hamilton created a 14-step problem-solving approach called the **Minnesota method**

FIGURE 2.1 Management problem-solving methods.

Drucker's 5 steps	McKinsey 7 steps	Design thinking method	Minnesota method
1. Define the problem 2. Analyze the problem 3. Develop alternative solutions 4. Decide upon the best solution 5. Convert decision into effective action	1. Structure the problem 2. Disaggregate the problem 3. Prioritize problem components 4. Plan analyses 5. Conduct analyses 6. Synthesize findings 7. Develop recommendations	• Empathize – Research users' needs • Define – State users' needs and problems • Ideate – Challenge assumptions and create ideas • Prototype – Start to create solutions • Test – Try the solutions out	• Define – Work with stakeholders, identify difficulties, group them into categories, and define problem statement. • Study – Search for the root causes, develop alternative solutions, and draw conclusions. • Act – Articulate recommendations, gain acceptance of solutions, and prepare for implementation.

(Plain, 2020). Sandra J. Potthoff et al. (2020) published the modern version of the Minnesota method, which is ideal for solving organizational-level problems. Also, McKinsey & Company consultants follow a 7-step **McKinsey approach** to solve client problems efficiently and effectively (Davis et al., 2007). Finally, the **design thinking method** emerged from various design fields over decades, and it entered the mainstream consciousness in the 1990s as a way to innovate products and services (Buchanan, 1992). Throughout the chapter, aspects from all three of these methods will be used to show how health services managers can solve problems using scientific thinking. More specialized problem-solving methods used in healthcare quality improvement projects, including Lean and Six Sigma, will be presented in Chapter 12, "Healthcare Quality Management."

DEFINE PROBLEMS

Stakeholder Analysis

First, health services managers must define the problem. This step begins with interviewing key people—stakeholders who have an interest in solving the problem or those who are impacted by the solution. Internal stakeholders include frontline clinicians; patients; top-level health services executives; and managers with expertise in finance, marketing, supply chain management, and others. External stakeholders can include suppliers, community organizations, regulators, and accreditors. In many problem-solving situations, the health services manager will be solving problems for themselves. In other instances, health services managers will be asked to solve problems for someone else, often referred to as the client (Potthoff et al., 2020).

> ⚠ **KEY IDEA**
>
> During the stakeholder analysis step, health services managers can borrow from the design thinking method, which places great importance on understanding the needs of the stakeholders, viewing empathy for "end users" as a vital part of problem-solving.

During the **stakeholder analysis** step, health services managers can borrow from the design thinking method, which places great importance on understanding the needs of the stakeholders, viewing empathy for "end users" as a vital part of problem-solving. According to this approach, a problem can only be effectively understood by prioritizing the needs of people most affected by the product, service, or experience (Mawer & Katz, 2019). Some questions that can be asked during the stakeholder interviews include the following (Perales, 2023; Turner, 1982):

- What do you want to achieve?
- How did you notice the problem?
- What do you think causes the problem?
- Why does that problem need to be solved?
- Which solutions have you attempted in the past? What were the results?
- How do you currently address the problem?
- What are some untried steps toward a solution?
- What solutions will not work and why?
- How would the work be different if the problem were solved?
- If the problem was solved, how would the solution be implemented?
- What can be done to ensure that people accept a solution?

During the problem definition phase, stakeholders may have very different views of the problem. So, effective health services managers seek out stakeholders with different perspectives, backgrounds, values, or professional training (Roberts et al., 2016). Varied perspectives can uncover contradictory information. Until the problem is fully investigated, health services managers should document stakeholder views about the problem (and solutions) as opinions, not facts (Potthoff et al., 2020). Stakeholder analysis means collecting all the facts from people who matter.

Problem Analysis

During the problem analysis step in the problem-solving process, effective health services managers resist the temptation to narrow the scope of the problem before the problem is fully analyzed. The Minnesota method problem definition step recommends that health services managers "make the problem bigger" (Potthoff et al., 2020, p. 34). This approach to problem analysis is often referred to as the Eisenhower principle, due to the quote attributed to Dwight D. Eisenhower: "Whenever I run into a problem I can't solve, I always make it bigger. I can never solve it by trying to make it smaller, but if I make it big enough, I can begin to see the outlines of a solution."

△ KEY IDEA
The Minnesota method problem definition step recommends that health services managers "make the problem bigger."

Widening the inquiry to encompass the larger context stimulates the imagination for new ways to define the problem that will lead to creative solutions. For example, consider a health services manager who wants to prevent patients from returning to the hospital again soon after being discharged from a previous hospital stay, occurrences referred to as **inpatient readmissions**. Enlarging the problem may uncover more effective solutions. In this case, the medical system may not be the major contributor to readmissions. If the problem is expanded beyond the medical system to include social risks, such as lack of food, unstable housing, or loneliness, then the solution to preventing readmissions may emerge to include food pantries, supportive housing, or social support (Emechebe et al., 2019).

While a problem may seem simple, it may be caused by multiple issues or something different entirely. **Root cause analyses** are a collection of techniques for discovering the underlying causes of a problem. Importantly, root cause analyses can be used to avoid mistaking a **consequence** as a problem. For example, patients waiting too long for care is a consequence of another issue, and not a problem itself. It is likely that there is at least one underlying problem causing patients to wait. These causes can be identified through root cause analysis. To begin a root cause analysis, health services managers conduct interviews, review documents, or analyze data to identify possible factors or events that contribute to the problem.

There are well-established root cause analyses methodologies. One approach is called **five whys**, whereby a problem can be uncovered by asking "why?" multiple times. The first question seldom finds the root cause of the problem, and it often takes multiple rounds of questions to uncover the real cause. So, health services managers repeatedly ask "why?" to each subsequent answer. Asking "why?" five times is not required, as the root cause might be identified after just three "whys." As illustrated in Figure 2.2, asking "why?" five times reveals that health services manager does not use patient volume patterns to predict nurse staffing needs.

Sometimes health services managers need to solve multifaceted problems that are so complicated that they require a more elaborate problem definition approach. These are known as

FIGURE 2.2 Five whys analysis.

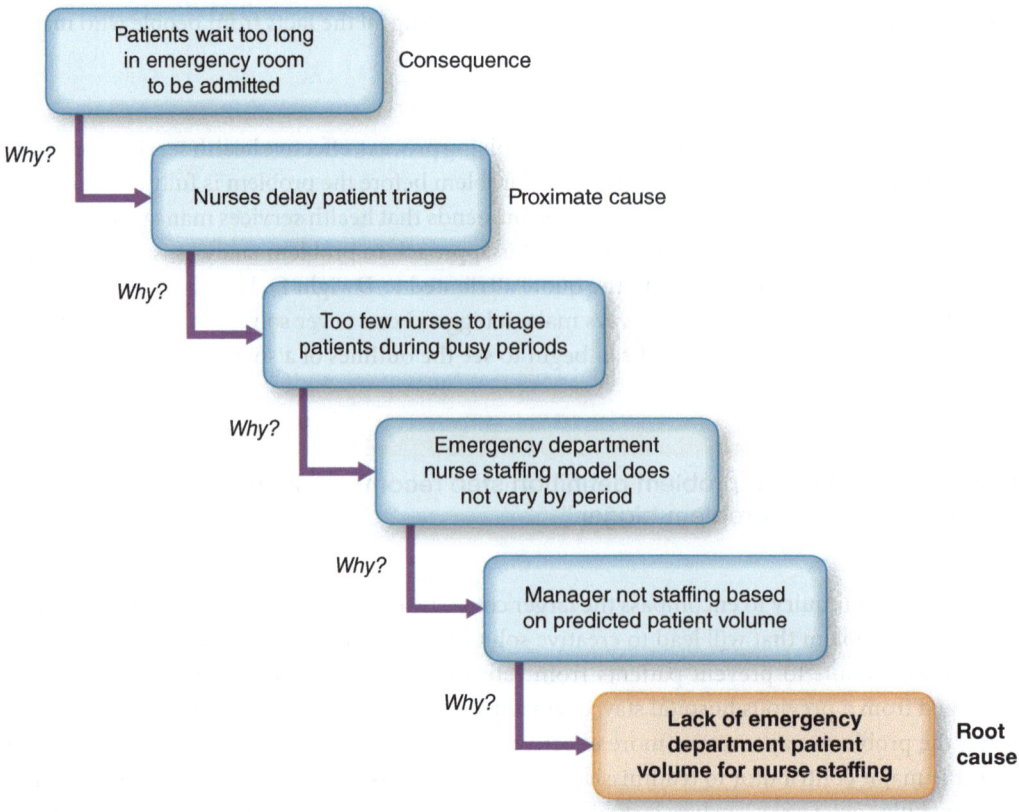

megaproblems. Health services delivery is full of complex, multifaceted, large-scale megaproblems for which systematic methods can make problem-solving more manageable (Warner & Holloway, 1978). When there are multiple root causes for a complex problem, the problem analysis can be expanded into a **logic tree** that illustrates multiple levels of megaproblems (London et al., 2019). Essentially, a logic tree is a multipronged root cause analysis that identifies multiple root causes to a complex problem. As Figure 2.3 shows, multiple root causes can be discovered at various iterations of asking "Why does that happen?" which creates a (sideways) tree of problems.

Another way to illustrate multiple causes of a problem is called the **fishbone diagram**, also known as an Ishikawa diagram or cause-and-effect diagram. The fishbone categorizes the various causes of a complex problem (i.e., effect) so that the graphic resembles a fish head with bones. To construct a fishbone diagram, one main branch is drawn through the center with several lines branching off of it. At one end of the main branch is the problem, effect, or "head of the fish." The branches that stem from the main branch are the categories of causes or fishbones. The categories are assigned to the different branches of the fishbone diagram. Categories can be named anything that groups the causes of the problem by similar concepts, such as people or process related. Sub-branches are then added to each cause until the fundamental root causes of the problem are identified. Figure 2.4 illustrates a fishbone diagram for the multiple causes of the patient no-show rate of 25% of all scheduled appointments.

For large organizational-level problems where dozens of interrelated problems are uncovered, an exhaustive list can be placed in categories based on their relatedness. By grouping complex problems around related concepts into a limited number of problem areas, health services managers can prioritize their problem-solving efforts. If there is an obvious critical problem area that needs to be solved before anything else, then the problem solver can begin there. If there are problem areas that will not be solved immediately, then those can be excluded from the project.

FIGURE 2.3 Root cause analysis logic tree.

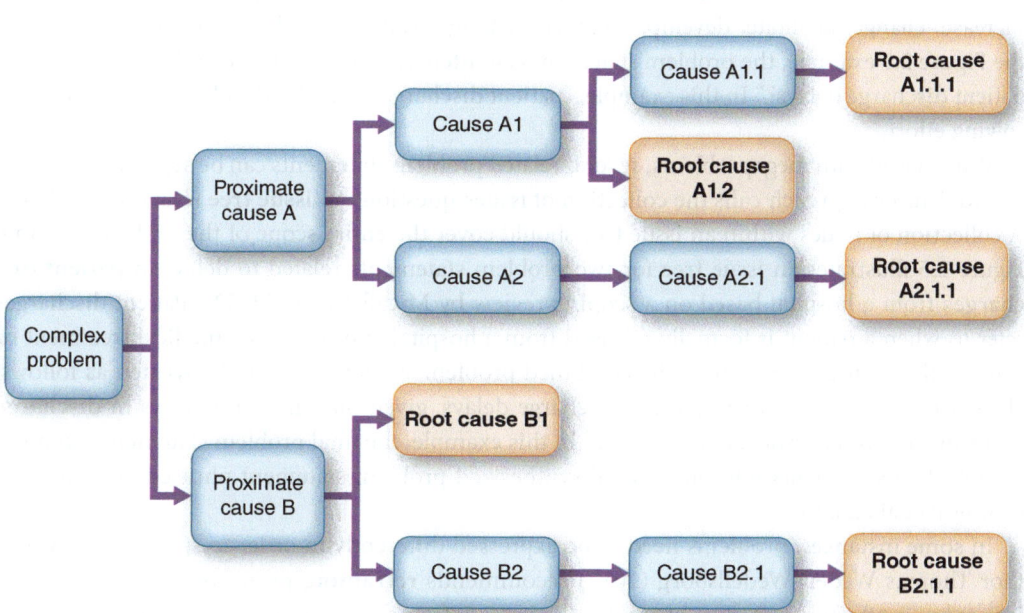

FIGURE 2.4 Fishbone analysis.

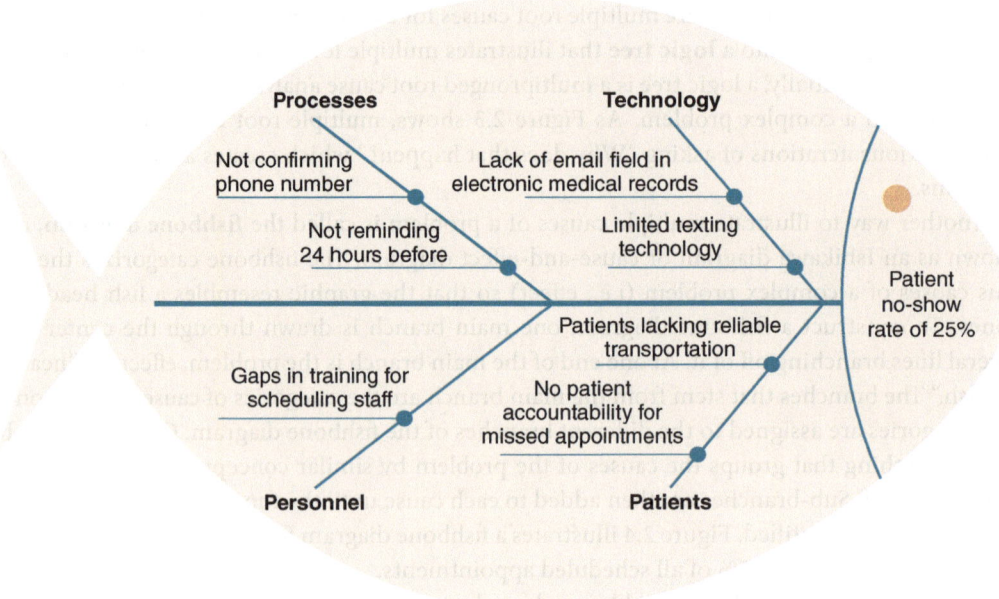

Framing and Reframing Problems

Once the root causes of complex problems are documented and grouped, the problem(s) should be explicitly defined. **Framing** a problem means to define and structure a problem in a way that makes it easier to understand, analyze, and solve. A **problem statement** is a definitive description of the problem that needs to be solved, usually phrased as a question. In other words, the problem statement is worded as a question. The format for simple problem statements is as follows: "How can [the organization] [action verb] [object of problem-solving effort]?" Action verbs include increase, change, facilitate, develop, organize, redesign, stabilize, and more (Lipuma, 2013). In the Figure 2.5 example, the problem statement is written as follows: "How can the HCO decrease patient discharge delays?" In this example, "patient discharge delays" is the object of the problem-solving effort.

When faced with megaproblems, several related problem statements can be separately defined. The McKinsey approach calls the collection of issues/questions an **issue tree** (Davis et al., 2007). A collection of issues within an issue tree should cover the entire scope of the problem at hand. Figure 2.5 illustrates an issue tree for two problem statements related to delays in **patient discharges** from a hospital based on a scoping review by Micallef et al. (2022). Patient discharges refer to when a patient is formally released from a hospital after receiving medical treatment or care. In the Figure 2.5 example, the combined problem statement would be written as follows: "How can the HCO decrease patient discharge delays, given that there are delays in **discharge planning** and transfer of care problems?" In this example, the final problem statement combines the problem statements into one overall synthesized problem statement phrased as a question (Potthoff et al., 2020).

In some instances, problems need to be expressed differently in order to spur creativity. Author Thomas Wedell-Wedellsborg (2017) recommends **reframing** problems to improve problem-solving effectiveness. For example, Figure 2.5 frames the problem as, "How can HCO

FIGURE 2.5 Issue tree with potential solutions.

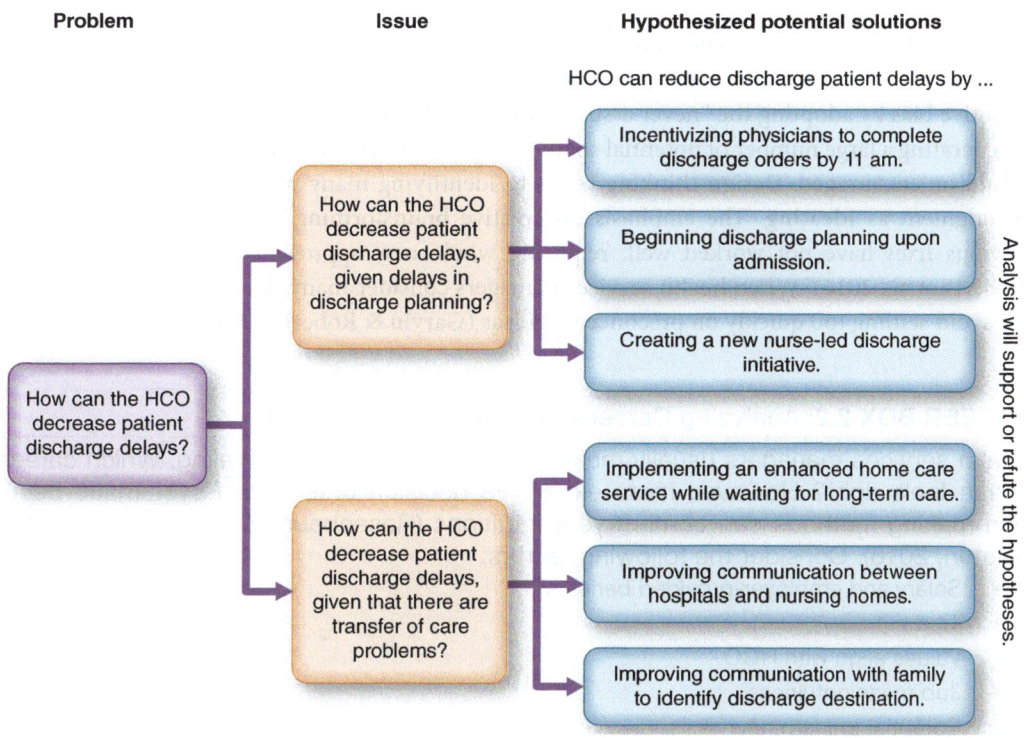

HCO, health care organization.

decrease patient discharge delays?" From this question, subsequent answerable questions are logically posed about discharge delays. But what if the problem were reframed? Instead of solving for delayed patient discharges, what if the question were posed about patients not occupying a hospital bed? By simply thinking about the issue differently, new potential solutions can be generated. For instance, would building a discharge lounge for patients to wait for discharges effectively allow admissions of other patients (Franklin et al., 2020)? A discharge lounge allows the patient to wait in comfort for prescriptions or transportation before the formal discharge is made, allowing the HCO to free up a hospital bed for another patient.

△ KEY IDEA

Without clear articulation of the problem, health services managers can waste time solving the wrong problem (or only part of the problem).

Most problem-solving methods encourage a final problem statement to be defined clearly and agreed to by all stakeholders to avoid miscommunication. Without clear articulation of the problem, health services managers can waste time solving the wrong problem (or only part of the problem). Agreement on the problem statement involves thorough deliberations and negotiation. When everyone shares an understanding of the problem and why the HCO should solve it, the problem-solving process will be more effective and efficient (Davis et al., 2007).

IDENTIFY POTENTIAL SOLUTIONS AND GENERATE HYPOTHESES

Health services managers should never advocate for a particular solution without systematically investigating all of the alternative solutions. The Minnesota method recommends avoiding cognitive bias by adopting the "never assume attitude" (Potthoff et al., 2020, p. 4). One approach to generating a large number of potential solutions is called **brainstorming**. In this step, creativity should be encouraged. Design thinking refers to identifying many potential solutions without prejudgment as **ideating**. The emphasis on creative brainstorming is especially useful when previous fixes have not worked well, requiring whole new approaches to solving problems (Roberts et al., 2016). When health services managers consider many alternative solutions, they can avoid settling too quickly on preconceived ideas (Garvin & Roberto, 2001).

CAREER BOX 2.2: Analyzing Career Alternatives

Health services managers usually make career decisions by gut feeling. Which career option feels right? However, more expansive decision criteria and systematic decision-making methods can confirm your intuitions (Rosenbaum & Rosenbaum, 2016; Salmon, 2018). Consider the following factors:
- Salary and employer-provided benefits
- Title
- Values align with HCO
- Job meaningfulness
- Potential to learn new skills
- Mobility and growth opportunities
- HCO size, location, or setting
- Workplace flexibility and schedule control
- Autonomy and self-direction

When there are multiple job options to compare, you can score each criterion, such as from 1 to 10. If some criteria are more important, then they can be weighted by multiplying by a factor, such as 1.5. This more rigorous evaluation of career options can be used to confirm your intuition about a job option and help you clarify the right decision.

Health services managers can discover ideas for alternative solutions from many different sources, including the following (Briner & Walshe, 2014; Kovner & Rundall, 2006; Pfeffer & Sutton, 2006):

- *Stakeholders:* Because they are knowledgeable about the problem, stakeholders may propose potential solutions.
- *Outside experts or consultants:* Experts or consultants with experience solving similar problems can offer ideas for solutions. However, these people often address the problem with a proprietary solution in mind. Their interest may involve selling products and services, not necessarily solving problems.
- *Professional contacts:* Ideas for alternative solutions can be borrowed from other HCOs, sometime gathered from personal contacts or professional associations
- *Past solutions:* Experience solving similar problems can be valuable sources of ideas. However, to protect against bias, other alternative solutions should be also identified and evaluated.
- *Scholarly publications or industry whitepapers:* For early careerists with fewer professional experiences or social networks upon which to draw, examples from journals or respected industry sources can be useful sources of alternative solutions.

- *No action:* Health services managers can also consider "doing nothing" as an alternative solution (Potthoff et al., 2020). However, like other alternate solutions, the impact of not acting needs to be analyzed and compared to the other solutions.

Once a comprehensive list of potential solutions has been produced for each category of problems, the health services manager narrows down the alternatives and eliminates infeasible, ineffective, or irrelevant options. Only the most promising potential solutions should be selected for deeper analysis and evaluation (Oliveira, Zancul, & Fleury, 2021). The goal of problem-solving is to converge on the best alternative solution for each problem or issue.

> △ **KEY IDEA**
>
> The goal of problem-solving is to converge on the best alternative solution for each problem or issue.

Hypothesis-Driven Thinking

The McKinsey Approach advocates **hypothesis-driven thinking**, in which each alternative is tentatively hypothesized as the best solution (Davis et al., 2007). Hypothesis-driven thinking focuses on making educated guesses about which alternative solutions may solve the problem, then evaluating and comparing them systematically. In this approach, no particular hypothesized solution is assumed to be the best choice. Rather, each is only a tentative solution that needs to be supported with critical thinking and evidence. For example, Figure 2.5 shows two problem statements, one of which is "How can the HCO's patients be discharged timely, given delays in discharge planning?" For this issue, three different hypothesized potential solutions are described, beginning with "HCO can reduce discharge patient delays by …." Each of these alternative solutions are plausibly the best solution, but each must be analyzed, evaluated, and compared (Cadel et al., 2021). Stating the alternative solutions as hypotheses leads to focused analysis of the problem. Instead of conducting interesting but aimless analysis, health services managers analyze only the information that will test the hypothesized solutions.

> △ **KEY IDEA**
>
> The McKinsey approach advocates hypothesis-driven thinking, in which each alternative is tentatively hypothesized as the best solution. Hypothesis-driven thinking focuses on making educated guesses about which alternative solutions may solve the problem, then evaluating and comparing them systematically.

Set Decision Criteria

To objectively evaluate alternative solutions, health services managers use **decision criteria**. The decision criteria are the predetermined set of principles by which alternative solutions are evaluated and compared (Potthoff et al., 2020). Decision criteria help to select the best solution according to the objectives of the HCO. Some decision criteria can be uncovered during stakeholder interviews. In some instances, interpersonal relations and historical conflict between stakeholders are important decision criteria to consider when evaluating alternative solutions.

Based on the decision criteria, a series of research questions are written. Each research question is posed and answered in order to assess the advantages of each of the alternative solutions. For example, if the problem is to reduce patient discharge delays, then the criteria should include timeliness. Table 2.2 includes example decision criteria and research questions for evaluating many common alternative solutions (Davis, et al., 2007; Drucker, 1954; Potthoff et al., 2020).

When there are only a few decision criteria for each problem, then the analytical step of problem solving can be completed rather quickly. Using Figure 2.5 as an example, the research

TABLE 2.2 Example Decision Criteria for Evaluating Alternative Solutions

DECISION CRITERION	RESEARCH QUESTION
Access to care	Which alternative most effectively increases access to care?
Clinician satisfaction	Which alternative most effectively increases clinician satisfaction? Which alternative increases patient referrals to the HCO?
Community need	To what extent do the alternatives meet the health services needs of the community? Which alternative makes the largest impact on community health?
Competitive advantage	Do the alternatives enable the HCO to create long-term value more effectively for customers in ways that competitors cannot? To what extent do the alternatives increase customer demand, prices, or market share?
Compliance	Do the alternatives comply with existing HCO policy, accreditation standards, or other requirements?
Cost	How much do the alternatives cost? Are the alternatives within the budget of the HCO?
Cost of care	Which alternative most effectively reduces the average costs per patient?
Culture/mission/values	To what extent are the alternatives consistent with HCO culture? Are the alternatives aligned with the HCO's stated mission and values?
Employee satisfaction	Which alternative most effectively increases employee satisfaction? Which alternative decreases employee intention to leave the HCO?
Ethics/laws/regulations	Are the alternatives ethical? Are the alternatives acceptable under the laws and regulations?
Functionality	To what extent do the alternatives meet performance needs? Which alternative is most reliable? usable? scalable? adaptable? compatible? customizable?
Innovative	To what extent do the alternatives introduce new processes, concepts, technologies, or approaches?
Patient experience	Do the alternatives improve patients' perception of experiences related to health service delivery?
Patient safety	To what extent do the alternatives keep patients safe?
Practical feasibility	How feasible are alternatives are to implement?

TABLE 2.2 Example Decision Criteria for Evaluating Alternative Solutions (*continued*)

DECISION CRITERION	RESEARCH QUESTION
Political feasibility	Do decision-makers or other stakeholders favor the alternatives? Will stakeholders object to the alternatives? Is there conflict among stakeholder groups that would make the alternatives unworkable?
Population health	Which alternative most effectively reduces unnecessary health services utilization?
Profit	Which alternative most effectively creates positive profit margins (revenues higher than costs)? What is the return on investment of the alternatives? payback period? cost-benefit? internal rate of return?
Risk	What are potential for losses associated with the alternatives?
Strategic objectives	To what extent are the alternatives consistent with the HCO's strategy?
Time	How much time will the alternatives take to implement? Will the alternatives meet the imposed deadline?

HCO, health care organization.

questions to "How can the HCO's patients be discharged timely, given delays in discharge planning?" could include the following:

- *Timeliness:* To what extent does the alternative solution decrease delays in discharge planning?
- *Cost:* How much will the alternative solution cost to implement?
- *Political feasibility:* Will the alternative solution be acceptable to stakeholders?

The aim of answering research questions is to test whether each hypothesized alternative solution would fix the problem, according to each objective decision criterion. In other words, when analyzing alternative solutions, health services managers should focus on generating answers to the questions, not simply generating analytical results (Davis et al., 2007). As described in evidence-based management principles, each of these questions should be answered by analyzing facts collected from the best available evidence and critically assessing the results.

ANALYZE ALTERNATIVE SOLUTIONS

Analytical Plan

Effective health services managers plan problem-solving analyses like scientists develop their study methodology. Proceeding without an analytical plan is a waste of time. Without a plan, health services managers will end up running unneeded analysis. Therefore, before beginning analysis, the following questions should be answered:

- *What evidence would answer the research question?* Describe the evidence that would most effectively test the hypothesized alternative solution.
- *What data is available?* All relevant, accessible, and useful facts should be considered. Quantitative results, such as numbers, statistics, and metrics, are the preferred evidentiary

form for the management profession. Nevertheless, qualitative results, gathered by interviews and surveys, can be meaningful, if presented logically.
- *What analytical tools can be used?* Ranging from simple to highly technical, there are numerous analytical tools available to skilled health services managers, many of which are addressed in this textbook. Examples include spreadsheet and data visualization software applications.
- *What are resources and time limits?* Ideal analysis may not be possible due to tight deadlines and/or limited resources.

With these questions answered, health services managers create an **analytical plan** that outlines the hypothesized alternative solutions, the research questions, the data sources, and the analytical tools. The analytical plan estimates how long each step will take and identifies the person responsible for completing the task. Related project management skills will be presented in Chapter 13.

Analysis of Alternative Solutions

As early as possible in the problem-solving process, basic statistics need to be generated to understand the shape and scope of the problem (London et al., 2019). Effective health services managers start with simple **descriptive statistics**, which includes producing summary tables of data frequencies, proportions, and averages, such as mean (average), median (middle value), and mode (most frequently occurring value). Descriptive statistics are useful for simplifying complex problems or revealing relationships between factors. In many instances, data visualization techniques, such as graphs and charts, can be used to make results easy to understand. Descriptive statistics can be used to evaluate alternative solutions, if more sophisticated analysis is not possible.

In many instances, however, more advanced analysis will be necessary to test hypothesized alternative solutions. **Analytics** refers to the use of computer software to quantitatively analyze large sets (Gavin, 2019). Successful health services managers are skilled in using analytical tools and translating evidence to improve their decision-making (Association of Universities and Programs in Health Administration [AUPHA], 2022). Table 2.3 describes the various terms, tools, and methods associated with analytical problem-solving skills (Glandon et al., 2021; Johri, 2022).

TABLE 2.3 Terms, Tools, and Methods Associated With Analytical Problem-Solving Skills

TERM, TOOL, OR METHOD	DEFINITION	APPLICATION TO TESTING HYPOTHESES
ALGORITHMS	Well-defined computational procedures that can be implemented through a series of logical and precise steps	Simulate experiments of real-world phenomena to test the predictions of a hypothesized alternative solutions.
ARTIFICIAL INTELLIGENCE	Simulation of human intelligence processes by computers to interpret events, predict outcomes, automate decisions, and recommend actions	Provide valuable insights that may not be apparent to human analysts. Hypotheses can be tested by simulating different scenarios and observing the outcomes.
BIG DATA	A collection of large and unstructured data sets that requires specialized data processing systems and software	Uncover relationships or model complex simulations.

TABLE 2.3 Terms, Tools, and Methods Associated With Analytical Problem-Solving Skills (*continued*)

TERM, TOOL, OR METHOD	DEFINITION	APPLICATION TO TESTING HYPOTHESES
CLINICAL DECISION SUPPORT SYSTEMS	Real-time, evidence-based information and recommendations to assist in clinical decision-making	Improve diagnostic accuracy, enhance treatment planning, and promote adherence to best practices and clinical guidelines.
COST-BENEFIT ANALYSIS	Comparison of the costs relative to the expected benefits, including both tangible and intangible factors	Determine whether the benefits alternatives outweigh the costs.
DATA MINING	Process of discovering statistical relationships within large data sets	As opposed to traditional hypothesis testing, data mining is a form of exploratory data analysis.
FORECASTING	Predicting future events, trends, or developments based on existing data using various statistical techniques, such as regression analysis	Provides insights into potential outcomes and implications of alternatives under different scenarios
INFERENTIAL STATISTICS	A type of statistics that involves using sample data to make predictions about a larger population. Includes linear regression analysis and correlation analysis	Facilitates the development of predictive models that can forecast outcomes. Statistical hypothesis tests can assess the significance of effects of interventions.
MACHINE LEARNING	A type of artificial intelligence in which a computer has the ability to learn without being preprogramed	Automatically analyze constantly changing data to automatically make decisions as trends evolve.
NATURAL LANGUAGE PROCESSING	A type of artificial intelligence that that enable computers to process and analyze vast amounts of natural human language	Enables the analysis from large volumes of textual data in computer systems, such as clinical notes or social medial posts
REGRESSION ANALYSIS	A type of statistical analysis used to understand how the change in one variable affects the change in another; can be used to make predictions based on relationships observed in data	Enables the identification of key factors that influence outcomes or to predict future results based on historical data
STATISTICAL MODELING	Any of a number of mathematical techniques that use sample data to make real-world predictions	Supports hypothesis testing by calculating the statistical significance of relationships between variables

Sources of Data

Health services managers use quantitative data from a variety of sources to analyze alternative solutions. The best evidence for testing hypothesized alternative solutions comes from internal sources, such as the following (Taylor et al., 2022):

- *Electronic health records (EHR):* Securely stores and manages patient health information, including medical history, diagnoses, medications, and treatment plans; contains data relevant to operations, quality, patient safety, resource utilization, gaps in care, and regulatory compliance
- *Health information exchanges:* Enables electronic transfer of health information between HCOs, according to nationally recognized standards, in order to analyze patient data, treatment outcomes, and healthcare utilization patterns
- *Data warehouses:* A centralized data repository from various clinical, operational, and financial sources; combines elements from multiple data sources into one accessible database
- *Knowledge management systems:* Specialized information systems designed to organize and share knowledge and expertise, including patient data, medical research, clinical guidelines, and policies, to support informed decision-making

Sometimes alternative solutions seem promising, but do not create the expected results, perhaps due to cognitive bias or unknown complexities (Kahneman, 2011). Therefore, health services managers can test out the alternative solutions at relatively low risk by running small-scale experiments (Pfeffer & Sutton, 2006; Rigby, 2021). Design thinking refers to testing small-scale solutions as **prototyping**, whereby the alternative solutions are tested in a limited manner to collect evidence (Roberts et al., 2016). This step is an example of how problem-solving actually involves iterative steps of testing and learning (London et al., 2019).

CAREER BOX 2.3: Prototyping Career Options

In their book, *Designing Your Work Life*, Bill Burnett and Dave Evans (2020) explain how design thinking can help create fulfilling careers. Prototyping is central to how designers develop new products. Instead of making career decisions based on little or no evidence, Burnett and Evans recommend prototyping career options to protect against fear of action or prevent rash decisions. Prototyping careers can include informational interviews, shadowing, interning, volunteering, or working on the weekends. If the prototyping experience is successful, investigate more; if not, then move to another career option. Prototyping allows you to make mistakes, revise, and try again.

To complement internal data, health services managers can also acquire, assess, and analyze several types of external data (Kovner & Rundall, 2006). First, management research published in scholarly journals can be used as evidence for evaluating alternative solutions. The most credible form of external evidence is a systematic review of published research (Briner, Denyer, & Rousseau, 2009). Compared to medical scholarship, there are few systematic reviews on health services management topics (Jaana et al., 2014). As such, health services managers may have to acquire evidence from single research studies. In these instances, health services managers need to appraise whether the context of the study is applicable to the HCO and/or problem at hand (Briner, Denyer, & Rousseau, 2009; Pfeffer & Sutton, 2006).

Synthesize Findings, Conclusions, and Recommendations

Consistent with the evidence-based management approach, health services managers systematically evaluate the hypothesized alternative solutions based on the collected evidence. **Findings** are the interpretation of the results generated after asking the research questions. In other words, findings summarize the relative strengths of the evidence for each alternative

TABLE 2.4 Example Findings for Alternative Solutions Regarding Delays in Discharge Planning

Issue: How can the HCO's patients be discharged timely, given delays in discharge planning?			
SOLUTION	**CRITERION: COSTS**	**CRITERION: TIMELINESS**	**CRITERION: FEASIBILITY**
Incentivizing physicians to complete discharge orders by 11 a.m.	Education campaign, physician training, and bonus pool estimated at $109 per discharge	No significant change in average discharge time, adjusted for patient factors ($p=0.65$)	Low. Challenges exist with resistant community-based physicians.
Beginning discharge planning upon admission	Education campaign and staff time estimated at $88 per discharge	Discharge time reduced from 4.9 hours to 4.1 hours, adjusted for patient factors ($p<0.05$)	Medium. Some resistance to paperwork and communication requirements at shift changes
Creating a new nurse-led discharge initiative	Development, training, and staff time estimated at $105 per discharge	Discharge time reduced from 4.9 hours to 3.2 hours, adjusted for patient factors ($p<0.01$)	High. Pilot initiative found that nurses developed unit-specific rules based on process improvement principles.

solution according to the established decision criteria. When the number of criteria is large, the criteria may be arranged from most to least important. Alternatively, a weighting system can be applied to each decision criteria to reflect their level of importance (Triantaphyllou, 2000). When there are relatively few criteria, health services managers can synthesize the results more subjectively. Table 2.4 shows the findings to the alternative solutions using the example regarding delays in discharge planning illustrated in Figure 2.5.

Health services managers should explain what the findings mean by stating their **conclusions**. In other words, conclusions are interpretations of the findings and judgments about the relative merits of the alternative solutions (Potthoff et al., 2020). Health services managers can take a variety of approaches to expressing conclusions but should always explicitly connect findings to the established decision criteria. In effect, the conclusions describe the pros and cons of each alternative solution.

Finally, once the findings have been interpreted and conclusions have been summarized, health services managers recommend preferred solutions. Effective **recommendations** are logical and actionable. The recommendations should explicitly state how and to what extent the solutions solve the defined problems. If none of the alternative solutions will effectively solve the problem, then health services managers can recommend that the HCO take no action. However, not acting should be evaluated for it potential impacts on organizational goals.

INFORMATIONAL INTERVIEW 2.2

Clinic Administrator

Access the informational interview online at http://connect.springerpub.com/content/book/978-0-8261-4807-0/chapter/ch00.

Transform Decisions Into Action

Once a final recommendation has been made, it must be put into action. Problem-solving recommendations that are not implemented (or poorly implemented) are a waste of time, money, and effort (London et al., 2019; Turner, 1982). To improve the likelihood of successful implementation, health services managers need to connect the recommendations to specific action by documenting the following elements:

- *Priorities:* Explain the actions that need to be implement in the short, medium, and long term. Sketch a timeline with key milestones for tracking success.
- *Roles and responsibilities:* Clarify which stakeholders, clients, or teams are responsible for specific actions.
- *Success measure:* Describe how the stakeholders will determine when the problem is solved.
- *Next steps:* Problem-solving is iterative. Seek out new ways to work or new problems to solve.

Health services managers need to communicate how the recommendations will be implemented. Completed problem-solving projects typically conclude with a written report and/or oral presentation. Chapter 3, "Managing Interpersonal Communications," describes these communication types in more detail.

FUTURE DIRECTIONS

Some problems are so complex, unpredictable, and intractable that they cannot be solved with the step-by-step approach described in this chapter. Urban planners Horst Rittel and Melvin Webber (1973) used the phrase **wicked problems** to describe society-level issues that are so messy that they cannot be systematic, science-based approaches (Ritchey, 2013). Wicked problems related to society's ills resist definition and analysis. Unlike problems about which there is general agreement, wicked problems are characterized by deep ambiguity. People debate the various issues but never really define the problem. By extension, there are no optimal solutions to wicked problems, only value-laden ideologies posing as objective decision criteria. Even when solutions are attempted, the complexity of the problem leads to unpredictable chain reactions of unintended consequences. So, wicked problems appear frustratingly unsolvable.

The U.S. healthcare system is a wicked problem—actually, a mess of interrelated, macro-level problems. More expensive than any other country in the world, the United States trails other countries in life expectancy, infant mortality, and maternal mortality and has the highest death rates for avoidable or treatable conditions (Centers for Disease Control and Prevention [CDC], 2022; Commonwealth Fund, 2023). The low-quality and high-expense challenge alone is a wicked problem, not to mention other issues that may be overlooked, including health inequities, health care inaccessibility, and workforce shortages. For health services managers with ambitions to improve the healthcare system, untangling these wicked problems may require bold and experimental solutions.

SUMMARY

- Problems exist when there are differences between a current situation and a future desired state. Problems are also called obstacles, challenges, complications, opportunities, issues, concerns, and predicaments.
- The basic problem-solving steps include identifying problems, understanding causes of problems, framing problems as answerable questions, developing multiple alternative solutions, comparing the merits of alternative solutions, drawing conclusions, and presenting recommendations logically and persuasively.

- Evidence-based management involves taking a more formal, explicit, and structured approach to using the best available evidence to solve problems and make decisions.
- Health services managers use quantitative data from a variety of sources to test hypothesized alternative solutions. Analytical approaches used to generate evidence include algorithms and statistical modeling.
- Based on findings, health services managers draw conclusions about the relative merits of alternative solutions by comparing them to objective decision criteria. Recommendations are made based on the most logically supported alternative solution.

END-OF-CHAPTER RESOURCES

KEY TERMS*

*For the full list of key terms, please see the online glossary at **http://connect.springerpub.com/content/book/978-0-8261-4807-0.**

analytical plan
analytics
artificial intelligence (AI)
brainstorming
big data
clinical decision support system
cognitive biases
conclusions
consequence
critical thinking
data warehouse
decision criteria
descriptive statistics
design thinking method
differential diagnosis
discharge planning
electronic health records
evidence-based management
evidence-based medicine
findings
fishbone diagram
five whys
framing
health informatics

health information exchange
heuristic
hypothesis-driven thinking
ideating
inpatient readmissions
issue tree
knowledge management
logic tree
machine learning
megaproblems
McKinsey approach
Minnesota method
patient discharges
problem
problem statement
prototyping
recommendations
reframing
root cause analyses
scientific method
stakeholder analysis
statistical modeling
truthiness
wicked problems

LEARNING ACTIVITIES

Professional Development and Reflection

1. Identify a career decision that you have made in the past or will make in the future. Reflect on how the application of hypothesis-driven thinking and use of decision criteria could enhance decision-making. Describe how you might analyze the career options.

2. Reframing changes how problems are defined to create alternative perspectives and produce new possible solutions. Imagine that you received the bad news that you did not get hired for the job you wanted. While you do not know why, you hypothesize that you did not get the job because you were not qualified. This is a negative framing. Reframe why you did not get the job from a positive perspective. For example, you could hypothesize that you did not get the job because the hiring manager was intimidated by your talent. Write at least three new positively framed hypotheses.

Discussion Questions

1. In what ways do factors such as frustration, fear, fatigue, ignorance, and distraction undermine critical thinking among health services managers? What are the best ways to effectively manage or minimize these factors to make better decisions?
2. In your opinion, what role should education and training play in equipping health services managers with the necessary skills to assess and apply evidence in decision-making? How can organizations encourage a culture of evidence-based management within their teams?
3. Which of the cognitive biases are most likely to lead health services managers to make bad decisions? Why?

RECOMMENDED READING AND MEDIA

Burnett, B., & Evans, D. (2020). *Designing your work life: How to thrive and change and find happiness at work*. Alfred A. Knopf.

Chevallier, A., & Enders, A. (2022). *Solvable: A simple solution to complex problems*. Pearson.

Conn, C., & McLean, R. (2019). *Bulletproof problem solving: The one skill that changes everything*. Wiley.

Kahneman, D. (2011). *Thinking fast and slow*. Farrar, Straus and Giroux.

London, S., Conn, C., & Sarrazin, H. (2019, September 13). *How to master the seven-step problem-solving process*. https://www.mckinsey.com/capabilities/strategy-and-corporate-finance/our-insights/how-to-master-the-seven-step-problem-solving-process

Potthoff, S. J., Mishek, J. H., & Hart, G. W. (2020). *Applied problem-solving in healthcare management*. Springer Publishing, Inc.

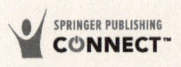

A robust set of instructor resources designed to supplement this text is located at http://connect.springerpub.com/content/book/978-0-8261-4807-0. Qualifying instructors may request access by emailing textbook@springerpub.com.

REFERENCES

Association of Universities and Programs in Health Administration. (2022, January). *AUPHA Environmental Scan and Trends Report (2021–2022)*. https://higherlogicdownload.s3.amazonaws.com/AUPHA/5c0a0c07-a7f7-413e-ad73-9b7133ca4c38/UploadedImages/benchmarking/AUPHA-2022-Trends-Report_Final.pdf

Begun, J. W., Butler, P. W., & Stefl, M. E. (2018). Competencies to what end? Affirming the purpose of healthcare management. *Journal of Health Administration Education, 35*(2), 133–155.

Briner, R. B., Denyer, D., & Rousseau, D. M. (2009). Evidence-Based Management: Concept Cleanup Time? *Academy of Management Perspectives, 23*(4), 19–32.

Briner, R. B., & Walshe, N. D. (2014). From passively received wisdom to actively constructed knowledge: Teaching systematic review skills as a foundation of evidence-based management. *Academy of Management Learning & Education, 13*(3), 415–432. https://doi.org/10.5465/amle.2013.0222

Buchanan, R. (1992). Wicked problems in design thinking. *Design Issues, 8*(2), 5–21.

Burnett, B., & Evans, D. (2020). *Designing your work life: How to thrive and change and find happiness at work*. Alfred A. Knopf.

Cadel, L., Guilcher, S. J., Kokorelias, K. M., Sutherland, J., Glasby, J., Kiran, T., & Kuluski, K. (2021). Initiatives for improving delayed discharge from a hospital setting: A scoping review. *BMJ Open, 11*(2), e044291. https://doi.org/10.1136/bmjopen-2020-044291

Centers for Disease Control and Prevention. (2022, December). *Mortality in the United States, 2021*. https://www.cdc.gov/nchs/data/databriefs/db456.pdf

Chevallier, A., & Enders, A. (2022). *Solvable: A simple solution to complex problems*. Pearson.

Commonwealth Fund. (2023, January). *U.S. health care from a global perspective, 2022: Accelerating spending, worsening outcomes*. https://www.commonwealthfund.org/publications/issue-briefs/2023/jan/us-health-care-global-perspective-2022

Davis, I., Keeling, D., Schreier, P., & Williams, A. (2007). *The McKinsey approach to problem solving*. McKinsey & Company, Inc.

Djulbegovic, B., & Guyatt, G. H. (2017). Progress in evidence-based medicine: A quarter century on. *The Lancet, 390*(10092), 415–423. https://doi.org/10.1016/s0140-6736(16)31592-6

Drucker, P. F. (1954). *The practice of management*. Harper & Row, Publishers, Inc.

Emechebe, N., Lyons Taylor, P., Amoda, O., & Pruitt, Z. (2019). Passive social health surveillance and inpatient readmissions. *American Journal of Managed Care, 25*(8), 388–95.

Ennis, R. H. (2015). Critical thinking: A streamlined conception. In M. Davies & R. Barnett (Eds.), *The palgrave handbook of critical thinking in higher education* (pp. 31–47). Palgrave Macmillan US.

Erwin, M. (2019, August 1). 6 reasons we make bad decisions, and what to do about them. *Harvard Business Review*. https://hbr.org/2019/08/6-reasons-we-make-bad-decisions-and-what-to-do-about-them

Franklin, B. J., Vakili, S., Huckman, R. S., Hosein, S., Falk, N., Cheng, K., Murray, M., Harris, S., Morris, C. A., & Goralnick, E. (2020). The inpatient discharge lounge as a potential mechanism to mitigate emergency department boarding and crowding. *Annals of Emergency Medicine, 75*(6), 704–714. https://doi.org/10.1016/j.annemergmed.2019.12.002

Garvin, D. A., & Roberto, M. (2001, September). What you don't know about making decisions. *Harvard Business Review*. https://hbr.org/2001/09/what-you-dont-know-about-making-decisions

Gavin, M. (2019, July 16). *Business analytics: What it is & why it's important*. Harvard Business School Online's Business Insights Blog. https://online.hbs.edu/blog/post/importance-of-business-analytics

Glandon, G. L., Smaltz, D. H., & Slovensky, D. J. (2021). *Information technology for healthcare managers* (9th ed.). Health Administration Press.

Guo, R., Hermanson, P. M., & Farnsworth, T. J. (2016). Study on hospital administrators' beliefs and attitudes toward the practice of evidence-based management. *Hospital Topics, 94*(3–4), 62–66. https://doi.org/10.1080/00185868.2016.1258886

Guyatt, G. H., & Rennie, D. (1993). Users' guides to the medical literature. *JAMA, 270*(17), 2096–2097. https://doi.org/10.1001/jama.1993.03510170086037

Hardman, D. (2009). *Judgment and decision making: Psychological perspectives*. Wiley-Blackwell.

Jaana, M., Vartak, S., & Ward, M. M. (2014). Evidence-based health care management: What is the research evidence available for health care managers? *Evaluation & the Health Professions, 37*(3), 314–334. https://doi.org/10.1177/0163278713511325

Johri, N. (2022). Health data analytics for population health management. In A. M. Hewitt, J. L. Mascari, & S. L. Wagner (Eds.), *Population health management: Strategies, tools, applications, and outcomes* (pp. 79–102). Springer Publishing.

Kahneman, D. (2011). *Thinking fast and slow*. Farrar, Straus and Giroux.

Kovner, A. R., & D'Aunno, T. (2016). *Evidence-based management in healthcare* (2nd ed.). Health Administration Press.

Kovner, A. R., & Rundall, T. G. (2006). Evidence-based management reconsidered. *Frontiers of Health Services Management, 22*(3), 3–22. https://doi.org/10.1097/01974520-200601000-00002

Lipuma, J. M. (2013). *Fundamentals of undergraduate education and learning*. Kendall Hunt Publishing Company.

London, S., Conn, C., & Sarrazin, H. (2019, September 13). *How to master the seven-step problem-solving process*. McKinsey podcast. https://www.mckinsey.com/capabilities/strategy-and-corporate-finance/our-insights/how-to-master-the-seven-step-problem-solving-process

Mawer, S., & Katz, B. (2019). Designing the future of healthcare. *Journal of Healthcare Management, 64*(5), 272–278.

Micallef, A., Buttigieg, S. C., Tomaselli, G., & Garg, L. (2022). Defining delayed discharges of inpatients and their impact in acute hospital care: A scoping review. *International Journal of Health Policy and Management, 11*(2), 103–111. https://doi.org/10.34172/ijhpm.2020.94

Moon, J. (2007). *Critical thinking: An exploration of theory and practice*. Routledge.

Oliveira, M., Zancul, E., & Fleury, A. L. (2021). Design thinking as an approach for innovation in healthcare: Systematic review and research avenues. *BMJ Innovations, 7*(2), 1–8. https://doi.org/10.1136/bmjinnov-2020-000428

Orasanu-Engel, J., & Mosier, K. L. (2019). Flight crew decision-making (pp. 139–183). In B. G. Kanki, J. Anca, & T. R (Eds.), *Crew resource management*. Academic Press

Payette, P., & Barnes, B. (2017, May). Teaching for critical thinking: Combatting the 'truthiness' tendencies. *The National Teaching & Learning Forum, 26*(4), 7–9. https://doi.org/10.1002/ntlf.30117

Perales, J. J. (2023, May 5). *Great questions lead to great design: A guide to the design-thinking process*. Toptal: Designers. https://www.toptal.com/designers/product-design/design-thinking-great-questions

Pfeffer, J., & Sutton, R. I. (2006). Evidence-based management. *Harvard Business Review, 84*(1), 62–74.

Plain, C. (2020, Winter). *Solving problems the Minnesota way: A new textbook shares the method*. Minnesota Advances. https://advances.umn.edu/winter-2020/solving-problems-the-minnesota-way

Potthoff, S. J., Mishek, J. H., & Hart, G. W. (2020). *Applied problem-solving in healthcare management*. Springer Publishing, Inc.

Quarantotto, D. (2020). Aristotle on science as problem solving. *Topoi, 39*(4), 857–868. https://doi.org/10.1007/s11245-018-9548-2

Rasiel, E. M., & Friga, P. N. (2001). *The Mckinsey mind*. McGraw Hill.

Rigby, D. (2021, August 13). 3 Questions to Help Your Team Solve Problems. *Harvard Business Review*. https://hbr.org/2021/08/3-questions-to-help-your-team-solve-problems

Ritchey, T. (2013). Wicked problems. *Acta Morphologica Generalis, 2*(1), 1–8.

Rittel, H. W., & Webber, M. M. (1973). Dilemmas in a general theory of planning. *Policy Sciences, 4*(2), 155–169.

Roberts, J. P., Fisher, T. R., Trowbridge, M. J., & Bent, C. (2016, March). A design thinking framework for healthcare management and innovation. *Healthcare, 4*(1), 11–14. https://doi.org/10.1016/j.hjdsi.2015.12.002

Rosenbaum, J., & Rosenbaum, J. (2016). Money isn't everything: Job satisfaction, nonmonetary job rewards, and sub-baccalaureate credentials. *Research in Higher Education Journal, 30*, 1–17.

Rynes, S. L., & Bartunek, J. M. (2017). Evidence-based management: Foundations, development, controversies and future. *Annual Review of Organizational Psychology and Organizational Behavior, 4*, 235–261. https://doi.org/10.1146/annurev-orgpsych-032516-113306

Sackett, D. L., Rosenberg, W. M., Gray, J. M., Haynes, R. B., & Richardson, W. S. (1996). Evidence based medicine: What it is and what it isn't. *BMJ, 312*(7023), 71–72. https://doi.org/10.1136/bmj.312.7023.71

Salmon, E. (2018, August 27). *Five elements of a good job*. Urban Institute. https://www.urban.org/urban-wire/five-elements-good-job

Simon, H. A. (1955). A behavioral model of rational choice. *The Quarterly Journal of Economics, 69*(1), 99–118. https://doi.org/10.2307/1884852

Stern, S. D. C., Cifu, A. S., & Altkorn, D. (2020). *Symptom to diagnosis: An evidence-based guide* (4th ed.). McGraw-Hill Medical.

Subbiah, V. (2023). The next generation of evidence-based medicine. *Nature Medicine, 29*(1), 49–58. https://doi.org/10.1038/s41591-022-02160-z

Taylor, H., Brumitt, G., Harle, C. A., Johnston, A., Williams, K. S., & Vest, J. R. (2022). Student perceptions of a teaching electronic medical record in Health Administration education. *Journal of Health Administration Education, 38*(4), 957–974.

Triantaphyllou, E. (2000). Multi-criteria decision making methods. In *Multi-criteria decision making methods: A comparative study. Applied Optimization* (Vol. 44). Springer Publishing Company.

Turner, A. N. (1982, September-October). Consulting is more than giving advice. *Harvard Business Review*. https://hbr.org/1982/09/consulting-is-more-than-giving-adviceTversky, A., & Kahneman, D. (1974). Judgment under uncertainty: Heuristics and biases. *Science, 185*(4157), 1124–1131. https://doi.org/10.1126/science.185.4157.1124

Warner, D. M., & Holloway, D. C. (1978). *Decision making and control for health administration: The management of quantitative analysis*. Health Administration Press.

Wedell-Wedellsborg, T. (2017, January-February). Are you solving the right problems? *Harvard Business Review*. https://hbr.org/2017/01/are-you-solving-the-right-problems

Whittlestone, J. (2013, May 17). *Biases: How they affect your career decisions, and what to do about them*. 80000 hours. https://80000hours.org/2013/05/biases-how-they-affect-your-career-decisions-and-what-to-do-about-them

Woods, D. R. (2000). An evidence-based strategy for problem solving. *Journal of Engineering Education, 89*(4), 443–459. https://doi.org/10.1002/j.2168-9830.2000.tb00551.x

CHAPTER 3

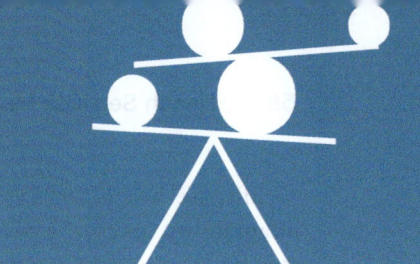

MANAGING INTERPERSONAL COMMUNICATIONS

Managing interpersonal communications involves exchanging information in spoken, written, or nonverbal forms for the purposes of building relationships and informing, persuading, and motivating people to achieve organizational goals.

COMPETENCIES

- Adapt interpersonal communication style and content to various management situations.
- Create psychological safety and interpersonal understanding by listening.
- Manage interpersonal and task conflict through dispute resolution and mediation.
- Negotiate contracts with vendors.
- Develop a respected professional reputation through executive presence, personal branding, and networking.
- Communicate with sensitivity when communicating to diverse audiences.
- Facilitate effective meetings and discussions.
- Write credible business communications, including email and reports.
- Deliver verbal presentations with confidence.

CHAPTER OUTLINE

- Interpersonal Communications
- Professional Reputation
- Communicating in Meetings
- Presentation Skills
- Written Communications

INTRODUCTION

Interpersonal communications refer to the exchange of information between individuals in spoken, written, or nonverbal forms for the purposes of building relationships and informing, persuading, and motivating people (Adler & Proctor, 2023). Communication is a mandatory management competency for goal attainment and career advancement (Drucker, 1954). Health care organizations (HCOs) value health services manager's communication competence above all others, and only those who develop outstanding interpersonal communication skills will progress to the executive ranks (Porter, Haberling, & Hohman, 2016; Tacconelli et al., 2020).

Effective health services managers communicate in many different ways. **Communication adaptability** refers to a person's ability to adjust their communications to a variety of circumstances (Duran, 1992). Adaptable communicators effectively convey meaning to people from various cultures or backgrounds, in different social situations, and through numerous methods (Spitzberg, 2013). Few people are naturally adept at all styles and modes of communication. Some people are strong writers, whereas others have an innate talent for public speaking (Hullman et al., 2010). Some work best in teams, while others excel in one-on-one settings. Nevertheless, anyone can improve every method in which they communicate (Morreale et al., 2013). This chapter focuses on interpersonal communications competencies that health services managers need to master in their careers, including developing relationships, building positive professional reputations, facilitating and participating in meetings, writing business reports and emails, and delivering verbal presentations.

INTERPERSONAL COMMUNICATIONS

Managing Interpersonal Relationships

Communication skills are fundamental to building and maintaining relationships with others (Adler & Proctor, 2023; Mikkelson et al., 2021). The more adept a person communicates, the greater their ability to build and sustain strong relationships with coworkers and the happier they are with their careers (Kundi et al., 2022; Spitzberg, 2013). Research shows that managers can reduce employee job stress and improve engagement, commitment, and trust by using basic communication approaches, such as the following (Fehr et al., 2020; Jiang & Luo, 2018; Mikkelson & Hesse, 2023; Mikkelson, Sloan, & Tietsort, 2021; Spitzberg, 2013):

- *Demonstrate concern for employees:* Show a desire for genuine relationships with others. Regardless of personal feelings about the person, show interest in understanding their needs and motivations.
- *Seek constant feedback:* Solicit input from employees through a variety of mechanisms, including one-on-one meetings, focus groups, anonymous surveys, and exit interviews with departing employees.
- *Express gratitude:* Recognize and appreciate the actions of others, especially those in less visible roles.
- *Reinforce strategic direction:* Constantly communicate the mission, vision, and values of the organization. Every interpersonal exchange serves as an opportunity to remind employees of what is important to organizational success.
- *Set clear expectations for results:* Communicate work objectives. Remind people of the importance of their individual contribution to team success.
- *Prioritize work:* Help employees understand what is most important. Provide them with resources, as needed.
- *Check in regularly:* Implement ways to regularly follow-up with employees on their goals. Supply necessary resources to support them.

These interpersonal communication techniques also apply to how health services managers relate to physicians and other clinicians. Mayo Clinic frequently convenes physician focus groups to identify ways to improve patient care and mitigate work-related stress (Swensen et al., 2016). Mayo Clinic managers practice what they call "participatory management principles" to learn what motivates each individual physician on their team. Based on each physician's input, managers arrange for them to spend at least 20% of their time working on work projects important to them (Shanafelt & Noseworthy, 2017). By showing concern for clinicians' well-being and supporting them with resources, managers can significantly prevent occupational **burnout**, a type of chronic stress typified by feelings of exhaustion, negativity, and powerlessness (World Health Organization [WHO], 2019).

> **△ KEY IDEA**
>
> **By showing concern for clinicians' well-being and supporting them with resources, managers can significantly prevent occupational burnout, a type of chronic stress typified by feelings of exhaustion, negativity, and powerlessness**

Creating Psychological Safety

People will not share confide in their managers if they feel threatened. **Psychological safety** is a shared belief among team members that taking risks would be supported by others at work (Edmondson, 1999). With a sense of psychological safety, employees point out errors to their managers, provide candid feedback, acknowledge disagreements, and admit mistakes (Newman et al., 2017). In HCOs, psychological safety is especially important to reducing patient errors. Clinicians need to trust that they can report patient safety issues without fear of reprisals from managers or other authorities (Leroy et al., 2012). When employees have psychological safety, they understand that most mistakes are not inherently bad, but they actually represent opportunities for improvement.

Because employees lower in the organizational hierarchy perceive that they know less than their superiors, they are less likely to speak up about issues (O'Donovan & McAuliffe, 2020). Therefore, effective managers spend significant effort helping people feel psychologically safe. Table 3.1 illustrates communication approaches for creating psychological safety among their employees (Cox, 2022; Nembhard & Edmondson, 2006; Nikita & Lordan, 2023; Rudolph et al., 2006; Weiss et al., 2018).

When health services managers demonstrate behaviors associated with psychological safety, such as speaking up about bad news, taking risks, and admitting mistakes, employees learn that they are also safe to express themselves (Newman et al., 2017). Employees watch how managers act, and if the manager is not willing to speak up to their bosses, then employees will learn that speaking up is neither safe nor useful (Bandura, 1977; Knight, 2014).

When people take risks to speak up about tough issues, effective managers listen. **Active listening** is a technique that requires the listener to pay close attention to the speaker, paraphrase their words to clarify understanding, make verbal affirmations (e.g., "tell me more"), and use other nonverbal cues to indicate engagement (e.g., nodding; Adler & Proctor, 2023). Because people are often too busy thinking about what they want to say instead of truly listening, active listening remains an underutilized skill. Managers can remember to listen by following Stephen R. Covey's recommendation from *7 Habits of Highly Effective People* which states, "First seek to understand, then to be understood" (Covey, 2013, p. 237). In other words, health services managers should listen with the intent of understanding the other person's perspective before attempting to convey their own viewpoint. This rule can also be stated as "Listen first, speak last" (Drucker & Maciariello, 2008).

> **△ KEY IDEA**
>
> **Because people are often too busy thinking about what they want to say instead of truly listening, active listening remains an underutilized skill.**

TABLE 3.1 Communication Approaches to Help People to Feel Psychologically Safe

APPROACH	SITUATIONS	SUPPORTIVE LANGUAGE
Refer to the team collectively.	Building team cohesion	"We have important goals to accomplish together."
Give people the benefit of the doubt.	Giving negative feedback	"From my point of view, this approach was problematic. What am I missing?" or "Help me understand your approach."
Seek reactions to events.	Requesting emotional perspective	"How did you feel?" or "What feels good?" or "What feels difficult?"
Invite ideas, comments, or opinions.	Persuading others to give unique perspective	"Do you have any ideas?" or "How will this impact your work?"
Immediately voice appreciation for input.	Demonstrating gratitude for others sharing ideas	"That's a great idea!" or "Interesting I'm writing that down."
Celebrate when others speak up.	Recognizing when others assert opinions or raise concerns	"Thank you for bringing up your concerns. Your willingness to voice your opinions demonstrates your commitment to our team."
Use respectful, identity-affirming language.	Demonstrating awareness and sensitivity to the diversity of identities and experiences	"My preferred pronouns are he/him."

Health services managers also create psychological safety by modeling inclusivity. Human beings place great value on social relationships and almost universally desire to feel recognized and valued (Seppälä & McNichols, 2022). **Inclusiveness** entails the words and deeds that managers use to invite collaboration and appreciate others' work contributions (Nembhard & Edmondson, 2006). Inclusiveness instills a sense of **belonging**, which is the feeling of connectedness to a team or organization. People who feel excluded and disconnected will not feel psychologically safe. Employees notice when health services managers respectfully collaborate with individuals of different ages, races, ethnicities, and professional backgrounds (Cox, 2022). When differences are embraced and all perspectives are considered, teams develop shared psychological safety.

> ### △ KEY IDEA
> **Promoting an open-door policy may not be enough. Employees need to regularly see managers within their own environment to feel comfortable talking about challenges.**

Health services managers can also create a sense of psychological safety among employees by enhancing their visibility and approachability. **Visibility** means the apparent presence of managers to employees, often associated with the ability to support work goals (Bailey et al., 2022). **Approachability** means that others, especially those people with less authority, perceive someone to be open, supportive, welcoming, warm, and accepting of ideas (Brown, 2016). If health services managers really want to hear genuine opinions, they need to increase the number and quality of interactions with employees and clinicians. Promoting an open-door policy may not be enough. Employees need to regularly see managers within their own environment to feel comfortable talking about challenges (Adelman, 2012). Managers gather feedback from employees by routinely visiting each department or unit of the HCO, a practice that improves visibility and approachability called **management rounds** (Adelman, 2012; Knight, 2014; Roussin, 2008). Clinicians commonly make the rounds in the hospital environment as a means to systematically assess each admitted patient, so when health services managers conduct management rounds, the behavior is familiar and respected.

Managing Conflict

Interpersonal conflict refers to disagreements between individuals and within groups about goals, expectations, or interests that are perceived to be incompatible (Boulding, 1963). HCOs are high-pressure work environments, where life-and-death stakes and occupational fatigue inevitably lead to conflict. Therefore, competent health services managers collaborate with clinical and administrative professionals to resolve unhealthy conflict (Begun et al., 2011).

In HCOs, conflict can be disruptive and dangerous, resulting in medical errors, poor patient satisfaction, and preventable deaths (The Joint Commission, 2021). Scholars distinguish between two main types of conflict in workplaces—task conflict and relationship conflict. **Task conflict** refers to disagreements among team members about goals and content of work (Jehn, 1995). Table 3.2 presents common causes of task-related conflicts that managers face in the workplace (Jehn, 1995; Laker & Pereira, 2022; Moisoglou et al., 2014).

Relationship conflict exists when there is tension, annoyance, and animosity between group members, usually arising from differences in personality, style, or professional background (Jehn, 1995). In HCOs, relationship conflict frequently occurs between professions, such as physicians,

TABLE 3.2 Common Causes of Task-Related Conflict in the Workplace

CONFLICT	DESCRIPTION	EXAMPLE
How to accomplish tasks	Debate, disagree, and argue about the content of the task needed to be performed, usually among people who do the same type of work	Individuals cannot agree to the best course of action among multiple options for action, each with merit
Who is responsible for tasks	Ambiguity, overlaps, or difference of opinion about roles, responsibilities, and work tasks	Disagreements about which department is responsible for a task, often accompanied by complaints about unfair workload and lack of clear job descriptions
How to allocate resources	Disagreements about distribution of assets, including financial resources, personnel, time, and other resources, to various projects, departments, or units	Limited resources must be divided up among teams or team members, and there are differences in goals and priorities.
When to complete work	Unreasonable time constraints or misalignment on timing or deadlines for collaborative tasks	Team members misunderstand or misinterpret the amount of time it takes for others to complete a task.

nurses, and health services managers, due to differences in professional cultures, which are exacerbated by disruptive organizational change (Kaissi, 2005; Keller et al., 2019). When organizational disruption threatens deeply held convictions, tensions intensify into animosity.

For example, conflict between physicians and health services managers is common in HCOs. Physicians and health services managers are often different types of people with very different education and training (Garman, Leach, & Spector, 2006). These differences can lead to faulty assumptions about each other's professions. Generally speaking, physicians and health services managers approach problem-solving differently, causing physicians to view health services managers as "indecisive and excessively bureaucratic" and health services managers to view physicians as "impulsive and less resilient to change" (Keller et al. 2019, p. 8). To preserve positive working relationships with physicians, health services managers help clinicians understand how wise decisions about money can support patient care. When physicians blame health services managers for not approving requested investments, managers should remain calm and composed. Saying no to physicians on occasion is part of the health services manager's job, and physician frustrations should not be taken personally.

> ⚠ **KEY IDEA**
>
> **Not all conflict in the workplace is bad. Conflict can actually improve performance, inspire innovation, and improve communication on teams.**

Not all conflict in the workplace is bad. Conflict can actually improve performance, inspire innovation, and improve communication on teams (A. Gallo, 2018). However, conflict often requires that managers intervene, a vital skill called **conflict management** (Bradley et al., 2015). Effective health services managers insist on respectfully and directly addressing conflict, instead of avoiding it (Weingart et al., 2014). Health services managers are responsible for either providing support so that individuals and teams can resolve their own conflicts or facilitating resolution of conflict directly. To support conflict resolution indirectly, health services managers can allocate resources to training and create procedures that enable conflicts to be resolved fairly (Oxenstierna et al., 2011; The Joint Commission, 2021). Conflict resolution can also be reached through **alternative dispute resolution** processes, including **mediation**, in which a neutral third party facilitates communication between disputing parties, or the more formal process of **arbitration**, which uses evidence, argumentation, and legally binding decisions (Sharma, 2021). When directly intervening, health services managers can reframe discussions as conflict of ideas (i.e., not personal), help the people understand the disagreements more clearly, identify common ground among the conflicting parties, and assist conflicting parties to collectively brainstorm solutions (Begun et al., 2011; Lencioni, 2002; Shonk, 2023).

Negotiating and Contracting

Negotiation is a form of decision-making in which two or more people engage in discussions to reach an agreement or resolve a dispute (Pruitt, 1981). In health services management, negotiations tend to be related to contracts for supplies, drugs, medical equipment, and insurance payment (American College of Healthcare Executives [ACHE], 2023). **Contracting** is the process of selecting a vendor, supplier, provider, or payer to deliver products or services; negotiating terms of a contract for services; and managing the relationship throughout the term of that contract (Curry & Smith, 2017). For mid-career health services managers, contracting is often stressful because mistakes can be financially costly and highly visible (Curry & Smith, 2017).

Later in their careers, health services managers negotiate outsourcing contracts, health insurance payment terms, and physician employment contracts. Executive health services managers will negotiate with union representatives or with other HCO executives on multibillion-dollar merger and acquisition deals. Health services managers are supported in most large-scale negotiations by lawyers and/or human resource professionals (Fottler et al., 2015).

The art and skill of contract negotiation is complex. Nevertheless, there are basic principles to follow when negotiating with vendors, suppliers, providers, and payers (Lewicki et al., 2011). Prior to negotiation, health services managers should conduct extensive research to determine a realistic price goal. This includes developing a **reservation price**, which is the highest amount that a buyer would be willing to pay. For the seller, their reservation price is the lowest amount that they would be willing to sell their products or services.

Improving negotiating power means having options. The concept known as **BATNA** (Best Alternative To a Negotiated Agreement) refers to the option a negotiator will pursue if the current negotiations do not result in an agreement (Dawson, 2021). In other words, the more attractive the fallback position is, the stronger the negotiating position will be for the negotiator. If the terms offered in the negotiation are better than the BATNA, then the price may be a good deal; if the price is worse, then the BATNA may be the preferred course of action. Buyers with stronger BATNAs are in better positions to offer a lower initial price, known as an **anchor price**. Skilled negotiators use the anchor price as a way to achieve a better price in the negotiation process. Both the buyer and sellers have BATNAs that, when considered together, determine the **Zone Of Possible Agreement (ZOPA)**, as illustrated in Figure 3.1.

> **CAREER BOX 3.1: Negotiating a Salary**
>
> Salary negotiations can be stressful, especially for early-career health services managers, because the employer typically holds more power in the negotiation process. You might fear that negotiating a higher salary may negatively impact their relationship with the employer or even get their job offer rescinded. Negotiation anxiety can be particularly acute if you are currently unemployed or dissatisfied with your current job. However, negotiating rarely causes negative feelings for the employer, especially if conducted with affability and professionalism. In fact, most recruiters and hiring managers will expect you to negotiate your salary and will respect you more if you do. The following are some common negotiating tips used following a job offer (Dawson, 2021; Maaravi & Levy, 2017):
>
> - *Identify alternatives:* The best way to increase your negotiating power is to develop a backup plan (i.e., BATNA) to improve the likelihood that you can walk away from a bad offer.
> - *Know your worth:* Always do research on the salary ranges for similar roles. The internet is a great source of information for salary expectations, as are acquaintances who work at the organization or in similar roles elsewhere.
> - *Let the employer make the first offer:* If you do not know the salary range, then let the employer make the first offer. This can give you information about how much to counteroffer to negotiate to achieve your salary goal. It is possible that their offer will be higher than you expect.
> - *Overstate your initial offer:* If you possess valid information about the salary range, then you should make the first offer. Do not be afraid to propose a high number because your offer will make subsequent counteroffers higher than they might be otherwise.
> - *Never say yes to the first offer:* Always counteroffer to an employer's offer or counteroffer. Respond with a salary higher than your preferred salary. When doing so, the final offer may settle closer to your salary goal.

FIGURE 3.1 BATNA negotiation diagram.

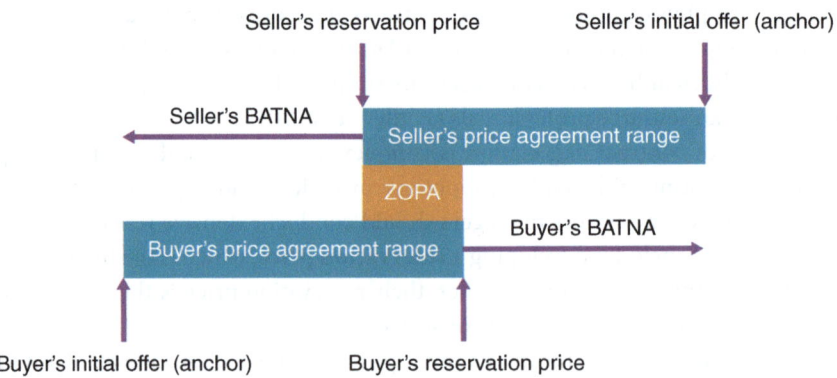

BATNA, Best Alternative To a Negotiated Agreement; ZOPA, Zone Of Possible Agreement.

For example, if a health services manager wants to negotiate a better price for a certain category of medical supplies, then they would need to identify the reservation price and secure a BATNA so that they can walk away from a bad deal with a supplier. Many HCOs belong to group purchasing organizations (GPOs), purchasing groups that negotiate discounts on medical supplies, equipment, and services by buying in bulk for cooperatives made up of many HCOs. A health services manager may aggressively negotiate with a supplier knowing that the GPO prices will serve as an adequate BATNA.

Of course, price is not the only element of purchasing negotiations. Health services managers can negotiate product quality, delivery time, payment terms, and customer service as part of the deal. In fact, considering multiple issues during negotiation will improve the likelihood of closing a deal that is mutually beneficial to the HCO and the supplier or payer. In *Getting to Yes: Negotiating Agreement Without Giving In*, the authors argue that negotiators do not need to resort to win-lose battles (Fisher et al., 2011). Instead, health services managers can develop cooperative relationships with suppliers and payers. Fisher and Ury recommend collaborating and focusing on meeting each other's interests with creative, win-win deals.

PROFESSIONAL REPUTATION

Executive Presence

Health services managers can also use their communication skills to manage their professional reputation. Health services managers who communicate with **executive presence** improve their chances for organizational influence and professional advancement (Hewlett, 2014). Managers with executive presence project confidence, authority, and credibility in a manner that inspires respect and appreciation of others. Communicating with executive presence means articulating messages in clear, convincing, and simple ways (Dagley & Gaskin, 2014). Executive presence also means that a person's voice sounds warm and relaxed (Crittenden, 2018). Finally, according to Dagley and Gaskin (2014), people who communicate with executive presence in social situations are able to gracefully engage with people with etiquette and poise.

Sylvia A. Hewlett has identified three domains that comprise executive presence: verbal communication (i.e., speech), gravitas (i.e., action), and appearance (i.e., grooming and polish; Hewlett, 2014). According to Hewlett's research, gravitas matters most to executives when perceiving someone as possessing an executive presence (Hewlett, 2024). **Gravitas** means projecting dignity in their physical bearing, deportment, and personal conduct. The most appreciated trait within the gravitas domain is **confidence**. Self-confidence enables a person to display composure in difficult, unpredictable situations (Beeson, 2012). **Confidence** means that a person trusts their own judgment and asserts one's opinions respectfully when working with other strong-willed executives (Spitzberg, 2013). A confident person may feel nervous but projects an outward sense of calm (Dagley & Gaskin, 2014).

Appearance, probably the least important domain of executive presence, is related to grooming and polish rather than physical attractiveness (Hewlett, 2014). Researchers Dagley and Gaskin (2014) found that physical stature, eye contact, style of walk, and posture also mattered to perceptions of executive presence. People with executive presence still follow the social norms of the workplace, including dressing appropriately, monitoring personal hygiene, and remembering that people often judged others based on their appearance (Baedke & Lamberton, 2018; Hewlett, 2024).

Personal Brand

Personal branding is a term of relatively recent invention that means communicating professional strengths to create a positive perception in the minds of people outside their immediate network (Gorbatov et al., 2023). Building a personal brand is a deliberate form of professional reputation management (National Center for Healthcare Leadership [NCHL], 2018). Personal branding is associated with increased visibility, improved employability, and higher salaries, especially in virtual work environments where face-to-face contact is limited (Golden & Eddleston, 2020; Gorbatov et al., 2018). According to the research, effective professional branding consists of the following aspects (Davis et al., 2020; Gorbatov et al., 2019, 2021; Kanter, 2009):

- *Communicate strategically:* Target messaging to specific audiences.
- *Convey value and uniqueness:* Create unique professional identity in the field.
- *Use technology to tell a story:* Leverage social media and well-designed visuals to enhance professional reputation. Research shows that the number of social media contacts does not benefit careers as much as the frequency of usage.
- *Do not mistake attention for reputation:* Brand recognition is different from brand appeal. Make sure personal branding communicates authenticity, not narcissism.
- *Track the reception:* Ask trusted people for feedback and make sure communications are interpreted as intended.

The ability to build a personal brand is positively related to whether a person is extraverted but negatively correlated with whether a person was perceived as honest and humble (Gorbatov et al., 2021). To avoid the costs of brazen self-promotion, it is important that health services managers conduct personal branding consistent with the culture of the profession (Parmentier et al., 2013). Professional reputations are built on providing value to HCOs, so any personal branding efforts should explain how professional achievements benefit patients, employers, communities, or the industry.

INFORMATIONAL INTERVIEW 3.1
CEO and Brand Strategist
Access the informational interview online at http://connect.springerpub.com/content/book/978-0-8261-4807-0/chapter/ch00.

Networking

Health services management reputations can be bolstered through professional **networking**, a method of building and maintaining professional relationships in order to exchange resources for the benefit of one's work and career (Porter et al., 2023). Some people hold the misperception that networking is a shallow endeavor only useful for people looking for a new job (Burnison, 2018). While it is true that those people who network are more likely to receive job offers, promotions, and higher salaries, people build professional networks for a variety of reasons, including the following (Burnison, 2018; NCHL, 2018; Porter et al., 2023; Ravishankar, 2023):

- *Satisfaction of making connections:* Some enjoy meeting new people with similar goals and interests. Social connections improve career satisfaction.
- *Helping others:* Professional colleagues can exchange professional resources.
- *Status and respect:* Perceptions of expertise can turn into career-building professional opportunities.
- *Learning and performance*: Facilitate personal or professional growth and learn knowledge and skills that advance careers.
- *Career development:* In cases where new career opportunities are needed, professional networks can make job searches more effective.
- *Professional obligation:* Many professionals, including health services managers, see networking as a responsibility to bring value to their organizations.

Networking does not necessarily mean attending professional networking events with associates and other business contacts in which everyone wears a name tag and informally mingles. For health services managers, every type of social interaction counts as networking. People often find that collaborating on projects together builds useful professional connections (Zack, 2019). Health services managers can volunteer to work for professional associations, such as local chapters of the American College of Health Care Executives or National Association of Health Services Executives. Networking can also include working on project teams or conducting one-on-one meetings, such informational interviews or before-work breakfasts.

CAREER BOX 3.2: Elevator Pitches

The idea of summarizing your professional career to strangers in 30 seconds probably makes you cringe. However, the professional elevator pitch is actually an excellent way to share your expertise and credentials quickly and effectively. Unfortunately, many people deliver stilted recitations of their résumé that come across as awkward or boastful. Of course, any strong elevator pitch needs to explain your professional background and abilities, but this should be kept as short as possible. To make an elevator pitch sound friendly, confident, and approachable, try sharing your motivations (Cenedella, 2010). For example, if you are attending a professional networking event to find a job, then tell people that. When people understand your motivations, they are more likely to trust you and offer to help you. Also, talk about what kind of work most excites you. This can give the other person insight into the value you bring to an organization and your ability to articulate a vision for the future. Finally, practice your elevator pitch enough so that it sounds smooth and natural. Making professional connections is much easier when you engage others in normal conversation.

COMMUNICATING IN MEETINGS

Participating in Meetings

Meetings are goal-directed collaborative interactions with two or more people (Allen et al., 2015). Some managers spend between 50% and 80% of their work time in meetings, including preparation, participation, and facilitation of meetings (Rogelberg et al., 2007). Meetings are where the management action happens (Mroz et al., 2018). As such, meeting-related communication skills are considered an essential competency for health services management career success (ACHE, 2023; Ortiz et al., 2016).

> △ **KEY IDEA**
>
> Meetings are where the management action happens. As such, meeting-related communication skills are considered an essential competency for health services management career success.

Unfortunately, workplace meetings tend to be ineffective and inefficient (Mroz et al., 2018). Many people dread going to meetings because they are often viewed as a waste of time (Allen et al., 2012). Some people pretend to participate in meetings by nodding, agreeing with another's viewpoint, or alternately tune out and speak up (Beck et al., 2024). Ideally, people would only attend meetings for which they are fully engaged. However, due to the high number of meetings a manager has in a given day, full participation in every meeting would be exhausting (Allen et al., 2022). **Meeting load** refers to the frequency and time spent in meetings. Employees with higher meeting loads struggle with interrupted workflow, less productivity, and overall work dissatisfaction (Allen et al., 2012). High-performing employees tend to engage more in meetings even though more meetings can also sap their energy and motivation (Romney et al., 2023 Sonnentag, 2001). Therefore, to make the most out of meetings without undermining the best employees, effective health services managers make each meeting as efficient and effective as possible.

Planning, Coordinating, and Facilitating Meetings

Effective and efficient meetings require detailed plans, coordination, and facilitation. An effectively planned meeting always includes a written **agenda** that is circulated in advance and presented verbally at the beginning of the meeting (Mroz et al., 2018). For meeting planners, agendas serve as a planning tool and as a meeting script (Butler, 2014). As reflected in Table 3.3, agendas need to define the **meeting purpose**, which is the objective or goal for the meeting. The purpose is usually a single objective statement related to informing, discussing, or deciding something. A clearly stated purpose will focus the participants on achieving the goal of the meeting (Porter & Baker, 2006). The meeting's topic is not the same thing as the meeting's purpose. The **meeting topic** is usually the name of a project or issue, not what the meeting is intended to accomplish. For example, in a meeting about an office space renovation project, the purpose might be to make a decision on the project vendor.

> △ **KEY IDEA**
>
> Effectively planned meetings always include a written agenda that is circulated in advance and presented verbally at the beginning of the meeting.

Agenda items refer to the specific issues that are scheduled to be discussed and addressed during a meeting. Each item is assigned to a person who is responsible for leading the discussion, a question that needs to be answered, and the time needed to discuss. Agendas also include the person who is responsible for facilitating a meeting, a role designed to assist participants to address the agenda items (Rogelberg, 2020). A **facilitator** actively encourages everyone to participate in meeting introductions and discussions. Meeting facilitators also guide the decision-making processes in meetings and make meetings productive by keeping the discussions on time and on topic. If the meeting gets off task with unrelated but worthy issues, then the facilitator can place the issue in a **parking lot**, which is the term used to describe the list of issues to be discussed at a later time (Butler, 2014). Table 3.3 is an example of an agenda, but agendas will vary depending on the meeting purpose (Porter & Baker, 2006).

When closing the meeting, an effective facilitator checks for achievement of the agenda purpose. In addition, the facilitator reviews any action items that emerged from the meeting and confirms participants' commitments on their new tasks. Any assignment of participants' tasks should be coupled with expressions of appreciation for their contributions (Axtell, 2020). Following a meeting, helpful meeting facilitators send meeting minutes and action items out immediately (Mroz et al., 2018).

Types of Meetings

Health services managers participate in many different types of meetings, from formal organization-wide meetings to informal conversations. Whether held in person or virtually, meetings provide a forum for sharing information, debating, discussing, brainstorming, and decision-making.

TABLE 3.3 Sample Meeting Agenda Template

MEETING TOPIC: Review of HCAHPS scores			
MEETING PURPOSE: Identify actions based on recent patient experience survey results.			
ATTENDEES: Elena Rodriguez, Jonathan Mercer, Angela Bennett, Marcus Thompson, Catherine Chen, and Derek Williams			
AGENDA ITEMS	**ITEM QUESTION**	**WHO**	**TIME**
News and notes	What updates does the team need since we last met?	Elena	5 minutes
Overview of HCAHPS scores	What summary of the results can be shared with HCO employees and other stakeholders?	Jonathan	10 minutes
Discuss positive feedback	What actions can be shared with others as best practices?	Jonathan	10 minutes
OFI	What actions can be implemented to address OFIs?	Jonathan	15 minutes
Action items and follow-up	What action items were assigned during the meeting? Responsible parties? Due dates?	Elena	5 minutes

HCAHPS, Hospital Consumer Assessment of Healthcare Providers and Systems; HCO, health care organization; OFI, opportunities for improvement.

No matter the purpose, meetings need to be delivered in the right format. Table 3.4 lists the various types of meeting and their respective frequencies, durations, and functions (Adelman, 2012; Beck et al., 2024; Fernandez, Landis, & Lee, 2023; Flinchum et al., 2023; Kello & Allen, 2020; Lencioni, 2004).

Early-career health services managers spend most of their meeting time in huddles and status meetings (Allen et al., 2014). As health services managers progress in their careers, they spend more time in staff, one-on-one, and debrief meetings tracking ongoing projects, solving problems, and addressing issues related to employee performance. Compared to other levels, executive health services managers conduct more offsite and town hall meetings.

TABLE 3.4 Types of Meetings in Health Care Organizations

MEETING TYPE	ALTERNATE TERM	FREQUENCY	DURATION	FUNCTION
HUDDLE	Daily check-in or stand-up meeting	Scheduled, administrative meetings	Usually lasting no more than 10 minutes	Discussion of day-to-day operations, such as daily HCO facilities activities
STATUS MEETING	Project update	Regularly on established cadence	Approximately 30 to 45 minutes	Present updates on activities followed by brief discussions about any open issues, risks, or concerns
STAFF MEETING	Team meeting	Regularly scheduled and recurring	Approximately 30 minutes	Focus on discussion and decision-making related to near-term objectives
DEBRIEF	Ad hoc, one-off meeting	Single topic meetings scheduled as needed, not recurring	As short as possible	Appropriate when decisions need to be made quickly. Disruptive and unproductive unless highly purposeful
ONE-ON-ONE MEETING	Conversation, dialogue	Frequently	Usually less than 30 minutes; meals last 1 hour	Nearly half of all meetings are between two people
OFFSITE MEETING	Retreat	Quarterly or annually, in person and outside the office	Half or full day	Team building and strategic planning; offsites can reduce distractions and enhance participant engagement
TOWN HALL MEETING	Site-wide, all-hands meeting	At least annually, scheduled, as needed	Approximately 60 to 90 minutes, balancing thoroughness with and respect for employee productivity	Senior managers share relevant, accurate, and timely information on operations and strategic direction of the HCO, then open the meeting to questions and comments from employees.

HCO, health care organization.

FIGURE 3.2 Types of meetings.

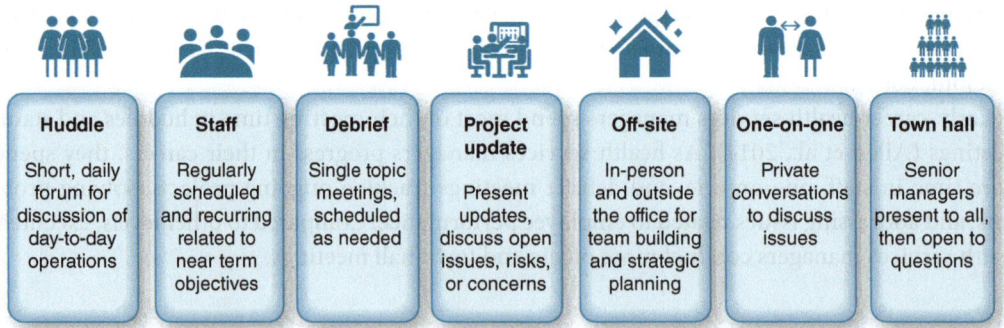

PRESENTATION SKILLS

Verbal Presentation Competency

Verbal presentation skills are critical to performance in the health services management profession. Professional presentations require significant planning, constructive feedback, iterative adjustments, and plenty of practice (Potthoff et al., 2020). Successful early-career health services managers need to demonstrate their ability to present to executives to be considered as possessing career advancement potential (Beeson, 2012). With concerted effort and growth in verbal communication skills, health services managers earn substantial professional credibility (NCHL, 2018).

Ancient philosopher Aristotle developed a formula for delivering speeches still used by the best public speakers today (Edinger, 2020). Memorable speakers express three rhetorical elements in their speeches: ethos (character), pathos (emotion), and logos (reason). Speakers combine credibility (ethos) and enthusiasm (pathos) with sound logic (logos) to persuade, inspire, or inform audiences. Compelling speeches balance these three rhetorical modes, depending on the audience, purpose, and context. For example, a speech can start with ethos to establish credibility, then convey logos to support the argument, and finally deliver pathos to inspire action. Table 3.5 illustrates Aristotle's three rhetorical modes using health services management presentation examples.

Politicians often make persuasive speeches that include ethos, pathos, and logos rhetorical elements. For example, President Barack Obama gave an important healthcare speech in 2009 where he advocated for healthcare reform legislation. To express ethos (credibility), Obama's speech downplayed any ideologically charged rhetoric in favor of language that made health reform sound like a fair compromise (Schimmel, 2016). Obama argued that healthcare reform was not about "big government" but rational policy intended to solve common problems (Obama, 2009). To draw upon pathos (emotion), Obama referred the feeling of "terror and helplessness" associated with not having health insurance and being unable to afford lifesaving health care for a child or parent. Finally, and most prominently, Obama relied on logos (logic), when he stated his case for reforming the healthcare system by highlighting startling stories about "middle-class Americans" who cannot afford health insurance. Ultimately, the speech was successful, as the Patient Protection and Affordable Care Act of 2010 became law.

TABLE 3.5 Aristotle Persuasive Rhetorical Modes in Presentations

RHETORICAL MODE	DEFINITION	HEALTH SERVICES EXAMPLES
Ethos (credibility, character)	Respect gained due to knowledge, integrity, and reputation of the speaker. Job titles are helpful, but credibility is most powerfully derived from confidently expressing expertise and morality. Presentations should be mistake-free and highly professional.	"This presentation is based on extensive analysis of our health services management team." "I can address any questions, doubts, or objections today." "Included in your resource packet are detailed analyses and resources."
Pathos (emotion, inspiration)	Connect feeling to action. Express excitement about achievements, frustration about failures, concern about poor performance, and/or enthusiasm about the future.	"This new service line will save lives and demonstrate our commitment to the health and well-being of the community."
Logos (reason, logic)	A sound argument, generated from evidence and evaluated through critical thinking, provides a clear rationale for recommendations. Articulate the link between facts and conclusions.	"I recommend that the HCO invest in this new services line due to the community need and attractive financial return on investment." "According to the analysis, the internal rate of return exceeds the established threshold for investment and outperforms similar projects in which the HCO previously invested."

HCO, health care organization.

Presentation Delivery

Communication delivery is the ability to verbally and nonverbally convey a message to an audience. The fundamental challenge of all public speaking engagements is to capture and hold the attention of audiences (Lawrence, 2015). Confident public speakers express themselves using three vocal elements: stress (volume), intonation (rising and falling tone), and rhythm (pacing). Like a musical instrument, the voice can be used to maintain interest, to stress certain words, and create or release dramatic tension. Varying vocal quality prevents the perceptions of a droning, monotone speech delivery.

However, most speakers tend to forget to use the vocal variations because they speak too quickly, usually due to anxiety (Arushi et al., 2023). Effective verbal communicators speak at a rate typical of most conversations at about 150 words per minute (wpm; Yuan et al., 2006). Popular Technology, Entertainment, and Design (TED) Talk speaking rates include Sir Ken Robinson at 165 wpm (76 million views), Brené Brown at 154 wpm (64 million views), and Simon Sinek at 170 wpm (64 million views; Barnard, 2022). In addition to speaking too rapidly, speakers should avoid these other self-defeating habits (Schreiber et al., 2012):

- *Fillers:* Common, short, but meaningless utterances, such as "like," "uh," and "you know"
- *Hedges:* Words that soften the assertiveness of speech, such as "kinda," "sort of," "I guess," and "I think"
- *Tag questions:* Ending statements with a question, such as "Right?" "Isn't it?" "Okay?" and "Don't you think?"

- *Uptalk:* Ending statements with questioning intonations that convey uncertainty when expressing confidence would be more appropriate.
- *Read the speech:* Reading from notes or the presentation screen renders most speakers monotonous and robotic. Teleprompters should be used by experts only.

Of course, stage fright makes public speaking exceedingly difficult and mistake prone. For many people, speaking in public is more feared than death (Dwyer & Davidson, 2012). Successful health services managers overcome their apprehension through preparation, which can help nervous speakers to recover quickly if flustered (Raja, 2017). Anxiety can also be reduced by breathing deeply when speaking. Not only does breathing calm the nerves, but it also allows speakers to create pauses in their speeches, a technique that conveys confidence (Zandan, 2018).

INFORMATIONAL INTERVIEW 3.2
Founder and CEO
Access the informational interview online at http://connect.springerpub.com/content/book/978-0-8261-4807-0/chapter/ch00.

Nonverbal communication can be equally effective at conveying meaning, including the use of facial expressions, professional appearance, and body language and movement (Spitzberg, 2013). Public speaking experts also provide the following nonverbal communication advice to improve speeches (Clarke et al., 2019; C. Gallo, 2018; Wezowski, 2017):

- *Make eye contact:* Eye contact is a powerful way to capture and maintain the audience's attention. Even when nervous, making eye contact creates the impression of confidence and control.
- *Stand strong:* Avoid swaying, crossing legs, or leaning on a podium. Stand with feet shoulder-width apart to indicate strength and stability.
- *Use open posture:* Avoid putting hands in pockets or folding arms across the chest.
- *Make metaphoric hand gestures:* Symbolize business ideas, such as increasing profits, with symbolic motions, such as pointing upward. Or use a pinching gesture to indicate marginal improvements, for example.
- *Use gestures:* Palms up indicate openness and honesty; palms down reflect authority and assertiveness.
- *Wear neat, professional attire:* Dress somewhat better than the audience.

Presentation Content

Presentation content includes the messages, data, visuals, and other elements that are used to convey information to an audience. To create effective presentation content, health services managers first need to understand the audience (Duarte, 2010). Knowing the audience allows the speaker to adapt the message, structure, length, and level of detail to be tailored to their level of interests, needs, and understanding. Empathizing with the audience helps the speaker to identify why the audience might care, what they need, and how they make decisions. When speakers create trust between them and the audience, the likelihood that the message will be accepted increases (Duarte, 2010). Many HCOs consist of people from many diverse backgrounds, professions, and experiences. As such, health services managers must develop presentation messages that are sensitive to diverse audiences (Broeckelman-Post & Ruiz-Mesa, 2018). For example, culturally sensitive presentations consider whether the audience's dominant culture appreciates humor and personal anecdotes or prefers formality and serious content.

> **△ KEY IDEA**
>
> Empathizing with the audience helps the speaker to identify why the audience might care, what they need, and how they make decisions.

Goals determine the structure and content of the presentation. What does the presentation seek to accomplish? Why is the presentation important? Does the presentation need to inform the audience? To entertain? Educate? Persuade? Inspire? Or create changes in behavior? According to Dan Roam's *Show and Tell: How Everybody Can Make Extraordinary Presentations*, there are four main narrative presentation types, as illustrated in Table 3.6.

Speeches structured with **storytelling** elements are more compelling and memorable (Duarte, 2010; Landrum et al., 2019). Human beings are naturally inclined to absorb information delivered through narrative structures. Schank and Ableson (1995) argued that virtually all human knowledge is based on stories and that humans interpret new experiences in terms of stories we already know. Therefore, effective speakers structure their presentations as stories. Even technical reports can be structured as stories. The **report** delivers content linearly, with each part addressed in a logical sequence. But like any good story, a report presentation must convey meaning by explaining cause and effect as well as the reason behind the relationship. In other words, "This happened, and, therefore, this happened, and this is why." For example, patient volume is down 10% because the largest cardiology group in the community is no longer referring their patients to the HCO.

TABLE 3.6 Presentation Types, Goals, and Rhetorical Devices With Examples

PRESENTATION TYPE	GOAL	RHETORICAL DEVICES	EXAMPLES
REPORT	Informational. Convey facts insightfully and memorably.	Answer why, who, what, where, when, how, and how much? Use examples.	Team status meeting, quarterly report, project review
EXPLANATION	Educational; teaches new abilities or knowledge. Explain complex ideas to nonexpert audiences.	Build new knowledge on existing concepts. Share examples through narratives or anecdotes.	Academic presentation, class lecture, training course, news report
PITCH	Identify problems, recommend solutions, and urge action. Construct persuasive message with credible evidence. Make call to action.	Connect problem and solution. Draw contrasts in current state and potential future state. Demonstrate advantages and disadvantages of alternatives.	Sales pitch, product launch, funding request, job interview
DRAMATIC	Inspire a new way of looking at the world.	Heroes, conflict, change, metaphors, and analogies	Vision setting, motivate change, keynote speech, TED talk

TED, Technology, Entertainment, and Design.

> **CAREER BOX 3.3: Tell a Story, Land the Job**
>
> Just like any good presentation or writing, you can tell a good story with your job application materials (Kurnoff & Lazarus, 2021). When applying for a job, identify the problem or set of problems the role is intended to solve. With the problem identified, a good story can be written with you as the hero, the problems as the obstacles, and your abilities to solve problems as the themes. The overarching themes on your résumé, in your cover letter, and during your interview should directly relate to how you can solve the organization's problems. For example, if applying for the position of assistant clinic administrator, a role that requires a broad range of people management abilities, then the job application theme could feature your strong interpersonal skills. This theme could be reinforced with stories that incorporate settings (e.g., school club), characters (e.g., fellow members), and conflict (e.g., how to plan an event). By connecting the job requirements to your stories, your application becomes more relevant and memorable to the hiring manager.

The **explanation** presentation structure, on the other hand, seeks to build knowledge or skills by starting with foundational knowledge and builds to more complex concepts. At each stage of explanation, the presentation checks for understanding. Effective explanations incorporate the power of story to engage audiences and help them remember key knowledge. Narrative "hooks," such as dramatic scenarios or anecdotes, create emotional connection to the content (McNett, 2016). Using classic story elements of conflict, drama, plot, and characterizations can turn otherwise dry material into memorable presentations. For example, when presenting a patient safety training program, a health services manager could incorporate a dramatic story about a narrowly avoided patient medication error and the steps taken to keep the patient safe.

The **pitch** is a persuasive presentation designed to remove barriers to accomplishing specified goals. Health services managers commonly use the pitch structure to persuade decision-makers (Potthoff et al., 2020). Health services managers are often called upon to define problems, analyze root causes, identify alternative solutions, and make recommendations to take certain action. The pitch story structure focuses on overcoming a problem, barrier, or hurdle of some kind. In addition, pitch underscores the "why" and the costs of not taking action. As illustrated in Figure 3.3, the pitch structure follows Dan Roam's seven steps that enable the speaker to tell a good story (Roam, 2016). In the pitch presentation, the speaker creates tension between problems and solutions, uses credible evidence to make the case, and persuades the audience to take action.

Effective speakers also communicate organizational vision, motivate change, and inspire new ideas using the **dramatic presentation** style. Nancy Duarte's *Resonate* (2010) recommends structuring dramatic presentations using a story pattern commonly used in mythical traditions and fairy tales to create dramatic tension. In a simple story of any kind, the hero is called to action, goes on an adventure, encounters obstacles, but emerges transformed. When structuring a speech in this dramatic fashion, the audience is the metaphorical hero, and dramatic tension is created by describing the gap between how the audience currently operates and the changes that need to happen. In this structure, the speaker anticipates that the audience resist recommended change, so explains how sacrifice and hard work will lead the audience to success. Table 3.7 demonstrates the structure of a health services manager's change presentation compared to a traditional story (Duarte, 2010).

FIGURE 3.3 The pitch narrative structure.

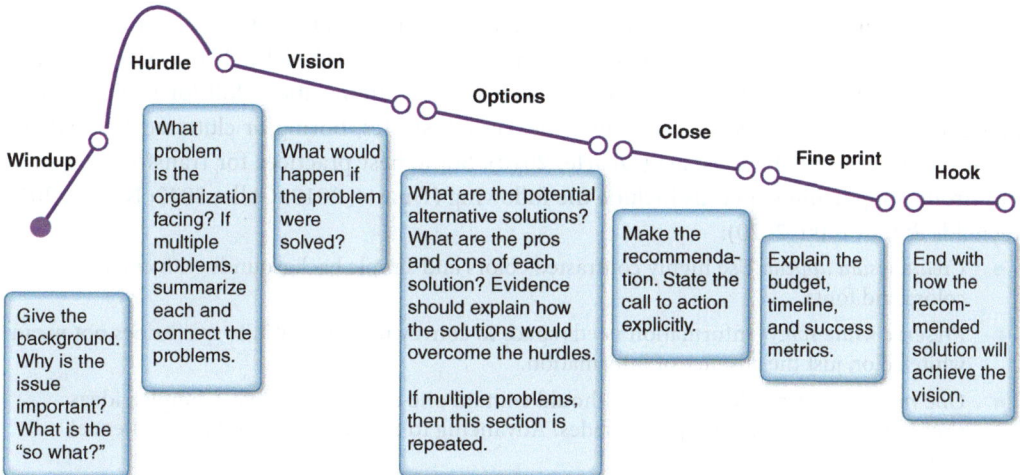

Source: Adapted from Roam, D. (2016). *Show and tell: How everybody can make extraordinary presentations*. New York: Porfolio/Penguin.

TABLE 3.7 Structure of a Change-Inspiring Presentation Compared to a Traditional Story

STORY	TRADITIONAL STORY	CHANGE INSPIRING PRESENTATION
Beginning	A long time ago, there was a young girl who did not know she was a princess. She loved her farm and her animals.	We aspire to become the leading provider of compassionate and innovative healthcare, transforming lives with safe, patient-centered, and evidence-based practices.
Call to action	One day, a mysterious old woman revealed that the farm girl was actually the long-lost heir to a kingdom in a distant land. The old woman urged the girl to embrace her destiny and embark on a journey to discover her true self.	We committed to creating a "zero-harm" culture. We hoped to create an open and nonpunitive environment where employees felt comfortable reporting patient safety errors.
Complication	Overwhelmed, the girl initially refused to leave her life behind, but her farm was destroyed by the same evil that was also threatening the kingdom.	Unfortunately, we have not yet achieved the goal. We still cause preventable adverse events when caring for our patients.
Proposed resolution	The girl agreed to journey to the kingdom and embrace her royal lineage, the powers she possessed, and the responsibilities that came with them.	New AI tools can transform our EHR systems to identify potential errors so that we can prevent patient harm.
Conflict	The girl and the old woman left the farm to journey to the kingdom and faced various obstacles, including dragons and giants.	AI tools are embedded in our EHR systems but are not used by clinicians.
End	With each challenge, the girl grew stronger. With new strengths, the girl confronted the evil forces, ensuring the kingdom's lasting peace.	If we change how clinicians use the EHR, it will reduce errors and save lives.

AI, artificial intelligence; EHR, electronic health record.

Presentation Materials

Competent health services managers effectively use electronic audiovisual media and printed presentation packets appropriate for the audience and occasion (NCHL, 2018). Mastering presentation software, such as PowerPoint, is a necessary communication skill for health services managers. While strong visuals can help a speaker tell stories, boring or cluttered PowerPoints can also detract from the message (Duarte, 2010). Some best practices for transforming slides into strong supporting materials include the following (Duarte, 2010; Gallo, 2022; Naegle, 2021; Reynolds & Kawasaki, 2020):

- *Create visual appeal:* Use highly contrasted colors and simple backgrounds with consistent colors and fonts.
- *Preserve white space:* Information needs space to convey meaning. White space does not mean white color, just the absence of information.
- *One main idea per slide:* Each slide should contain one central objective. Complex ideas should be conveyed with separate slides. Advancing to a new slide helps keep audiences engaged.
- *Less is more:* If information cannot be deciphered in 3 seconds, then the slide is too busy and confusing. Practice visual restraint.
- *Limit text:* If text is required, use large fonts only (28 points and above). Limit word count to 10 words per slide maximum.
- *Short bullets statements, not sentences*: Minimize text, as audience cannot listen and read at the same time. Effective speakers never read from slides.

WRITTEN COMMUNICATIONS

Business Writing Style

Effective health services managers use a variety of written communication skills and styles, depending on the circumstances. In general, health services managers write in a clear and concise business style (NCHL, 2018). The book, *Smart Brevity: The Power of Saying More with Less*, explains the value of strong business writing (VandeHei et al., 2022). People are overwhelmed with information, the authors argue, so business writing must accommodate how people read. This requires that health services managers write to make the main points obvious to the reader. If people have to expend too much energy to understand writing, then they will simply avoid reading it.

Business Reports

Even detailed business reports can be written in a readable style. A **business report** is a formal document written to provide stakeholders with information. Health services managers write many types of business reports, including proposals, project charters, consulting reports, analytical reports, progress reports, policies and procedures, and more. The ability to clarify business objectives, explain logic of a persuasive argument, or simplify technical matters are all necessary skills of managers. Health services managers incorporate the following elements of business writing to create effective reports (Canavor, 2022; Garner, 2013; McInerney, 2023; Selingo, 2017):

- *Write to accomplish objectives:* Every business report should be written to accomplish something. Identify that goal and write to achieve it.
- *Use attention-grabbing title:* Understandable titles attract readers; complicated, pretentious titles repel them.

- *Avoid **fluff***: Unnecessary words, repetitive points, or extraneous words are considered fluff.
- *Eliminate **jargon***: Highly technical language is confusing and annoying to readers.
- *Write literally*: Avoid clichés, idioms, and overused metaphors.
- *Use graphics*: Tables, charts, and figures break up blocks of text. Simple visuals supplement writing with context, comparisons, and trends.
- *Minimize **passive voice***: Passive voice usually includes a version of the verb "to be" plus a past tense verb (i.e., He was promoted). Instead, active voice employs strong verbs with the subject-verb-object construction. For example, managers (subject) write (verb) strong sentences (object).
- *Edit, edit, edit*: Strong writing requires repeated rounds of planning, drafting, revising, editing, and feedback. Complete a draft, print it out, wait a day, then revise.

Extensive business reports often include an executive summary after the title page and before the table of contents. An **executive summary** provides an overview of the report to readers who do not have the time to read the full report details. Instead of blocks of text, the summary should incorporate bullets, headings, or other visual elements to break up the page and make the writing easier to read. Following the *Smart Brevity* approach, the executive summary invites the executive to access more details within the report, if desired. Table 3.8 lists key elements of an executive summary (VandeHei et al., 2022). To keep the executive summary no longer than two pages, each element should be limited to a few sentences each.

TABLE 3.8 Key Elements of a Business Report Executive Summary

ELEMENT	DESCRIPTION	QUESTION TO ANSWER
Goal or vision	With a strong opening sentence, directly and succinctly explain what the report intends to accomplish.	What is the goal of the report? Why does the report matter?
Problem or need	Describe the problem or need that the report aims to address. Provide context that explains why the problem must be solved.	Why is the problem important to the organization?
Analytical approach	Brief summary of the analysis, investigation, or other approach.	How were the potential solutions evaluated? Why are the subsequent recommendations credible?
Recommended solution(s)	Outline the proposed solution(s). Use numbering or bullets to break up the text.	What recommended approaches or strategies will solve the problem?
Supporting evidence	Briefly summarize major findings that support solution or solutions	What are the key findings that logically support the recommendation?
Conclusion	Wrap up the summary	How will the goal be accomplished by implementing the recommended solution(s)? How will it benefit the organization or project?

Emails and Collaboration Tools

Computer scientist Cal Newport (2021) argued in his book, *A World Without Email: Reimagining Work in an Age of Communication Overload*, that email makes people miserable. Workers exchange too many poorly written emails that are then amplified, misunderstood, or ignored. Health services managers have a responsibility for writing better emails that reduce stress and improve productivity (Stich, 2023). The overall goal of a successfully written emails is to structure the content so that it is easy for the reader to understand. Tips for better email communication that improve timely replies and/or action include the following (Harmon, 2017; McNitt, 2021; Stein, 2022; Stich, 2023):

- *Tailor the subject line:* A succinct but meaningful subject line gains attention.
- *Always BLUF:* Bottom Line Up Front (BLUF) is a military communication method in which the main point comes first, then the context is provided later in the message.
- *Call to action:* Be specific about how people need to act. Use phases such as "Decision:" or "Action Required:" depending on the message.
- *Always state the deadline:* Include due dates for tasks or requests.
- *Use short paragraphs:* No one reads email paragraphs of more than two to three sentences.
- *Break up text with visual elements:* Use bullet points, bold text, highlights, and italics to bring attention to important points, tasks, or requests.
- *Limit one topic per email thread:* A different topic addressed later in a message thread will get lost.

Many of these recommendations apply to other electronic collaboration tools, such as calendar invites, instant messaging, corporate messaging systems, SMS text messaging, and social media posts. Spending time to communicate clearly is more efficient than fixing any miscommunications that occur from sloppy written communications.

FUTURE DIRECTIONS

Hybrid work arrangements, which entail a combination of office-based and work-from-home workdays, are common in many health services management jobs, especially in middle and executive positions (Barrero et al., 2023). Therefore, videoconferencing applications, such as Microsoft Teams, WebEx, or Zoom, are likely to become the preferred modes for business meetings. While virtual meeting platforms can offer conveniences, they can also bring major distractions which can leave people feeling mentally and physically exhausted, the so-called "Zoom fatigue" effect (Nesher Shoshan & Wehrt, 2022). In addition to instituting meeting management best practices, such as distributing agendas, health services managers can improve the productivity and perceptions of virtual meetings by following these pieces of advice (Karl et al., 2022; Reed & Allen, 2021):

- Insist that people turn on their cameras in small meetings.
- Invest in good microphones that improve sound quality.
- Mute microphones when not speaking to reduce echo and interruptions.
- Choose a good camera angle that frames only the head and upper torso.
- Select good lighting, preferably natural light, but ring lights also work.
- Make eye contact with the camera when speaking.
- Mute the microphone when eating.
- Discourage multitasking by holding short and effective virtual meetings.

Using these communication skills will enhance health services managers' professional reputations and improve meeting effectiveness in the increasingly virtual workplace.

SUMMARY

- Interpersonal communication entails the fundamental set of skills that managers use to inform, persuade, and motivate people. Health services managers communicate using various methods, depending on the needs of the situation.
- Effective managers spend significant effort helping people feel safe to speak up without fear of negative consequences in order to elicit candid feedback and learn from mistakes.
- Health services managers work with clinicians and others to resolve unhealthy conflict. Conflict resolution can be reached through forms of alternative dispute resolution, such as mediation or arbitration.
- Health services managers build positive professional reputations by acting with executive presence, managing their professional brand, and networking with other healthcare professionals.
- Planning, participating, coordinating, and facilitating meetings are essential competencies for health services management career success.
- Effective public speaking builds professional credibility and shared understanding. Health services managers deliver speeches to persuade and inspire employees to accomplish HCO goals.
- Health services managers communicate through a variety of written formats, including business reports and emails. Business writing is characterized by a succinct, clear, direct, and readable style.

END-OF-CHAPTER RESOURCES

KEY TERMS*

*For the full list of key terms, please see the online glossary at **http://connect.springerpub.com/content/book/978-0-8261-4807-0.**

active listening
agenda
agenda items
alternative dispute resolution
anchor price
appearance
approachability
arbitration
Best Alternative To a Negotiated Agreement (BATNA)
Bottom Line Up Front (BLUF)
belonging
burnout
business report
communication adaptability
Confidence
conflict management
contracting
debrief meeting
dramatic presentation
executive presence
executive summary
explanation
facilitator
fluff
gravitas
huddle
inclusiveness
interpersonal communication
interpersonal conflict
jargon
management rounds
mediation
meeting load
meeting purpose
meeting topic
negotiation
networking
offsite meeting
one-on-one meeting
parking lot
passive voice
personal branding
pitch
psychological safety
relationship conflict
reservation price
status meeting
storytelling
task conflict
town hall meeting
visibility
Zone Of Possible Agreement (ZOPA)

LEARNING ACTIVITIES

Professional Development and Reflection

1. Reflect on each of the elements of executive presence outlined in the chapter. In what ways are these elements of executive presence considered crucial for professional advancement?
2. Reflect on your experiences with public speaking. How has stage fright or anxiety associated with public speaking shaped your approach to developing effective communication skills? What strategies from the chapter do you find most helpful in overcoming apprehensions related to public speaking?

Discussion Questions

1. Authenticity refers to the quality of being genuine, real, and true to one's own identity, values, and beliefs. How do the concepts of executive presence, personal brand, and networking relate to authenticity? In what ways can these concepts conflict with authenticity? Should authenticity be the goal of executive presence, personal brand, and networking? Why or why not?
2. What strategies have been effective in making workplace meetings more productive and engaging? How can meeting-related communication skills be enhanced for better collaboration?
3. Examine the storytelling element that occurs when the hero faces resistance in their journey toward change. What are some examples of this in HCOs? How can health services managers address an audience's potential resistance to change in their presentations?

RECOMMENDED READING AND MEDIA

Allen, J. A., & Reed, K. M. (2022). *Running effective meetings for dummies*. John Wiley & Sons, Inc.

Baedke, L., & Lamberton, N. (2018). *The emerging healthcare leader: A field guide* (2nd ed.). Health Administration Press.

Burnison, G. (2018). *Lose the resume: Land the job*. John Wiley & Sons, Inc.

Carnegie, D. (1936). *How to win friends and influence people*. Simon & Schuster.

Covey, S. R. (2013). *The 7 habits of highly effective people: Powerful lessons in personal change* (25th anniversary ed.). Simon & Schuster.

Dawson, R. (2021). *Secrets of power salary negotiating: Inside secrets from a master negotiator* (25th anniversary ed.). Career Press.

Fisher, R., Ury, W., & Patton, B. (2011). *Getting to yes: Negotiating agreement without giving in*. Penguin Books.

Grenny, J., Patterson, K., McMillan, R., Switzler, A., & Gregory, E. (2022). *Crucial conversations: Tools for talking when stakes are high*. McGraw Hill.

Hewlett S. A. (2014). *Executive presence: The missing link between merit and success*. Harper Business.

Liu, C. (2020, October 9). How to speak up in meetings. *Harvard Business Review*. https://hbr.org/video/6199861287001/how-to-speak-up-in-meetings

VandeHei, J., Allen, M., & Schwartz, R. (2022). *Smart Brevity: The power of saying more with less*. Workman Publishing.

Zack, D. (2019). *Networking for people who hate networking: A field guide for introverts, the overwhelmed, and the underconnected* (2nd ed.). Berrett-Koehler Publishers.

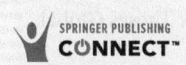 A robust set of instructor resources designed to supplement this text is located at http://connect.springerpub.com/content/book/978-0-8261-4807-0.
Qualifying instructors may request access by emailing textbook@springerpub.com.

REFERENCES

Adelman, K. (2012). Promoting employee voice and upward communication in healthcare: The CEO's influence. *Journal of Healthcare Management, 57*(2), 133–148. http://doi.org/10.1097/00115514-201203000-00009

Adler, R. B., & Proctor, R. F. (2023). *Interplay: The process of interpersonal communication* (16th ed.). Oxford University Press.

Allen, J. A., Beck, T., Scott, C. W., & Rogelberg, S. G. (2014). Understanding workplace meetings: A qualitative taxonomy of meeting purposes. *Management Research Review, 37*(9), 791–814. http://doi.org/10.1108/MRR-03-2013-0067

Allen, J. A., Lehmann-Willenbrock, N., & Rogelberg, S. G. (Eds.). (2015). *The Cambridge handbook of meeting science*. Cambridge University Press.

Allen, J. A., Sands, S. J., Mueller, S. L., Frear, K. A., Mudd, M., & Rogelberg, S. G. (2012). Employees' feelings about more meetings: An overt analysis and recommendations for improving meetings. *Management Research Review, 35*(5), 405–418. http://doi.org/10.1108/01409171211222331

Allen, J. A., Thiese, M. S., Eden, E., & Knowles, S. E. (2022). Why am I so exhausted?: Exploring Meeting-to-Work Transition Time and Recovery from Virtual Meeting Fatigue. *Journal of Occupational and Environmental Medicine, 64*(12), 1053–1058.

American College of Healthcare Executives. (2023). *ACHE Healthcare Executives 2023 Competencies Assessment Tool*. https://www.ache.org/-/media/ache/career-resource-center/cat_2023.pdf

Arushi, Dillon, R., Teoh, A. N., & Dillon, D. (2023, March). Detecting public speaking stress via real-time voice analysis in virtual reality: A review. In *Sustainability, economics, innovation, globalisation and organisational psychology conference* (pp. 117–152). Springer Nature.

Axtell, P. (2020). *Make meetings matter: How to turn meetings from status updates to remarkable conversations*. Simple Truths, an imprint of Sourcebooks.

Baedke, L., & Lamberton, N. (2018). *The emerging healthcare leader: A field guide*. Health Administration Press.

Bailey, K. D., Losty, L. S., Albert, D., Rodenhausen, N., & De Santis, J. P. (2022, November). Leadership presence: A concept analysis. *Nursing Forum, 57*(6), 1069–1079. https://doi.org/10.1111/nuf.12784

Bandura, A. (1977). *Social learning theory*. Prentice Hall.

Barnard, D. (2022, November 8). *Average speaking rate and words per minute*. Virtual Speech. https://virtualspeech.com/blog/average-speaking-rate-words-per-minute

Barrero, J. M., Bloom, N., & Davis, S. J. (2023). The evolution of work from home. *Journal of Economic Perspectives, 37*(4), 23–49. http://doi.org/10.1257/jep.37.4.23

Beck, S. J., Paskewitz, E. A., & Allen, J. A. (2024). Toward a strategic perspective of meeting participation. *Organizational Psychology Review*. http://doi.org/10.1177/20413866231226405

Beeson, J. (2012, August 22). Deconstructing executive presence. *Harvard Business Review*. https://hbr.org/2012/08/de-constructing-executive-pres

Begun, J. W., White, K. R., & Mosser, G. (2011). Interprofessional care teams: The role of the healthcare administrator. *Journal of Interprofessional Care, 25*(2), 119–123. https://doi.org/10.3109/13561820.2010.504135

Boulding, K. E. (1963). *Conflict and defense: A general theory*. Harper & Row.

Bradley, B. H., Anderson, H. J., Baur, J. E., & Klotz, A. C. (2015). When conflict helps: Integrating evidence for beneficial conflict in groups and teams under three perspectives. *Group Dynamics: Theory, Research, and Practice, 19*(4), 243.

Broeckelman-Post, M., & Ruiz-Mesa, K. (2018). *Measuring college learning in public speaking*. Social Science Research Council.

Brown, C. G. (2016). *Leader approachability: What is it, what is it good for, and who needs it?* (Publication No. 101466050) [Doctoral dissertation: The University of Tulsa]. ProQuest Dissertations & Theses Global.

Burnison, G. (2018). *Lose the resume: Land the job*. John Wiley & Sons, Inc.

Butler, A. S. (2014). *Mission critical meetings: 81 practical facilitation techniques*. Wheatmark.

Canavor, N. C. (2022). *Business writing today: A practical guide*. (4th ed.). SAGE Publications.

Cenedella, M. (2010, August 19). How not to embarrass yourself doing the elevator pitch. *The ladders*. https://www.theladders.com/career-newsletters/how-not-to-embarrass-yourself-doing-elevator-pitch

Clarke, J. S., Cornelissen, J. P., & Healey, M. P. (2019). Actions speak louder than words: How figurative language and gesturing in entrepreneurial pitches influences investment judgments. *Academy of Management Journal, 62*(2), 335–360. http://doi.org/10.5465/amj.2016.1008

Covey, S. R. (2013). *The 7 habits of highly effective people: Powerful lessons in personal change*. (25th anniversary ed.). Simon & Schuster.

Cox, G. (2022). *Leading inclusion: Drive change your employees can see and feel*. Page Two.

Crittenden, J. K. (2018). *Executive Presence Questionnaire*. The Discreet Guide. https://www.discreetguide.com/wp1/wp-content/uploads/EPQuestionnaireDG.pdf

Curry, N., & Smith, J. (2017). Purchasing healthcare. In K. Walshe & J. Smith (Eds.), *Healthcare management* (2nd ed.). McGraw-Hill Open University Press.

Davis, J., Wolff, H. G., Forret, M. L., & Sullivan, S. E. (2020). Networking via LinkedIn: An examination of usage and career benefits. *Journal of Vocational Behavior, 118*, 103396. https://doi.org/10.1016/j.jvb.2020.103396

Dawson, R. (2021). *Secrets of power negotiating: Inside secrets from a master negotiator* (25th anniversary ed.). Career Press.

Drucker, P. F. (1954). *The practice of management*. Harper & Row, Publishers, Inc.

Drucker, P. F., & Maciariello, J. A. (2008). Management (rev. ed.). New York: HarperCollins.

Duran, R. L. (1992). Communicative adaptability: A review of conceptualization and measurement. *Communication Quarterly, 40*(3), 253–268. https://doi.org/10.1080/01463379209369840

Dwyer, K. K., & Davidson, M. M. (2012). Is public speaking really more feared than death? *Communication Research Reports, 29*(2), 99–107. https://doi.org/10.1080/08824096.2012.667772

Edinger, S. (2020, October 15). *An ancient formula for executive presence that works today*. Forbes. https://www.forbes.com/sites/scottedinger/2020/10/15/an-ancient-formula-for-executive-presence-that-works-today

Edmondson, A. C. (1999). Psychological safety and learning behavior in work teams. *Administrative Science Quarterly, 44*(2), 350–383. https://doi.org/10.2307/2666999

Fehr, R., Zheng, X., Guo, Y., Song, L., & Ni, D. (2020). Thanks for everything: A quasi-experimental examination of gratitude in organizations. In *Academy of Management Proceedings* (Vol. 2020, No. 1, p. 18312). Academy of Management.

Fernandez, J., Landis, K., & Lee, J. (2023, January 18). Helping Gen Z Employees Find Their Place at Work. *Harvard Business Review*. https://hbr.org/2023/01/helping-gen-z-employees-find-their-place-at-work

Fisher, R., Ury, W., & Patton, B. (2011). *Getting to yes: Negotiating agreement without giving in*. Penguin Books.

Flinchum, J. R., Kreamer, L. M., Rogelberg, S. G., & Gooty, J. (2023). One-on-one meetings between managers and direct reports: A new opportunity for meeting science. *Organizational Psychology Review, 13*(4), 478–505. https://doi.org/10.1177/20413866221097570

Fottler, M. D., Malvey, D., Hyde, J. C., & Deschamp, C. (2015). Human resources management. In *Handbook of Healthcare Management* (pp. 127–152). Edward Elgar Publishing.

Gallo, A. (2018, January 3). Why we should be disagreeing at work. *Harvard Business Review*. https://hbr.org/2018/01/why-we-should-be-disagreeing-more-at-work

Gallo, C. (2018, May 28). 5 ways to project confidence in front of an audience. *Harvard Business Review*. https://hbr.org/2018/05/5-ways-to-project-confidence-in-front-of-an-audience

Gallo, C. (2022, April 27). What the best presenters do differently. *Harvard Business Review*. https://hbr.org/2022/04/what-the-best-presenters-do-differently

Garman, A. N., Leach, D. C., & Spector, N. (2006). Worldviews in collision: Conflict and collaboration across professional lines. *Journal of Organizational Behavior: The International Journal of Industrial, Occupational and Organizational Psychology and Behavior. 27*(7), 829-849.

Garner, B. A. (2013). *HBR guide to better business writing: Engage readers, tighten and brighten, make your case.* Harvard Business Review Press.

Golden, T. D., & Eddleston, K. A. (2020). Is there a price telecommuters pay? Examining the relationship between telecommuting and objective career success. *Journal of Vocational Behavior, 116,* 103348.

Gorbatov, S., Khapova, S. N., & Lysova, E. I. (2018). Personal branding: Interdisciplinary systematic review and research agenda. *Frontiers in Psychology, 9,* 2238.

Gorbatov, S., Khapova, S. N., Oostrom, J. K., & Lysova, E. I. (2021). Personal brand equity: Scale development and validation. *Personnel Psychology, 74*(3), 505–542. https://doi.org/10.1111/peps.12412

Gorbatov, S., Oostrom, J. K., & Khapova, S. N. (2023). Work does not speak for itself: Examining the incremental validity of personal branding in predicting knowledge workers' employability. *European Journal of Work and Organizational Psychology, 33*(1), 1–14. https://doi.org/10.1080/1359432X.2023.2276533

Harmon, S. (2017, February 6). How to make sure your emails give the right impression. *Harvard Business Review.* https://hbr.org/2017/02/how-to-make-sure-your-emails-give-the-right-impression

Hewlett, S. A. (2014). *Executive presence: The missing link between merit and success.* Harper Business.

Hewlett, S. A. (2024, January–February). The new rules of executive presence. *Harvard Business Review.* https://hbr.org/2024/01/the-new-rules-of-executive-presence.

Hullman, G. A., Planisek, A., McNally, J. S., & Rubin, R. B. (2010). Competence, personality, and self-efficacy: Relationships in an undergraduate interpersonal course. *Atlantic Journal of Communication, 18*(1), 36–49. http://doi.org/10.1080/15456870903340506

Jehn, K. A. (1995). A multimethod examination of the benefits and detriments of intragroup conflict. *Administrative Science Quarterly, 40,* 256–282. http://doi.org/10.2307/2393638

Jiang, H., & Luo, Y. (2018). Crafting employee trust: From authenticity, transparency to engagement. *Journal of Communication Management, 22*(2), 138–160. http://doi.org/10.1108/JCOM-07-2016-0055

Kaissi, A. (2005). Manager-physician relationships: An organizational theory perspective. *The Health Care Manager, 24*(2), 165–176. https://doi.org/10.1097/00126450-200504000-00010

Kanter, R. M. (2009, July 23). The downsides of branding. *Harvard Business Review.* https://hbr.org/2009/07/the-downsides-of-branding

Karl, K. A., Peluchette, J. V., & Aghakhani, N. (2022). Virtual work meetings during the COVID-19 pandemic: The good, bad, and ugly. *Small Group Research, 53*(3), 343–365. https://doi.org/10.1177/%2F10464964211015286

Keller, E. J., Giafaglione, B., Chrisman, H. B., Collins, J. D., & Vogelzang, R. L. (2019). The growing pains of physician-administration relationships in an academic medical center and the effects on physician engagement. *PLoS One, 14*(2), e0212014. https://doi.org/10.1371/journal.pone.0212014

Kello, J. E., & Allen, J. A. (2020, March). The staff meeting . . . and beyond. . . . In *Managing meetings in organizations* (Vol. 20, pp. 27–43). Emerald Publishing Limited.

Knight, R. (2014, October 10). How to get your employees to speak up. *Harvard Business Review.* https://hbr.org/2014/10/how-to-get-your-employees-to-speak-up

Kundi, Y. M., Soomro, S. A., & Kamran, M. (2022). Does social support at work enhance subjective career success? The mediating role of relational attachment. *International Journal of Organizational Analysis, 30*(6), 1491–1507. http://doi.org/10.1108/IJOA-08-2020-2379

Kurnoff, J., & Lazarus, L. (2021, May 13). The key to landing your next job? Storytelling. *Harvard Business Review.* https://hbr.org/2021/05/the-key-to-landing-your-next-job-storytelling

Laker, B., & Pereira, V. (2022, May 31). 4 triggers cause the majority of team conflicts. *Harvard Business Review.* https://hbr.org/2022/05/conflict-is-not-always-bad-but-you-should-know-how-to-manage-it

Landrum, R. E., Brakke, K., & McCarthy, M. A. (2019). The pedagogical power of storytelling. *Scholarship of Teaching and Learning in Psychology, 5*(3), 247. http://doi.org/10.1037/stl0000152

Lawrence, S. G. (2015). Waking up audiences: Lessons in rhetorical devices. *Communication Teacher, 29*(4), 212–218. http://doi.org/10.1080/17404622.2015.1058965

Lencioni, P. (2002). *The five dysfunctions of a team: A leadership fable.* Jossey Bass.

Lencioni, P. (2004). *Death by meeting: A leadership fable about solving the most painful problem in business.* Jossey-Bass.

Leroy, H., Dierynck, B., Anseel, F., Simons, T., Halbesleben, J. R. B., & McCaughey, D. (2012). Behavioral integrity for safety, priority of safety, psychological safety, and patient safety: A team-level study. *Journal of Applied Psychology, 97*, 1273–1281. https://doi.org/10.1037/a0030076

Lewicki, R. J., Saunders, D. M., Minton, J. W., Roy, J., & Lewicki, N. (2011). *Essentials of negotiation.* McGraw-Hill.

Maaravi, Y., & Levy, A. (2017). When your anchor sinks your boat: Information asymmetry in distributive negotiations and the disadvantage of making the first offer. *Judgment and Decision Making, 12*(5), 420–429. https://doi.org/10.1017/S193029750000646X

McInerney, E. (2023, October 23). *Tips to eliminate fluff in your writing.* Eleven Writing. https://www.elevenwriting.com/blog/fluff-writing

McNett, G. (2016). Using stories to facilitate learning. *College Teaching, 64*(4), 184–193. http://doi.org/10.1080/87567555.2016.1189389

McNitt, A. (2021, January–February). Leadership and military writing. *Military Review,* 122–128. https://www.armyupress.army.mil/Portals/7/military-review/Archives/English/JF-21/McNitt-Military-Writing.pdf

Mikkelson, A. C., & Hesse, C. (2023). Conceptualizing and validating organizational communication patterns and their associations with employee outcomes. *International Journal of Business Communication, 60*(1), 287–312. http://doi.org/10.1177/2329488420932299

Mikkelson, A. C., Sloan, D., & Tietsort, C. J. (2021). Employee perceptions of supervisor communication competence and associations with supervisor credibility. *Communication Studies, 72*(4), 600–617. http://doi.org/10.1080/10510974.2021.1953093

Moisoglou, I., Panagiotis, P., Galanis, P., Siskou, O., Maniadakis, N., & Kaitelidou, D. (2014). Conflict management in a Greek public hospital: Collaboration or avoidance. *International Journal of Caring Sciences, 7*(1), 75–82.

Morreale, S. P., Spitzberg, B. H., & Barge, J. K. (2013). *Communication: Motivation, knowledge, skills.* Peter Lang Inc.

Mroz, J. E., Allen, J. A., Verhoeven, D. C., & Shuffler, M. L. (2018). Do we really need another meeting? The science of workplace meetings. *Current Directions in Psychological Science, 27*(6), 484–491. http://doi.org/10.1177/0963721418776307

Naegle, K. M. (2021). Ten simple rules for effective presentation slides. *PLoS Computational Biology, 17*(12), e1009554. https://doi.org/10.1371%2Fjournal.pcbi.1009554

National Center for Healthcare Leadership. (2018). *Healthcare leadership competency model 3.0.* https://nchl.member365.org/publicFr/store/item/19

Nembhard, I. M., & Edmondson, A. C. (2006). Making it safe: The effects of leader inclusiveness and professional status on psychological safety and improvement efforts in health care teams. *Journal of Organizational Behavior: The International Journal of Industrial, Occupational and Organizational Psychology and Behavior, 27*(7), 941–966. http://doi.org/10.1002/job.413

Nesher Shoshan, H., & Wehrt, W. (2022). Understanding "Zoom fatigue": A mixed-method approach. *Applied Psychology, 71*(3), 827–852. https://doi.org/10.1111/apps.12360

Newman, A., Donohue, R., & Eva, N. (2017). Psychological safety: A systematic review of the literature. *Human Resource Management Review, 27*(3), 521–535. http://doi.org/10.1016/j.hrmr.2017.01.001

Newport, C. (2021). *A world without email: Reimagining work in an age of communication overload.* Portfolio

Nikita, & Lordan, G. (2023, February 2). 7 small ways to be a more inclusive colleague. *Harvard Business Review.* https://hbr.org/2023/02/7-small-ways-to-be-a-more-inclusive-colleague

Obama, B. (2009, September 9). Obama's health care speech to Congress. *The New York Times.* https://www.nytimes.com/2009/09/10/us/politics/10obama.text.html

O'Donovan, R., & McAuliffe, E. (2020). A systematic review of factors that enable psychological safety in healthcare teams. *International Journal for Quality in Health Care, 32*(4), 240–250. https://doi.org/10.1093/intqhc/mzaa025

Ortiz, L. A., Region-Sebest, M., & MacDermott, C. (2016). Employer perceptions of oral communication competencies most valued in new hires as a factor in company success. *Business and Professional Communication Quarterly, 79*(3), 317–330. http://doi.org/10.1177/2329490615624108

Oxenstierna, G., Hanson, L. L. M., Widmark, M., Finnholm, K., Stenfors, C., Elofsson, S., & Theorell, T. (2011). Conflicts at work—The relationship with workplace factors, work characteristics and self-rated health. *Industrial Health, 49*(4), 501–510. https://doi.org/10.2486/indhealth.ms1171

Parmentier, M. A., Fischer, E., & Reuber, A. R. (2013). Positioning person brands in established organizational fields. *Journal of the Academy of Marketing Science, 41*, 373–387. http://doi.org/10.1007/s11747-012-0309-2

Pruitt, D. G. (1981). *Negotiation behavior*. Academic Press.

Porter, C. M., Woo, S. E., Alonso, N., & Snyder, G. (2023). Why do people network? Professional networking motives and their implications for networking behaviors and career success. *Journal of Vocational Behavior, 142*(2), 103856. http://doi.org/10.1016/j.jvb.2023.103856

Porter, J., & Baker, E. L. (2006). Meetings, meetings, and more meetings. *Journal of Public Health Management and Practice, 12*(1), 103–106. https://doi.org/10.1097/00124784-200601000-00017

Porter, J. A., Haberling, K., & Hohman, C. (2016). Employer desired competencies for undergraduate health administration graduates entering the job market. *Journal of Health Administration Education, 33*(3), 355–375.

Potthoff, S. J., Mishek, J. H., & Hart, G. W. (2020). *Applied problem-soling in healthcare management*. Springer Publishing, Inc.

Raja, F. (2017). Anxiety level in students of public speaking: Causes and remedies. *Journal of Education and Educational Development, 4*(1), 94–110. http://doi.org/10.22555/joeed.v4i1.1001

Ravishankar, R. A. (2023, March 22). A beginner's guide to networking. *Harvard Business Review*. https://hbr.org/2023/03/a-beginners-guide-to-networking.

Reed, K. M., & Allen, J. A. (2021). *Suddenly virtual: Making remote meetings work*. Wiley.

Reynolds, G., & Kawasaki, G. (2020). *Presentation Zen 3: Simple ideas on presentation design and delivery*. (3rd ed.). New Riders.

Roam, D. (2016). *Show & tell: How everybody can make extraordinary presentations*. Portfolio/Penguin.

Rogelberg, S. G. (2020, February 26). How to create the perfect meeting agenda. *Harvard Business Review*. https://hbr.org/2020/02/how-to-create-the-perfect-meeting-agenda

Rogelberg, S. G., Scott, C., & Kello, J. (2007). The science and fiction of meetings. *MIT Sloan Management Review, 48*(2), 18–21.

Romney, A. C., Allen, J. A., & Heydarifard, Z. (2023). Meeting load paradox: Balancing the benefits and burdens of work meetings. *Business Horizons*. https://doi.org/10.1016/j.bushor.2023.10.002

Roussin, C. J. (2008). Increasing trust, psychological safety, and team performance through dyadic leadership discovery. *Small Group Research, 39*(2), 224–248. https://doi.org/10.1177/1046496408315988

Rudolph, J. W., Simon, R., Dufresne, R. L., & Raemer, D. B. (2006). There's no such thing as "nonjudgmental" debriefing: A theory and method for debriefing with good judgment. *Simulation in Healthcare, 1*(1), 49–55. https://doi.org/10.1097/01266021-200600110-00006

Schank, R. C., & Abelson, R. P. (1995). Knowledge and memory: The real story. In R. S. Wyer Jr. (Ed.), *Knowledge and memory: The real story—Advances in social cognition* (Vol. VIII, pp.1–86). Erlbaum.

Schimmel, N. (2016). Barack Obama's September 9, 2009 Healthcare Speech to Congress. In *Presidential Healthcare Reform Rhetoric: Continuity, Change & Contested Values from Truman to Obama* (pp. 217–253). http://doi.org/10.1007/978-3-319-32960-4_7

Schreiber, L. M., Paul, G. D., & Shibley, L. R. (2012). The development and test of the public speaking competence rubric. *Communication Education, 61*(3), 205–233. https://doi.org/10.1080/03634523.2012.670709

Selingo, J. J. (2017, August 11). *Why can't college graduates write coherent prose?*. Washington Post. https://www.washingtonpost.com/news/grade-point/wp/2017/08/11/why-cant-college-graduates-write

Seppälä, E., & McNichols, N. K. (2022, June 21). The power of healthy relationships at work. *Harvard Business Review.* https://hbr.org/2022/06/the-power-of-healthy-relationships-at-work

Shanafelt, T. D., & Noseworthy, J. H. (2017, January). Executive leadership and physician well-being: Nine organizational strategies to promote engagement and reduce burnout. In *Mayo Clinic Proceedings* (Vol. 92, No. 1, pp. 129–146). Elsevier.

Sharma, A. (2021). Role of ADR in the healthcare sector on resolving medical malpractice disputes. *International Journal of Law Management & Humanities, 4*(6), 1019–1028. https://doi.org/10.10000/IJLMH.112351

Shonk, K. (2023, December 14). *3 Types of conflict and how to address them.* Harvard Law School Program on Negotiation. https://www.pon.harvard.edu/daily/conflict-resolution/types-conflict

Sonnentag, S. (2001). High performance and meeting participation: An observational study in software design teams. *Group dynamics: Theory, Research, and Practice, 5*(1), 3–18. https://doi.org/10.1037/1089-2699.5.1.3

Spitzberg, B. H. (2013). (Re) Introducing communication competence to the health professions. *Journal of Public Health Research, 2*(3), e23. https://doi.org/10.4081%2Fjphr.2013.e23

Stein, S. (2022, August 10). 5 tips for writing professional emails. *Harvard Business Review.* https://hbr.org/2022/08/5-tips-for-writing-professional-emails

Stich, J. F. (2023). Towards a sustainable and supportive email culture. *Psychology of sustainability and sustainable development in organizations* (pp. 159–171). Routledge

Swensen, S., Kabcenell, A., & Shanafelt, T. (2016). Physician-organization collaboration reduces physician burnout and promotes engagement: The Mayo Clinic experience. *Journal of Healthcare Management, 61*(2), 105–127.

Tacconelli, S., DeLellis, N., Ankomah, S., Nowak, A., & Zikos, D. (2020). Health administration graduates: Responsibilities expected by Michigan employers. *Journal of Health Administration Education, 37*(1), 335–348.

The Joint Commission. (2021, June 18). *Sentinel Event Alert, Issue 40.* https://www.jointcommission.org/-/media/tjc/documents/resources/patient-safety-topics/sentinel-event/sea_40.pdf

VandeHei, J., Allen, M., & Schwartz, R. (2022). *Smart Brevity: The power of saying more with less.* Workman Publishing.

Weingart, L., Behfar, K., Bendersky, C., Todorova, G., & Jehn, K. (2014). The directness and oppositional intensity of conflict expression. *Academy of Management Review, 40*(2), 235–262. http://doi.org/10.5465/amr.2013.0124

Weiss, M., Kolbe, M., Grote, G., Spahn, D. R., & Grande, B. (2018). We can do it! Inclusive leader language promotes voice behavior in multi-professional teams. *The Leadership Quarterly, 29*(3), 389–402.

Wezowski, K. (2017, April 06). 6 ways to look more confident during a presentation. *Harvard Business Review.* https://hbr.org/2017/04/6-ways-to-look-more-confident-during-a-presentation

World Health Organization. (2019). *Burn-out an "occupational phenomenon": International Classification of Diseases.* https://www.who.int/news/item/28-05-2019-burn-out-an-occupational-phenomenon-international-classification-of-diseases

Yuan, J., Liberman, M., & Cieri, C. (2006). Towards an integrated understanding of speaking rate in conversation. In *Ninth International Conference on Spoken Language Processing.*

Zandan, N. (2018, August 1). How to stop saying "um," "ah," and "you know." *Harvard Business Review.* https://hbr.org/2018/08/how-to-stop-saying-um-ah-and-you-know

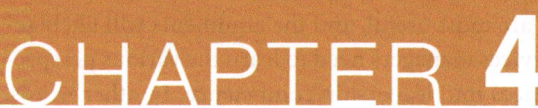
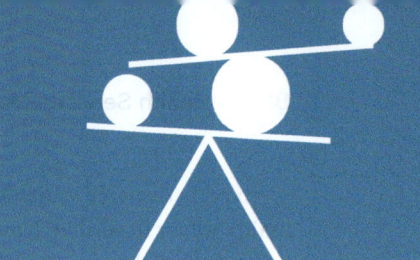

CHAPTER 4

LEADERSHIP AND CHANGE MANAGEMENT

Leadership involves envisioning the future and influencing people to act in order to create organizational change. Change management is the planned process of initiating, implementing, and maintaining organizational change.

COMPETENCIES

- Construct and communicate a shared vision.
- Role model behaviors beneficial to building a strong organizational culture.
- Assemble effective teams and engage in shared leadership practices.
- Motivate individuals and teams to achieve goals.
- Employ appropriate leadership style depending on organizational circumstances.
- Develop emotional and social intelligence.
- Acquire and utilize power to influence others or gain commitment for resources.
- Promote and manage processes that create organizational change and innovation.
- Develop leaders using organizational resources, such as training and leadership development programs.

CHAPTER OUTLINE

- Vision Setting
- Leadership and Organizational Culture
- Emotional and Social Intelligence
- Power and Influence
- Change Management

INTRODUCTION

Leadership entails envisioning the future and influencing followers' actions in order to create organizational change. Leadership is conceptually simple but exceedingly difficult in practice. To understand what makes an effective leader and how to develop people into leaders, popular leadership gurus and relatively obscure scholars have proposed dozens of leadership theories, competency models, and styles, some of which are supported by strong evidence and some not. Some leadership texts focus on more aspirational behaviors, such as integrity, authenticity, and kindness. Others advance personal development of emotional and social intelligence as key to becoming an effective leader. Some authors, contrary to prominent leadership theories, insist that leadership effectiveness actually derives from power and political skill.

Experts disagree which leadership concepts are most useful, and the arguments will likely remain forever unsettled. Nevertheless, health services managers need to learn the various perspectives, so that they can turn on-the-job experiences into leadership competence. In other words, leadership is learned through experimentation, failure, reflection, and growth, but the first step in leadership development is learning the essential concepts associated with effective leadership. This chapter reviews five fundamental competency domains necessary for effective leadership and successful health services management careers: (1) creating and communicating vision, (2) modeling behaviors to create and reinforce organizational culture, (3) demonstrating emotional and social intelligence, (4) utilizing power and influence, and (5) initiating and maintaining organizational change.

VISION SETTING

Management and Leadership

While managers often act as leaders, effective leadership requires a separate set of skills, knowledge, and attitudes from management. Managers seek to create order, whereas leaders seek to produce change (Northouse, 2021). Managers think analytically, methodically, rationally and logically and favor planning, organizing, and controlling. Leaders think creatively, strategically, and adaptively and prefer experimenting with new ways of working and convincing others to change (Cerni et al., 2014; Mumford et al., 2015). Managers are necessary for organizational effectiveness, but when the future is in doubt and change is needed, organizations need skilled leaders. Health care organizations (HCOs) value health services managers with both management and leadership skills (Begun & Thygeson, 2015). Fortunately, people can learn to become both managers and leaders.

> △ **KEY IDEA**
>
> Managers are necessary for organizational effectiveness, but when the future is in doubt and change is needed, organizations need skilled leaders.

Figure 4.1 contrasts leadership and management using Northouse's Functions of Management and Leadership.

FIGURE 4.1 Northouse's functions of management and leadership.

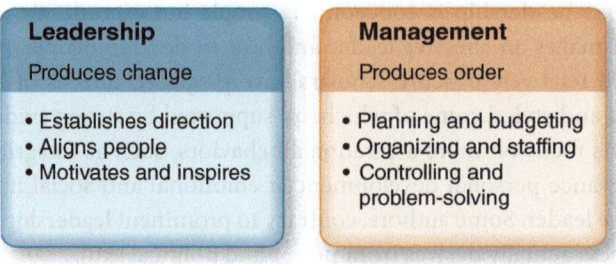

Source: Adapted from Northouse, P. G. (2021). *Leadership: Theory and practice* (9th ed.). Sage Publications, Inc.

Imagining the Future

Leadership is fundamentally about imagining the future for the organization (Bennis & Nanus, 1985). The strength of a leader's **vision** is determined by their capacity to imagine the future, describe this future to followers, and influence their organization to make that future happen (Lovelace et al., 2019). Vision setting is one of the most sought-after competencies for executive-level healthcare leaders because of the rate of change occurring in the healthcare sector (Dye & Garman, 2015). For example, health services financing is rapidly changing. After the Patient Protection and Affordable Care Act of 2010 (ACA), new value-based payment models began to reward HCOs for providing more value-conscious care (Young & Cosgrove, 2012). Dr. Toby Cosgrove, the former CEO of Cleveland Clinic, realized that for his organization to become competitive in the future, the health system needed to reorganize health services delivery to focus on medical care quality and positive patient experiences (Austin, 2023). Cosgrove envisioned a future with integrated medical specialties in patient-friendly, physically colocated institutes. Today, the trend toward value-based financing models seems unstoppable, and Cosgrove successfully reorganized Cleveland Clinic to succeed in value-based health care (Agba et al., 2022; Emanuel, 2023).

> **INFORMATIONAL INTERVIEW 4.1**
> *Director of Programming/Operations*
> Access the informational interview online at http://connect.springerpub.com/content/book/978-0-8261-4807-0/chapter/ch00.

Gaining Commitment to a Shared Vision

However, effective leadership is more than creating a compelling vision. Leaders must convince people that the vision is worth achieving (Kouzes & Posner, 2017). For a vision to be attractive to followers, the leader's vision must promise a solution to a relevant problem. In other words, an appealing vision addresses challenges, uncertainties, and dissatisfactions with how things are (Seyranian, 2014). A vision without a warranted justification for change will likely be ignored. In other words, leadership is a transparent, two-way discussion between leaders and followers that creates a clear vision for the future. Gaining commitment to a shared vision in HCOs requires leaders to deliver evidence-supported messaging (Chatfield et al., 2017).

> **△ KEY IDEA**
>
> Effective leadership is more than creating a compelling vision. Leaders must gain shared commitment throughout an organization to turn the vision into a reality.

To increase the likelihood of gaining commitment of followers, an effective leader explains how the vision is compatible with shared values. **Shared values** are commonly accepted principles, beliefs, or ideals that provide meaning to work (Chatfield et al., 2017). For health services managers to gain commitment from clinicians and other healthcare workers, the shared vision must be more than data, charts, and business-speak. People working in HCOs rally around visions that focus on helping patients, patients' families, and their communities. For example, if a healthcare leader wants to prevent an HCO from getting financial penalties from Medicare associated with inpatient readmissions, the vision cannot be to "avoid penalties by reducing readmissions by 10 per month." Instead, an effective vision is framed more meaningfully as "We will change the lives of 10 people and their families" (Chatfield et al., 2017).

Planning Future Action

Effective leaders connect shared vision to action and describe in practical terms how their vision will be realized (Seyranian, 2014). By connecting the envisioned future to what can be realistically implemented, leaders empower followers to use their own discretion to carry out the vision (Hickman, 1992). In this manner, effective leaders are also competent managers who can create mutual understanding and motivate people to transform the vision into reality, which underscores the notion that leadership and management are complementary skill sets.

CAREER BOX 4.1: Envisioning Career Success

A vision is a mental image of the future that inspires, energizes, and motivates. A career vision is a statement about what your career will become, your major accomplishments, and the impacts you will make on your world. The following are considerations for developing your career vision (LiveCareer, 2023):

- *Know your values:* A career vision statement puts your values into action. How do you define career success? What is important to you?
- *Paint a vivid picture:* Use visual language. What does your workspace look like? Is the space quiet or does your environment feature a lot of action? What do you wear?
- *Consider culture:* What kind of organizational culture are you a part of? How do you feel about the people you work with? Who do you talk with on a regular basis? How is conflict handled? What does the organization value?
- *Connect to emotions:* Feelings can be powerful motivators. How do you feel when you imagine yourself achieving your career vision? Excited? Satisfied? Fulfilled?
- *Tell a story:* Imagine your future and write a story that describes how you will make your career vision a reality. What obstacles did you overcome? What strengths did you rely on?
- *Find a role model:* Imagine yourself with a career similar to someone you respect. Whose career do you most respect and how can your vision emulate their career?
- *Think big:* Anything is possible in a career vision, so try not to filter out impractical ideas. What would you do if you had relatively unlimited money?

Once you set a vision, the next step is action. Take advantage of every opportunity to move you closer to your vision. With a strong career vision, it will be easier to overcome various obstacles on your way to success (Bielaszka-DuVernay, 2009).

LEADERSHIP AND ORGANIZATIONAL CULTURE

Role Modeling

Modern leadership theories recognize the ability to influence organizational culture as a core competency of leadership (Bass & Avolio, 1993; Xenikou, 2022). **Organizational culture** entails the learned values, assumptions, rules, attitudes, traditions, and expectations for behaviors in an organization (Northouse, 2021). Leaders influence organizational culture when they set strategic priorities, allocate resources, decide who to hire, reward certain behaviors, and punish actions that violate organizational norms (Bass & Riggio, 2006; Zhu et al., 2015). Shaping organizational culture, especially in large HCOs, takes significant time and effort. Through **role modeling**, health services managers can influence organizational culture. **Social learning theory** holds that new behaviors are learned through direct experience or by observing the behavior of role models (Bandura, 1971). How leaders behave—not necessarily what they say—offers cues for how followers should act.

△ KEY IDEA

How leaders behave—not necessarily what they say—offers cues for how followers should act.

Acting as a role model, a leader's behavior influences organizational culture—for better or worse. When behaviors are inconsistent with the HCO's stated values, it may signal a failure of leadership (Brinkley, 2013). On the other hand, when leaders model behaviors consistent with cultural values—even when the actions require sacrifice—people are more likely to follow. For example, when CEO Michael Fisher eliminated employee raises at Cincinnati Children's Hospital in the face of COVID-related financial pressures, he coupled the announcement with the fact that he and the senior management team were also taking significant pay cuts (Chopra & Keller, 2020).

Role modeling HCO culture is crucial for leaders because of healthcare's unique blend of highly trained professionals, life-and-death circumstances, and high-stress working environments (Kaplan, 2020). Subcultures of professions within the HCO—physicians, nurses, allied health professionals, and health services managers—commonly hold opposing views on what is best for the HCO, which can lead to disagreements (Garman et al., 2006). To reduce the negative impacts of conflict on HCO culture, health services managers can role model collaborative behaviors that contribute to positive organizational cultures, such as the following (Begun, White, & Mosser, 2011; Couris, 2022; Sullivan et al., 2016):

- Recognize professional limitations and consult with others who have relevant knowledge and skills.
- Treat all professions with respect while acknowledging substantial differences in education, training, and responsibilities.
- Acknowledge the social risk of discussing opposing views.
- Embrace healthy conflict as opportunity for change.
- Create and follow organizational rules for openly resolving power struggles.
- Avoid making conflict personal. Attack bad ideas, not people.
- Discourage passive-aggressive behaviors, such as procrastination or sabotage.
- Celebrate conflict resolution and collaboration successes.

Teamwork and Collaborative Leadership

Health services delivery is an extensive network of teams that work together to care for patients and families. **Teamwork** involves coordinating efforts among a group of people who possess a common purpose, shared workload, and collective accountability for achieving performance goals (Belbin et al., 2022). In healthcare, teams who engage in teamwork processes are more likely to achieve high medical care quality and patient satisfaction (Schmutz et al., 2019).

The ability for health services managers to work in teams can accelerate health services management careers. For example, early in her career, Agnes Therady collaborated on teams as a care coordinator at a long-term care facility (Therady, 2022). Her superiors recognized her abilities to influence others, so she was asked to lead more teams, which furthered her abilities to motivate, engage, and influence others. By steadily building leadership skills, Therady progressed through the management ranks to become senior vice president and chief nursing officer of Franciscan Health in Indiana.

> **CAREER BOX 4.2: Teamwork Promotes Leadership Skills**
>
> Early in your health services management careers, you are unlikely to be offered formal leadership roles. Instead, you will work on a variety of teams. To showcase your leadership skills and earn promotions, you should be recognized as an effective team member. Many behaviors associated with teamwork are also related to effective leadership. For example, strong interpersonal skills and the ability to collaborate are often seen as essential skills for effective leaders. To be a leader on a team, you do not need to be formally assigned authority. According to one typology of collective leadership roles, each team member can influence the team in these four unique ways (Contractor et al., 2012):
>
> - *Navigator:* Set the vision. Enable the team to establish and maintain a clear purpose and direction.
> - *Engineer role:* Act as project manager. Coordinate team task assignments and workflow.
> - *Social integrator:* Mediate conflict. Create harmony among the team members. Maintain positive social interactions on the team.
> - *Liaison:* Link team to external stakeholders. Maximize information and resources for the team.
>
> Each of these roles involve skills related to leadership that many employers look for in candidates for promotions. By demonstrating leadership in teams, early-career health services managers can prove that they deserve more responsibility and authority associated with higher level management positions.

Team leadership is an important competency for health services managers. The main function of a team leader is to ensure that the team can work together effectively to accomplish their goals. Team leaders are responsible for removing barriers to success, in the form of interpersonal conflict, lack of coordination, or external resistance. In other words, a team leader is a social problem solver (Zaccaro et al., 2001). Effective team leadership includes the following actions (Mayo, 2020; National Center for Healthcare Leadership [NCHL], 2018; Sullivan et al., 2016):

- Define team members and clarify the roles of each position.
- Reinforce commitment to the team purpose and organizational values.
- Orient team to one another and confirm shared understanding of the goals.
- Encourage detailed planning of team actions.
- Share information among team members.
- Facilitate commitment and accountability for results.
- Motivate or minimize the impact of negatively performing individuals.

In some HCOs, the leadership responsibilities are shared among the team members. **Collaborative leadership** involves sharing, distributing, or rotating roles and responsibilities for leadership among multiple people at different times (De Brún et al., 2019). For example, Texas Health Resources health system implemented a triad structure for the executive leadership of its hospitals (Berdan, 2016). In this model, the chief medical officer, the chief nursing officer, and the president shared responsibilities for operations, medical quality, patient satisfaction, and the hospital's financial performance. All major functions for the HCOs were distributed among the three leaders, and each leader could influence the others regarding their areas of responsibility.

Positive Theories of Leadership

Over the last 3 decades, a series of positive leadership theories have suggested that ethical and moral behaviors inspire followers and create positive employee **morale** (Avolio & Gardner, 2005). Such positive leadership perspectives are consistent with the social missions central to many HCOs (American College of Healthcare Executives [ACHE], 2022; Griffith, 1993; Healthcare Financial Management Association [HFMA], 2022). Leaders who behave in ways inconsistent with the organizational culture undercut their ability to lead effectively. Without **moral legitimacy**, healthcare leaders lose followers and will not remain leaders for very long (Sidani & Rowe, 2018). In the sense that leaders serve as role models, then positive leadership theories—with their focus on core values and beliefs—are important for health services managers to understand. Table 4.1 describes prominent positive leadership theories, their descriptions, and key citations.

TABLE 4.1 Prominent Positive Leadership Theories

THEORY	DEFINITION	KEY CITATIONS
AUTHENTIC LEADERSHIP	Leaders rely on self-awareness, transparency, judicious displays of emotions, and an openness to views that challenge deeply held positions. Leaders act consistently with internal moral code.	Gardner et al. (2011)
CHARISMATIC LEADERSHIP	Leaders justify the organizational mission by appealing to values that distinguish right from wrong, demonstrate passion for the mission using positive emotional displays, and communicate with symbolism to make the message vivid.	Antonakis et al. (2016)
ETHICAL LEADERSHIP	Leaders demonstrate behaviors consistent with organizational values in ways that are perceived to be conscientious, agreeable, emotional stable, and consistent with clear ethical standards.	Den Hartog (2015)
SERVANT LEADERSHIP	Leaders prioritize the needs, development, and well-being of followers so that employees are more engaged and effective in their work, leading to improved organizational performance.	Eva et al. (2019)
TRANSFORMATIONAL LEADERSHIP	Leaders inspire followers, engage them intellectually, and view them as trustworthy and unique contributors to the organization. Contrasted with transactional style of leadership, in which leaders motivate followers with tangible rewards	Bass & Avolio (1993)

Moreover, many highly regarded values associated with positive leadership theories, such as humility, kindness, generosity, authenticity, and vulnerability, are also captured in various health services management professional codes of conduct (ACHE, 2022; Couris, 2022; Kaissi, 2018; Wymer, 2023; Yoder, 2019). As such, positive leadership theories are critical for health services managers to embrace when building organizational cultures, including the following (Avolio & Gardner, 2005; Couris, 2020; Bass, 2019; Den Hartog, 2015; Wymer, 2023; Zambrano, 2019):

- *Inspire and motivate:* Connect to a higher purpose and convey optimism and hope.
- *Distinguish right from wrong:* Serve moral goals of the HCO and advocate for social justice. Enable others to pursue righteous and meaningful goals.
- *Show vulnerability:* Encourage criticism, admit mistakes, and be open to learning.
- *Empower others:* Make followers feel confident enough to take the initiative.
- *Build trust:* Lead with empathy and warmth. Emphasize relationships with people and value their input.
- *Promote diversity, equity, and inclusion:* Advocate for policies that improve health equity. Fostering inclusive structures, especially for underrepresented racial and ethnic minorities. Diverse teams better serve diverse patients.

Finally, there is considerable evidence that positive leadership behaviors promote healthy work environments for staff, increase job satisfaction, build trusting leader-follower relationships, and decrease staff turnover (Alilyyani et al., 2018; Hussain, & Khayat, 2021; Langhof & Güldenberg, 2020). In effect, when health services managers lead positively, they create working environments where caregivers can effectively collaborate, communicate, and care for others. Creating environments where clinicians can care for others is unique to the health services management profession and a fundamental role of health services managers (Couris, 2022).

Leadership Styles

There is no one best way to lead. Leadership styles refer to the different approaches or behaviors that leaders adopt to guide and influence their team or organization (Cerni et al., 2014). Some situations call for using an **autocratic style**, a top-down, command-and-control approach in which leaders command the work for followers (Billig, 2015). For example, leading during emergencies requires decisive action where the leader makes all decisions without necessarily taking into account the opinion of the staff. In emergencies, autocratic leadership is ideal because of the clarity and efficiency they bring to decision-making. Autocratic leadership was once common in healthcare, where physician orders were dutifully carried out by clinical staff without question (Thorne, 2006). Today's health services delivery environment, however, more commonly features the **participative style** of leadership, whereby followers are given freedom to act and are included in shared decision-making processes.

> △ **KEY IDEA**
>
> **Leading during emergencies requires decisive action where the leader makes all decisions without necessarily taking into account the opinion of the staff.**

In a **laissez-faire style**, the leader delegates control over the decision-making process and allows followers to solve problems and make decisions independently. In healthcare, the laissez-faire style can be an effective leadership approach, if followers are supported with resources they need for the successful performance of their tasks (López-Cabarcos et al., 2021). However, the passive or avoidant leadership behaviors associated with laissez-faire style can lead to lower employee retention and organizational commitment (Perez, 2021).

Leadership style can also be determined by a leader's assumptions about employees. According to Douglas McGregor's famous book, *The Human Side of Enterprise*, **Theory X** assumes that employees need to be controlled, coerced, or directed by external forces to motivate them to achieve organizational objectives. When leaders expect employees to be lazy and incapable, they lead in an autocratic style. Conversely, McGregor's **Theory Y** posits that employees are self-motivated, self-directed, creative, and capable of taking responsibility for their own work. When leaders operate under Theory Y, they tend to engage in participative style of leadership.

Some leadership experts insist that leadership is less about the personal traits, behaviors, or characteristics of leaders and more about their interactions with followers and the environment in which they lead (Johns, 2023). In the leadership theories that adopt this view, leadership depends on the interaction among the leader, followers, and the organizational context. A variety of leadership theories and models have emerged to account for interactions with followers and environmental contexts, as described in Table 4.2.

For these theories and models, the most important consideration of a leader is the match between their approaches and the requirements of the circumstances. Is there significant resistance to change? How much authority does the leader possess? For health services managers, these

TABLE 4.2 Leadership Models and Theories Incorporating Interactions Among Leaders, Followers, and the Organizational Context

THEORY	DEFINITION	KEY CITATIONS
AMBIDEXTROUS LEADERSHIP	Leaders adopt complementary leadership behaviors, such as positive and autocratic, to exploit current conditions and to affect organizational change.	Rosing et al. (2011)
CONTINGENCY LEADERSHIP	Leadership effectiveness is dependent upon how well a leader's leadership style matches a given situation.	Fiedler & Chemers (1984)
LEADER-MEMBER EXCHANGE (LMX)	Focuses on dynamics of leader and team member relationships, emphasizing that leaders should build positive relationships with each team member. Leaders do not treat all followers equally but instead form unique relationships based on follower individual performance, contribution, and other factors.	Erdogan & Liden (2002)
PRAGMATIC LEADERSHIP	Leaders carefully observe people and the social environment to identify and use problem-solving skills to address organizational problems. Pragmatic leaders patiently await opportunities to propose solutions according to the needs of people involved and the circumstances of the environment.	Mumford & Van Doorn (2001)
SITUATIONAL LEADERSHIP	Leaders provide varying amounts of direction to followers depending on the amount of support needed and the readiness level that followers exhibit. Leadership styles include delegating, supporting, coaching, and directing.	Hersey et al. (1979)

leadership theories and models recommend adopting many different leadership approaches in order to improve the chances of success, depending on the circumstances.

EMOTIONAL AND SOCIAL INTELLIGENCE

Emotional Intelligence Model

Because context greatly impacts leadership effectiveness, leaders who are able to interpret environmental and social cues are more likely to improve organizational performance. High-performing leaders tend to be more socially attuned than poor leaders (Joseph et al., 2015). **Emotional intelligence** (EI) emerged in the 1990s as a model of various abilities used to monitor the emotions of oneself and others, to discriminate among the emotions, and to control one's thinking and action (Mayer et al., 1999). EI is an important component to career success and leadership competence, perhaps even more important than a person's overall intelligence (Goleman et al., 2002). Health services managers can develop or strengthen their EI competencies (Mattingly & Kraiger, 2019). Daniel Goleman and Richard E. Boyatzis (2017) created a popular EI model with four competency domains: self-awareness, self-management, social awareness, and relationship management. As illustrated by Figure 4.2, twelve separate competencies are within those four domains.

Self-Awareness

The first domain of Goleman & Boyatzis's EI model is **self-awareness**, which entails understanding one's emotions, values, motives, strengths, and weaknesses (Goleman & Boyatzis, 2017). Self-awareness is also the ability to understand oneself in different roles and situations and how one is perceived by others (Eurich, 2018). According to Goleman and Boyatzis (2017), the

FIGURE 4.2 Emotional intelligence domains and competencies.

Self-awareness	Self-management	Social awareness	Relationship management
Emotional self-awareness	Emotional self-control	Empathy	Influence
	Adaptability		Coach and mentor
	Achievement orientation		Conflict management
	Positive outlook	Organizational awareness	Teamwork
			Inspirational leadership

Source: Goleman, D. & Boyatzis, R. E. (2017). Emotional Intelligence Has 12 Elements. Which Do You Need to Work On? Harvard Business Review. https://hbr.org/2017/02/emotional-intelligence-has-12-elements-which-do-you-need-to-work-on

more accurately a leader assesses themselves compared to how others see them, the better their organizations tend to perform. For example, if a leader sees themselves as patient and kind but their followers are intimidated by the leader's brusque commands, they will be less likely to seek guidance and the leader will be mystified by why followers avoid them.

One way to increase self-awareness is to seek constructive criticisms from others. Feedback can reveal how one's behaviors impact others and emphasize differences in self-perception compared to others' perceptions. Early in one's health services management career, feedback will be abundant. However, as health services managers ascend the organizational hierarchy, people may be less willing to give honest feedback for fear of reprisal. Moreover, people tend to avoid uncomfortable feelings or quickly forget negative feedback when it corresponds to personal insecurities, such as not being good enough, smart enough, or likable enough (London et al., 2023). Goleman et al. (2002, p. 92) call this isolation from feedback the *CEO disease*. To prevent this, effective executive managers seek out negative critiques from credible sources, reflect honestly about any differences between others' perceptions compared to their self-perception, and use the feedback to improve their performance. Self-aware leaders constructive criticism as an opportunity for self-improvement, not as an indictment on their worth as a professional.

△ KEY IDEA

Effective executive managers seek out negative critiques from credible sources, reflect honestly about any differences between others' perceptions compared to their self-perception, and use the feedback to improve their performance.

Self-Management

Self-management skills allow a person to think clearly and avoid sabotaging their performance with disruptive emotions, such as fear, frustration, anxiety, and anger (Goleman et al., 2002). Within this domain, **emotional self-control** is the skill of regulating negative emotions, resisting temptations, or using emotions purposefully. Outbursts of emotion are not considered emotionally intelligent. However, the ability to show emotion in the appropriate circumstance can help build relationships with others. John Couris, the CEO of Tampa General Hospital, recommends acknowledging one's emotions, especially when the leaders sense similar emotions in others. For example, fear during the height of the COVID-19 pandemic was a natural emotional response. Couris wrote, "[I]t is the responsibility of healthcare leaders to listen to the fears of their teams.... If I get emotional, I show it. If I feel fear, I own it. We are in this together" (Couris, 2020, p. 250).

Self-management EI domain also includes the competency of **adaptability**. Health services managers who are adaptable show the ability to adjust to changing circumstances and modify their approach based on new information (Sampson, 2023). High-pressure situations often trigger strong emotions that stifle innovation, which can lead to a condition that Jacqueline Brassey and her colleagues call the *adaptability paradox* (Brassey et al., 2021). In such cases, the need for change is stressful, so people tend to retreat to old behaviors and miss out on opportunities to innovate. However, when leaders approach challenges with curiosity and flexibility, they often find innovative solutions to problems.

> ⚠ **KEY IDEA**
>
> When leaders approach challenges with curiosity and flexibility, they often find innovative solutions to problems.

An **achievement orientation**, which is the drive to improve, accomplish goals, or meet established standards, is another competency in the EI self-management domain (Goleman & Boyatzis, 2017). Achievement-oriented leaders accept accountability and motivate themselves and others to improve. Achievement orientation entails focusing on meeting or exceeding a standard of excellence and appreciating feedback on performance. The desire to achieve propels action toward needed changes.

> **CAREER BOX 4.3: Ambition or Dissatisfaction**
>
> Research on achievement has found that smart, talented, ambitious managers attain higher levels of career success. However, ambition can be an impediment to long-term career satisfaction. Amdurer and colleagues (2014) speculate that when high achievers get promoted, they immediately set their sights on the next promotion. When someone always seeks the next big thing without appreciating their success, it can lead to perpetual career dissatisfaction, which is ultimately self-defeating. To achieve both career success and career satisfaction, you should combine achievement orientation with other highly developed EI competencies, such as emotional self-awareness and positive thinking.

A **positive outlook** is seeing the positive in people, situations, and events. As a competency within the EI self-management domain, a positive outlook allows people to transform negative thoughts into positive ones. One tactic to improve positivity is to compare the challenges of life to successful past experiences to draw problem-solving ideas (Bekhet & Zauszniewski, 2013). This approach implies that adopting a positive outlook is not a personal disposition but a way of thinking that can be developed. Practicing positive thinking does not mean leaders should fake positivity, however. Suppressing negative thoughts without questioning their validity may distort one's perception of reality. Worse still, imposing optimism on others may force them to fake positivity, which is detrimental to leadership effectiveness (Garayeva, 2022).

Social Awareness

The social awareness domain of the EI model includes **empathy**, which is the ability to understand other people's needs, feelings, perspectives, and problems. Critically important to positive social interactions, empathy enables leaders to sense an organization's shared values and act and speak appropriately (Goleman et al., 2002). The social awareness domain also includes **organizational awareness**, which is the ability to understand the formal and informal decision-making structures and processes, the power dynamics among decision-makers, and the unspoken rules of the social networks. Organizational awareness includes interpreting office politics and grasping underlying interpersonal dynamics, which are crucial to career success, especially in large HCOs (NCHL, 2018).

> ⚠ **KEY IDEA**
>
> Organizational awareness includes interpreting office politics and grasping underlying interpersonal dynamics, which are crucial to career success, especially in large HCOs.

Relationship Management

According to Goleman et al. (2002) relationship management is the most important EI domain of leadership. In fact, these competencies are addressed elsewhere in this chapter and featured in established health services management competency models (Dye & Garman, 2015; Goleman et al., 2002; NCHL, 2018):

- *Influence:* Persuade, convince, or impress others to gain support for a specific course of action. It is best achieved by understanding others' interests and motivations to have a specific impact, effect, or impression on them and/or convince them to take action.
- *Coach and mentor:* Coaches listen to people and reflect back to confirm understanding and support self-discovery. Mentors give advice and guide professional development.
- *Conflict management:* Understand various perspectives and collaborate to find common interests among individuals and groups. Provide supporting mechanisms for conflict resolution. Engage conflict constructively to stimulate creativity.
- *Teamwork:* Coordinate groups of people who have a common purpose, shared workload, and collective accountability for achieving results.
- *Inspirational leadership:* Rouse people to action with a compelling vision that is connected to shared values.

In summary, emotional and social intelligence competencies are associated with professional and organizational success (O'Boyle et al., 2011; Pirsoul et al., 2023). Therefore, health services managers who develop competencies in self-awareness, self-management, and relationship management will be more likely to be promoted to leadership positions in HCOs.

POWER AND INFLUENCE

Dark-Side Leaders

Dark personality traits and behaviors, such as lying, selfishness, or overconfidence, may also lead to promotions and financial rewards (Forsyth et al., 2012). **Narcissism** is a characteristic that, along with psychopathy and Machiavellianism, are called the dark triad.

Narcissism is characterized by self-importance, overconfidence, aggressive interpersonal style, and a hypersensitivity to criticism. However, narcissists also have skills related to EI, such as the ability to perceive and regulate emotions that can be used to manipulate others (Walker et al., 2021). Narcissistic individuals benefit from their personality when advancing their careers to leadership positions (Rovelli & Curnis, 2021). While narcissistic leaders may be unjustifiably impressed with themselves, other people commonly misinterpret displays of confidence as a sign of competence, meaning that dark-side leaders attain unfair promotions (Chamorro-Premuzic, 2013).

Unfortunately, leadership positions can attract people who are callous, selfish, and malevolent in their interpersonal relationships (Forsyth et al., 2012). Manipulation, domination, and coercion may be common and even beneficial, at least for their careers, even though toxic leadership behaviors create stressful work environments with unhappy workers (Pfeffer, 2021). Dark-side leaders engage in abusive relationships with their subordinates and attain their performance goals through unethical means (Day et al., 2021). Even in benevolent, mission-driven HCOs, ambitious people will act aggressively because they are driven to achieve organizational results and career success (Couris, 2022). The financial rewards associated with leadership positions, especially at the highest levels of HCOs, make career advancement attractive to dark-side leaders. As such, some HCO leaders achieve career success through malevolent means, despite their behaviors running counter to the stated organizational values.

> ⚠ **KEY IDEA**
>
> The financial rewards associated with leadership positions, especially at the highest levels of HCOs, make career advancement attractive to dark-side leaders. As such, some HCO leaders achieve career success through malevolent means, despite the work behaviors running counter to stated organizational values.

While most people would prefer admirable leadership qualities (e.g., integrity, competence, and inspiration), there is evidence that a minority of individuals prefer leaders who are tough, manipulative, and somewhat tyrannical (Day et al., 2021). People voluntarily follow so-called toxic leaders (Pfeffer, 2021). Even if they want to avoid dark-side leaders, it is not always easy for people to distinguish the good leaders from the bad. Dark-side leaders can pretend to care for others, tell the truth, and follow the rules because they are good liars and skilled at managing how people view them (Den Hartog, 2015).

Self-Protective Behaviors

Recognizing the usefulness of dark-side traits, some scholars warn against promoting positive leadership theories that exclude bad behaviors as potentially effective in attaining leadership positions (Gardner et al., 2021; Hoch et al., 2018; Pfeffer, 2015). Instead, these scholars recommend studying these nefarious leadership behaviors so that people can recognize them and develop countermeasures to protect themselves (and their organizations). Aspiring leaders can adopt sound self-defense mechanisms to protect their interests and careers, including the following (Alvesson & Einola, 2019; Chamorro-Premuzic, 2013; Miller, 1999; Pfeffer, 2015):

- *Watch actions, not words:* Dark-side leaders know that bad behavior will disappoint some followers, so they will verbally support positive leadership values, but they lie, bully, and scheme.
- *Do not be surprised:* Bad behaviors are common. While perhaps more prevalent in some industries than others, dark-side leadership behaviors can be found everywhere.
- *Assume a norm of self-interest:* Most people care about others and often act altruistically, especially in HCOs. However, dark-side leaders will probably assume others are only acting in self-interest, a common misconception about human nature. When acting selfishly, dark-side leaders may rationalize their actions as "do unto others as they would have done to me."
- *Distrust attraction to leader archetypes:* Resist the seduction of charismatic or overconfident leaders. Instead of bravado, evaluate leaders based on performance. Be willing to change opinion of leaders based on new evidence.
- *Be guarded about who to trust:* It is not necessary to be cynical, but be cautious about trusting others. Not everyone will be a confidant; let them earn trust.
- *Develop a well-honed set of personal values:* Pressures to achieve results will test leadership ethics. Without knowing if the ends justify the means, a leader cannot determine when they have crossed the line between toughness and unethical behavior.

Jeffrey Pfeffer (2021) argues that toxic leaders are common enough to justify using more value-neutral descriptions of their behaviors. Thus, using overly moralistic terms to describe dark-side leaders' lies or displays of overconfidence are misplaced. Instead of a preoccupation with calling out dark-side leaders' behaviors as morally reprehensible, managers can realize that these behaviors can be strategically adopted or dropped according to the circumstances. For example, when a health services manager engages in business negotiations with a supplier, "the truth can get in the way of a good deal" (Strudler, 1995, p. 805). According to ethics professor Alan Strudler, despite the moral repugnancy of deceptive behaviors, more generally, some deception during negotiations may be morally acceptable (Strudler, 1995). When managers are unaware of the full range of leadership behaviors, they miss the opportunity to influence others and affect organizational change, which is the essence of leadership.

Sources of Power

Successful health services management careers depend on understanding the realities of the workplace (Pfeffer, 2015). To get things done, a leader needs **power**, especially more power than those who oppose them (Pfeffer, 1992). Early conceptions of power and leadership focused on how to control individuals, but later studies examine how leaders use power to achieve goals (Fennell, 2021). According to Jeffrey Pfeffer's *7 Rules of Power* (2022), power is acquired by controlling resources that other people need. Effective leadership involves incrementally acquiring power and willingly exercising power to overcome resistance to goals (Pfeffer, 1992). To achieve the shared vision of the HCO, employees, patients, and communities, health services managers need to learn how to accumulate and use power to influence others.

> ⚠ **KEY IDEA**
>
> To achieve the shared vision of the HCO, employees, patients, and communities, health services managers need to learn how to accumulate and use power to influence others.

Research by French and Raven (1959) advanced one of the most influential and lasting theories on the sources of power, which is called the Five Forms of Power and includes the following (Fennell, 2021; French & Raven, 1959; Pfeffer, 2005, 2022):

- *Legitimate power:* Formal authority that comes with the position in the organization. It isoften based on a hierarchical structure where certain individuals or roles grant authority over others.
- *Referent power:* An informal type of power that is earned through respect and admiration. Managers with referent power are liked and seen as role models, so followers achieve results in order to be accepted by them.
- *Expert power:* Knowledge is power. Performing at a high level becomes a resource that people need to their work-related goals. A reputation for being powerful and effective also becomes an important source of power.
- *Reward power:* The most common type of power, rewards, can include budget control, promotions, and bonuses. Even if other types of power do not work, people will respond to leaders who are able to offer rewards for action.
- *Coercive power:* The opposite of reward power. People comply with leaders due to their ability to take things away or punish.

Successful health services managers can (and do) acquire, develop, and use power for the good of their organizations, employees, patients, and communities. Their intelligence, hard work, and performance frequently result in promotions to increasingly powerful leadership positions.

Political Skill

Political skill is the savviness to get things done within an organization and the willingness to force the issue when necessary (Pfeffer, 1992). All HCOs—especially large ones—are fundamentally political entities. To influence change in HCOs, one needs to engage in organizational politics. In fact, responsible leaders continually assess the political dynamics throughout organizations to determine their impacts on performance, morale, and interdepartmental collaborations (Yoder-Wise et al., 2020). The failure to recognize how political skills impact organizational performance will render a leader less influential in accomplishing important goals, such as those related to protecting employees or improving patient care.

INFORMATIONAL INTERVIEW 4.2

Chief Development Officer
Access the informational interview online at http://connect.springerpub.com/content/book/978-0-8261-4807-0/chapter/ch00.

In addition, career success is sometimes determined by factors unrelated to job performance. All things being equal, demonstrating political skill can make the difference between career advancement and stagnation (Blickle et al., 2018). Political behaviors that advance the personal agenda are inherently risky because they often involve the risk of personal relationships and reputation (Treadway et al., 2013). However, political skill also gives people a sense of control over events at work (Ahearn et al., 2004). For health services managers, the scholarly literature shows that those with high degrees of political skill tend to have higher levels of confidence, job satisfaction, and career success (Waring et al., 2022). Figure 4.3 illustrates the four important concepts that constitute political skill: social astuteness, networking ability, apparent sincerity, and interpersonal influence (Ferris et al., 2005).

While some people are more naturally political, certain aspects of political skill can be developed through practice (Ahearn et al., 2004). As health services managers advance in their careers, the need for a wider range of political skills will increase. Fortunately, if they demonstrate the desire to improve, people tend to build their political skills with age and experience (Maher et al., 2021).

Checks on Power and Abusive Behaviors

Political skill can conceal abusive behavior and unbridled accumulation of power (Maher et al., 2021). This does not mean, however, that nothing can be done to compel leaders to act with integrity and kindness (Pfeffer, 2015). In fact, organizational checks can control nefarious behaviors (Day et al., 2021). For one, executive leaders can prevent toxic leadership within their organizations by acting as role models and enforcing policies against incivility, bullying, and harassment (Hodgins et al., 2020). A lack of commitment to preventing abusive behaviors—even by powerful individuals—will result in employee complaints, absenteeism, and staff turnover.

FIGURE 4.3 Elements of political skill.

Social astuteness
- Sense the motivations and hidden agendas of others.
- Present professional demeanor to others.
- Say or do the right things to influence others.
- Pay close attention to people's facial expressions.

Networking ability
- Spend time and effort networking with others.
- Build relationships with influential people, colleagues, and associates.
- Use connections to support goals and to make things happen.

Apparent sincerity
- Be genuine in word and action.
- Make people believe presence of sincerity.
- Show genuine interest in other people.

Interpersonal influence
- Make people feel at ease.
- Communicate effectively with others.
- Develop good rapport with people.
- Exhibit likability.

Source: Adapted from Ferris, G. R., Treadway, D. C., Kolodinsky, R. W., Hochwarter, W. A., Kacmar, C. J., Douglas, C., & Frink, D. D. (2005). Development and validation of the political skill inventory. *Journal of Management, 31*(1), 126–152. https://doi.org/10.1177/0149206304271386

△ KEY IDEA

Top leaders can also energetically act against toxic leadership within the organization by creating and enforcing policies against incivility, bullying, and harassment.

When a CEO abuses others or allows toxic leadership from other executives, the board of directors can address the bad behavior and hold the CEO accountable (Center for Healthcare Governance, 2009). However, the challenge for board members is to determine when the line has been crossed between hard-driving leaders who are difficult to work with and toxic leadership behaviors (Epstein & Shelton, 2019). If the board misguidedly equates the CEO's dark leadership with tough leadership, then the HCO culture will likely suffer (Self, 2013). Effective boards prevent CEOs from wielding unchecked power and acting abusively without consequences (Jesper et al., 2022).

CHANGE MANAGEMENT

A Leadership Process

Instead of traits, characteristics, or behaviors associated with leadership, some scholars prefer to frame leadership as a process that can be managed (Kotter, 2012; Northouse, 2021). In healthcare, leaders need to be responsive to the changing environment and consistently drive and prioritize change initiatives (Herd et al., 2016). **Change management** is the planned process of initiating, implementing, and maintaining organizational change (Kotter, 2012). Change management is an ever-present focus of a leader's work, from large-scale transformations to department-level enhancements to individual performance improvement (Herd et al., 2016).

One well-known change management model was developed by Jeffrey Hiatt, called the AD-KAR® model (Hiatt, 2006). **ADKAR** stands for **A**wareness, **D**esire, **K**nowledge, **A**bility, and **R**einforcement, representing the five phases people undergo as they experience change. The following are the ADKAR phases and change management actions related to each phase:

- *Awareness:* Convey the need for the change. Change will be resisted if the person is satisfied with the status quo.
- *Desire:* Evaluate readiness to support the change. In response to resistance to change, focus on the benefits to individuals and the organization.
- *Knowledge:* Provide the appropriate education and training to ensure people have the skills to perform the expected behaviors that are part of the change effort.
- *Ability:* Turn knowledge into change and ensure the team can implement the new process at the required performance level.
- *Reinforcement:* Establish processes and systems to sustain the new process and behaviors.

Kotter's 8 Steps of Change

Another well-regarded change model is **Kotter's 8 Steps of Change**, developed by John P. Kotter, a management professor (Kotter, 2012). The model specifies health services managers with a step-by-step method of initiating, managing, and maintaining change. The eight steps can be used as a planning tool and a guide to be removing obstacles (Appelbaum et al., 2012). Figure 4.4 illustrates Kotter's 8-Step Change Model.

Step 1: Create a Sense of Urgency

The first step in Kotter's change model is to describe the urgent need for change in a manner that everyone can understand. To create a sense of urgency, leaders describe the status quo as a crisis that needs to be fixed to avoid dire consequences. Instead of simply explaining the business case for change, effective leaders convey an emotional message (Kotter, 2012). The greater the feeling of urgency for change, the higher the chances for successful implementation. Kotter (2008) identified creating a sense of urgency as the most important step and failing to do so as the biggest obstacle to change.

> ### △ KEY IDEA
> **Instead of simply explaining the business case for change, effective leaders convey an emotional message. The greater the feeling of urgency for change, the higher the chances for successful implementation.**

According to Kotter's 2008 book, *A Sense of Urgency*, one way to create urgency—especially in the absence of a crisis—is to communicate a sense of urgency every day. This requires that leaders repeatedly deliver the message of change and prioritize the needed change actions above other less urgent matters. Also, sometimes an actual crisis creates opportunities to implement change more rapidly. For example, the President and CEO of Carilion Clinic, Nancy Howell Agee, hoped to implement telemedicine services throughout the health system within 2 years. But when the

FIGURE 4.4 Kotter's 8-step change model.

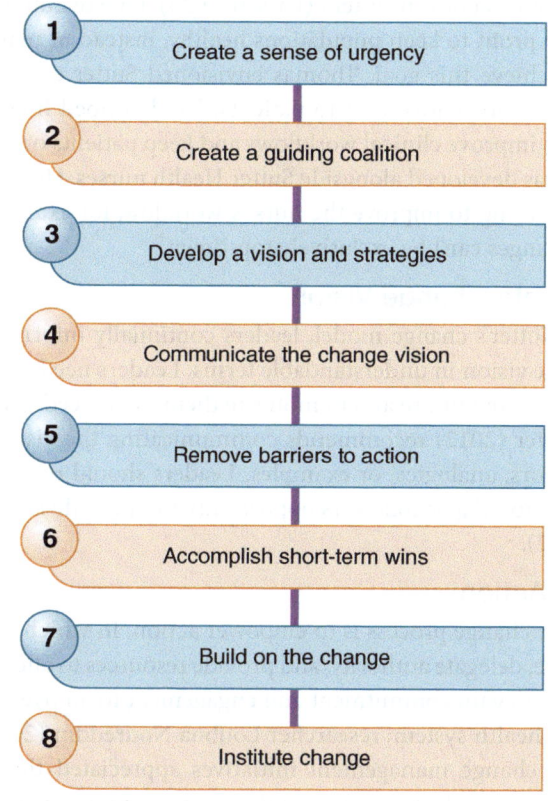

Source: Adapted from Kotter, J. P. (1996). *Leading change: An action plan from the world's foremost expert on business leadership*. Harvard Business Press.

COVID-19 pandemic emerged, Agee used the crisis to create urgency. Due to the need for infection control, the pandemic created a *burning platform* to motivate Carilion Clinic managers to transition 75% outpatient care service to virtual channels in a matter of months (Agee, 2020). This is an example of Winston Churchill's famous saying, "Never let a good crisis go to waste."

Step 2: Build a Guiding Coalition

The second step in Kotter's model is to build a coalition of enthusiastic and authoritative people who can guide the organization through the change. For example, at the beginning of the COVID-19 pandemic, Albert Wright, the CEO of West Virginia University Hospitals and Health Systems, delegated authority for COVID-19 response to a physician leader. Dr. Steve Hoffman immediately became known as the leader of the COVID-19 response who was responsible for recruiting over 30 experts to serve as the health system's guiding coalition. The guiding coalition discussed and resolved any disagreements and communicated unanimous decisions about policy throughout the HCO.

Step 3: Develop a Vision and Strategy

As discussed in this chapter, creating a vision is one of the most important leadership competencies. In the third step of Kotter's change model, the leaders must describe a clear, consistent, and motivating vision that explains why change needs to occur (Kotter, 2012). Kotter recommends that leaders conceive an initial draft of the vision and then improve it alongside the guiding coalition.

For example, CEO Warner Thomas developed a vision for digital transformation for Sutter Health, a Northern California health system (Larsen, 2023). One of Sutter's strategic goals was to contract with payers to profit to keep populations healthy, instead of making money only when patients got sick. To achieve this goal, Thomas envisioned Sutter embracing digital tools that could assist in delivering preventive care to patients. He described how Sutter would use new technology solutions to improve clinical workflows and keep patients out of the hospital. He reiterated that the vision was developed alongside Sutter Health nurses. He said, "We have more than 15,000 nurses. If we're trying to improve the nurse's workflow, for example, where is the nurse's working group? . . . Changes can't be exclusively top-down."

Step 4: Communicate Change Vision
In the fourth step of Kotter's change model, leaders continually inform people of the need for change and describe the vision in understandable terms. Leaders need to ensure that all involved are able to clearly imagine the future and to motivate them to proceed with the necessary actions to achieve change. Kotter (2012) recommends communicating the vision as simply as possible using imagery, metaphors, analogies, or examples. Leaders should repeatedly communicate the vision. Finally, leaders should give followers opportunities to provide feedback and ask questions (Appelbaum et al., 2012).

Step 5: Empower Action
Kotter's fifth step in the change process is to empower action, in which leaders clarify priorities, empower independence, delegate authority, and provide resources to affect change (Kotter, 2012). Empowerment is a way to gain commitment and engagement to an overall change goal (Herd et al., 2016). At a Florida health system, researcher Loubna Noureddin (2018) found that frontline managers involved in change management initiatives appreciated the latitude to implement change independently. One study participant said, "Vision from my leader; implementation from me. I completely believed in the benefits of the change initiative. . . . It worked because we owned it" (Noureddin, 2018, p. 166).

Moreover, it is the responsibility of the leaders to remove barriers to change. Obstacles to change will frustrate employees who will then abandon change effort (Kotter, 2012). Effective change management entails confronting individuals who actively resist change management as soon as possible. Naysayers can be prevented from stalling change by motivating them, removing them from the action, or counseling them out of the organization.

Step 6: Generate Short-Term Wins
The sixth step of Kotter's change model recommends creating quick wins to demonstrate that the change effort is worth it (Kotter, 2012). For example, at St. Michael's Hospital in Toronto, the accreditation inspection for the department responsible for decontaminating medical devices and instruments identified several areas of concern (Chadwick, 2014). The health services managers initiated a change management process to improve performance, absenteeism, and morale. One early initiative provided the management with a quick win. Within the first 3 months, a new shift schedule balanced the workload among staff, positively impacting employees' attitudes. Once this win was achieved, the managers gradually made incremental changes, eventually leading to the department's exemplary accreditation report. Quick wins made the St. Michael's employees willing to go along with other initiatives related to the department's vision for change.

Step 7: Consolidate Gains and Produce More Change
In step seven of Kotter's change model, leaders consolidate gains and produce more change. Once the difficult effort of initiating the change toward the ultimate goal, the forward momentum is

easier to maintain. In other words, change is hard to start, but once in action, the direction of change becomes much easier to steer (Maxwell, 2022). Building on increased credibility from the short-term wins, a leader incorporates the early changes into systems, structures, and policies that formalize change initiatives into established organizational processes. Well-defined systems, structures, and policies convert forward momentum into lasting change and prevent organizations from sliding back into old ways (Kotter, 2012). Resistance to change never fully disappears, and naysayers will use any opportunity to reverse the changes. Momentum can be used to recruit new people to the change process with exciting new initiatives related to the overall change goals.

Step 8: Anchor New Approaches in the Culture

The eighth and final step of Kotter's change model is to incorporate changes into the organizational culture. To make the changes stick, leaders constantly communicate how hard-won changes positively impact organizational performance. Also, the change must be consistently taught to new and existing hires in training sessions. For example, Mayo Clinic founded Time's Up Healthcare to end sexual harassment and gender inequity in the workplace, a longstanding problem with increased exposure during 2017's #MeToo movement (Rihal et al., 2020). Mayo Clinic updated and clarified its policies regarding sexual harassment, which were reinforced by training every prehire, new hire, and employee regularly. Mayo Clinic continues to sustain the changes in culture by tracking incidents in HCO's sexual harassment dashboard and by setting expectations for zero tolerance for disrespectful behavior of any kind.

FUTURE DIRECTIONS

Mastery of leadership, like most challenging skills, emerges through consistent practice. However, some health services managers do not have enough self-awareness to learn from mistakes or the ability to turn feedback from advisors into new leadership skills (Kragt & Day, 2020). To account for this, many HCOs provide **leadership training** programs that teach leadership competencies (Careau et al., 2014). Training typically includes opportunities to practice and receive constructive feedback. However, short-term job-based training alone may not be enough to develop effective leaders. Leadership training courses may attempt to teach the importance of traits such as kindness, integrity, and authenticity, but it is unlikely that participants will truly learn positive leadership behaviors unless behaviors were practiced over a long-term period (Day et al., 2021).

To supplement training, some HCOs provide **leadership development** programs designed to turn workplace challenges into leadership competencies. Leadership development programs are long-term professional development initiatives that are personalized, collaborative, and intensive (Day, Bastardoz, Bisbey, Reyes, & Salas, 2021). Leadership development programs aim to create greater leadership capacity to solve issues in the real-world context (Gurdjian et al., 2014). When leadership development programs integrate actual workplace situations, leaders build relevant skills by immediately applying them to their jobs. These experiences force developing leaders to try various styles and skills to learn which work for them and under which situations.

The future of leadership development will be technology enabled. A growing assortment of online courses, social media applications, and learning tools enable personalized and interactive leadership development (Moldoveanu & Narayandas, 2019). While traditional leadership development programs typically include only high-potential senior leaders, these lower cost tools will permit HCOs to invite early- and mid-career individuals to participate. Technology-enabled leadership development programs will encourage colleagues to collaborate with each other in real work situations, allowing the application of leadership competencies. It is unclear whether these new tools will be a passing fad or an effective combination of convenient training programs and personalized leadership development programs (Day et al., 2021). Nevertheless, developing leadership competencies takes persistent effort, meaningful feedback, deep reflection, and plenty of practice.

SUMMARY

- Leaders create a vision for new ways of operating, gain support from teams, acquire resources, or influence action. To develop a vision for the future, leaders take their knowledge of the past, analyze the present-day context, and create vivid images of the future.
- Through role modeling, health services managers can strengthen organizational culture. When leaders model behaviors consistent with cultural values, others are more likely to follow them.
- Emotional and social intelligence competencies are critical to professional and organizational success. Health services managers who develop competencies in self-awareness, self-management, social awareness, and relationship management will be more likely to be promoted to leadership positions in HCOs.
- Aspiring leaders can adopt sound self-defense mechanisms to protect their interests and careers from leaders who demonstrate dark personality traits and behaviors, such as lying, selfishness, or overconfidence.
- Becoming an effective leader involves acquiring power and the willingness exercise that power to overcome resistance to professional or organizational goals. To achieve a vision for HCOs, health services managers need to learn how to accumulate and use power.
- To succeed in large HCOs, health services managers must build political skills, including social astuteness, networking ability, apparent sincerity, and interpersonal influence. Those with high degrees of political skill tend to have higher levels of confidence, job satisfaction, and career success.
- Change management is the planned process of initiating, implementing, and maintaining organizational change. Kotter's 8 Steps of Change is a model that specifies a step-by-step method of change management.

END-OF-CHAPTER RESOURCES

KEY TERMS*

*For the full list of key terms, please see the online glossary at **http://connect.springerpub.com/content/book/978-0-8261-4807-0.**

achievement orientation
adaptability
ADKAR
ambidextrous leadership
authentic leadership
autocratic style
charismatic leadership
collaborative leadership
coercive power
conflict management
contingency leadership
change management

empathy
emotional intelligence
ethical leadership
emotional self-control
expert power
Kotter's 8 Steps of Change
laissez-faire style
leadership
leadership development
leadership training
legitimate power
moral legitimacy

narcissism	self-awareness
organizational awareness	servant leadership
organizational culture	shared values
participative style	situational leadership
political skill	social learning theory
positive outlook	teamwork
power	Theory X
pragmatic leadership	Theory Y
referent power	transformational leadership
reward power	vision
role modeling	

LEARNING ACTIVITIES

Professional Development and Reflection

1. Social and emotional intelligence influence career success. Reflect on Goleman and Boyatzis's EI model by choosing your three most developed EI competencies and three least developed competencies. How will your EI strengths and weakness boost and hinder your career? How can you improve your least developed EI competencies? Ask your network of friends, family, colleagues for feedback about your EI competency strengths and weaknesses. Compare your self-assessment to the feedback you receive.

2. The strength of a leader's vision is determined by their capacity to imagine the future and to influence make the future happen. In vivid terms, describe your vision for your career. Write two versions of your career vision—one for 3 to 5 years in the future and another for 20 years in the future. See Career Box 4.1, Envisioning Career Success.

Discussion Questions

1. This chapter presented at least 20 leadership and change management theories and models. Which theories and models are most useful for an early-career health services management to develop as a leader?

2. According to comedian George Burns (1980), "The key to success is sincerity. If you can fake that, you've got it made." How is this witticism consistent with the following theories and models: various positive leadership theories, dark-side leadership, political skills, and EI?

3. Why are health services managers with developed EI more likely to be promoted to leadership positions. Choose at least one competency from Goleman and Boyatzis's EI model domains and describe how each competency would influence career advancement. Consider the impacts of both high competence and low competence.

RECOMMENDED READING AND MEDIA

Baedke, L., & Lamberton, N. (2018). *The emerging healthcare leader: A field guide* (2nd ed). Health Administration Press.

Brown, B. (2021). *Atlas of the heart: Mapping meaningful connection and the language of human experience*. Random House.

Christensen, C. (2013). *The innovator's dilemma: When new technologies cause great firms to fail.* Harvard Business Review Press.

Chamorro-Premuzic, T. (2020, March 12). *How to stop promoting incompetent men (Quick Study)* [Video]. YouTube. https://www.youtube.com/watch?v=5XikR_aN0Hk

Dye, C. (2022). *Leadership in healthcare: Essential values and skills* (4th ed). Health Administration Press.

Eurich, T. (2018). What self-awareness really is (and how to cultivate it). *Harvard Business Review.* https://hbr.org/2018/01/what-self-awareness-really-is-and-how-to-cultivate-it

George, B. (2010). *True north: Discover your authentic leadership.* John Wiley & Sons.

Gregersen, H. (2020, March 19). Stay or go? *Harvard Business Review.* https://hbr.org/podcast/2020/03/stay-or-go

Kotter, J. P., & Rathgeber, H. (2016). *Our iceberg is melting: Changing and succeeding under any conditions.* Portfolio.

Maxwell, J. C. (2022). *The 21 irrefutable laws of leadership: Follow them and people will follow you.* (25th anniversary edition). HarperCollins.

Pfeffer, J. (2015). *Leadership BS: Fixing workplaces and careers one truth at a time.* Harper Business.

Pfeffer, J. (2022). *7 rules of power: Surprising—but true—advice on how to get things done and advance your career.* Matt Holt Books.

Sinek, S. (2011). *Start with why.* Portfolio/Penguin.

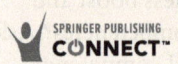

A robust set of instructor resources designed to supplement this text is located at http://connect.springerpub.com/content/book/978-0-8261-4807-0.
Qualifying instructors may request access by emailing textbook@springerpub.com.

REFERENCES

Agba, C. O., Snowden-Bahr, J. D., Kadakia, K. T., Chaker, S. A., Young, J. B., & Forystek, A. G. (2022). Global horizons for value-based care: Lessons learned from the Cleveland Clinic. *NEJM Catalyst Innovations in Care Delivery, 3*(3).

Agee, N. H. (2020, May 13). *COVID-19 pandemic gives new sense of urgency to the need for regulatory reform.* Becker's Hospital Review. https://www.beckershospitalreview.com/hospital-management-administration/covid-19-pandemic-gives-new-sense-of-urgency-to-the-need-for-regulatory-reform.html

Ahearn, K. K., Ferris, G. R., Hochwarter, W. A., Douglas, C., & Ammeter, A. P. (2004). Leader political skill and team performance. *Journal of Management, 30*(3), 309–327. https://doi.org/10.1016/j.jm.2003.01.004

Alilyyani, B., Wong, C. A., & Cummings, G. (2018). Antecedents, mediators, and outcomes of authentic leadership in healthcare: A systematic review. *International Journal of Nursing Studies, 83*, 34–64. https://doi.org/10.1016/j.ijnurstu.2018.04.001

Alvesson, M., & Einola, K. (2019). Warning for excessive positivity: Authentic leadership and other traps in leadership studies. *The Leadership Quarterly, 30*(4), 383–395. https://doi.org/10.1016/j.leaqua.2019.04.001

Amdurer, E., Boyatzis, R. E., Saatcioglu, A., Smith, M. L., & Taylor, S. N. (2014). Long term impact of emotional, social and cognitive intelligence competencies and GMAT on career and life satisfaction and career success. *Frontiers in Psychology, 5*, 1447. https://doi.org/10.3389/fpsyg.2014.01447

American College of Healthcare Executives. (2022). *ACHE code of ethics.* https://www.ache.org/about-ache/our-story/our-commitments/ethics/ache-code-of-ethics

Antonakis, J., Bastardoz, N., Jacquart, P., & Shamir, B. (2016). Charisma: An ill-defined and ill-measured gift. *Annual Review of Organizational Psychology and Organizational Behavior, 3*, 293–319. https://doi.org/10.1146/annurev-orgpsych-041015-062305

Appelbaum, S. H., Habashy, S., Malo, J. L., & Shafiq, H. (2012). Back to the future: Revisiting Kotter's 1996 change model. *Journal of Management Development, 31*(8), 764–782. https://doi.org/10.1108/02621711211253231

Austin, J. (2023). Strategic healthcare change: Balancing change and stability. *Journal of Healthcare Management, 68*(1), 9–14. https://doi.org/10.1097/JHM-D-22-00228

Avolio, B. J., & Gardner, W. L. (2005). Authentic leadership development: Getting to the root of positive forms of leadership. *The Leadership Quarterly, 16*(3), 315–338. https://doi.org/10.1016/j.leaqua.2005.03.001

Bandura, A. (1971). *Social learning theory*. General Learning Press.

Bass, B. L. (2019). What is leadership? *Leadership in Surgery*. https://doi.org/10.1007/978-3-030-19854-1_1

Bass, B. M., & Avolio, B. J. (1993). Transformational leadership and organizational culture. *Public Administration Quarterly, 17*(1), 112–121.

Bass, B. M., & Riggio, R. E. (2006). Transformational leadership. Psychology press.

Begun, J. W., & Thygeson, M. (2015). Managing complex healthcare organizations. In *Handbook of healthcare management* (pp. 1–17). Edward Elgar Publishing.

Begun, J. W., White, K. R., & Mosser, G. (2011). Interprofessional care teams: The role of the healthcare administrator. *Journal of Interprofessional Care, 25*(2), 119–123.

Bekhet, A. K., & Zauszniewski, J. A. (2013). Measuring use of positive thinking skills: Psychometric testing of a new scale. *Western Journal of Nursing Research, 35*(8), 1074–1093. https://doi.org/10.1177/0193945913482191

Belbin, M., Tuckman, B., Katzenbach, J., Smith, D., Janis, I., & Gibson, C. (2022). Managing groups and teams. In D. King & S. Lawley (Ed.), *Organizational behaviour*. Oxford University Press.

Bennis, W., & Nanus, B. (1985). *Leaders: The strategies for taking charge*. Harper & Row.

Berdan, B. E. (2016). Physician leadership in a changing healthcare environment. *Frontiers of Health Services Management, 32*(3), 27–32.

Bielaszka-DuVernay, C. (2009, February 11). Staying focused on your career goals in Today's Turmoil. *Harvard Business Review*. https://hbr.org/2009/02/interview-with-tim-butler

Billig, M. (2015). Kurt Lewin's leadership studies and his legacy to social psychology: Is there nothing as practical as a good theory? *Journal for the Theory of Social Behaviour, 45*(4), 440–460. https://doi.org/10.1111/jtsb.12074

Blickle, G., Schütte, N., & Wihler, A. (2018). Political will, work values, and objective career success: A novel approach–The Trait-Reputation-Identity Model. *Journal of Vocational Behavior, 107*, 42–56. https://doi.org/10.1016/j.jvb.2018.03.002

Boyatzis, R. E., & Goleman, D. (2007). *Emotional and social competency inventory*. Hay Group.

Brassey, J., De Smet, A., Kothari, A., Lavoie, J., Mugayar-Baldocchi, M., & Zolley, S. (2021). Future proof: Solving the 'adaptability paradox' for the long term. McKinsey & Company. https://www.mckinsey.com/capabilities/people-and-organizational-performance/our-insights/future-proof-solving-the-adaptability-paradox-for-the-long-term.

Brinkley, R. W. (2013). The case for values as a basis for organizational culture. *Frontiers of Health Services Management, 30*(1), 3–13. https://doi.org/10.1097/01974520-201307000-00002

Burns, G. (1980). *The third time around*. Putnam.

Careau, E., Biba, G., Brander, R., Van Dijk, J. P., Verma, S., Paterson, M., & Tassone, M. (2014). Health leadership education programs, best practices, and impact on learners' knowledge, skills, attitudes, and behaviors and system change: A literature review. *Journal of Healthcare Leadership*, 39–50.

Center for Healthcare Governance. (2009). *The guide to good Governance for hospital boards*. American Hospital Association.

Cerni, T., Curtis, G. J., & Colmar, S. H. (2014). Cognitive-experiential leadership model: How leaders' information-processing systems can influence leadership styles, influencing tactics, conflict management, and organizational outcomes. *Journal of Leadership Studies, 8*(3), 26–39. https://doi.org/10.1002/jls.21335

Chadwick, J., Knapp, M., Sinclair, D., & Arshoff, L. (2014, April). Effect of a change management program in a medical device reprocessing department: A mixed methods study. *Healthcare Management Forum, 27*(1), 20–24. https://doi.org/10.1016/j.hcmf.2013.12.001

Chamorro-Premuzic, T. (2013, August 22). Why do so many incompetent men become leaders? *Harvard Business Review*. https://hbr.org/2013/08/why-do-so-many-incompetent-men

Chatfield, J. S., Longenecker, C. O., Fink, L. S., & Gold, J. P. (2017). Ten CEO imperatives for healthcare transformation: Lessons from top-performing academic medical centers. *Journal of Healthcare Management, 62*(6), 371–383. https://doi.org/10.1097/JHM-D-16-00003

Chopra, M., & Keller, S. (2020, July 23). *Making a daily 'to be' list: How a hospital system CEO is navigating the coronavirus crisis*. The McKinsey Quarterly. https://www.mckinsey.com/capabilities/strategy-and-corporate-finance/our-insights/making-a-daily-to-be-list-how-a-hospital-system-ceo-is-navigating-the-coronavirus-crisis

Contractor, N. S., DeChurch, L. A., Carson, J., Carter, D. R., & Keegan, B. (2012). The topology of collective leadership. *The Leadership Quarterly, 23*(6), 994–1011. https://doi.org/10.1016/j.leaqua.2012.10.010

Couris, J. (2022). Leading with a culture of authenticity. In J. F. Quinn & B. A. A. White (Eds.), *Cultivating leadership in medicine*. Kendall Hunt Publishing Company.

Couris, J. D. (2020). Vulnerability: The secret to authentic leadership through the pandemic. *Journal of Healthcare Management, 65*(4), 248–251.

Day, D., Bastardoz, N., Bisbey, T., Reyes, D., & Salas, E. (2021). Unlocking human potential through leadership training & development initiatives. *Behavioral Science & Policy, 7*(1), 41–54.

Day, D. V., Riggio, R. E., Tan, S. J., & Conger, J. A. (2021). Advancing the science of 21st-century leadership development: Theory, research, and practice. *The Leadership Quarterly, 32*(5), 101557. https://doi.org/10.1016/j.leaqua.2021.101557

De Brún, A., O'Donovan, R., & McAuliffe, E. (2019). Interventions to develop collectivistic leadership in healthcare settings: A systematic review. *BMC Health Services Research, 19*, 1–22. https://doi.org/10.1186/s12913-019-3883-x

Den Hartog, D. N. (2015). Ethical leadership. *Annual Review of Organizational Psychology and Organizational Behavior, 2*(1), 409–434. https://doi.org/10.1146/annurev-orgpsych-032414-111237

Dye, C. F., & Garman, A. N. (2015). *Exceptional leadership: 16 critical competencies for healthcare executives*. Health Administration Press.

Emanuel, E. J. (2023, May 10). *Nine health care megatrends, part 2: System reconfiguration*. Health Affairs Forefront. https://www.healthaffairs.org/content/forefront/nine-health-care-megatrends-part-2-system-reconfiguration

Epstein, M. J., & Shelton, R. (2019). When the CEO is a brilliant jerk. *Strategic Finance, 101*(3), 22–29.

Erdogan, B., & Liden, R. C. (2002). Social exchanges in the workplace. *Leadership, 65*(114), 175–186.

Eurich, T. (2018). What self-awareness really is (and how to cultivate it). *Harvard Business Review*. https://hbr.org/2018/01/what-self-awareness-really-is-and-how-to-cultivate-it

Eva, N., Robin, M., Sendjaya, S., Van Dierendonck, D., & Liden, R. C. (2019). Servant leadership: A systematic review and call for future research. *The Leadership Quarterly, 30*(1), 111–132. https://doi.org/10.1016/j.leaqua.2018.07.004

Ferris, G. R., Treadway, D. C., Kolodinsky, R. W., Hochwarter, W. A., Kacmar, C. J., Douglas, C., & Frink, D. D. (2005). Development and validation of the political skill inventory. *Journal of Management, 31*(1), 126–152. https://doi.org/10.1177/0149206304271386

Fennell, K. (2021). Conceptualisations of leadership and relevance to health and human service workforce development: A scoping review. *Journal of Multidisciplinary Healthcare, 14*, 3035–3051. https://doi.org/10.2147/JMDH.S329628

Fiedler, F. E., & Chemers, M. M. (1984). *Improving leadership effectiveness: The leader match concept* (2nd ed.). John Wiley & Sons.

Forsyth, D. R., Banks, G. C., & McDaniel, M. A. (2012). A meta-analysis of the Dark Triad and work behavior: A social exchange perspective. *Journal of Applied Psychology, 97*(3), 557. https://doi.org/10.1037/a0025679

French, J., & Raven, B. (1959). The bases of social power. In D. Cartwright (Ed.), *Studies in social power* (pp. 150–167). Institute for Social Research.

Garayeva, S. (2022). *Can thinking positive go wrong? A mixed-method study of positive thinking at work* [Doctoral dissertation, Birkbeck, University of London].

Gardner, W. L., Cogliser, C. C., Davis, K. M., & Dickens, M. P. (2011). Authentic leadership: A review of the literature and research agenda. *The Leadership Quarterly, 22*(6), 1120–1145. https://doi.org/10.1016/j.leaqua.2011.09.007

Gardner, W. L., Karam, E. P., Alvesson, M., & Einola, K. (2021). Authentic leadership theory: The case for and against. *The Leadership Quarterly, 32*(6), 101495. https://doi.org/10.1016/j.leaqua.2021.101495

Garman, A. N., Leach, D. C., & Spector, N. (2006). Worldviews in collision: Conflict and collaboration across professional lines. *Journal of Organizational Behavior, 27*(7), 829–849. https://doi.org/10.1002/job.394

Goleman, D., & Boyatzis, R. E. (2017, February 6). Emotional intelligence has 12 elements. Which do you need to work on? *Harvard Business Review*. https://hbr.org/2017/02/emotional-intelligence-has-12-elements-which-do-you-need-to-work-on

Goleman, D., Boyatzis, R. E., & McKee, A. (2002). *Primal leadership: Learning to lead with emotional intelligence*. Harvard Business School Press.

Griffith, J. R. (1993). *The moral challenges of health care management*. Health Administration Press.

Gurdjian, P., Halbeisen, T., & Lane, K. (2014, January 1). Why leadership-development programs fail. McKinsey Quarterly. https://www.mckinsey.com/featured-insights/leadership/why-leadership-development-programs-fail

Healthcare Financial Management Association. (2022, December 22). *Bylaws and code of ethics*. https://www.hfma.org/about-hfma/bylaws-and-code-of-ethics

Herd, A. M., Adams-Pope, B. L., Bowers, A., & Sims, B. (2016). Finding what works: Leadership competencies for the changing healthcare environment. *Journal of Leadership Education, 15*(4), 217–233. https://doi.org/10.12806/V15/I4/C2

Hersey, P., Blanchard, K. H., & Natemeyer, W. E. (1979). Situational leadership, perception, and the impact of power. *Group & Organization Studies, 4*(4), 418–428. https://doi.org/10.1177/105960117900400404

Hiatt, J. M. (2006). *ADKAR: A model for change in business, government, and our community*. Prosci Learning Center Publications.

Hickman, C. R. (1992). *Mind of a manager, soul of a leader*. Wiley.

Hoch, J. E., Bommer, W. H., Dulebohn, J. H., & Wu, D. (2018). Do ethical, authentic, and servant leadership explain variance above and beyond transformational leadership? A meta-analysis. *Journal of Management, 44*(2), 501–529. https://doi.org/10.1177/0149206316665461

Hodgins, M., Lewis, D., MacCurtain, S., McNamara, P., Hogan, V., & Pursell, L. (2020). "… A bit of a joke": Policy and workplace bullying. *SAGE Open, 10*(2), 2158244020934493.

Hussain, M. K., & Khayat, R. A. M. (2021). The impact of transformational leadership on job satisfaction and organisational commitment among hospital staff: A systematic review. *Journal of Health Management, 23*(4), 614–630. https://doi.org/10.1177/09720634211050463

Jesper, H., Fredrik, H., & Dennis, S. (2022). Ruthless Exploiters or Ethical Guardians of the Workforce? Powerful CEOs and their Impact on Workplace Safety and Health. *Journal of Business Ethics, 177*(3), 641–663. https://doi.org/10.1007/s10551-021-04740-4

Johns, G. (2023). The context deficit in leadership research. *The Leadership Quarterly, 35*(1), 101755. https://doi.org/10.1016/j.leaqua.2023.101755

Joseph, D. L., Jin, J., Newman, D. A., & O'Boyle, E. H. (2015). Why does self-reported emotional intelligence predict job performance? A meta-analytic investigation of mixed EI. *Journal of Applied Psychology, 100*(2), 298–342. https://doi.org/10.1037/a0037681

Kaissi, A. (2018). *Intangibles: The unexpected traits of high-performing healthcare leaders*. Health Administrative Press.

Kaplan, G. S. (2020). Defining a new leadership model to stay relevant in healthcare. *Frontiers of Health Services Management, 36*(3), 12–20. https://doi.org/10.1097/HAP.0000000000000077

Kotter, J. P. (2008). Force for change: How leadership differs from management. Simon and Schuster.

Kotter, J. P. (2012). *Leading change*. Harvard Business Press.

Kouzes, J. M., & Posner, B. Z. (2017). *The leadership challenge: How to make extraordinary things happen in organizations* (6th ed.). Leadership Challenge, A Wiley Brand.

Kragt, D., & Day, D. V. (2020). Predicting leadership competency development and promotion among high-potential executives: The role of leader identity. *Frontiers in Psychology, 11*, 1816. https://doi.org/10.3389/fpsyg.2020.01816

Langhof, J. G., & Güldenberg, S. (2020). Servant Leadership: A systematic literature review—toward a model of antecedents and outcomes. *German Journal of Human Resource Management, 34*(1), 32–68. https://doi.org/10.1177/2397002219869903

Larsen, E. (2023). *CEO Warner Thomas' vision for digital transformation at Sutter Health*. Advisory Board. https://www.advisory.com/topics/strategy-planning-and-growth/2023/07/digital-transformation-at-sutter-health

LiveCareer. (2023, May 22). *Creating a career vision for your life: Envisioning your ideal career*. https://www.livecareer.com/resources/careers/planning/creating-a-career-vision

London, M., Sessa, V. I., & Shelley, L. A. (2023). Developing self-awareness: Learning processes for self-and interpersonal growth. *Annual Review of Organizational Psychology and Organizational Behavior, 10*, 261–288. https://doi.org/10.1146/annurev-orgpsych-120920-044531

López-Cabarcos, M. Á., López-Carballeira, A., & Ferro-Soto, C. (2021). How to moderate emotional exhaustion among public healthcare professionals? *European Research on Management and Business Economics, 27*(2), 100140. https://doi.org/10.1016/j.iedeen.2020.100140

Lovelace, J. B., Neely, B. H., Allen, J. B., & Hunter, S. T. (2019). Charismatic, ideological, & pragmatic (CIP) model of leadership: A critical review and agenda for future research. *The Leadership Quarterly, 30*(1), 96–110. https://doi.org/10.1016/j.leaqua.2018.08.001

Maher, L. P., Ejaz, A., Nguyen, C. L., & Ferris, G. R. (2021). Forty years of political skill and will in organizations: A review, meta-theoretical framework and directions for future research. *Career Development International, 27*(1), 5–35. https://doi.org/10.1108/CDI-07-2021-0191

Mattingly, V., & Kraiger, K. (2019). Can emotional intelligence be trained? A meta-analytical investigation. *Human Resource Management Review, 29*(2), 140–155. https://doi.org/10.1016/j.hrmr.2018.03.002

Maxwell, J. C. (2022). *The 21 irrefutable laws of leadership: Follow them and people will follow you*. (25th anniversary edition). HarperCollins.

Mayer, J. D., Caruso, D. R., & Salovey, P. (1999). Emotional intelligence meets traditional standards for an intelligence. *Intelligence, 27*, 267–298. https://doi.org/10.1016/S0160-2896(99)00016-1

Mayo, A. T. (2020). Teamwork in a pandemic: Insights from management research. *BMJ Leader, 4*(2), 53–56. https://doi.org/10.1136/leader-2020-000246

Miller, D. T. (1999). The norm of self-interest. *American Psychologist, 54*(12), 1053–1060. https://doi.org/10.1037/0003-066X.54.12.1053

Moldoveanu, M., & Narayandas, D. (2019). The future of leadership development. *Harvard Business Review, 97*(2), 40–48.

Mumford, M. D., & Van Doorn, J. R. (2001). The leadership of pragmatism: Reconsidering Franklin in the age of charisma. *The Leadership Quarterly, 12*(3), 279–309. https://doi.org/10.1016/S1048-9843(01)00080-7

Mumford, M. D., Watts, L. L., & Partlow, P. J. (2015). Leader cognition: Approaches and findings. *The Leadership Quarterly, 26*(3), 301–306. https://doi.org/10.1016/j.leaqua.2015.03.005

National Center for Healthcare Leadership. (2018). *Healthcare leadership competency model 3.0*. https://nchl.member365.org/publicFr/store/item/19

Northouse, P. G. (2021). *Leadership: Theory and practice* (9th ed.). Sage Publications, Inc.

Noureddin, L. (2018). *Enabling organizational change: How first-level managers influence and commit to implementing and sustaining change in a healthcare system* [Doctoral dissertation, Grand Canyon University].

O'Boyle Jr, E. H., Humphrey, R. H., Pollack, J. M., Hawver, T. H., & Story, P. A. (2011). The relation between emotional intelligence and job performance: A meta-analysis. *Journal of Organizational Behavior, 32*(5), 788–818.

Pirsoul, T., Parmentier, M., Sovet, L., & Nils, F. (2023). Emotional intelligence and career-related outcomes: A meta-analysis. *Human Resource Management Review, 33*(3), 100967. https://doi.org/10.1016/j.hrmr.2023.100967

Perez, J. (2021). Leadership in healthcare: Transitioning from clinical professional to healthcare leader. *Journal of Healthcare Management, 66*(4), 280–302. https://doi.org/10.1097/JHM-D-20-00057

Pfeffer, J. (1992). *Managing with power: Politics and influence in organizations.* Harvard Business School Press.

Pfeffer, J. (2015). *Leadership BS: Fixing workplaces and careers one truth at a time.* Harper Business.

Pfeffer, J. (2021). The dark triad may be not so dark: Exploring why 'toxic' leaders are so common—with some implications for scholarship and education. *Psychoanalytic Inquiry, 41*(7), 540–551. https://doi.org/10.1080/07351690.2021.1971470

Rihal, C. S., Baker, N. A., Bunkers, B. E., Buskirk, S. J., Caviness, J. N., Collins, E. A., Copa, J. C., Hayes, S. N., Hubert, S. L., Reed, D. A., Wendorff, S. R., Fraser, C. H., Farrugia, G., & Noseworthy, J. H. (2020, April). Addressing sexual harassment in the# MeToo era: An institutional approach. *Mayo Clinic Proceedings, 95*(4), 749–757. https://doi.org/10.1016/j.mayocp.2019.12.021

Rosing, K., Frese, M., & Bausch, A. (2011). Explaining the heterogeneity of the leadership-innovation relationship: Ambidextrous leadership. *The Leadership Quarterly, 22*(5), 956–974. https://doi.org/10.1016/j.leaqua.2011.07.014

Rovelli, P., & Curnis, C. (2021). The perks of narcissism: Behaving like a star speeds up career advancement to the CEO position. *The Leadership Quarterly, 32*(3), 101489. https://doi.org/10.1016/j.leaqua.2020.101489

Sampson, C. J. (2023). How Agile Leadership Can Sustain Innovation in Healthcare. *Frontiers of Health Services Management, 40*(2), 1–3. https://doi.org/10.1097/HAP.0000000000000186

Schmutz, J. B., Meier, L. L., & Manser, T. (2019). How effective is teamwork really? The relationship between teamwork and performance in healthcare teams: A systematic review and meta-analysis. *BMJ Open, 9*(9), e028280. https://doi.org/10.1136/bmjopen-2018-028280

Self, J. G. (2013, May 8). *Five reasons hospital CEOs get fired.* John G. Self. https://johngself.com/2013/05/08/five-reasons-hospital-ceos-get-fired-2

Seyranian, V. (2014). Social identity framing. In R. E. Riggio & S. J. Tan (Eds.), *Leader interpersonal and influence skills: The soft skills of leadership* (pp. 207–242). Routledge, Taylor & Francis Group.

Sidani, Y. M., & Rowe, W. G. (2018). A reconceptualization of authentic leadership: Leader legitimation via follower-centered assessment of the moral dimension. *The Leadership Quarterly, 29*(6), 623–636. https://doi.org/10.1016/j.leaqua.2018.04.005

Strudler, A. (1995). On the ethics of deception in negotiation. *Business Ethics Quarterly, 5*(4), 805–822.

Sullivan, E. E., Ibrahim, Z., Ellner, A. L., & Giesen, L. J. (2016). Management lessons for high-functioning primary care teams. *Journal of Healthcare Management, 61*(6), 449–465. https://doi.org/10.1097/00115514-201611000-00011

Therady, A. M. (2022). A leadership lesson learned: Employees come first. *Journal of Healthcare Management, 67*(2), 71–74. https://doi.org/10.1097/JHM-D-22-00013

Thorne, M. (2006). What kind of leader are you? *Advanced Emergency Nursing Journal, 28*(2), 104–109.

Treadway, D. C., Breland, J. W., Williams, L. M., Cho, J., Yang, J., & Ferris, G. R. (2013). Social influence and interpersonal power in organizations: Roles of performance and political skill in two studies. *Journal of Management, 39*(6), 1529–1553. https://doi.org/10.1177/0149206311410887

Walker, S. A., Double, K. S., & Birney, D. P. (2021). The complicated relationship between the dark triad and emotional intelligence: A systematic review. *Emotion Review, 13*(3), 257–274. https://doi.org/10.1177/17540739211014585

Waring, J., Bishop, S., Clarke, J., Exworthy, M., Fulop, N. J., Hartley, J., Ramsay, A. I. G., Black, G., & Roe, B. (2022). Healthcare Leadership with Political Astuteness and its role in the implementation of major system change: The HeLPA qualitative study. *Health and Social Care Delivery Research, 10*(11), 1–148. https://doi.org/10.3310/FFCI3260

Wymer, J. A. (2023). Positive leadership behaviors empower teams and effect change. *Journal of Healthcare Management, 68*(5), 307–311. https://doi.org/10.1097/JHM-D-23-00146

Xenikou, A. (2022). Leadership and organizational culture. In A. Xenikou & A. Furnham (Eds.), *Handbook of research methods for organisational culture* (pp. 23–38). Edward Elgar Publishing Limited.

Yoder, L. M. (2019). Purpose in place: Communicating the corporate soul. *Frontiers of Health Services Management, 36*(1), 30–35. https://doi.org/10.1097/HAP.0000000000000067

Yoder-Wise, P. S., Kowalski, K., & Sportsman, S. (2020). *The leadership trajectory: Developing legacy leadership.* Elsevier Health Sciences.

Young, J. B., & Cosgrove, D. M. (2012). Commentary: Change we must: Putting patients first with the institute model of academic health center organization. *Academic Medicine, 87*(5), 552–554. https://doi.org/10.1097/ACM.0b013e31824d5960

Zaccaro, S. J., Rittman, A. L., & Marks, M. A. (2001). Team leadership. *The Leadership Quarterly, 12*(4), 451–483. https://doi.org/10.1016/S1048-9843(01)00093-5

Zambrano, R. H. (2019). The value and imperative of diversity leadership development and mentoring in healthcare. *Journal of Healthcare Management, 64*(6), 356–358. https://doi.org/10.1097/JHM-D-19-00209

Zhu, W., He, H., Treviño, L. K., Chao, M. M., & Wang, W. (2015). Ethical leadership and follower voice and performance: The role of follower identifications and entity morality beliefs. *The Leadership Quarterly, 26*(5), 702–718. https://doi.org/10.1016/j.leaqua.2015.01.004

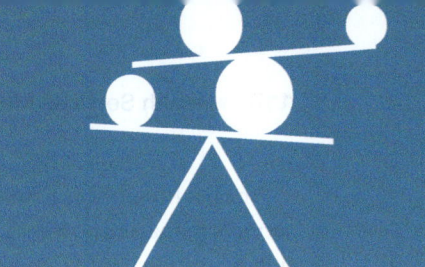

CHAPTER 5

PROFESSIONALISM AND ETHICS

Professionalism involves the behaviors, values, attitudes, and commitments that are common to health services managers. Ethics refers to the standards of moral conduct that guide the decision-making process when confronted with dilemmas about the right thing to do.

COMPETENCIES

- Follow professional and ethical standards of behavior.
- Contribute to the health services management profession and the community.
- Promote diversity, equity, and inclusion for patients, employees, and the community.
- Build and maintain effective professional connections with other health services managers, including membership in professional associations.
- Engage lifelong learning and career development.
- Apply principles of ethical analysis to issues of health services management.
- Guide ethical conduct based on professional and organizational values, codes of ethics, and other sources of ethical standards.
- Recognize ethical issues related to health information privacy, security, and confidentiality.
- Enable multidisciplinary ethics committees and institutional research boards to function.

CHAPTER OUTLINE

- Professionalism
- Professional Ethics
- Organizational Ethics
- Clinical and Research Ethics

INTRODUCTION

A profession is not just a job but a responsibility to serve the public. In exchange for commitment to service, professionals earn special benefits, such as independence in their work and certain economic protections (Khurana et al., 2004). In healthcare, professions include physicians, registered nurses, pharmacists, physical therapists, dentists, respiratory therapists, and many other clinician types. As **licensed independent professionals**, these clinicians are permitted by law to provide patient care services within the scope of their licenses and without direct supervision (Collins, 2019). Professional licensure signals that practitioners possess exclusive knowledge and skills, which conveys respect and status (Begun et al., 2018).

The health services management role enjoys many of the characteristics of a profession. Health services managers possess a distinct knowledge, expectations for conduct, a specialized accreditation educational body, and professional credentialing processes (Begun, 1986). Unlike clinicians, however, health services managers are not required to have licenses to work in most types of health care organizations (HCOs). Because the health services management role is not licensed, health services managers face the risk of being mistakenly perceived by clinicians as lacking professional legitimacy (Begun et al., 2011).

Irrespective of whether the health services management role is technically a profession, when health services managers fail to behave respectably, boards of directors, medical staff, and donors seize power and control of the HCO. Effective healthcare managers, therefore, preserve their organizational (and moral) authority in the HCO by conducting themselves professionally and ethically (Begun et al., 2018; National Center for Healthcare Leadership [NCHL], 2018; Sakowski, 2020). **Professionalism** refers to the traits, behaviors, values, attitudes, and commitments common to health services managers. **Ethics** are the standards of moral conduct that guide the decision-making process when confronted with dilemmas about what is the right thing to do (Falcone, 2022). This chapter describes how professional and ethical conduct of health services managers guides organizational culture; earns the trust of clinicians; and fulfills the duty to serve patients, employees, clinicians, the profession, the HCO, and society.

PROFESSIONALISM

Trusting Relationships

Professional legitimacy depends on health services managers building and sustaining the trust of other health professionals, patients, and the public (Begun et al., 2018). **Trust** happens when people are willing to rely on others because their behaviors are consistent and predictable (Currall & Judge, 1995). To gain professional trust of colleagues and clinicians, health services managers demonstrate the following characteristics (Austin et al., 2020; Collins, 2015; Darr, 2019; Tucker & Singer, 2015; Varga, Spehar, & Skirbekk, 2023):

- *Supportiveness:* Show concern for the interests and well-being of clinical professionals and other staff.
- *Approachability:* Ensure visibility and accessibility through face-to-face interaction with the staff, often called **management by walking around**. Seek to interact with the intention of solving problems.
- *Fairness:* Apply rules consistently and allocate resources equitably.
- *Service*: Prioritize patients and clinicians first, then address the financial needs of the HCO.
- *Competence:* Above all, be useful. Apply management discipline-specific knowledge, skills, and abilities to help others.

Education

There is no educational requirement to work as a health services manager, with the exception of nursing home administrators who must earn undergraduate degrees and obtain licenses (NAB, 2022). In all other healthcare settings, managers can have a variety of educational backgrounds, including high school education, an undergraduate degree, a master's degree, or a doctorate (Abbott, 1988; Khurana et al., 2004). Senior-level management positions in HCOs often require Master of Health Administration (MHA) or Master of Business Administration (MBA) degrees (Garman et al., 2020). In some instances, law or medical degrees are acceptable educational credentials for high-level management positions. Some clinicians who aspire to transition to health services management executive positions need to learn management skills, often by earning graduate-level degrees (Frich et al., 2015). HCOs value these professionals, as they understand both the clinical and management sides of healthcare.

To distinguish graduate programs in healthcare management, the Commission on Accreditation of Healthcare Management Education (CAHME) accredits programs that meet certain educational quality standards. Over 100 CAHME-accredited graduate programs teach the fundamentals of management applied to the healthcare industry and facilitate internships and other kinds of field-based experiences that prepare students for health services management positions (CAHME, 2023).

Credentials

Beyond formal education, successful health services managers seek continuous professional training to keep their competencies relevant and current. Professional associations offer opportunities to earn advanced credentials that distinguish them in the healthcare management field. Among the Healthcare Leadership Alliance consortium, the oldest professional association is the American College of Healthcare Executives (ACHE) with over 48,000 members, student

FIGURE 5.1 Elements of health services management professionalism.

Trusting relationships	Education	Credentials	Adapting to organizational norms
• Supportiveness • Approachability • Fairness • Service • Competence	• High school • Technical school • Undergraduate • Graduate school	• Professional association certifications • Advanced credentials	• Professional demeanor • Authenticity • Embrace multiculturalism

Work ethic	Self-management	Lifelong learning	Contribute to the community
• Hard work • Delay gratification • Self-reliance • No wasted time	• Time management • Stress management • Self-evaluation • Career planning	• Courses and workshops • Learn from experts • Read voraciously • Participate in thought leadership	• Stewardship • Fidelity • Enlightened self-interest • Volunteerism and philanthropy

Build professional connections	Valuing diversity, equity, and inclusion	Integrity
• Networking • Informational interviews • Mentorship • Advising • Coaching	• Listen to others • No discrimination • Hold self and others accountable • Commit to long-term action	• Transparency • Disclosure • Keep promises or explain reasoning with honesty

associates, and faculty associates (ACHE, 2023). The ACHE Board Certification in Healthcare Management credentialing program recognizes qualified individuals as ACHE Fellows, who use the FACHE® credential (Fellow of the American College of Healthcare Executives; ACHE, 2022c). Candidates become eligible to take the ACHE Board of Governors Exam when they attain a master's degree or its equivalent, hold a position of authority, and acquire sufficient continuing education credits. Other professional credentialing associations for health services manager that are a part of the Healthcare Leadership Alliance include the following (Garman & Johnson, 2006):

- *Healthcare Financial Management Association (HFMA):* Among other certifications, HFMA offers healthcare finance specialists with the Fellow of HFMA credential.
- *American Health Information Management Association (AHIMA):* A variety of certifications are offered for management specialists in healthcare information technology.
- *Medical Group Management Association (MGMA)*: Among other certifications, MGMA offers physician practice managers with the Fellow of the American College of Medical Practice Executives credential.
- *American Association for Physician Leadership (AAPL):* For physician executives, AAPL offers the Certified Physician Executive certification.
- *American Organization for Nursing Leadership (AONL):* For nurse executives, AONL offers two certification programs: Certified Nurse Manager and Leader and Certified in Executive Nursing Practice.

> ### △ KEY IDEA
> **Candidates become eligible to take the ACHE Board of Governors Exam when they attain a master's degree or its equivalent, hold a position of authority, and acquire sufficient continuing education credits.**

Adapting to Organizational Norms

Professionalism also means knowing how to interact with colleagues and the appropriate ways to present oneself to others, including dress, hairstyles, grooming, and others. Many early careerists do not present themselves professionally in the workplace, even though it is very important to employers (Gray, 2022). Fortunately, like other competencies, looking and acting professionally are learned skills (NCHL, 2018). Professionalism sometimes requires that health services managers play a role, such as the authority figure, mediator, or problem solver, requiring their professional demeanor to match people's expectations (Baedke & Lamberton, 2018). Behaving in a manner consistent with the expectations of the management role is sometimes called **executive presence**. While a somewhat vague concept, executive presence reflects how others perceive a health services manager's professional competence (Smith, 2021).

However, there are no hard-and-fast rules for what is deemed professional behavior. The nature of professionalism can vary based on the role, type of organization, and the region of the country (McCluney et al., 2019). As such, adapting to norms and expectations while also presenting a professional demeanor that is authentic and comfortable is a key professional skill (Agris et al., 2018; Fielding, 2023). Professionalism requires balancing one's personal and professional selves in the workplace (Baedke & Lamberton, 2018). While authenticity at work helps build professional relationships that enrich careers, not every situation demands sharing personal uniqueness and not all professional contacts will become work friends (McPherson, 2021). The key is to act authentically as possible but to also maintain a level of decorum expected in the workplace (Fielding, 2023). In this regard, professionalism requires making others feel more confident in health services managers' competence.

> ⚠ **KEY IDEA**
> While authenticity at work helps build professional relationships that enrich careers, not every situation demands sharing personal uniqueness and not all professional contacts will become work friends.

Unfortunately, the need to adapt to the HCO culture places an unfair burden on those with minority racial, religious, or sexual identities. Those who do not identify with the dominant culture of the workplace may feel the need to relentlessly monitor their appearance, speech, and behaviors while at work so that they do not face discrimination. Switching back and forth between work and personal identities can be exhausting, possibly contributing to work dissatisfaction and ineffectiveness (McCluney et al., 2019). Senior-level health services managers, therefore, can embrace multiculturalism and actively shape what personal characteristics, such as hairstyles, grooming, tattoos, clothing, and communication styles, are deemed professionally appropriate (Gray, 2019).

Work Ethic

Work ethic refers to the value someone places on work, a notion that has its roots in what sociologist Max Weber termed the "Protestant work ethic" (Weber, 1958). In this view, work ethic can be described as the desire to become a better person through working hard at a meaningful job. Despite its religious overtones, Weber associated the concept of work ethic with capitalism's individualistic ethos that believes that hard work and personal discipline can improve anyone's condition in life. Based on Weber's work, researchers Miller et al. (2002) sought to understand the various dimensions of the concept of work ethic, as presented in Table 5.1.

TABLE 5.1 Statements That Identify the Dimensions of the Work Ethic Concept

DIMENSION	SAMPLE STATEMENT
Importance of work	"A hard day's work is fulfilling." "I feel content when I have spent the day working."
Hard work	"Working hard is the key to becoming successful." "Hard work makes one a better person."
Delay of gratification	"The best things in life are those you have to wait for." "The only way to get anything worthwhile is to save for it."
Self-reliance	"It is important to control one's destiny by not being dependent on others." "Having a great deal of independence from others is very important to me."
Wasted time	"Time should not be wasted; it should be used efficiently." "I constantly look for ways to productively use my time."

Source: Adapted from Miller, M. J., Woehr, D. J., & Hudspeth, N. (2002). The meaning and measurement of work ethic: Construction and initial validation of a multidimensional inventory. *Journal of Vocational Behavior*, 60(3), 451–489. http://doi.org/10.1006/jvbe.2001.1838

> **CAREER BOX 5.1: Effort Counts Twice**
>
> To underscore the importance of work ethic to your career success, consider the formula that Angela Duckworth (2016) proposed in her book, *Grit: The Power of Passion and Perseverance*. Duckworth argued that talent is important to achievement, but it is not as important as hard work. Talent is how fast a person can learn new skills. When talent is applied through effort, skills are developed. This idea implies that even if you have little talent, you can work very hard and develop a skill (although immense talent makes acquiring skill much easier). However, Duckworth emphasized that neither talent nor skill is enough to succeed. You must apply their skill with grit—a blend of tenacity and persistence—to achieve anything worthwhile. Therefore, in Duckworth's formula for success, there are two parts to success: (1) talent times effort equals skill and (2) skill times effort equals achievement. So, in the final formulation, talent and skill are important components of success, but to really succeed, "effort counts twice" (Duckworth, 2016, p. 35).

Older generations seem to perpetually argue that work ethic has declined among the younger generations, while others think that there is little empirical difference in work ethic among the generations (Meriac et al., 2010; Zabel et al., 2017). Nevertheless, successful health services managers—especially those in the baby boomer generation—often sacrificed family time and other personal endeavors to put in long hours at the office (Brown, 2012). As such, executives with established successful health services management careers sometimes hold narrow views of what constitutes a strong work ethic. Stories of long workweeks should be taken with a grain of salt, however, as most people do not work as much as they claim. If people claim they work about 80 hours per week, they probably only work 60 hours per week, which is still more than most people's 41.5-hour average workweek (Vanderkam, 2011).

> **INFORMATIONAL INTERVIEW 5.1**
>
> *System Leader, Supplier Diversity*
> Access the informational interview online at http://connect.springerpub.com/content/book/978-0-8261-4807-0/chapter/ch00.

Still, because people tend to compare the work ethic of others based on themselves, executive health services managers will have a favorable view of early careerists who demonstrate a commitment to the HCO and make personal sacrifices (Woehr et al., 2023). Work hour expectations aside, successful health services managers demonstrate competencies that can be characterized as a strong work ethic, and these qualities are often associated with professionalism and career success (Duckworth, 2016; NCHL, 2018; Taygerly, 2022). These qualities include the following:

- *Positivity:* Express upbeat attitudes about work. Accept assignments with enthusiasm.
- *Dependability:* Be punctual, follow through, and meet deadlines.
- *Perseverance:* Set goals and work to achieve them with deliberate practice.
- *Ambitiousness:* Show commitment and motivation to accomplish goals.
- *Resourcefulness:* Take the initiative. Identify needed change and proactively develop solutions. Embrace responsibility and work independently.
- *Productivity:* Prioritize important tasks, use time efficiently, and deliver high-quality results.

Self-Management

One of the features of professionalization is the degree to which the person is empowered to perform their work in a manner they see fit (Begun, 1986). With relatively minimal oversight comes the requirement that health services managers learn how to prioritize work, handle stress, develop professionally, and plan for future career advancement. In other words, management professionals must excel at self-management skills that include the following (Griffith, 1993; Drucker, 2005; Vanderkam, 2011):

- *Time management:* Most people claim to be busy, but being overscheduled and overcommitted is a symptom of poor self-management skills. Effective and efficient self-management requires organizing goals, scheduling work, prioritizing tasks, minimizing distractions, and adjusting to interruptions.
- *Stress management:* Nurturing oneself bolsters the ability to respond to stress in ways that align with professional and organizational values. Learning to recover after stressful events is called **resilience**.
- *Self-evaluation:* Discover strengths and weaknesses. Identify career aspirations and set goals for acquiring new knowledge, skills, or experience.
- *Career planning:* Identify interests, values, and aspirations, and create structured plans for achieving career goals.

Lifelong Learning

Professionalism in health services management requires a lifelong commitment to acquiring new competencies (ACHE, 2018). Some people believe that being smart can act as a substitute for learning and self-improvement (Drucker, 2005). This is not true. Due to the rapid changes in the healthcare industry—artificial intelligence, medical technologies, and genetic therapies, to name a few—health services managers have an obligation to themselves and the profession to engage in lifelong learning. Fortunately, the health services management profession offers a variety of options to engage in professional development, such as the following (ACHE, 2018; HFMA, 2012):

- *Obtain credentials or certifications:* Demonstrate commitment to professional development and earn recognition from colleagues by earning professional credentials or certifications.
- *Take courses and workshops:* Engage in continuing education through employers, professional associations, and other offerings.
- *Learn from experts:* Seek insights from others who possess special knowledge or skills. Actively interact with colleagues at professional association events.
- *Read voraciously:* Subscribe to healthcare journals, newsletters, and newsfeeds to identify trends and challenges affecting health services management. Read popular career and professional development books. (See Recommended Reading and Media sections of each chapter of this textbook.)
- *Participate in thought leadership:* Develop professional content that demonstrates expertise and support other health services managers' professional development. Write articles, join speaker panels, or teach a class.

Contribute to the Community

Health services managers have a professional responsibility to serve their communities. **Stewardship** is the motivation to carefully manage the organizational resources for long-term benefit of the patients, the HCO, and the community (Davis et al., 2007). Even when they disagree, management colleagues and clinicians acknowledge the professional obligation of health services managers to make decisions that protect the HCO resources for future generations (Lear et al., 2016). **Fidelity** means the loyal execution of duties, especially in the context of allocating resources, in the best interests of the HCO and the community. Stewardship and fidelity do not mean self-sacrifice for health services managers. Doing well financially by doing good for the community, health services managers can engage in **enlightened self-interest**. By contributing to the well-being of the community, health services managers can ultimately benefit themselves because a healthy community and prosperous HCO translates into personal success in the form of promotions and other rewards (Karpoff, 2021).

> ### △ KEY IDEA
> By contributing to the well-being of the community, health services managers can ultimately benefit themselves because a stable and prosperous HCO can create personal success in the form of promotions and other rewards.

Health services managers are also expected to give back to the community through volunteerism and philanthropy (ACHE, 2021). Health services managers have the responsibility to volunteer in community programs that address the most prevalent health and social issues and concerns. Health services management professionals invest their time and energy in activities that improve access to affordable health care and improve community well-being (Begun et al., 2018). They can also donate to HCOs and/or other organizations intended to help others. By setting the example for philanthropy, health services managers can create the expectation that supporting community initiatives through giving of time or money is important to the HCO (Taylor, 2012).

Build Professional Connections

Health services managers serve the profession through mentoring, advising, sponsoring, and coaching (ACHE, 2019; NCHL, 2018). Executive health services managers have a professional responsibility to give back to people at all career levels. In addition, those seeking professional support have a responsibility to actively engage with higher level executives with respect and professionalism (ACHE, 2018). The practice of creating professional connections is known as **networking**. Savvy health services managers start networking long before they need a job because reaching out to people only when they are job hunting can come across as desperate (Burnison, 2018). One way that early careerists develop a network of contacts is through **informational interviews**, which are 15- to 30-minute informal discussions—not job inquiries—with individuals who work in an attractive career or organization. This kind of networking enables early-career health services managers to connect to potential hiring managers, increase their understanding of career possibilities, and prepare for future job interviews.

> ### △ KEY IDEA
> Savvy health services managers start networking long before they need a job because only reaching out to people when job hunting can come across as desperate.

Table 5.2 describes the ways that health services managers can contribute to their profession and the questions that early-career health services managers can ask for professional development support (ACHE, 2018; Baedke, 2023; Johnson & Smith, 2019; Omadeke, 2021; Walker, 2020).

TABLE 5.2 Mentoring, Advising, Coaching, and Other Forms of Supporting Professional Development Provided by Health Services Managers

SUPPORT TYPE	DESCRIPTION	PROFESSIONAL INQUIRY
Formal or informal **mentorship**	Many HCOs offer formal mentoring programs with structured curricula to support the development of high-potential managers. Informal mentorship relationships can also be formed in more spontaneous situations.	"I admire your career achievements. Would you consider being my mentor? I need help with developing a plan for my career."
Professional development **advising**	Even the busiest health services managers can find time to give advice to others. One-on-one "informational interviews" can be virtually or in person. These meetings are not job interviews but ways to learn about real-life experiences of managers working in a field.	"I am exploring a career in health services management. Your role is very interesting to me. Do you have 15 or 20 minutes to answer some questions about career possibilities?"
Career **sponsorship**	As higher level of mentorship, a manager with significant influence can advocate for a protégé and create opportunities for their career advancement. The sponsor stakes their reputation that the protégé will perform at a high level.	"Your support would help me to reach the next level of my career. Can you recommend me to lead an important project?"
Political guidance	More experienced health services managers can give guidance on how to navigate office politics with positivity and integrity.	"I know you've successfully managed interpersonal conflict in the office. Can you help me figure out how I should address a situation?"
Career **coaching**	Coaches do not give advice or guidance to others but ask clarifying questions that help build self-awareness. Health services managers can act as informal coaches to others by listening and reflecting back what they hear the coachee say.	"I need help thinking through my career options. Will you act as a sounding board for me?"
Succession planning	Succession planning is an investment in professional development of high-potential future health services executives. Senior health services managers have the responsibility to prepare potential successors for their own and other key positions.	"Here is the impact I've already made on the HCO. What can I do to be ready for a more senior position?"
College internships and postgraduate fellowships	Senior health services managers can create programs to identify and recruit talent through field-based learning, as part of academic training or postgraduate professional development.	"I am building my health services management career, and I would appreciate any information on how to get involved with your HCO."

HCO, health care organization.

Moreover, health services managers have responsibility to the profession to remove barriers to career success faced by women and minorities. This obligation extends to everyone practicing health services management, not just representative members from those communities. For example, the onus does not just fall on women to help other women but also on men, who currently hold a majority of health services management executive positions (Berlin et al., 2019). Representatives of the majority (i.e., straight White men) may be reluctant to initiate professional relationships with others of a different gender, sexuality, and race because they fear they lack cultural competence to build effective relationships (Johnson & Smith, 2019). However, health services managers, especially those in positions of power, have the professional responsibility to actively advocate for different genders, sexual orientations, races, and ethnicities (ACHE, 2022b; Chow, 2023).

Valuing Diversity, Equity, and Inclusion

Addressing diversity, equity, and inclusion are ethical and professional imperatives for health services managers, not only because of the ethics related to fairness and justice but also because diversity, equity, and inclusion create stronger work cultures, improve decision-making, and create a competitive advantage (ACHE, 2022b). Professionalism means actively seeking to increase diversity within the executive ranks, as appropriate for the community and population being served. Health services managers can actively increase diversity, equity, and inclusion through behaviors that typify professionalism, such as the following (Cox, 2022; Gurchiek, 2018; Wilkinson, 2021):

- *Seek professionalism, not conformity:* Expand the idea of professionalism to be more inclusive while still promoting positive and productive work culture.
- *Listen to others without defensiveness:* Help people feel safe to express their experiences with exclusion and injustice.
- *Consistently apply antidiscrimination rules:* Constantly seek ways to prevent bias on the basis of race, ethnicity, religion, gender, sexual orientation, age, and disability.
- *Hold self and others accountable for progress:* Relevant metrics can be measured, monitored, and improved.
- *Commit to long-term action:* Creating an organization that embraces different perspectives does not mean the occasional one-off initiatives.

In addition, professionalism means understanding the existence of health disparities among certain communities and the roles of socioeconomic, environmental, and other population-level determinants of health on the health status of populations (Agris et al., 2018). Professionalism obligates health services managers to address health disparities through investment in training clinicians to deliver culturally competent care; reducing barriers to health care access; supporting social service programs that address poverty, housing, education, food needs, and other resources for underserved communities; and more (ACHE, 2021).

Integrity

Integrity is a fundamental component of professionalism that includes honesty and transparent communications with others. **Transparency** implies a proactive commitment to being open and forthcoming about actions, decisions, and motives. A lack of transparency—secret motives, hidden agendas, double standards, shifting blame, vague statements—is never professional. When health services managers are transparent, they explain the process and rationale for their decisions. **Disclosure** is the act of revealing, providing, or making information, facts, or details known to others. However, health services managers can be transparent but not disclose certain information. In fact, disclosure is sometimes inappropriate or illegal. Privileged information, such as competitively sensitive information, should only be disclosed if the other person has the ability to act on the information (Moore, 2022). For example, the CEO may share detailed information related to a financial crisis with the board of directors but not to employees. The board can influence a decision about the right actions to address financial concerns, but disclosure to employees may only serve to worry them. Health services management professionalism means balancing discretion and disclosure.

△ KEY IDEA

Health services management professionalism means balancing discretion and disclosure.

However, certain circumstances require full disclosure. The **Lexington model** is the ethical and professional imperative of disclosing adverse events due to medical errors. The name for this disclosure approach stems from a Veterans Health Administration (VHA) discovery in Lexington, Kentucky, where a patient died due to a medical mistake. The Lexington VHA proactively accepted responsibility for severe patient harm and apologized to patients. This model of "extreme honesty" was adopted as an organizational policy at the Lexington VHA because the administrators believed it was "the right thing to do" for their patients (Kraman & Hamm, 1999, p. 964). Their research showed that disclosure reduces the filing of baseless lawsuits, which saves money for doctors and insurers.

INFORMATIONAL INTERVIEW 5.2

Market Director of Oncology
Access the informational interview online at http://connect.springerpub.com/content/book/978-0-8261-4807-0/chapter/ch00.

Integrity also means keeping promises. Because integrity is a hallmark of professionalism, promise making, keeping, and rescinding require considerable reflection. **Promise-making** is the act of committing to someone with the intention of adhering to the pledge (ACHE, 2021). Due to changing circumstances, health services managers are often faced with the need to revise or rescind past promises made by them or others. To change or break a promise, health services managers need to explain the circumstance and the reasoning with honesty and transparency.

PROFESSIONAL ETHICS

Ethics for Health Services Managers

Morals are the rules that distinguish right from wrong. While morality is specific to a community's values, there are principles that most cultures follow, such as honesty, fairness, justice, compassion, and respect for others. Some argue that people simply know the difference between right and wrong, as the foundations are constructed in early childhood through interactions with parents, teachers, religion, and secular society (Thompson, 2012). However, good people can disagree about what constitutes moral behavior and take opposite positions on health services management topics, not to mention controversial issues, such as abortion and euthanasia. As such, there is plenty of ambiguity in healthcare for debate about how to behave morally. When the right choice of action is unclear, people need to make judgment calls that are thoughtful, informed, and rational. **Ethics** describes the analysis of moral principles by which people judge the actions and behaviors of themselves and others (Falcone, 2022).

> **CAREER BOX 5.2: Save Up and Head Out**
>
> There may come a time when your HCO asks you to perform a work task that you consider unethical. Before taking action, clarify with your boss that there are no misunderstandings about the request. If you still have ethical concerns, review your HCO's policies, professional codes of ethics, and any relevant guidelines. Ready with the facts, apply the ethical analysis and decision-making process. You may need to escalate the issue to higher level management or to the compliance officer. If you believe that unethical behavior is widespread, you may need to report the issues to authorities. However, there could be career consequences to whistleblowing, such as minimized involvement in key projects or lack of promotions (Victor, 2017).
>
> If faced with an ethical issue, you may need to quit your job. However, quitting a job, especially without another one lined up, can be frightening. Therefore, it is crucial that you have savings in the bank to help you bridge the gap between jobs. Creating a financial cushion—at least a few months of your budget—will empower you to make ethical decisions without feeling obligated to an unethical employer. When looking for a new job, you can simply say that you are looking for an HCO that aligns with your values and ethics.

Within the health services management profession, there are commonly held expectations for what is considered ethical behavior. For one, health services managers willingly accept the moral duty to prioritize patient health outcomes over financial interests (Darr, 2019; Griffith, 1993). **Deontology** emphasizes the need to abide by certain duties, moral principles, and codes of behaviors when making moral decisions (Kagan, 2018). Health services managers who belong to the various professional associations pledge to follow a **code of ethics**, which is a set of guidelines that outline the expected behavior and ethical standards for individuals within a particular profession. In other words, the codes of ethics supply principles for what is right and wrong, according to the standards of the profession. Table 5.3 excerpts key language from the codes of ethics for health services management professional associations.

TABLE 5.3 Codes of Ethics for Health Services Management Associations

PROFESSIONAL ASSOCIATION	CODE OF ETHICS EXCERPT
American College of Healthcare Executives	"Healthcare executives have an obligation to act in ways that will merit the trust, confidence and respect of healthcare professionals, staff and the general public" (ACHE, 2022a).
Healthcare Financial Management Association	"As a member of the Healthcare Financial Management Association, I will endeavor to promote the highest standards of professional conduct . . ." (HFMA, 2022).
American Health Information Management Association	"The AHIMA Code of Ethics establishes a set of ethical principles to be used to guide decision-making and actions" (AHIMA, 2019).
Medical Group Management Association	"Members' professional conduct shall remain consistent with the mission, goals and objectives of the Association" (MGMA, 2015).

AHIMA, American Health Information Management Association.

Ethical Analysis and Decision-Making

In addition to the codes of ethics, there are theories to consider when determining the appropriate course of action when faced with a moral decision that is not obvious, called an **ethical dilemma**. Ethical theories provide different perspectives for evaluating ethical dilemmas and, depending on the circumstances, may inform ethical judgments and actions. The following concepts can be used to make better, more ethical decisions:

- *Utilitarianism:* Promotes social benefit with the goal of creating the greatest good for the greatest number (e.g., most life-years saved)
- *Moral rights approach:* Emphasizes the importance of recognizing and respecting the inherent individual rights
- *Egalitarianism:* Seeks to minimize or eliminate inequalities based on factors such as wealth, social status, race, gender, or other characteristics (e.g., allocation by lottery)
- *Communitarianism:* Maintains that individuals are inseparable from community life and that no one person can ever be completely self-determining

In ethical decision-making, following the law is a necessary but not sufficient condition. The **law fallacy** is the mistake characterized by asking a legal question, such as "Is this legal?" when a person should be asking an ethical question, such as "What is the right thing to do?" (Falcone, 2022). Identifying the right course of action requires that health services managers engage in thoughtful ethical analysis of the issues involved. **Casuistry** is the approach in which ethics principles are applied to practical cases. The following six steps support a systematic approach to making ethical decisions in real-world situations (Nelson, 2015):

1. *Identify all the relevant facts:* Gather documents and speak to individuals involved in the situation to understand all perspectives in conflict. Differentiate between facts and opinions.
2. *Consider relevant ethical concepts:* Identify and analyze all ethical theories, professional codes, and/or HCO values that are related to the situation.
3. *Determine the ethical principles in conflict:* Agree on which ethical principles, professional codes, and/or HCO values conflict with each other.
4. *Determine potential alternative actions:* Review the arguments for and against an action. Collaborate and discuss among stakeholders. If needed, consult with experts.
5. *Recommend action:* Provide justification for one particular action and clearly communicate the decision to all affected parties.
6. *Prevent recurrence of ethical conflict:* Examine how future conflicts can be prevented. Develop guidelines that can diminish the impact of similar ethical conflicts.

Ethical Dilemmas in Business of Healthcare

Ethical dilemmas are prevalent in the business of healthcare due to the interaction of complex medical, economic, and social issues. One of the most prominent ethical dilemmas that health services managers face is the need to control costs while enabling the delivery of safe patient care. Questions of how to allocate resources are the responsibility of health services managers that happen in the budgeting, staffing, purchasing, and facilities planning functions.

> ⚠ **KEY IDEA**
> One of the most prominent ethical dilemmas that health services managers face is the need to control costs while enabling the delivery of safe patient care.

For example, when HCOs experience workforce shortages, health services managers have an ethical obligation to ensure that enough staff is available to provide patient care that is safe and effective (Lesandrini & Reis, 2022). This requires that the existing staff are not unduly burdened with caring for too many patients. Understaffing can lead to clinicians experiencing **moral distress**, which is "When one knows the right thing to do, but institutional constraints make it nearly impossible to pursue the right course of action" (Jameton, 1984, p. 6). Unfortunately, when short staffed, clinicians may provide less care than patients need, delay care, or may simply omit the care altogether (Scott, 2019). Extreme stress is sometimes called **moral injury**, a condition where clinicians are not able to provide care consistent with their professional oath to put the needs of patients first (Dean et al., 2019). To address critical labor shortages, health services managers can hire expensive temporary staff, close patient units, or divert patients to other HCOs if it is impossible to safely staff patient care units.

Leaving the underlying ethical conflicts unresolved cannot exist within HCOs without creating rifts among managers and clinicians. Frustrated or outraged clinicians will blame the health services manager (or the health system more generally) for leaving ethical dilemmas unresolved and accuse them of being solely motivated by profit or lacking compassion for patients (Damania, 2019). To avoid this, health services managers need to develop HCO systems and procedures designed to encourage staff to act ethically (Griffith, 1993). Other ethical dilemmas in the business of healthcare are described in Table 5.4 (Alhazmi, 2019; Komesaroff et al., 2019; Saini et al., 2022).

> **CAREER BOX 5.3: Practice Responding to Ethical Dilemmas**
>
> Conducting yourself ethically takes concerted effort and practice. If your boss asks you to do something unethical, it may be difficult to do the right thing in the moment. However, if you practice first, then you will know how to respond. Forethought will allow you to develop a habit of noticing ethical dilemmas, analyzing them, and determining the right course of action. Based on the psychological principle of implementation intentions, you can link anticipated ethical dilemmas with predetermined actions (Gollwitzer, 1999). You can say, "Whenever ethical dilemma X arises, I will respond with Y." For example, you can practice ethical decision-making with the following scenarios:
> - If I see racist behavior, I will respond with "That's not how we do things here."
> - If I witness a violation of a patient's privacy, I will report it to the HCO privacy officer.
> - If I witness conflict of interest violation, I will seek guidance from an ethics adviser.

TABLE 5.4 Examples of Ethical Dilemmas in the Business of Healthcare

ETHICAL ISSUE	DEFINITION	EXAMPLE
CONFLICT OF INTEREST	Occurs when two coexisting interests directly conflict with each other and could compromise judgment, decisions, and actions in the workplace. Even the appearance of conflicts of interest should be avoided.	Medical equipment suppliers host vacations with health services managers to influence purchase of their products for use in the HCO.
SELF-DEALING	Use of corporate funds contrary to the best interest of the HCO or patients.	Using HCO funds for personal expenses, such as a party to host friends and business associates.

TABLE 5.4 Examples of Ethical Dilemmas in the Business of Healthcare (*continued*)

ETHICAL ISSUE	DEFINITION	EXAMPLE
EXCESSIVE PAY	Executive pay that is out of line with the performance and value they bring to the organization can be viewed as unethical.	Bonus awarded to the CEO even as other employees' pay were slashed because of HCO's financial losses.
WORKFORCE REDUCTIONS	Layoffs, furloughs, and other workforce reductions should be the option of last resort and should consider quality and safety of patient care delivered by the HCO.	Employees are laid off to achieve short-term financial gains instead of creating long-term strategic change.
TORTIOUS INTERFERENCE	When someone intentionally damages another's business relationship with a third party, causing economic harm.	An HCO revokes a surgeon's admitting privileges without cause because the physician is planning to start a competing surgery center that threatens the HCO's revenues.
BREACH OF CONTRACT	Occurs when a party has failure to fulfill their obligations by the due date or performed duties incompletely or improperly.	A medical equipment supplier fails to deliver product within specific timeframes, causing delays in patient care.
UNRELATED BUSINESS INCOME	Nonprofit HCOs are granted tax-exempt status to serve the public, but when engaged in businesses unrelated to providing patient care, it can raise ethical issues.	An HCO develops a medical-entertainment district that requires significant staff time and financial investment. Real estate development is an ethically questionable use of resources that may not be aligned with the HCO mission.
PREFERENTIAL TREATMENT	When HCOs prioritize the interests of financial donors, it creates ethical concerns about equity and access to health care services.	A health services manager asks staff to provide extra attention to a wealthy donor, potentially at the expense of other patients.
IMPAIRED HEALTH SERVICES MANAGERS	Abstain from all professional activities if impaired, including alcohol and substance abuse, incapacitating mental physical illnesses, and cognitive impairment.	A dependency on prescription drugs caused a drastic change in the CEO's demeanor and performance.

HCO, health care organization.

ORGANIZATIONAL ETHICS

Creating Ethical Cultures

Health services managers, in partnership with the board of governors and medical staff, are responsible for setting the standards for ethical behavior of individuals throughout the HCO. Through policy, formal training, and establishing consequences for violations, health services managers communicate which behaviors are appropriate in the HCO and which behaviors are unacceptable. By setting the ethical norms and practices for the organization, health services managers create organizational cultures in which staff and clinicians can make ethical business decisions and deliver high-quality patient care.

> ⚠ **KEY IDEA**
> When respected health services managers demonstrate ethical behaviors through personal actions, people around them are more likely to follow their example.

The most impactful way that health services managers can promote ethical cultures is through **modeling** of the behaviors. When respected health services managers demonstrate ethical behaviors through personal actions, people around them are more likely to follow their example (Bandura, 1997). However, it is not necessary to be perfect. Effective health services managers must acknowledge that they can make mistakes when confronting ethical dilemmas. Ethical oversights are inevitable parts of management practice, and demonstrating tolerance and humility will strengthen ethical culture (Griffith, 1993). Learning from failure establishes an environment where difficult ethical issues can be discussed, and consistent rules of behavior can be reinforced.

Health services managers are responsible for creating **culturally competent** HCOs, which refers to the capacity to understand and meet the needs of diverse employees, patients, families, and communities (Dreachslin et al., 2017). Cultural competency is incompatible with **discrimination**, which means the unfair treatment based on negative attitudes of a group or individual. Discrimination can be expressed in a variety of unethical (and sometimes illegal) behaviors, including **racism** and **sexual harassment** (ACHE, 2015; Cox, 2022). Figure 5.2 provides examples of discrimination that are incompatible with culturally competent HCOs.

Compliance Programs

Health services managers operate **compliance programs** that train employees on ethical behaviors and provide processes for reporting ethical lapses and concerns (Hussein et al., 2021). Compliance training can cover a range of topics, including laws and regulations, ethical standards and expectations, and HCO policies and procedures. Anonymous compliance hotlines allow employees to report compliance concerns without disclosing their identity.

> ⚠ **KEY IDEA**
> Whistleblowing is considered to be morally courageous act, and laws protect whistleblowers from retribution.

Compliance programs are also designed to prevent healthcare **fraud and abuse**, which is intentional deception, misrepresentation, or falsification to realize financial gain. The **False Claims Act** addresses fraud and abuse in government healthcare programs, such as Medicare and Medicaid. The law encourages individuals with knowledge of fraudulent activities to come forward as whistleblowers to file lawsuits on behalf of the government. **Whistleblowing** is considered to be morally courageous act, and laws protect whistleblowers from retribution, such as **retaliatory discharge** (i.e., firing without cause) after reporting fraud and abuse. In addition to whistleblowers, false claims can be discovered through the **Medicare Recovery Audit Program** (RAC), a federal program designed to identify and recover improper payments. Such fraud can include instances where patients' diagnoses are **upcoded**, a falsification of claims where billing codes for more severe and expensive diagnoses or procedures are documented to overcharge payers (Coustasse, 2021).

FIGURE 5.2 Examples of discrimination incompatible with culturally competent HCOs.

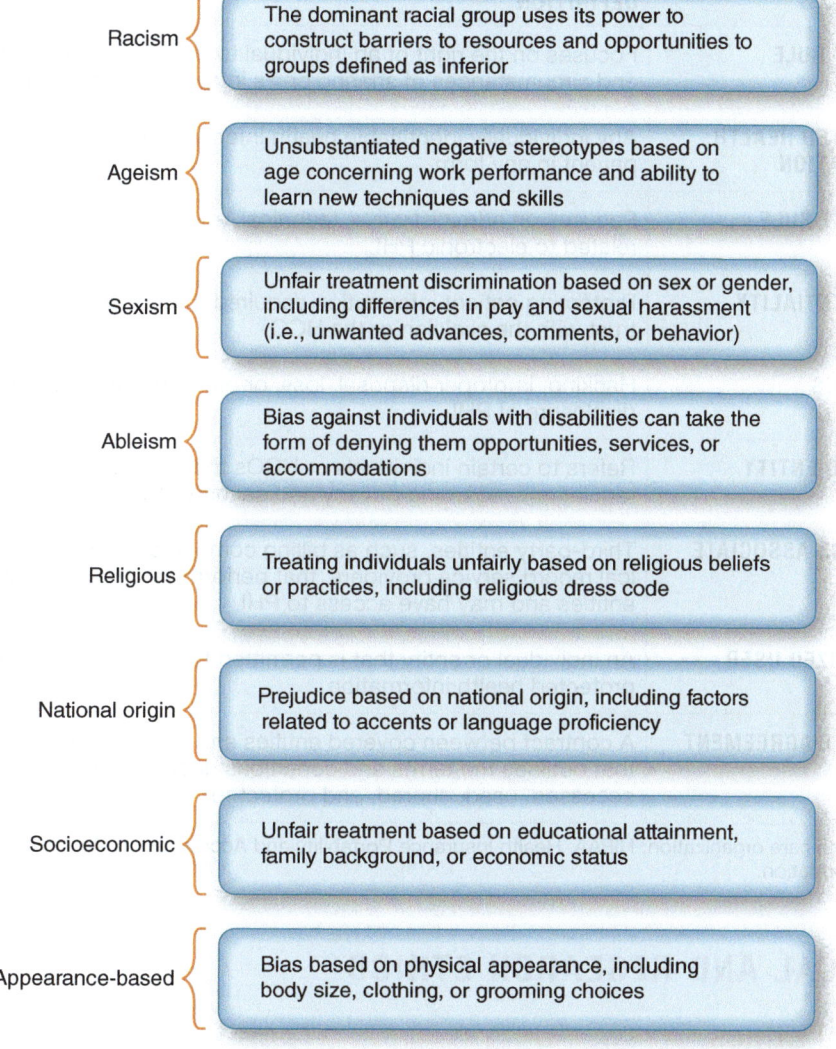

HCO, health care organization.

One key compliance initiative includes ensuring patient privacy and confidentiality protections afforded by the **Health Insurance Portability and Accountability Act** of 1996 (HIPAA). Health services managers are responsible for overseeing compliance with HIPAA regulations and preventing significant financial penalties. The **Health Information Technology for Economic and Clinical Health** (HITECH) Act of 2009 significantly increased the penalties for violations of HIPAA's privacy and security rules. Table 5.5 lists key terms and definitions related to HIPAA (Alder et al., 2017).

Finally, compliance programs attempt to prevent unethical or illegal behaviors associated with clinical care. For example, the **Emergency Medical Treatment and Labor Act** (EMTALA) requires that all emergency department patients receive a medical screening examination and stabilization regardless of ability to pay. Intended as an antidumping law, HCO emergency departments can be fined for EMTALA deficiencies, such as not providing appropriate medical screening exam before transferring a patient to another HCO (Terp et al., 2017).

TABLE 5.5 HIPPA Key Terms

KEY TERM	DEFINITION
PRIVACY RULE	Focuses on the right of an individual to control the extent, timing, and circumstances of sharing one's information without intrusion.
PROTECTED HEALTH INFORMATION	Any individually identifiable health information collected from patient in any form.
SECURITY RULE	Focuses on administrative, technical, and physical safeguards related to electronic PHI.
CONFIDENTIALITY	Protecting patient information acquired through a relationship of trust with the clinician or the HCO.
BREACHES	Hacking, improper disposal, loss, or other unauthorized access or disclosure of PHI.
COVERED ENTITY	Refers to certain individuals or HCOs that are subject to HIPAA regulations regarding privacy and security PHI.
BUSINESS ASSOCIATE	Third-party entities, such as billing companies or electronic medical record service providers, that perform services for covered entities and may have access to PHI.
AUTHORIZED USER	An individual or entity that is permitted to access, use, or disclose protected health information.
DATA USE AGREEMENT	A contract between covered entities and their business associates that outlines the terms and conditions under which data can be accessed, used, shared, and protected.

HCO, health care organization; HIPAA, Health Insurance Portability and Accountability Act; PHI, protected health information.

CLINICAL AND RESEARCH ETHICS

Clinical Ethics

Clinical ethics refers to the complex ethical considerations of clinical practice and provides a framework for clinicians, patients, and their families for making decisions about patient care. One of the main principles of clinical ethics is the respect for **autonomy**. This ethical principle emphasizes an individual's right to make rational choices about their life, body, and medical care preferences (Varkey, 2021). Autonomy involves obtaining **informed consent** for medical or surgical procedures and ensuring the freedom for people to make decisions without coercion. Many HCOs write and share the **patient rights and responsibilities** documentation to promote patients' right to make informed decisions about their medical care. These documents also acknowledge that patients have certain responsibilities, such as following treatment plans, treating others with respect and courtesy, and participating in decision-making. Patients also have a right to create an **advance directive**, a legal document that provides instructions for medical care in cases where patients become unable to communicate decisions due to illness. If a patient's preferences are not known, a **proxy** (also known as a representative, surrogate, or agent) makes the medical decision that most benefits the patient, called the **best interests standard**.

When there is ethical uncertainty in clinical practice, an **ethics committee** assists with making clinical decisions. The ethics committee is made up of an interdisciplinary team with expertise in law, ethics, medicine, and sometimes external experts from a variety of fields. Medical ethical dilemmas are reviewed on a case-by-case basis, called **case consultations**. In such instances, clinicians can request support for a pending decision about an ethical dilemma to obtain a recommendation for action. Retrospective reviews of previously made clinical decisions are also common and can confidentially review consequences or serve as the basis for setting clinical policy for the HCO (Post & Blustein, 2021).

For example, **end-of-life care** presents many ethical dilemmas for which an ethics committee can provide guidance. In cases of **medical futility**, where families request lifesaving medical care but additional treatment would be ineffective and wasteful, physicians may request that an ethics committee clarify legitimate differences of opinion. The ethics committee would make recommendations by applying an ethical decision-making process (Donnellan, 2013).

Research Ethics

Many larger and academically affiliated medical centers actively engage in a wide range of research activities. Research ethics refers to the set of laws, rules, regulations, and policies that guide an HCO in research activities (Donnellan, 2013). When conducting research funded by U.S. federal departments and agencies, HCOs must follow certain ethics regulations. **Federalwide Assurance of Compliance** is a commitment made by HCOs that engage in research with human subjects. The **Common Rule** refers to a set of federal regulations governing the ethical conduct of research involving human subjects for which **Institutional Review Boards** (IRBs) review research protocols and protect research participant rights and welfare (Post & Blustein, 2021).

Federal research ethics regulations are based in international guidelines developed in the 20th century in response to historic tragedies occurring in the name of scientific research (Post & Blustein, 2021). The **Nuremberg Code** is a set of ethical principles and guidelines for conducting human experimentation that was developed in response to atrocities committed by Nazi Germany during World War II. The **Declaration of Helsinki** is the international ethical rules for human research that prevents future wrongful or illegal conduct, particularly by persons in a position of authority, an act known as **malfeasance**. The **Tuskegee Syphilis Study** was another notorious ethical lapse—among the most egregious in the history of medical research—in which experiments were conducted on African American men without their consent.

△ KEY IDEA

Federal research ethics regulations are based in international guidelines developed in the 20th century in response to historic tragedies occurring in the name of scientific research.

In response to these grievous ethical lapses, the **Belmont Report** outlined three ethical principles pertaining to human participants in research in the United States: (1) respect for persons, (2) beneficence, and (3) justice (National Commission for the Protection of Human Subjects of Biomedical and Behavioral Research, 1979). **Respect for persons** recognizes that individuals possess autonomy and require informed consent to participate in research studies. **Beneficence** protects the well-being of research participants and ensures that the benefits of research are greater than the risks. When any action that decreases the welfare of any research participant, it is called

maleficence, and the opposite is called **nonmaleficence**. The principle of **justice** refers to whether the benefits and burdens are distributed fairly and whether affected groups have the opportunity to participate in making decisions. These principles guide ethical conduct when conducting research with human subjects.

FUTURE DIRECTIONS

As private equity investors and for-profit corporations control larger portions of the U.S. healthcare delivery system (Goddard, 2022), health services managers will need to confront demands for increased profit margins by asking, "How much margin is enough to meet our mission?" (Culbertson, 2019). The pressure to balance mission and margin is not unique to health services businesses, nor is it a new phenomenon for health services managers. Management scholars have debated the ethics of profit maximization for at least 50 years. Milton Friedman wrote, "there is one and only one social responsibility of business—to use its resources and engage in activities designed to increase its profits so long as it . . . engages in open and free competition without deception or fraud" (Friedman, 1970, p. 427). In contrast, Peter Drucker wrote that "the business enterprise . . . exists for the sake of the contribution which it makes to the welfare of society as a whole" (Drucker, 1990, p. 208).

Contradictory forces have clashed in healthcare for decades, such as when charity hospitals transitioned into large nonprofit corporations in the 1980s. At that time, tension between business and service to patients was in the hands of the Catholic sisters running the HCOs, who popularized the maxim, "No margin, no mission" (Newport, 1991). Today, balancing margin and mission is the responsibility of the health services management profession. Going forward, it will not be easy for health services managers to uphold professional obligations and guide an ethical HCO while confronting intensifying profit pressures of the evolving healthcare environment. Nonetheless, with a commitment to ethics and professionalism, health services managers will be able to strengthen their profession and authority in the HCO to support functions related to high-quality patient care.

SUMMARY

- Health services managers have largely succeeded in claiming privileges of professionalism through education, credentials, and commitments to professionalism and ethics.
- Professionalism in health services management means embracing motivations, such as helping patients, empowering clinicians, building community ties, and serving society, while controlling costs as good stewards of scarce HCO resources.
- Professionalism includes appropriate presentation oneself to others; a strong work ethic; self-management skills; lifelong learning; acting with integrity; connections to community and the profession; and valuing diversity, equity, and inclusion.
- Since health services managers are responsible for the systems and procedures of the HCO, they have the ethical obligation for addressing challenges associated with allocating resources.
- Identifying ethical decision requires that health services managers engage in systematic analysis of relevant facts, ethical theories, professional codes, and/or HCO values, and collaborating with others to evaluate potential alternative actions and justifications.
- Health services managers create organizational cultures that foster ethical behaviors by modeling appropriate behaviors and creating ethics structures, such as compliance programs, ethics committees, and institutional review boards.

END-OF-CHAPTER RESOURCES

KEY TERMS*

*For the full list of key terms, please see the online glossary at **http://connect.springerpub.com/content/book/978-0-8261-4807-0**.

advance directive
authorized user
autonomy
Belmont report
beneficence
best interests standard
breach of contract
business associate
case consultation
casuistry
clinical ethics
coaching
code of ethics
common rule
communitarianism
compliance programs
confidentiality
conflict of interest
covered entity
data use agreement
Declaration of Helsinki
deontology
disclosure
discrimination
Emergency Medical Treatment and Labor Act (EMTALA)
end-of-life care
enlightened self-interest
ethics
ethics committee
ethical dilemma
executive presence
fidelity
False Claims Act
federal-wide assurance of compliance
fraud and abuse
Health Information Technology for Economic and Clinical Health (HITECH) Act
Health Insurance Portability and Accountability Act (HIPAA)
informational interviews
informed consent
Institutional Review Boards (IRBs)
integrity
justice
law fallacy
licensed independent professional
Lexington Model
malfeasance
management by walking around
medical futility
Medicare recovery audit program
mentoring
modeling
moral distress
moral injury
morality
morals
networking
nonmaleficence
Nuremberg Code
patient rights and responsibilities
preferential treatment
privacy rule
professionalism
promise-making
protected health information
proxy
racism
resilience
respect for persons
security
sexual harassment
sponsorship
tortious interference
transparency
trust
Tuskegee Syphilis Study
unrelated business income
upcoded
utilitarianism
whistleblowing
work ethic

LEARNING ACTIVITIES

Professional Development and Reflection

1. In *The Road to Character*, David Brooks distinguishes between résumé virtues and eulogy virtues. Your résumé contains job titles and professional successes. Your eulogy will include stories about your character, such as kindness, integrity, empathy, and trustworthiness. Brooks argues that we are too worried about our career accomplishments and not nearly concerned enough with what people say about us when we are gone. When faced with an ethical dilemma, which virtue will you be considering? Résumé virtues or eulogy virtues? Write some examples of eulogy virtues that you believe will be or have been valuable in your professional career.

2. Health services managers create professional connections with others to support their own and other's career development. For the following professional relationships, identify one person you can ask to serve in the role. If you do not know anyone, describe a plan to identify a person that could fulfill the role.
   a. Formal or informal mentor
   b. Professional development advisor
   c. Career sponsor
   d. Political guide
   e. Career coach

Discussion Questions

1. What role does work ethic play in the perception of early careerists by executive health services managers? Can a strong work ethic sometimes lead to unhealthy work hours or an imbalance between work and personal life? How can this be managed effectively?

2. The chapter describes the expectation for health services managers to give back to the community through volunteerism and philanthropy. Why is volunteerism and philanthropy considered part of health services management professionalism?

3. How can early-career health services managers effectively network with executive-level health services managers? What strategies can they employ to make the most out of these networking opportunities? How might these approaches enhance professional relationships and opportunities for career development? Discuss the consequences of networking in ways perceived as unprofessional.

RECOMMENDED READING AND MEDIA

American College of Healthcare Executives. (2022). *ACHE code of ethics*. https://www.ache.org/about-ache/our-story/our-commitments/ethics/ache-code-of-ethics

American College of Healthcare Executives. (2023). *ACHE policy statements*. https://www.ache.org/about-ache/our-story/our-commitments/policy-statements

Baedke, L., & Lamberton, N. (2018). *The emerging healthcare leader: A field guide*. Health Administration Press.

Baedke, L. (2023). *Mentor, coach, lead to peak professional performance*. American College of Healthcare Executives.

Brooks, D. (2015). *The road to character*. Random House.

Brooks, D. (2023). How America got mean. *The Atlantic*. https://www.theatlantic.com/magazine/archive/2023/09/us-culture-moral-education-formation/674765

Duckworth A. (2016). *Grit: The power of passion and perseverance*. Scribner.

Falcone, P. (2022). *Workplace ethics: Mastering ethical leadership and sustaining a moral workplace*. HarperCollins Leadership.

Fielding, J. (2023). *All pride, no ego: A queer executive's journey to living and leading authentically*. John Wiley and Sons, Inc.

McPherson, S. (2021, February 12). How much of your "authentic self" should you really bring to work?. *Harvard Business Review*. https://hbr.org/2021/02/how-much-of-your-authentic-self-should-you-really-bring-to-work

Meacham, M. R. (2015). *From backpack to briefcase*. Cengage Learning.

Sandberg, S. (2014). *Lean in*. Random House.

Stanford Life Design Lab. (2017, September 30). *Designing your career: The informational interview*. YouTube. https://www.youtube.com/watch?v=m6Pa4ZB4mvQ

Wilkinson, B. (2021) *The diversity gap: Where good intentions meet true cultural change*. HarperCollins Leadership.

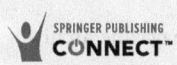

A robust set of instructor resources designed to supplement this text is located at http://connect.springerpub.com/content/book/978-0-8261-4807-0. Qualifying instructors may request access by emailing textbook@springerpub.com.

REFERENCES

Abbott, A. (1988). *The system of professions*. University of Chicago Press.

Agris, J., Brichto, E., Meacham, M., & Louis, C. (2018). Developing professionalism in healthcare management programs: An examination of accreditation outcomes. *Journal of Health Administration Education, 35*(2), 187–203.

Alder, S., Kelleher, A., & Greene, S. (2017). HIPAA compliance guide. *HIPAA Journal*, 2–65.

Alhazmi, F. (2019). *The ethical challenge of conflicts of interest in healthcare*. [Doctoral dissertation, Duquesne University]. https://dsc.duq.edu/etd/1780

American College of Healthcare Executives. (2015). *Considering the value of experienced healthcare executives regardless of age*. https://www.ache.org/about-ache/our-story/our-commitments/policy-statements/considering-the-value-of-experienced-healthcare-executives-regardless-of-age

American College of Healthcare Executives. (2018). *Lifelong learning and the healthcare executive*. https://www.ache.org/about-ache/our-story/our-commitments/policy-statements/lifelong-learning-and-the-healthcare-executive

American College of Healthcare Executives. (2019, November 18). *Responsibility for mentoring*. https://www.ache.org/about-ache/our-story/our-commitments/policy-statements/responsibility-for-mentoring

American College of Healthcare Executives. (2021). *Promise making, keeping and rescinding*. https://www.ache.org/about-ache/our-story/our-commitments/ethics/ache-code-of-ethics/promise-making-keeping-and-rescinding

American College of Healthcare Executives. (2022a). *ACHE code of ethics*. https://www.ache.org/about-ache/our-story/our-commitments/ethics/ache-code-of-ethics

American College of Healthcare Executives. (2022b). *ACHE statement on diversity*. https://www.ache.org/about-ache/our-story/our-commitments/policy-statements/statement-on-diversity

American College of Healthcare Executives. (2022c). *Board Certification in Healthcare Management*. https://www.ache.org/about-ache/our-story/our-commitments/policy-statements/board-certification-in-healthcare-management

American College of Healthcare Executives. (2023). *Membership*. https://www.ache.org/membership

American Health Information Management Association. (2019, April 29). *AHIMA Code of Ethics*. https://bok.ahima.org/doc?oid=105098

Austin, T., Chreim, S., & Grudniewicz, A. (2020). Examining health care providers' and middle-level managers' readiness for change: A qualitative study. *BMC Health Services Research, 20*(1), 1–14. https://doi.org/10.1186/s12913-020-4897-0

Baedke, L. (2023). *Mentor, coach, lead to peak professional performance*. American College of Healthcare Executives.

Baedke, L., & Lamberton, N. (2018). *The emerging healthcare leader: A field guide*. Health Administration Press.

Bandura, A. (1997). *Self-efficacy: The exercise of control*. W.H. Freeman and Company.

Begun, J. W. (1986). Economic and sociological approaches to professionalism. *Work and occupations, 13*(1), 113–129. https://doi.org/10.1177/0730888486013001008

Begun, J. W., Butler, P. W., & Stefl, M. E. (2018). Competencies to what end? Affirming the purpose of healthcare management. *Journal of Health Administration Education, 35*(2), 133–155.

Begun, J. W., White, K. R., & Mosser, G. (2011). Interprofessional care teams: The role of the healthcare administrator. *Journal of Interprofessional Care, 25*(2), 119–123. https://doi.org/10.3109/13561820.2010.504135

Berlin, G., Darino L., Greenfield M., Starikova I. (2019). *Women in the healthcare industry*. McKinsey & Co. https://www.mckinsey.com/~/media/McKinsey/Industries/Healthcare%20Systems%20and%20Services/Our%20Insights/Women%20in%20the%20healthcare%20industry/Women-in-the-healthcare-industry-FINAL.pdf

Brooks, D. (2023). How America got mean. *The Atlantic*. https://www.theatlantic.com/magazine/archive/2023/09/us-culture-moral-education-formation/674765

Brown, S. E. (2012). Attracting, challenging, and leading a multigenerational workforce: A perspective. *Frontiers of Health Services Management, 29*(1), 29–33. https://doi.org/10.1097/01974520-201207000-00004

Burnison, G. (2018). *Lose the résumé: Land the job*. John Wiley & Sons, Inc.

Chow, R. (2023, February 14). Don't just sponsor women and people of color—defend them. *Harvard Business Review*. https://hbr.org/2023/02/dont-just-sponsor-women-and-people-of-color-defend-them

Collins, J. (2015). Foreword. In Drucker, P. F., *The effective executive*. HarperBusiness.

Collins, R. (2019). *The credential society: An historical sociology of education and stratification*. Columbia University Press.

Comfort, L. K., Boin, A., & Demchak, C. C. (2010). *Designing resilience: Preparing for extreme events*. University of Pittsburgh Press.

Commission on Accreditation of Healthcare Management Education. (2023). *Accredited programs search*. https://cahme.org/advance/

Coustasse, A. (2021). Upcoding medicare: Is healthcare fraud and abuse increasing? *Perspectives in Health Information Management, 18*(4), 1f.

Cox, G. (2022). *Leading inclusion: Drive change your employees can see and feel*. Page Two.

Culbertson, R. (2019). Reflections on the Pattullo Lecture: An Ethics Perspective. *The Journal of Health Administration Education, 36*(1), 27.

Currall, S. C., & Judge, T. A. (1995). Measuring trust between organizational boundary role persons. *Organizational Behavior and Human Decision Processes, 64*(2), 151–170. https://doi.org/10.1006/obhd.1995.1097

Damania, Z. (2019, March 8). *It's not burnout, it's moral injury*. YouTube.com. https://www.youtube.com/watch?v=L_1PNZdHq6Q&t=18s

Darr, K. (2019). *Ethics in health services management*. (6th ed.). Health Professions Press.

Davis, J. H., Schoorman, F. D., & Donaldson, L. (2007). Toward a stewardship theory of management. In A. E. Singer (Ed.), *Business ethics and strategy, Volumes I and II* (pp. 473–500). Routledge.

Dean, W., Talbot, S., & Dean, A. (2019). Reframing clinician distress: Moral injury not burnout. *Federal Practitioner, 36*(9), 400–402.

Donnellan, J. J., Jr. (2013). A moral compass for management decision making: A healthcare CEO's reflections. *Frontiers of Health Services Management, 30*(1), 14–26.

Dreachslin, J. L., Weech-Maldonado, R., Gail, J., Epané, J. P., & Wainio, J. A. (2017). Blueprint for sustainable change in diversity management and cultural competence: Lessons from the National Center for Healthcare Leadership diversity demonstration project. *Journal of Healthcare Management, 62*(3), 171–183. https://doi.org/10.1097/jhm-d-15-00029

Drucker, P. F. (1990). *Managing the nonprofit organization: Practices and principles.* New York: HarperCollins.

Drucker, P. F. (2005, January). Managing oneself. *Harvard Business Review.* https://hbr.org/2005/01/managing-oneself

Duckworth, A. (2016). *Grit: The power of passion and perseverance.* Scribner.

Falcone, P. (2022). *Workplace ethics: Mastering ethical leadership and sustaining a moral workplace.* HarperCollins Leadership.

Fielding, J. (2023). *All pride, no ego: A queer executive's journey to living and leading authentically.* John Wiley and Sons, Inc.

Frich, J. C., Brewster, A. L., Cherlin, E. J., & Bradley, E. H. (2015). Leadership development programs for physicians: A systematic review. *Journal of General Internal Medicine, 30*(5), 656–674. https://doi.org/10.1007/s11606-014-3141-1

Friedman, M. (1970, September, 13). A Friedman doctrine—The social responsibility of business is to increase its profits. *New York Times.* https://www.nytimes.com/1970/09/13/archives/a-friedman-doctrine-the-social-responsibility-of-business-is-to.html

Garman, A. N., Boren, S., Masuda, D., & Shah, S. C. (2020). Mapping national center for healthcare leadership competencies to the CAHME accreditation competency domains. *The Journal of Health Administration Education, 37*(1), 349–354.

Garman, A. N., & Johnson, M. P. (2006). Leadership competencies: An introduction. *Journal of Healthcare Management, 51*(1), 13–17.

Goddard, R. (2022, September 14). *Healthcare vertical integration: Back to the future.* Lumeris. https://www.lumeris.com/healthcare-vertical-integration-back-to-the-future

Gollwitzer, P. M. (1999). Implementation intentions: Strong effects of simple plans. *American Psychologist, 54*(7), 493.

Gray, A. (2019, June 4). The bias of 'professionalism' standards. *Stanford Social Innovation Review.* https://ssir.org/articles/entry/the_bias_of_professionalism_standards

Gray, K. (2022, March 4). *Addressing the shifting standards of professionalism.* National Association of Colleges and Employers. https://www.naceweb.org/career-readiness/competencies/addressing-the-shifting-standards-of-professionalism

Griffith, J. R. (1993). *The moral challenges of health care management.* Health Administration Press.

Gurchiek, K. (2018, August 17). "Managers Play Significant Role in Creating Diverse Teams." SHRM. https://www.shrm.org/topics-tools/news/inclusion-equity-diversity/managers-play-significant-role-creating-diverse-teams.

Healthcare Financial Management Association. (2022, December 22). *Bylaws and code of ethics.* https://www.hfma.org/about-hfma/bylaws-and-code-of-ethics

Hussein, M., Pavlova, M., Ghalwash, M., & Groot, W. (2021). The impact of hospital accreditation on the quality of healthcare: A systematic literature review. *BMC Health Services Research, 21*(1), 1–12. https://doi.org/10.1186/s12913-021-07097-6

Jameton, A. (1984). *Nursing practice: The ethical issues.* Prentice-Hall.

Johnson, W. B., & Smith, D. G. (2019, December 30). Real mentorship starts with company culture, not formal programs. *Harvard Business Review.* https://hbr.org/2019/12/real-mentorship-starts-with-company-culture-not-formal-programs

Kagan, S. (2018). *Normative ethics.* Routledge/Taylor & Francis.

Karpoff, J. M. (2021). On a stakeholder model of corporate governance. *Financial Management, 50*(2), 321–343. https://doi.org/10.1111/fima.12344

Khurana, R., Nohria, N., & Penrice, D. (2004). *Management as a profession.* Centre for Public Leadership.

Kraman, S. S., & Hamm, G. (1999). Risk management: Extreme honesty may be the best policy. *Annals of Internal Medicine, 131*(12), 963–967. https://doi.org/10.7326/0003-4819-131-12-199912210-00010

Komesaroff, P. A., Kerridge, I., & Lipworth, W. (2019). Conflicts of interest: New thinking, new processes. *Internal Medicine Journal, 49*(5), 574–577. https://doi.org/10.1111/imj.14233

Lear, J. L., Fleig-Palmer, M. M., Hodge, K. A., Fleig, M. J., & Arensdorf, A. (2016). Business fundamentals for healthcare providers: Ensuring effective practice management and good stewardship. *Journal of Health Administration Education, 33*(1), 141–162.

Lesandrini, J., & Reis, D. (2022). Ethical challenges in staffing: The importance of building moral muscle. *Frontiers of Health Services Management, 38*(4), 33–38. https://doi.org/10.1097/hap.0000000000000140

McCluney, C. L., Robotham, K. J., Lee, S., Smith, R. E., II., & Durkee M. I. (2019). The costs of code-switching. *Harvard Business Review*. https://hbr.org/2019/11/the-costs-of-codeswitching

McPherson, S. (2021, February 12). How much of your "authentic self" should you really bring to work?. *Harvard Business Review*. https://hbr.org/2021/02/how-much-of-your-authentic-self-should-you-really-bring-to-work

Medical Group Management Association. (2015, September 29). *Code of ethics*. https://mgma.com/MGMA/media/files/about/Code-of-Ethics-Approved.pdf

Meriac, J. P., Woehr, D. J., & Banister, C. (2010). Generational differences in work ethic: An examination of measurement equivalence across three cohorts. *Journal of Business and Psychology, 25*(2), 315–324. http://doi.org/10.1007/s10869-010-9164-7

Miller, M. J., Woehr, D. J., & Hudspeth, N. (2002). The meaning and measurement of work ethic: Construction and initial validation of a multidimensional inventory. *Journal of Vocational Behavior, 60*(3), 451–489. http://doi.org/10.1006/jvbe.2001.1838

Moore, M. G. (2022, August 16). *5 rules of thumb for leadership transparency*. https://www.linkedin.com/pulse/5-rules-thumb-leadership-transparency-martin-g-moore

National Association of Long Term Care Administrator Boards [NAB]. (2022). "State Licensure Requirements." https://nabweb.org/seeking-licensure/state-licensure-requirements.

National Center for Healthcare Leadership. (2018). *Health leadership competency model 3.0*. https://nchl.member365.org/publicFr/store/item/19

National Commission for the Protection of Human Subjects of Biomedical and Behavioral Research. (1979). *The Belmont Report: Ethical principles and guidelines for the protection of human subjects of research*. U.S. Department of Health, Education, and Welfare.

Nelson, W. A. (2015, July-August). Making ethical decisions. *Healthcare executive*. https://www.ache.org/-/media/ache/about-ache/ja15_ethic_reprint.pdf

Newport, J. P. (1991, June 9). Health care; mission + margin: The nun as C.E.O. *The New York Times*. https://www.nytimes.com/1991/06/09/magazine/health-care-mission-margin-the-nun-as-ceo.html

Omadeke, J. (2021, October 20). What's the difference between a mentor and a sponsor? *Harvard Business Review*. https://hbr.org/2021/10/whats-the-difference-between-a-mentor-and-a-sponsor

Post, L. F., & Blustein, J. (2021). *Handbook for health care ethics committees*. JHU Press.

Saini, V., Garber, J., & Brownlee, S. (2022, February 10). *Nonprofit hospital CEO compensation: How much Is enough?*. Health Affairs Forefront. https://www.healthaffairs.org/content/forefront/nonprofit-hospital-ceo-compensation-much-enough

Sakowski, J. A., Hewitt, A. M., Johri, N., & Wagner, S. L. (2020). Implementing an incremental approach for developing leadership and professionalism skills among early careerists in the health administration curriculum. *Journal of Health Administration Education, 37*(2), 89–104.

Scott, P. A., Harvey, C., Felzmann, H., Suhonen, R., Habermann, M., Halvorsen, K., Christiansen, K., Toffoli, L., & Papastavrou, E. (2019). Resource allocation and rationing in nursing care: A discussion paper. *Nursing Ethics, 26*(5), 1528–1539. https://doi.org/10.1177/0969733018759831

Smith, D. D. (2021, June 30). If you want to lead, master this skill. *Harvard Business Review*. https://hbr.org/2021/06/if-you-want-to-lead-master-this-skill

Taygerly, T. (2022, September 14). How to develop a strong work ethic. *Harvard Business Review*. https://hbr.org/2022/09/how-to-develop-a-strong-work-ethic

Taylor, B. (2012). *Healthcare philanthropy*. Health Administration Press.

Terp, S., Seabury, S. A., Arora, S., Eads, A., Lam, C. N., & Menchine, M. (2017). Enforcement of the Emergency Medical Treatment and Labor Act, 2005 to 2014. *Annals of Emergency Medicine, 69*(2), 155–162. https://doi.org/10.1016/j.annemergmed.2016.05.021

Thompson, R. A. (2012). Whither the preconventional child? Toward a life-span moral development theory. *Child Development Perspectives, 6*(4), 423–429. http://doi.org/10.1111/j.1750-8606.2012.00245.x

Tucker, A. L., & Singer, S. J. (2015). The effectiveness of management-by-walking-around: A randomized field study. *Production and Operations Management, 24*(2), 253–271.

Vanderkam, L. (2011). *168 hours: You have more time than you think*. Portfolio/Penguin.

Varkey, B. (2021). Principles of clinical ethics and their application to practice. *Medical Principles and Practice, 30*(1), 17–28. https://doi.org/10.1159/000509119

Varga, A. I., Spehar, I., & Skirbekk, H. (2023). Trustworthy management in hospital settings: A systematic review. *BMC Health Services Research, 23*(1), 662.

Victor, D. (2017, July 6). When the boss wants you to do something unethical. *New York Times*. https://www.nytimes.com/2017/07/06/smarter-living/work-ethics-advice.html

Walker, A. M. (2020). Strategic succession planning for a hopeful future. *Frontiers of Health Services Management, 36*(4), 31–36. https://doi.org/10.1097/hap.0000000000000085

Weber, M. (1958). *The Protestant ethic and the spirit of capitalism*, trans. T. Parsons. Charles Scribner's Sons.

Wilkinson, B. (2021). *The diversity gap: Where good intentions meet true cultural change*. HarperCollins Leadership.

Woehr, D. J., Arciniega, L. M., González, L., & Stanley, L. J. (2023). Live to work, work to live, and work as a necessary evil: An examination of the structure and stability of work ethic profiles. *Group & Organization Management*. https://doi.org/10.1177/10596011221146363

Zabel, K. L., Biermeier-Hanson, B. B., Baltes, B. B., Early, B. J., & Shepard, A. (2017). Generational differences in work ethic: Fact or fiction?. *Journal of Business and Psychology, 32*(3), 301–315. http://doi.org/10.1007/s10869-016-9466-5

CHAPTER 6

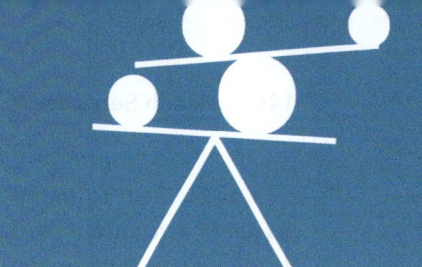

POPULATION HEALTH AND COMMUNITY COLLABORATION

Population health means that health care organizations accept financial responsibility for keeping a group of patients healthy. Community collaboration entails engaging with external organizations to improve the health, social, and economic strength of the community.

COMPETENCIES

- Innovate health services delivery in response to trends in healthcare policy and financing.
- Assess population health status and respond to changing needs of patient populations.
- Invest in population health management functions, such as risk-based financing, staff reorganization, and health information technology, to improve quality and reduce costs.
- Innovate health services operations with public health approaches, such as epidemiology and program planning and evaluation.
- Integrate social care with medical care to address social determinants of health, such as housing, food, and transportation.
- Collaborate with community organizations to improve population health and respond to emergencies.
- Advocate for patients, families, and communities by influencing healthcare policy at the local, state, and national levels.
- Promote health care organizations as community anchors for economic, ecological, and social development.
- Volunteer for community events, programs, and initiatives.

CHAPTER OUTLINE

- Population Health Assessment
- Population Health Management
- Community Collaboration

INTRODUCTION

The U.S. healthcare system spends too much on short-term interventions for individual patients and not enough on long-term prevention for populations. The healthcare system is commonly described using the upstream parable in which a physician is standing at the shore of a rapidly flowing river when a drowning person floats by (McKinlay, 1979). The physician jumps into the river, pulls them to shore, and resuscitates them. Then the physician sees a second drowning person to save, then a third person, then a fourth, and so on. Too busy saving people one by one, the physician could not go upstream to help people who were falling into the river in the first place. The U.S. healthcare system is designed to address downstream problems, not upstream causes.

When clinicians diagnose and treat individual patients in order to cure or prevent progression of disease, it is known as the **medical model** (Nash et al., 2021). As the upstream parable describes, the medical model emphasizes interventions within health care facilities after a patient is already sick. In many ways, Americans have access to the best clinicians in the world, but they cannot overcome the behavioral, social, and economic factors that cause sickness (Schneider et al., 2021). Recognizing the need to move upstream, government payers and health insurance companies are changing how they pay for health services. The **population health model** requires that health care organizations (HCOs) accept financial responsibility for the health of a group of patients (Atkins et al., 2020). The Institute of Medicine (IOM) popularized the term population health in their **Triple Aim** framework for U.S. healthcare system improvement. In addition to population health, the Triple Aim calls for improving patient experience and reducing overall costs of care to the system (IOM, Berwick, Nolan, & Whittington, 2008).

Clinicians, otherwise burdened with caring for an ever-increasing number of individual patients, need assistance from health services managers to address population health. As this chapter describes, the population health model requires that health services managers adapt HCO workforce and organizational processes to address the upstream causes of sickness. To improve population health, managers must understand the underlying causes of disease in the communities they serve and make significant but judicious investments in new health services management functions.

POPULATION HEALTH ASSESSMENT

Community Health Needs Assessments

To address the health of populations, health services managers first need to understand the communities that they serve. The **community health needs assessment** (CHNA) is a process of analyzing the health needs of a defined population, the services available to them, and the interventions required to meet their needs. In other words, CHNAs serve to identify gaps between the current health of the population and their community health goals. Health services managers use the CHNAs to prioritize health needs, set population health goals, and develop programs that address the gaps in community health and well-being (Burns et al., 2023). According to regulations mandated by the Affordable Care Act (ACA), all not-for-profit hospitals and health systems must conduct CHNAs every 3 years and implement interventions intended to improve population health (Institute for Healthcare Improvement [IHI], 2018). The Internal Revenue Service (IRS) evaluates the written CHNAs submitted by not-for-profit HCOs to justify their tax-exempt status with valuable benefits to communities (Pennel et al., 2016). Figure 6.1 illustrates the elements of CHNAs.

Community Stakeholders

Stakeholders collaborate to identify and prioritize the most critical community health problems. Common CHNA collaborators include local health departments, physicians, community health centers, public schools, academic institutions, faith-based organizations, local elected officials,

FIGURE 6.1 Elements of community health needs assessments.

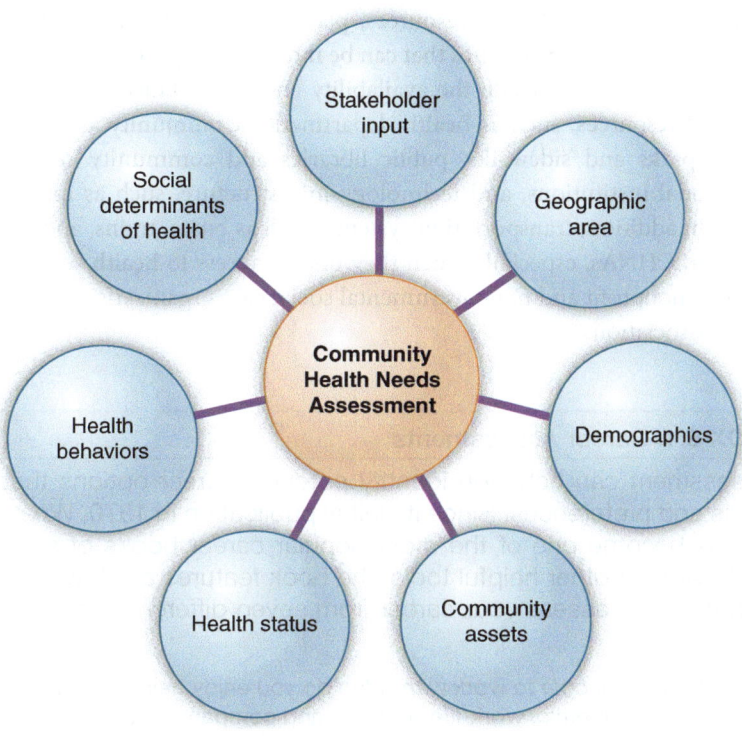

and nonprofit organizations that represent underserved populations. Health services managers and public health professionals collect data from community stakeholders through surveys, interviews, and focus groups (Pennel et al., 2016). Effective CHNA collaborations frequently turn into sustained population health partnerships (Hilts et al., 2021).

△ KEY IDEA
Effective CHNA collaborations frequently turn into sustained population health partnerships.

Geographic and Demographic Characteristics

When developing CHNAs, health services managers need to define the geographic area of the HCO, known as the **catchment area**. Generally, the catchment area includes the zip codes, census tracks, or counties that surround the HCO from which a certain proportion of patients obtain care from their facility (Ravaghi et al., 2023). For example, a zip code might be included in the catchment area if more than 50% of the patients obtained care from the HCO. Health services managers also use geographic information system (GIS) software to create maps of where a current or potential patient residences by distance from the HCO. CHNAs document the demographic composition of the population living in the catchment area, especially those factors related to morbidity and mortality, such as age, race, ethnicity, gender, and poverty. Also, CHNAs incorporate relevant community occupations, especially dangerous jobs that impact health status, such as loggers or migrant farmworkers. Demographics also include the health insurance types and rates of the community.

Community Assets

Community assets are the collective resources, places, businesses, organizations, and people available to individuals and communities that can be mobilized to promote health and well-being (Ravaghi et al., 2023). Assets include the availability and accessibility of clinical care facilities and other medical resources, such as health departments. Community assets also include the local employers, parks and sidewalks, public libraries and community centers, recreational facilities, educational institutions, and technology infrastructure, such as internet and mobile phone coverage. In addition, transportation systems, such as buses, trains, and highway systems are documented in CHNAs, especially when they impact access to health services. Community assets also include nonprofit and nongovernmental social care organizations, faith communities, and community associations.

CAREER BOX 6.1: Career Assessments

A career assessment can help you identify potential career options that would align with your skills and preferences. Since its initial publication in 1970, *What Color Is Your Parachute?* has become one of the most popular career books of all time (Bolles & Brooks, 2021). Among other helpful tools, the book features a "Flower Diagram" exercise that can help you assess your career from seven different perspectives (Bolles & Brooks, 2021):

- *Preferred kinds of people to work with:* Who do you enjoy being around? Who motivates you? Consider work ethic, work-life balance, and company culture.
- *Preferred working conditions:* Under which working conditions are you most productive? Consider office setting, virtual or hybrid work arrangements, number of meetings, and work-related socializing.
- *Skills and competencies:* What skills do you enjoy using? Consider the competencies listed at the beginning of each chapter of this book.
- *Values:* What things are important to you? What values do you live your life by? What do you act on repeatedly and consistently? How will those motivate your career choices?
- *Fields of knowledge:* What knowledge areas interest you most? What do you know from previous jobs? Consider your favorite subjects, courses, or experiences from college or graduate school.
- *Level of responsibility:* Are you seeking a leadership role, or do you prefer a team member role? What level of responsibilities do you want in 5 years? 20 years?
- *Salary and level of lifestyle:* What are your financial and lifestyle goals? Higher salaries have practical benefits but consider potential trade-offs.

The flower diagram is a practical tool for visualizing your professional preferences, skills, and aspirations that will enable you to make more informed decisions about your career.

Health Status

The CHNA needs to define the current health status of the community. **Epidemiology**, defined as the study of the distribution and determinants of disease in populations, is a fundamental health services management competency used in developing CHNAs. Two epidemiology concepts are crucial to defining the health status of a community—prevalence and incidence. **Prevalence** is

TABLE 6.1 Example *Healthy People 2030's* High-Priority Health Status Measures

HEALTH STATUS MEASURES	MEASURE DEFINITION	MOST RECENT DATA	2030 GOAL
Diabetes	Incidence per 1,000 adults aged 18 to 84	5.5	4.8
Hypertension	Percentage of adults aged 18 and over with hypertension under control	16.1	18.9
Maternal mortality	Maternal deaths per 100,000 live births	32.9	15.7
Infant deaths	Infant deaths per 1,000 live births	5.4	5.0
Suicide	Suicides per 100,000 population	14.1	12.8
Drug overdose deaths	Drug overdose deaths per 100,000 population	32.4	20.7

the proportion of a disease found to have been affecting a particular population, usually for a period of time. **Incidence** is the measure of new developments of a given disease in a population within a specified period of time. In other words, prevalence indicates how many people are currently diagnosed with the disease, whereas incidence conveys information about the rate at which people are contracting the disease.

Health outcomes are quantifiable indicators of health used to describe a population's health status. There are many sources of health outcomes data, including the Centers for Disease Control and Prevention, American Community Survey, Dartmouth Atlas of Health Care, and U.S. National Center for Health Statistics (Steifel et al., 2021). In addition, the U.S. Office of Disease Prevention and Health Promotion publishes more than 350 population health measures in the *Healthy People 2030* framework that sets health goals for the nation. Table 6.1 provides examples of *Healthy People 2030's* high-priority health status measures (Office of Disease Prevention and Health Promotion [ODPHP], 2021).

The University of Wisconsin's County Health Rankings' model emphasizes four categories of factors related to the health outcomes of populations (County Health Rankings & Roadmaps, 2022). As shown in Figure 6.2, the County Health Rankings' model employs a scientifically informed methodology that weighs the factors impacting health outcomes. These factors include social and economic factors (40%), health behaviors (30%), clinical care (20%), and physical environment (10%). Genetic causes of sickness are not included because the model focuses on the factors that can be changed in order to improve population health. Measures from the County Health Rankings' model can be used to write CHNAs and prioritize investments in population health interventions (Purtle et al., 2019).

Health Behaviors

Health behaviors are the personal actions that impact health and well-being positively or negatively, including smoking, exercise, and vaccinations. Public health practitioners have traditionally placed intense focus on the unhealthy behaviors (Marmot & Allen, 2014). The assumption underlying this approach is that individuals are largely responsible for their own health and can improve health through better health behaviors, such as exercising, eating sensibly, and not smoking. Table 6.2 provides examples of *Healthy People 2030's* high-priority health behavior measures (ODPHP, 2021).

FIGURE 6.2 County Health Rankings model with the weighted impacts on health outcomes.

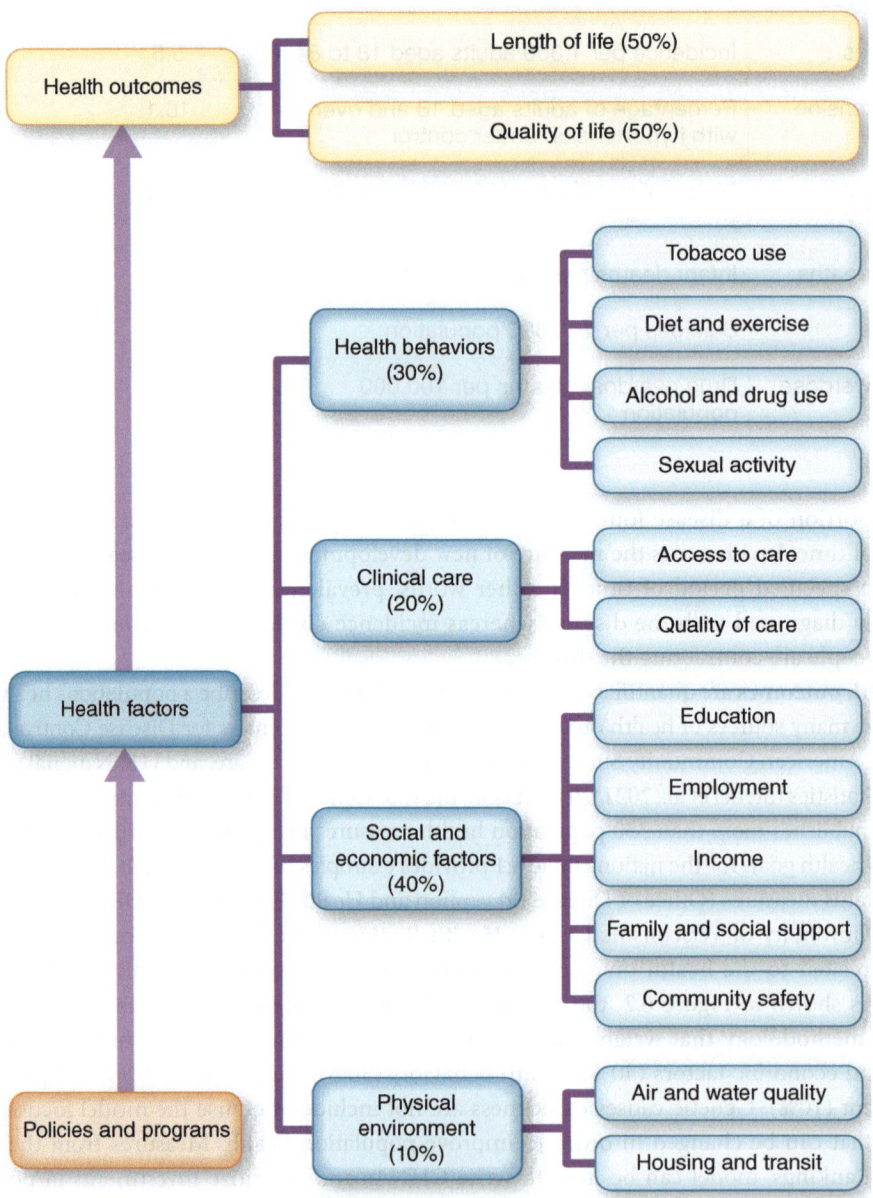

Source: Adapted from County Health Rankings Model. https://www.countyhealthrankings.org/explore-health-rankings/measures-data-sources/county-health-rankings-model. Copyright 2024 by County Health Rankings.

In addition to *Healthy People 2030*, other national surveys collect data on health-related risk behaviors and use of preventive services, including the American Community Survey, Behavioral Risk Factor Surveillance Survey, and National Center for Health Statistics (Steifel et al., 2021). The County Health Rankings & Roadmaps program compiles many of these measures on their website (County Health Rankings & Roadmaps, 2022).

TABLE 6.2 Example *Healthy People 2030's* **High-Priority Health Behavior Measures**

HEALTH BEHAVIOR MEASURES	MEASURE DEFINITION	MOST RECENT DATA	GOAL
Cigarette smoking	Percentage of adults aged 18 and over, current cigarette smokers	11.7	6.1
Binge drinking	Percentage of adults engaging in binge drinking of alcoholic beverages during the past 30 days	26.0	25.4
Exercise	Percentage of adults aged 18 years and over who met the guidelines for aerobic physical activity and muscle-strengthening activity during their leisure time	25.3	29.7
Calories from added sugars	Mean percentage of calories from added sugars consumed	13.2	11.5
Colorectal screening	Percentage of adults aged 45 to 75 years who received a colorectal cancer screening within year	58.7	68.3
Influenza vaccines	Percentage of people vaccinated against seasonal influenza within the last flu season	49.8	70.0

Physical Environment

CHNAs also commonly include factors related to the physical environment, such as air pollution, water quality, and lead exposure (Thomas, 2022). These measures are especially important to document in the CHNA given the relationship between toxic environments and poor population health (Fuller et al., 2022). Examples of measures from the County Health Rankings website include the density of fine particulate matter and the presence of health-related drinking water violations (County Health Rankings & Roadmaps, 2022).

Social and Economic Factors

According to the County Health Rankings' model, social and economic factors have the largest influence on health and well-being, accounting for 40% of the underlying causes of morbidity and mortality (County Health Rankings & Roadmaps, 2022). **Social determinants of health** are the conditions in which people are born, grow, live, work, and age, and the wider set of forces and systems shape the conditions of daily life impact health and well-being (World Health Organization [WHO], n.d.). Substantial research demonstrates how social determinants of health, such as healthy food, safety, stable housing, quality education, and gainful employment, impact health over a person's lifespan (Gottlieb et al., 2019). **Social risks**, such as poverty, food insecurity, housing instability, unreliable transportation, and lack of education, are associated with poor health outcomes in patients and health inequities among communities (Alderwick & Gottlieb, 2019). Health services managers and public health professionals now recognize the significant extent to which social determinants of health contribute to poor health (Bradley, Sipsma, & Taylor, 2017). In response, health services managers mobilize HCO resources to address social determinants of health that may exist outside of the HCO's facilities.

> **INFORMATIONAL INTERVIEW 6.1**
> *Manager of Population Health*
> Access the informational interview online at http://connect.springerpub.com/content/book/978-0-8261-4807-0/chapter/ch00.

△ KEY IDEA

Health services managers mobilize HCO resources to address social determinants of health that may exist outside of the HCO's facilities.

Sources of population-level social determinants of health measures include the U.S. Agency for Healthcare Research and Quality's database on Social Determinants of Health, Behavioral Risk Factor Surveillance Survey, and National Center for Health Statistics (Adler & Stead, 2015; Agency for Healthcare Research and Quality [AHRQ], 2023; Steifel et al., 2021). The County Health Rankings & Roadmaps program combines measures from these and other sources on their website (County Health Rankings & Roadmaps, 2022). Table 6.3 provides examples of social determinants of health within various categories included in the County Health Rankings & Roadmaps website. County Health Rankings categorize a food insecurity social risk as a "health behavior" and housing and transportation factors as "physical environment," whereas they are included as social and economic factors in other published research articles (Gottlieb et al., 2024; Pruitt, Taylor, et al., 2018).

TABLE 6.3 Example County Health Rankings Measures for Social Determinants of Health

SOCIAL DETERMINANTS	SOCIAL RISK MEASURES	DEFINITION	U.S. METRICS
Education	High school completion	Percentage of adults ages 25 and over with a high school diploma or equivalent	89
Employment	Unemployment	Percentage of population ages 16 and older unemployed but seeking work	5.4
Nutrition	Food insecurity	Percentage of population who lack adequate access to food	12
Income	Children in poverty	Percentage of people under age 18 in poverty	17
Family and social support	Social support	Number of membership associations per 10,000 people	9.1
Community safety	Injury death	Number of deaths due to injury per 100,000 population	76
Housing	Severe housing problems	Percentage of households with at least one of four housing problems: overcrowding, high housing costs, lack of kitchen facilities, or lack of plumbing facilities	17
Transit	Long commute driving alone	Among workers who commute in their car alone, the percentage that commute more than 30 minutes	37

POPULATION HEALTH MANAGEMENT

Management Functions in Population Health

Under the population health model, HCOs accept financial responsibility for reducing overall costs, enhancing patient experience, and improving health outcomes. Health services managers use the results of CHNA analysis to prioritize community health needs, set goals for population health improvement, and implement population health interventions (Hewitt & Dykstra, 2022). Adopting the population health model requires a new set of management practices called **population health management**. Figure 6.3 illustrates the population health management functions for which health services managers are responsible under the population health model, including financial management, organizational design, health information technology, cost control, and operations restructuring.

The population health model changes how health services managers operate HCOs. For example, under the medical model, hospital-based health services managers attract patients by marketing to specialist physicians who admit patients. In this model, health systems rely on physicians to generate a majority of their revenues through patient referrals, the so-called "heads in beds" incentive (Allen, 2020; Saini et al., 2022). However, under the population health model, health services managers need to reduce expensive hospital care in favor of lower cost medical services. Instead of more patients in the hospital, physicians need to be given resources to keep patients out of the hospital. This model requires a new set of management competencies.

Population Health Financial Management

The traditional financing of the U.S. healthcare system, still predominant today, is called **fee for service** because HCOs are paid a fee for each service provided. The fee-for-service methodology incentivizes clinicians to increase the volume and intensity of care provided to patients. Increasingly, the U.S. government and most commercial health insurance companies pay for health services through new financing methods called **advanced payment models** or **alternative payment models** (Nussbaum et al., 2018). In most advanced payment models, HCOs are paid a predetermined amount of money in advance to cover the total costs of caring for groups of patients. To prevent HCOs from accepting money for patients but not delivering appropriate care, payers also require that HCOs meet certain medical quality standards, a concept known as **pay for performance**.

FIGURE 6.3 Population health management functions.

Financial management	Organizational design	Health information technology	Operations redesign
• Advanced payment models • Pay-for-performance • Value-based healthcare • Risk-based financing	• Management accountability • Patient-centered medical homes • Accountable care organizations	• Care coordination • Risk stratification • Risk adjustment • Health services utilization • Cost of care	• Program planning and evaluation • Control costs • Change health behaviors • Integrate medical and social care

⚠ KEY IDEA

The concept of value in health care means achieving the best health outcomes and patient experiences at the lowest cost.

The term **value-based health care** is used to distinguish the population health financing model from the volume-based incentives associated with fee for service. In healthcare, **value** means better health outcomes at a lower cost to the entire system (Porter & Teisberg, 2006). Mathematically, value is defined as the levels of health care quality and patient experience achieved divided by the amount for the total costs, as illustrated in Figure 6.4. Total costs include the money spent by the patient, government, and health insurance companies. As a ratio of quality and patient experience to costs, there are many ways to improve healthcare value. An HCO can improve health care value by increasing health care outcomes and patient experience while keeping costs the same. Value can also be created by reducing costs while achieving the same health outcomes and patient experience.

There are several common types of advanced payment models, all designed to control costs and improve quality but each varying in terms of financial risk (Bethke et al., 2020). Under value-based contracts, HCOs risk losing money if the costs of medical care exceed the predetermined payments, a concept known as **risk-based financing**. Financial risk involves the potential for financial losses due to unexpected costs, such as unplanned increases in salaries or unanticipated health services utilization. Health services managers can negotiate varying degrees of risk when they enter into value-based contracts with payers (Pruitt & Moseley, 2018). As presented in Table 6.4, some advanced payment models may be used to share risk between HCO and payer (Bethke et al., 2020).

For example, the ACA created a landmark value-based health care program, called the **Medicare Shared Savings Program** (MSSP; Huang et al., 2023). To participate in MSSP, HCOs are required to create legal entities called **Accountable Care Organizations** (ACOs), which are formal partnerships between hospitals, physicians, long-term care, and other providers. ACOs can opt to share risk with Medicare or to take on full risk with a chance for a bigger bonus. An **upside risk** means that the HCO only risks losing the potential bonus, not more. In effect, HCOs need to meet quality goals and reduce costs in order to get a bonus, without risking financial losses. In upside and **downside risk** contracts, the HCO would be paid a set amount per patient and risk losing money if the cost-saving targets or quality goals are not met. In exchange for taking on risk, a shared savings value-based contract could deliver significant financial returns.

⚠ KEY IDEA

In exchange for taking on risk, a shared savings value-based contract could deliver significant financial returns, if costs are below the predetermined benchmark and the quality of care goals are met.

FIGURE 6.4 Value equation for value-based health care.

$$\text{Value} = \frac{\text{Health care quality} + \text{Patient experience}}{\text{Total costs}}$$

Source: Adapted from Porter, M. E., & Teisberg, E. O. (2006). *Redefining health care: Creating value-based competition on results*. Harvard Business School Press.

TABLE 6.4 Value-Based Health Care Payment Types

PAYMENT ARRANGEMENT	DESCRIPTION	RISK LEVEL	LEVEL OF SERVICES
Pay for performance	Fee-for-service payments with incentives for achieving certain health outcome performance metrics (quality of care). A percentage of the fee-for-service payments is diverted into a bonus pool that would be paid to the HCO only if meeting certain quality targets.	Low	Variable
Bundled	Episode-based payment covering physician and facility fees for defined care pathway (i.e., diagnosis to therapy)	Medium	Specific diagnosis
Shared savings—upside risk only	If the HCO meets patient care quality targets, any savings below a certain benchmark spending amount is shared as a bonus. If above spending benchmark, the HCO does not lose money.	Medium	For defined population
Shared savings—upside and downside risk	Paid a fixed amount for set period for each patient (e.g., per patient per month). If the HCO meets patient care quality targets, any savings below a certain benchmark spending amount is shared as a bonus. If above spending benchmark, the HCO loses money.	High	For defined population
Global capitation	Paid a fixed amount for set period for each patient (e.g., per patient per month) with strict rules for delivering care according to quality standards.	High	All or primary care only

HCO, health care organization.

In recent years, most ACOs have entered into two-sided risk contracts (i.e., upside and downside risk). According to one study, among the almost 300 ACOs that faced downside risk in 2022, almost two thirds generated a bonus from Medicare (Wang et al., 2023). While some ACOs lost as much as $3,700 per Medicare patient per year, the average earnings were $192 per patient per year. On average, each ACO managed about 21,000 Medicare patients in the MSSP, so the upside financial benefits could be in the millions of dollars. While these upside bonuses are attractive to health services managers, ACOs must also invest in population health initiatives, so even with the bonuses, the HCO may not generate overall profits (Huang et al., 2023).

Table 6.4 also describes the level of services associated with the value-based health care payment types. A **bundled payment** structure pays a lump sum amount for a single episode of care for specifically defined diagnoses. For example, a patient diagnosed with osteoarthritis of the hip might need joint replacement surgery and rehabilitation. Medicare would pay a bundled payment for the episode of care beginning at qualified diagnoses and ending with successful rehabilitation after surgery (Agarwal et al., 2020). The bundled payment model incentivizes cost-efficient care for a well-defined set of treatments without compromising quality. To succeed, the surgeons and facilities would need to lower costs by streamlining care processes, reducing wasted supplies, and other efficiency-increasing methods.

Value-Based Health Care Organizational Design

Population health initiatives benefit from strong executive-level support and dedicated workforce to carry out management functions (Begun & Potthoff, 2017). Because HCOs typically need to make significant investments in redesigning jobs and reporting structures, HCOs that commit to population health innovations are typically large, not-for-profit, teaching-affiliated health systems (Atkins et al., 2020). These HCOs commonly assign responsibility for population health management actions to dedicated health services managers who have the authority to make organizational decisions. For example, Cambridge Health Alliance, a Connecticut-based health system, assigned two executive health services managers to accomplish population health initiatives—one executive responsible for bolstering primary care services and the other responsible for coordinating services across health care settings (Hacker et al., 2014).

CAREER BOX 6.2: Lifelong Learning

Value-based health care, telehealth, and artificial intelligence (AI) are changing healthcare, requiring health services managers to acquire new competencies. In fact, newly acquired knowledge will be required throughout your professional career. Changes in healthcare will require you to develop new competencies. In response to the rapid pace of change, you need to commit to lifelong learning to stay relevant. The following are key aspects of building lifelong learning habits (Coleman, 2017; Hagel, 2021):

- *Commit to sustained effort:* Learning new competencies requires deep concentration. Make time and remove distractions for learning throughout your career.
- *Take risks at work:* Try something new, fix something broken, and pitch a big idea.
- *Embrace unexpected challenges:* Problems are opportunities to learn. Learning makes you adaptable and resilient in the face of change.
- *Have fun learning:* Discovering new things can be exciting and engaging. Learning builds confidence and leads to professional and personal growth.
- *Seek out experts:* Connect with others to get answers to your questions. Experts often share their experience and expertise willingly.
- *Use all available learning tools:* Learn from brilliant people with the added commitment of class participation by signing up for massive open online courses (e.g. Coursera). Take advantage of your local library, podcasts, audiobooks, and YouTube.
- *Join professional associations:* Groups of like-minded professionals, such as the American College of Healthcare Executives, can build connections as you learn new competencies.

Lifelong learning will allow you to enhance your skills, stay up-to-date with new knowledge, explore new career opportunities, and stay competitive in the job market.

At Cambridge Health Alliance, the executive responsible for outpatient care led the implementation of a **patient-centered medical home** (PCMH) model. The PCMH model creates interdisciplinary primary care teams who coordinate preventive, acute, mental health, and chronic care. The Cambridge Health Alliance moved responsibilities for managing high-risk patients out of centralized hospital-based locations and into the community-based primary care clinics (Hacker et al., 2014). More effective care coordination by these clinic-based teams reduced patient hospital admissions and emergency department visits (Allen, 2020). When health services managers allocate resources to primary care, HCOs are more likely to earn financial bonuses in value-based healthcare programs (Coyne et al., 2024).

Successful population health management also requires that HCOs reorganize how care is delivered across health care settings, such as hospitals, rehabilitation centers, and nursing homes. By integrating these organizations, ACOs improve patient care transitions from one setting of care to another and reduce duplication of services or the need for very expensive services. Under the leadership of a chief administrative officer over the ACO, Cambridge Health Alliance ACO partnered with the hospital, elder service agencies, and post-acute care providers to improve transitions of Medicare patients between the hospital and post-acute care. For example, the ACO restructured their inpatient discharge processes and identified specific personnel to improve the transitions between hospitals and post-acute rehabilitation, changes that were designed to reduce readmissions (Hacker et al., 2014).

Health Information Technology

Successful population health management also requires significant investment in health information technology systems (Atkins et al., 2020; Schario et al., 2024). Before entering into value-based purchasing contracts, health services managers need to assess whether the HCO's electronic health records (EHRs) systems can support advanced technology functions required to enable population health management. With the appropriate investments in health information technologies, health services managers can conduct a wide range of population health management activities, including the following (Coran et al., 2022; Hunt et al., 2015; Pandya et al., 2021; Schario et al., 2024):

- *Data analytics:* Apply various statistical techniques used to generate reports and make predictions about future events, such as emergency department use.
- *Risk stratification:* Using statistics, categorize subsets of the overall population by their risk of mortality, morbidity, and costs of care. By risk level, match patients to the most appropriate types of care based on their health and social needs.
- *Risk adjustment:* Patients with multiple comorbidities would be expected to cost more than healthy patients. Health information technology is used to track and report the diagnoses to payers so the value-based payments can be adjusted to reflect the severity of illness and the expected costs associated with patients.
- *Health service utilization:* Summarize utilization patterns compared to goals and gain insights into whether evidence-based interventions can reduce inappropriate or avoidable health services use.
- *Cost of care:* Identify factors related to increased costs to create cost reduction initiatives.

Technology is also needed to collect and report risk factors related to health disparities. Using these data, health services managers can effectively allocate resources to population health interventions that reduce health inequities. **Health equity** aims to eliminate differences in health outcomes by race, ethnicity, gender, ability status, or neighborhood (Bhatt & Reh, 2023).

△ KEY IDEA
When social risk factors are identified, health services managers fund interventions designed to improve health equity.

Program Planning and Evaluation

Health services managers also need to adjust the HCO operations to support population health models, engaging in a process called **program planning and evaluation** (National Center for Healthcare Leadership [NCHL], 2018). When planning programs, health services managers use **logic models** to document the evidence-based reasoning behind the interventions and the succinct goals to impose discipline on the plan (Knowlton & Phillips, 2012). Logic models visually

FIGURE 6.5 Logic model for population health intervention example.

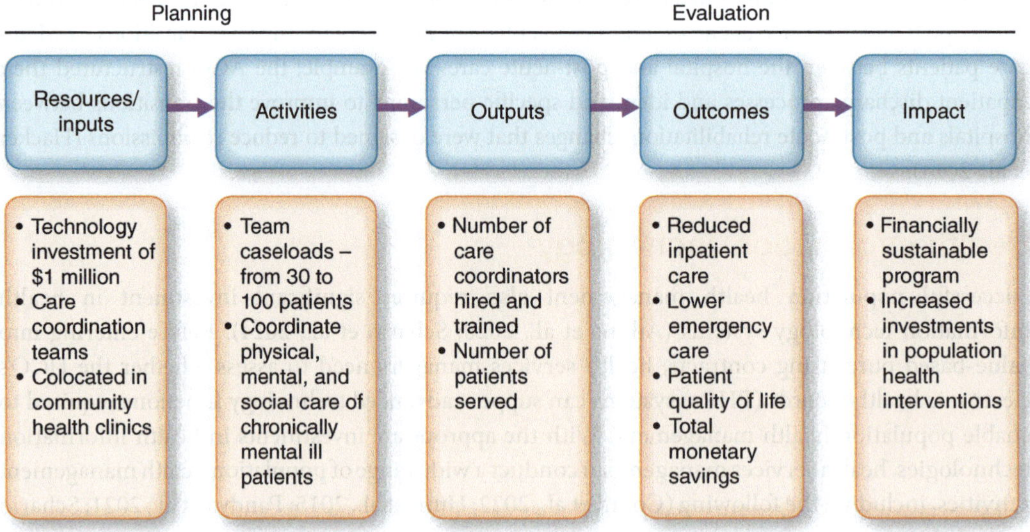

Planning		Evaluation		
Resources/inputs →	Activities →	Outputs →	Outcomes →	Impact
• Technology investment of $1 million • Care coordination teams • Colocated in community health clinics	• Team caseloads – from 30 to 100 patients • Coordinate physical, mental, and social care of chronically mental ill patients	• Number of care coordinators hired and trained • Number of patients served	• Reduced inpatient care • Lower emergency care • Patient quality of life • Total monetary savings	• Financially sustainable program • Increased investments in population health interventions

Source: Adapted from Kellogg Foundation (2001). *Logic model development guide.* https://wkkf.issuelab.org/resource/logic-model-development-guide.html

explain the causal relationships between the program interventions and expected outcomes using the following components (Kellogg Foundation, 2001):

- *Inputs:* Resources necessary to support program
- *Activities:* Interventions, services, and programs that serve patients or populations
- *Outputs:* Short-term measures within (1 to 3 years) of the program success
- *Outcomes:* Short- and long-term (3 to 10 years) effects of program activities
- *Impact:* Long-term effect of a sustained program

Figure 6.5 illustrates the logic model for an example population health intervention managed by health services managers. In this example, one outcome of the program is cost savings of the care coordination intervention, an important measure of success for many population health initiatives (Pruitt, Emechebe, et al., 2018).

Cost-Efficient Care

Population health management requires the ability to effectively control costs. There are a variety of methods that health services managers employ to reduce wasteful spending. First, **utilization management** is an approach that requires clinicians to gain approval to deliver certain services. Health insurance companies commonly require that hospitals obtain permission before admitting patients, so HCOs are accustomed to asking for preservice authorizations. In value-based health care, health services managers become responsible for instituting utilization management practices to control costs. Of course, any preservice authorization rules must adhere to **community standards of care**, which are accepted norms, expectations, and practices of the medical field. Effective health services managers follow the direction of clinicians regarding medical treatment protocols when instituting cost-saving methods associated with utilization management.

> ⚠ **KEY IDEA**
> In value-based health care, health services managers become responsible for instituting utilization management practices to control costs.

Health Promotion

Population health management interventions also seek to change the health behaviors of groups of patients, including screenings, community outreach, and other wellness initiatives. **Health promotion** activities typically focus on individuals with chronic conditions, such as diabetes, congestive heart failure, or asthma. For example, clinicians can also support behavior change by referring patients to chronic disease self-management education and support programs designed to help patients to manage their health on their own (Baer et al., 2020). The results of these health promotion programs, such as the number of patients who control their diabetes, can be tracked over time to determine their impact on population health.

Integrating Medical and Social Care

Compared to clinical interventions, addressing social risks may be the most efficient way to improve population health (Frieden, 2010). Connecting patients to needed social services, such as food pantries, housing support, and transportation, reduces health care spending compared to those whose social care needs remain unmet (Pruitt et al., 2018). However, health services managers should not expect physicians alone to address social determinants of health when they are already overburdened with handling patients' medical needs (Garg et al., 2016). Instead, health services managers support physicians by investing in population health management resources that lessen the need for sick care. Population health management investments designed to integrate medical and social care include the following (Gottlieb et al., 2019, 2024; Lewis et al., 2022; Perlin & Plough, 2023; (Pruitt, Taylor, & Bryant, 2018).

- *Use social health navigators:* Create organizational units staffed with individuals responsible for social needs screening and service linkages, tasked to connect patients to community-based services. Navigators can be nurses, social workers, or community health workers.
- *Enhance EHR systems:* Social risks need to be documented, tracked, and connected to social or medical care interventions in the patients' records.
- *Redesign workflows:* Positive screens for social risks require efficient referral processes to connect patients to appropriate social services.
- *Build social care partnerships:* Partner with community-based social services organizations that provide specialized social care services.
- *Monitor performance:* Track metrics related to activities and adjust interventions as needed.

Federal policies motivate health services managers to integrate social care into well-established medical care processes. Under the Centers for Medicare & Medicaid's Hospital Readmissions Reduction Program, HCOs can be penalized for readmitting patients to the hospital within 30 days of being discharged (Lachar et al., 2023). While excellent care may have been provided throughout the hospital stay and the discharge process may have been effective, social risks may lead to readmissions (Emechebe et al., 2019). To avoid significant financial penalties for readmissions, HCOs seek to identify social risks upon discharge (Gottlieb et al., 2024). For example, Hennepin Health ACO of Minneapolis, a partnership between Hennepin Healthcare System, Medicaid health plan, and the public health department, had hospital case managers screen patients for social risks during their hospital stay (Rhodes et al., 2021). For patients at risk of homelessness, the hospital case managers connected patients to homeless shelters and supportive services in the community.

> ⚠ **KEY IDEA**
> **Health services managers support physicians by investing in population health management resources that lessen the need for sick care.**

COMMUNITY COLLABORATION

Community Engagement

Successful health services managers build community partnerships, a competency known as "context management" or "boundary spanning" (International Hospital Federation [IHF], 2023; NCHL, 2018). HCOs community engagement activities seek to improve population health by making direct financial investments in community-based organizations (Gottlieb et al., 2019). A growing body of evidence shows that these community relationships improve overall perceptions of HCOs, leading to the following benefits (Chaiyachati et al., 2020; Grande et al., 2013; Hilts et al., 2021; Key et al., 2019; Nakielski, 2023; Rozier, 2020):

- *Enhanced responsiveness:* Ensure appropriate interventions for specific populations to meet community health needs.
- *Increased efficiency:* Complementary social services organizations can help HCOs share resources and avoid duplication of investments.
- *Higher workforce retention:* Positive perceptions of the HCO help recruit and retain employees.
- *Greater patient revenues:* Increased favorable brand awareness persuades patients to choose one HCO over another.
- *Improved population health:* Resources spent in the community, including time, workforce, and donations, are associated with improved community health.

Value-based health care incentives encourage HCOs to form partnerships with public health agencies, educational institutions, social service organizations, and other HCOs whose population health goals overlap (Gamache et al., 2018). Health services managers are responsible for negotiating collaborative relationships with complementary organizations that may improve population health (American College of Healthcare Executives [ACHE], 2021). Examples of HCO partnerships and collaborations with external entities are illustrated in Table 6.5 (ACHE, 2021; Cronin et al., 2021; Hacker et al., 2014; Hilts et al., 2021; Huppertz et al., 2014; Kindig et al., 2013; Lewis, 2023).

Health Policy Advocacy

Health services managers also advocate for population health policies to ensure equitable allocation of resources in the community (ACHE, 2021). For example, Alabama was one of only 11 states as of 2023 that had not expanded Medicaid with funds allocated by the ACA. On March 21, 2023, Cover Alabama, a coalition of over 100 HCOs and community organizations, rallied in front of the Alabama State House to urge lawmakers to expand Medicaid to cover more low-income individuals without health insurance (Willis, 2023). On the same day, representatives from the Alabama Hospital Association, a group of over 100 hospitals and health systems, and

TABLE 6.5 Examples of Health Care Organization Partnerships and Collaborations

COLLABORATIVE ENTITY	EXAMPLE GOAL	EXAMPLE ACTIVITY
Public health agencies	Acquire epidemiological resources and expertise.	Collaborate on writing community health needs assessment reports.
Social service organizations	Increase access to food for patients discharged from the hospital.	Contract with Area Agency on Aging to deliver hot meals to discharged patients at home.
Government (local, state, and national)	Engage in value-based health care contracts that incentivize population health.	Obtain funding for population health through value-based health care contracts.
Religious organizations	Reduce poverty.	Contribute to churches that provide financial support and education.
Educational institutions	Improve access to qualified nurses to work in underserved communities.	Provide clinical training to local nursing students to help recruit them directly from nursing schools.
Businesses	Reduce unemployment.	Attract employers to community with supportive health and wellness programs. Businesses want healthy, productive workers.
Foundations	Funds for population health research projects	Financially support pilot programs designed for population health improvement.
Other HCOs	Plan for operational continuity during emergencies.	Create plans that anticipate potential disasters and arrange for access to critical resources.

HCO, health care organization.

Blue Cross Blue Shield of Alabama, the state's largest health insurance company, spoke to state legislators in public hearings about the benefits of Medicaid expansion (Rocha, 2023). As major employers in their communities, many HCOs wield significant political clout, which can persuade legislators to endorse certain healthcare policies.

INFORMATIONAL INTERVIEW 6.2
Chief Executive Officer, Community Health Center
Access the informational interview online at http://connect.springerpub.com/content/book/978-0-8261-4807-0/chapter/ch00.

Anchor Institutions

Many HCOs leverage their financial and political influence to serve as **anchor institutions** that facilitate social, ecological, and economic development in their communities (Gottlieb et al., 2019). Recognizing that their success is intertwined with the communities in which they operate, HCOs implement business-related anchor strategies to strengthen local economies, such as the following (ACHE, 2021; Cronin et al., 2023; Koh et al., 2020):

- *Employ local workforce:* Provide stable employment to community members and promote employees from within the organization, when possible.
- *Buy local:* Contract with locally owned vendors to purchase supplies, services, and equipment.
- *Support rural community:* Explore remote working opportunities for people in rural areas.
- *Place-based investing:* Invest in projects that meet community needs and generate a modest financial return, such as building low-income housing units.
- *Environmental sustainability:* Reduce resource consumption and environmental impact to improve air quality, decrease water usage, handle chemical pollutants, and reduce carbon emissions.

Health services managers who advance their HCOs as anchor institutions can improve HCOs' medical care quality and cost-effectiveness while simultaneously benefiting society (Norris & Howard, 2016). This requires more than just doing good deeds but applying management competencies to community collaboration. Effective health services managers measure and report on the impact of their actions, such as reducing social risks, environmental impact, and economic challenges, and hold themselves and others accountable for effectively deploying resources that maximize community health and well-being (ACHE, 2021).

CAREER BOX 6.3: Superconnectors

Collaborative professional networks can help health services managers solve many of the ongoing and emerging healthcare challenges. When faced with career or professional obstacles, health services managers can reach out to "superconnectors" to get referrals to people with expertise or resources. Such highly connected professionals build networks of people with a variety of skills and backgrounds because they realize the professional referrals increase productivity and success for both the helper and the helped (Grant, 2014). Superconnectors often report higher career satisfaction because they earn personal satisfaction from helping others (Snow, 2013). Superconnectors are typically open to meeting new people and expanding their networks. Eager to help, they willingly share their insights, make introductions, and provide guidance to those who reach out to them. If you approach them respectfully and demonstrate genuine interest in building a mutually beneficial relationship, superconnectors are likely to be receptive to your outreach. So, when faced with a problem, reach out to a superconnector. Or better yet, become a superconnector yourself.

Emergency Preparedness and Response

Health services managers also collaborate with community partners when planning for operational continuity during emergencies. The **National Incident Management System** (NIMS) was created to guide government agencies, HCOs, and the private sector to work together during emergencies. NIMS sets requirements and expectations for emergency planning, such as the development of **emergency operations plan**, which details the HCO's emergency response procedures, roles, and responsibilities during various types of incidents. NIMS also requires a **Hospital Incident Command System (HICS)**, which establishes a clear chain of command and defines roles and responsibilities for HCO personnel, ensuring a coordinated and effective response to incidents (Hendrickx et al., 2016).

Contingency plans document the HCO preparations for emergencies or disasters to either reduce the probability that the problem will occur or prevent the occurrence altogether. An **all-hazards approach** involves planning and response strategies that can be applied to a wide range of potential incidents. The all-hazards approach incorporates plans to ensure that information systems continuity so that patient data are protected and that systems are functioning during and after disasters. This includes identifying key technology systems, establishing backup procedures, and ensuring data recovery in the event of natural disasters or intentional cyberattacks.

Community Volunteerism

Most health services managers personally contribute to the community (Weil & Kimball, 2010). Volunteerism is the practice of offering time, skills, and services for the benefit of nonprofit organizations, community groups, charities, or religious institutions without expecting financial compensation. HCOs frequently encourage employees to volunteer in their communities, through activities such as the United Way and American Heart Association fundraisers. Health service managers at all career levels possess a professional obligation to volunteer and to support employees who serve their communities (ACHE, 2021). Volunteerism provides health services managers with opportunities to express their humanitarian values, learn about their communities, and meet like-minded people.

> **△ KEY IDEA**
>
> Volunteerism provides health services managers with opportunities to express their humanitarian values, learn about their communities, and meet like-minded people.

FUTURE DIRECTIONS

The powerful incentives of value-based purchasing drive HCOs to integrate social care services into their regular medical care operations. However, it can be challenging to identify patients whose social risks could cause them to need expensive forms of medical care (Ong et al., 2024). HCOs possess large amounts of data, but these data are not currently standardized within EHR systems nor aggregated in a way that is readily useful. To improve the usefulness of the various forms of data, billions of dollars of funding have been invested in companies seeking to extract social determinants of health data from EHRs and other sources (Goldberg & Nash, 2022).

For example, AI technologies, including natural language processing, machine learning, and large language models, can be used to interpret EHR clinical notes and identify unmet social needs (Stewart de Ramirez et al., 2022). AI can also be used to predict health outcomes, such as patient hospitalizations, from diagnoses and social risks stored in EHRs (Kino et al., 2021). Finally, AI-based large language models, such as ChatGPT, can be used to refer patients to social services based on a positively screened social risk assessment and then flag these referrals in patients' EHRs for clinician follow-up. To take advantage of the benefits of AI, health services managers will need to understand how new technologies can reduce overall costs, enhance patient experience, and improve health outcomes.

SUMMARY

- Community health needs assessments serve to identify gaps between the current health of the population and to guide health services managers in allocating resources, implementing programs, and developing community partnerships.
- When developing community health needs assessments, health services managers define the geographic area and analyze demographics, community assets, health status, health behaviors, physical environment, and social and economic factors.

- Under the population health model, HCOs accept financial responsibility for reducing overall costs, enhancing patient experience, and improving health outcomes. Health services managers need to transform their management practices to meet the demands of new value-based healthcare policies and financing models.
- Risk-based contracting means that HCOs risk losing money if the costs of medical care exceed the predetermined payments. Taking on financial risk can generate significant financial bonuses if medical care quality standards are met and costs are kept below certain benchmarks.
- Population health management emphasizes preventive primary care, intensive care coordination across health care settings, and avoidance of unnecessary health care. Population health management functions, such as health information technologies, cost control processes, and health promotion initiatives, require HCOs to make significant investments in workforce reorganization and process redesign.
- Value-based health care incentives encourage HCOs to form partnerships with community organizations, such as public health agencies, educational institutions, social service organizations, and other HCOs with similar population health goals.
- HCOs act as anchor institutions to facilitate social, ecological, and economic development in their communities. Anchor institutions implement business-related strategies to strengthen local economies, such as hiring local workers and investing in projects that meet community needs.

END-OF-CHAPTER RESOURCES

KEY TERMS*

*For the full list of key terms, please see the online glossary at **http://connect.springerpub.com/content/book/978-0-8261-4807-0**.

Accountable Care Organization
advanced payment models
all-hazards approach
alternative payment models
anchor institutions
catchment area
community assets
community health needs assessment
community engagement
community standards of care
contingency plans
bundled payment
data analytics
downside risk
emergency operations plan
epidemiology
fee-for-service
health equity
health outcomes
health promotion
Hospital Incident Command System (HICS)
incidence
logic model
medical model
Medicare Shared Savings Program
National Incident Management System
Patient-centered medical home
pay-for-performance
population health model
population health management
program planning and evaluation
prevalence
risk-based financing
risk adjustment
risk stratification
shared savings
social determinants of health
social risks
Triple Aim
upside risk
utilization management
value
value-based health care

LEARNING ACTIVITIES

Professional Development and Reflection

1. Identify and list the career assets that can help you develop your career. Examples include university career service offices, professors or teachers, professional associations, personal friends, and work colleagues.
2. Using Career Box 6.1, complete the "Flower Exercise" from *What Color is My Parachute?* A free printable template can be found online. By completing the diagram and reflecting on its insights, you can gain clarity about your career preferences and improve your career decision-making.

Discussion Questions

1. What are the risks for health services managers who fail to recognize and adapt to the shifting financial policies toward population health management?
2. What challenges might health services managers encounter during the community health needs assessment process? How can they overcome these challenges to ensure effective community health improvement initiatives?
3. What challenges might health services managers face in transitioning from a fee-for-service model to a value-based health care financing model?
4. What strategies can be implemented to encourage collaboration between clinicians and health services managers in advancing population health management initiatives?
5. What are the potential benefits and challenges of HCOs engaging in health policy advocacy, both at the state and national levels?

RECOMMENDED READING AND MEDIA

Bard, M. (2011). *Accountable care organizations: Your guide to strategy, design, and implementation.* Health Administration Press.

Bolles, R. N., & Brooks, K. (2021). *What color is your parachute? 2022: Your guide to a lifetime of meaningful work and career success.* Ten Speed Press.

Center for Medicare & Medicaid Innovation. *The fundamental shift to value-based care* [YouTube.com]. https://www.youtube.com/watch?v=Yz4VO2s01cs

County Health Rankings & Roadmaps. (2022). *Explore health topics.* https://www.countyhealthrankings.org/what-impacts-health/county-health-rankings-model

Hendrickx, C., D'Hoker, S., Michiels, G., & Sabbe, M. B. (2016). Principles of hospital disaster management: An integrated and multidisciplinary approach. B-ENT, 12(26/2), 139-148.

Hewitt, A. M., Mascari, J. L., & Wagner, S. L. (2022). *Population health management: Strategies, tools, applications, and outcomes.* Springer Publishing Company.

National Committee for Quality Assurance. *Population health management: A primer.* [YouTube.com]. https://www.youtube.com/watch?v=vgMDIrjGDJ4

Norris, T., & Howard, T. (2016). *Can hospitals heal America's communities?* Democracy Collaborative.

Russell, C., & McKnight, J. (2022). *The connected community: Discovering the health, wealth, and power of neighborhoods.* Berrett-Koehler Publishers.

Schein, E. H., Van Maanen, J., & Schein, P. A. (2023). *Career anchors reimagined: Finding direction and opportunity in the changing world of work* (5th ed.). Wiley.

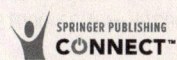

A robust set of instructor resources designed to supplement this text is located at http://connect.springerpub.com/content/book/978-0-8261-4807-0.
Qualifying instructors may request access by emailing textbook@springerpub.com.

REFERENCES

Adler, N. E., & Stead, W. W. (2015). Patients in context—EHR capture of social and behavioral determinants of health. *Obstetrical & Gynecological Survey, 70*(6), 388–390. https://doi.org/10.1097/01.ogx.0000465303.29687.97

Agarwal, R., Liao, J. M., Gupta, A., & Navathe, A. S. (2020). The impact of bundled payment on health care spending, utilization, and quality: A systematic review. *Health Affairs, 39*(1), 50–57. https://doi.org/10.1377/hlthaff.2019.00784

Agency for Healthcare Research and Quality. (2023, June). *Social determinants of health database.* https://www.ahrq.gov/sdoh/data-analytics/sdoh-data.html

Alderwick, H., & Gottlieb, L. M. (2019). Meanings and misunderstandings: A social determinants of health lexicon for health care systems. *The Milbank Quarterly, 97*(2), 407–419. https://doi.org/10.1111/1468-0009.12390

Allen, R. W. (2020). Reimagining ambulatory care as a key to population health. *Frontiers of Health Services Management, 37*(2), 3–10. https://doi.org/10.1097/hap.0000000000000099

American College of Healthcare Executives. (2021, December 6). *Healthcare executives' responsibility to their communities.* https://www.ache.org/about-ache/our-story/our-commitments/policy-statements/healthcare-executives-responsibility-to-their-communities

Atkins, D. N., Gabriel, M. H., Cortelyou-Ward, K., & Rotarius, T. (2020). Population health initiatives among hospitals: Associated hospital characteristics. *Journal of Healthcare Management, 65*(3), 187–200. https://doi.org/10.1097/jhm-d-19-00025

Baer, H. J., Rozenblum, R., De La Cruz, B. A., Orav, E. J., Wien, M., Nolido, N. V., Metzler, K., McManus, K. D., Halperin, F., Aronne, L. J., Minero, G., Block, J. P., & Bates, D. W. (2020). Effect of an online weight management program integrated with population health management on weight change: A randomized clinical trial. *JAMA, 324*(17), 1737–1746. https://doi.org/10.1001/jama.2020.18977

Begun, J. W., & Potthoff, S. (2017). Moving upstream in US hospital care toward investments in population health. *Journal of Healthcare Management, 62*(5), 343–353. https://doi.org/10.1097/jhm-d-16-00010

Berwick, D. M., Nolan, T. W., & Whittington, J. (2008). The triple aim: care, health, and cost. *Health affairs, 27*(3), 759-769.

Bethke, M., Guest, D., Lowry, A., Bailey, R., Fleisher, D., & Weger, J. (2020, December). *Value-based care models in a shifting economy.* Deloitte Consulting, LLP. https://www2.deloitte.com/content/dam/Deloitte/us/Documents/life-sciences-health-care/us-lshc-value-based-health-care-models-in-a-shifting-economy-december-2020.pdf

Bhatt, J., & Reh, G. (2023). Health equity is key to better population health. *Population Health Management, 26*(4), 215–216. https://doi.org/10.1089/pop.2023.0109

Bolles, R. N., & Brooks, K. (2021). *What color is your parachute? 2022: Your guide to a lifetime of meaningful work and career success.* Ten Speed Press.

Bradley, E. H., Sipsma, H., & Taylor, L. A. (2017). American health care paradox—high spending on health care and poor health. *QJM: An International Journal of Medicine, 110*(2), 61–65.

Burns, A., Yeager, V. A., Cronin, C. E., & Franz, B. (2023). Community engagement in nonprofit hospital community health needs assessments and implementation plans. *Journal of Public Health Management and Practice, 29*(2), E50–E57. https://doi.org/10.1097/phh.0000000000001663

Chaiyachati, K. H., Qi, M., & Werner, R. M. (2020). Nonprofit hospital community benefit spending and readmission rates. *Population Health Management, 23*(1), 85–91. https://doi.org/10.1089%2Fpop.2019.0003

Coleman, J. (2017, January 24). Make learning a lifelong habit. *Harvard Business Review.* https://hbr.org/2017/01/make-learning-a-lifelong-habit

Coran, J. J., Schario, M. E., & Pronovost, P. J. (2022). Stratifying for value: An updated population health risk stratification approach. *Population Health Management, 25*(1), 91–99. https://doi.org/10.1089/pop.2021.0096

Coyne, J., Gutman, R., Ferraro, C., & Muhlestein, D. (2024). Financial performance of accountable care organizations: A 5-year national empirical analysis. *Journal of Healthcare Management, 69*(1), 74–86. https://doi.org/10.1097/jhm-d-22-00141

Cronin, C. E., Choyke, K. L., & Franz, B. (2023). For-profit hospital reflections on community relationships in the time of COVID-19. *Journal of Healthcare Management, 68*(1), 25–37. https://doi.org/10.1097/jhm-d-22-00015

Cronin, C. E., Franz, B., & Garlington, S. (2021). Population health partnerships and social capital: Facilitating hospital-community partnerships. *SSM-Population Health, 13*, 100739. https://doi.org/10.1016/j.ssmph.2021.100739

Emechebe, N., Amoda, O., Taylor, P. L., & Pruitt, Z. (2019). Passive social health surveillance systems may identify individuals at risk of inpatient readmissions. *American Journal of Managed Care, 25*(8), 388–395.

Frieden, T. R. (2010). A framework for public health action: The health impact pyramid. *American Journal of Public Health, 100*(4), 590–595. https://doi.org/10.2105/ajph.2009.185652

Fuller, R., Landrigan, P. J., Balakrishnan, K., Bathan, G., Bose-O'Reilly, S., Brauer, M., Caravanos, J., Chiles, T., Cohen, A., Corra, L., Cropper, M., Ferraro, G., Hanna, J., Hanrahan, D., Hu, H., Hunter, D., Janata, G., Kupka, R., Lanphear, B., … Yan, C. (2022). Pollution and health: A progress update. *The Lancet Planetary Health, 6*(6), e535–e547. https://doi.org/10.1016/s2542-5196(22)00090-0

Gamache, R., Kharrazi, H., & Weiner, J. P. (2018). Public and population health informatics: The bridging of big data to benefit communities. *Yearbook of Medical Informatics, 27*(1), 199–206. https://doi.org/10.1055/s-0038-1667081

Garg, A., Boynton-Jarrett, R., & Dworkin, P. H. (2016). Avoiding the unintended consequences of screening for social determinants of health. *JAMA, 316*(8), 813–814. https://doi.org/10.1001/jama.2016.9282

Goldberg, Z. N., & Nash, D. B. (2022). For profit, but socially determined: The rise of the SDOH industry. *Population Health Management, 25*(3), 392–398. https://doi.org/10.1089/pop.2021.0231

Gottlieb, L., Fichtenberg, C., Alderwick, H., & Adler, N. (2019). Social determinants of health: What's a healthcare system to do? *Journal of Healthcare Management, 64*(4), 243–257. https://doi.org/10.1097/jhm-d-18-00160

Gottlieb, L. M., Hessler, D., Wing, H., Gonzalez-Rocha, A., Cartier, Y., & Fichtenberg, C. (2024). Revising the logic model behind health care's social care investments. *The Milbank Quarterly*. https://doi.org/10.1111/1468-0009.12690

Grande, D., Shea, J. A., & Armstrong, K. (2013). Perceived community commitment of hospitals: An exploratory analysis of its potential influence on hospital choice and health care system distrust. *INQUIRY: The Journal of Health Care Organization, Provision, and Financing, 50*(4), 312–321. https://doi.org/10.1177/0046958013516585

Grant, A. (2014). *Give and take: Why helping others drives our success*. Penguin Random House.

Hacker, K., Mechanic, R., & Santos, P. (2014). *Accountable care in the safety net: A case study of the Cambridge Health Alliance*. Commonwealth Fund.

Hagel, J., III. (2021, October 11). What motivates lifelong learners. *Harvard Business Review*. https://hbr.org/2021/10/what-motivates-lifelong-learners

Hewitt, A. M., & Dykstra, D. (2022). Assessing population health: Community health needs assessments. In A. M. Hewitt, J. L. Mascari, & S. L. Wagner (Eds.). *Population health management: Strategies, tools, applications, and outcomes*. Springer Publishing Company.

Hilts, K. E., Yeager, V. A., Gibson, P. J., Halverson, P. K., Blackburn, J., & Menachemi, N. (2021). Hospital partnerships for population health: A systematic review of the literature. *Journal of Healthcare Management, 66*(3), 170–198. https://doi.org/10.1097/jhm-d-20-00172

Huang, H., Zhu, X., Ullrich, F., MacKinney, A. C., & Mueller, K. (2023). The impact of Medicare shared savings program participation on hospital financial performance: An event-study analysis. *Health Services Research, 58*(1), 116–127. https://doi.org/10.1111/1475-6773.14085

Hunt, J. S., Gibson, R. F., Whittington, J., Powell, K., Wozney, B., & Knudson, S. (2015). Guide for developing an information technology investment road map for population health management. *Population Health Management, 18*(3), 159–171. https://doi.org/10.1089/pop.2014.0092

Huppertz, J. W., Strosberg, M., Burns, S., & Chaudhri, I. (2014). The uniqueness of US healthcare management: A linguistic analysis of competency models and application to health administration education. *Journal of Health Administration Education, 31*(3), 197–214.

Institute for Healthcare Improvement. (2018, April). *Pathways to population health framework*. http://pathways2pophealth.org/files/Pathways-to-Population-Health-Framework-April-2018.pdf

International Hospital Federation. (2023, July 2023). *Global healthcare leadership competency model*. https://healthmanagement.org/s/global-healthcare-leadership-competency-model

Kellogg Foundation. (2001). *Logic model development guide.* https://wkkf.issuelab.org/resource/logic-model-development-guide.html

Key, K. D., Furr-Holden, D., Lewis, E. Y., Cunningham, R., Zimmerman, M. A., Johnson-Lawrence, V., & Selig, S. (2019). The continuum of community engagement in research: A roadmap for understanding and assessing progress. *Progress in Community Health Partnerships: Research, Education, and Action, 13*(4), 427–434. https://doi.org/10.1353/cpr.2019.0064

Kindig, D. A., Isham, G. J., & Siemering, K. Q. (2013, August 8). *The business role in improving health: Beyond social responsibility.* NAM Perspectives.

Kino, S., Hsu, Y. T., Shiba, K., Chien, Y. S., Mita, C., Kawachi, I., & Daoud, A. (2021). A scoping review on the use of machine learning in research on social determinants of health: Trends and research prospects. *SSM-Population Health, 15*, 100836. https://doi.org/10.1016/j.ssmph.2021.100836

Knowlton, L. M., & Phillips, C. C. (2012). *Logic model guidebook: Better strategies for great results* (2nd ed.). SAGE Publications.

Koh, H. K., Bantham, A., Geller, A. C., Rukavina, M. A., Emmons, K. M., Yatsko, P., & Restuccia, R. (2020). Anchor institutions: Best practices to address social needs and social determinants of health. *American Journal of Public Health, 110*(3), 309–316. https://doi.org/10.2105/ajph.2019.305472

Lachar, J., Avila, C. J., & Qayyum, R. (2023). The long-term effect of financial penalties on 30-day hospital readmission rates. *The Joint Commission Journal on Quality and Patient Safety, 49*(10), 521–528. https://doi.org/10.1016/j.jcjq.2023.06.001

Lewis, A. L. (2023). *A qualitative study describing how black pastors approach meeting the socioeconomic needs of congregants* [Doctoral dissertation, Grand Canyon University]. ProQuest Dissertations & Theses Global.

Lewis, C., Abrams, M. K., Seervai, S., Horstman, C., & Blumenthal, D. (2022, April 28). *The impact of the payment and delivery system reforms of the affordable care act.* The Commonwealth Fund. https://www.commonwealthfund.org/publications/2022/apr/impact-payment-and-delivery-system-reforms-affordable-care-act

Marmot, M., & Allen, J. J. (2014). Social determinants of health equity. *American Journal of Public Health, 104*(S4), S517–S519. https://doi.org/10.2105/ajph.2014.302200

McKinlay, J. B. (1979). A case for refocusing upstream: The political economy of illness. In E. G. Jaco (Ed.), *Patients, physicians and illness: A sourcebook in behavioral science and health* (3rd ed., pp. 9–25). The Free Press.

Nakielski, M. L. (2023). Moving forward with ESG, sustainability, and corporate responsibility. *Frontiers of Health services Management, 40*(1), 33–39. https://doi.org/10.1097/hap.0000000000000178

Nash, D. B., Fabius, R. J., Skoufalos, A., & Oglesby, W. H. (2021). *Population health: Creating a culture of wellness.* Jones & Bartlett Learning.

National Center for Healthcare Leadership. (2018). *Healthcare leadership competency model 3.0.* https://nchl.member365.org/publicFr/store/item/19

Norris, T., & Howard, T. (2016). *Can hospitals heal America's communities?* Democracy Collaborative.

Nussbaum, S., McClellan, M., & Metlay, G. (2018). Principles for a framework for alternative payment models. *JAMA, 319*(7), 653–654. https://doi.org/10.1001/jama.2017.20226

Office of Disease Prevention and Health Promotion. (2021, September). *Healthy people 2030: Leading health indicators.* https://health.gov/healthypeople/objectives-and-data/leading-health-indicators

Ong, J. C. L., Seng, B. J. J., Law, J. Z. F., Low, L. L., Kwa, A. L. H., Giacomini, K. M., & Ting, D. S. W. (2024). Artificial intelligence, ChatGPT, and other large language models for social determinants of health: Current state and future directions. *Cell Reports Medicine, 5*(1).

Pandya, C. J., Chang, H. Y., & Kharrazi, H. (2021). Electronic health record-based risk stratification: A potential key ingredient to achieving value-based care. *Population Health Management, 24*(6), 654–656. https://doi.org/10.1089/pop.2021.0131

Pennel, C. L., McLeroy, K. R., Burdine, J. N., Matarrita-Cascante, D., & Wang, J. (2016). Community health needs assessment: Potential for population health improvement. *Population Health Management, 19*(3), 178–186. https://doi.org/10.1089/pop.2015.0075

Perlin, J., & Plough, A. (2023). Health systems need to transform data collection to advance health equity. *Population Health Management, 26*(2), 128–131. https://doi.org/10.1089/pop.2023.0005

Porter, M. E., & Teisberg, E. O. (2006). *Redefining health care: Creating value-based competition on results.* Harvard Business School Press.

Pruitt, Z., Emechebe, N., Quast, T., Taylor, P. L., & Bryant, K. B. (2018). Expenditure reductions associated with a social service referral program. *Population Health Management, 21*(6), 469–476. https://doi.org/10.1089/pop.2017.0199

Pruitt, Z., Emechebe, N., Quast, T., Taylor, P. L., & Bryant, K. B. (2018). Expenditure reductions associated with a social service referral program. *Population health management.* 21(6), 469-476.

Pruitt, Z., & Moseley, M. (2018). Interprofessional problem-based learning activity: A value-based contracting decision. *The Journal of Health Admin Education, 35*(3), 401–419.

Pruitt, Z., Taylor, P. L., & Bryant, K. M. (2018). A managed care organization's call center-based social support role. *American Journal of Accountable Care, 6*(1), e16–e22.

Purtle, J., Peters, R., Kolker, J., & Diez Roux, A. V. (2019). Uses of population health rankings in local policy contexts: A multisite case study. *Medical Care Research and Review, 76*(4), 478–496. https://doi.org/10.1177/1077558717726115

Ravaghi, H., Guisset, A. L., Elfeky, S., Nasir, N., Khani, S., Ahmadnezhad, E., & Abdi, Z. (2023). A scoping review of community health needs and assets assessment: Concepts, rationale, tools and uses. *BMC Health Services Research, 23*(1), 44. https://doi.org/10.1186/s12913-022-08983-3

Rhodes, H. M., Simon, H. L., Hume, H. G., Strief, D., Knutson, A., Webber, M. C., & Robertshaw, D. C. (2021). Safety-net accountable health model partnership drives inpatient connection to outpatient social services, reducing readmissions in a population experiencing homelessness. *Professional Case Management, 26*(3), 150–155.

Rocha, A. (2023, March 22). *Alabama hospitals pitch Medicaid expansion to House committee.* Alabama Reflector. https://alabamareflector.com/2023/03/22/alabama-hospitals-pitch-medicaid-expansion-to-house-committee

Rozier, M. D. (2020). Nonprofit hospital community benefit in the US: A scoping review from 2010 to 2019. *Frontiers in Public Health, 8*, 72. https://doi.org/10.3389/fpubh.2020.00072

Saini, V., Garber, J., & Brownlee, S. (2022, February 10). *Nonprofit hospital CEO compensation: How much is enough?* Health Affairs Forefront.

Schario, M. E., Pronovost, P. J., Runnels, P., Corder-Palko, T., Carson, B., & Szubski, M. (2024). A path to risk: Critical elements of a structured approach. *Population Health Management, 27*(1), 49–54. https://doi.org/10.1089/pop.2023.0197

Schneider, E. C., Shah, A., Doty, M. M., Tikkanen, R., Fields, K., & Williams, R. D. II. (2021). *Mirror, mirror 2021: Reflecting poorly.* The Commonwealth Fund. https://www.commonwealthfund.org/publications/fund-reports/2021/aug/mirror-mirror-2021-reflecting-poorly

Snow, S. (2013, April 2). The rise of the superconnector. *Fast Company.* https://www.fastcompany.com/3007657/rise-superconnector

Stewart de Ramirez, S., Shallat, J., McClure, K., Foulger, R., & Barenblat, L. (2022). Screening for social determinants of health: Active and passive information retrieval methods. *Population Health Management, 25*(6), 781–788. https://doi.org/10.1089/pop.2022.0228

Stiefel, M. C., Straszewski, T., Taylor, J. C., Huang, C., An, J., Wilson-Anumudu, F. J., & Cheadle, A. (2021). Using the county health rankings framework to create national percentile scores for health outcomes and health factors. *The Permanente Journal, 25.*

Thomas, R. K. (2022). Data needs for the population health model. In *Population Health and the Future of Healthcare* (pp. 299–334). Springer International Publishing.

Wang, A., Debab, S., Muhlestein, D., McStay, F., Bleser, W. K., McClellan, M. B., & Saunders, R. S. (2023). Medicare accountable care organizations in 2022: Renewed growth and improved savings show small rebound from the COVID-19 pandemic. *Health Affairs Forefront.*

Weil, P. A., & Kimball, P. A. (2010). The volunteer activities of healthcare executives. *Journal of Healthcare Management, 55*(2), 115–131.

Willis, A. (2023, March 22). *Dozens rally at Alabama State House demanding Medicaid expansion.* Alabama Daily News. https://aldailynews.com/dozens-rally-at-alabama-state-house-demanding-medicaid-expansion

World Health Organization. [WHO]. (n.d.). *Social determinants of health.* https://www.who.int/health-topics/social-determinants-of-health AQ: author, adjusted year to match ref entry, OK?

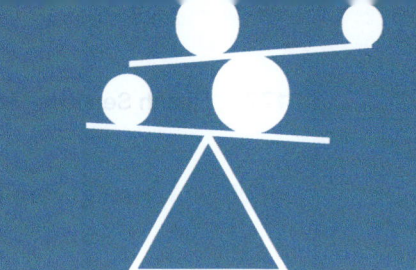

CHAPTER 7

HEALTHCARE GOVERNANCE

Healthcare governance involves the structures and processes used to share power, make collective decisions, and hold managers and clinicians accountable for performance.

COMPETENCIES

- Influence organizational strategy and policy through collaborative relationships with the board of directors, medical staff, nurses, and patients.
- Use governance structures and processes to enhance organizational performance, patient experience, and clinical quality.
- Allocate organizational assets and resources to support effective governance.
- Advocate for sound governance practices, including the commitment to fiduciary, legal, and ethical responsibilities.
- Build physician leadership capacity to ensure effective medical staff governance.
- Enable shared governance to ensure clinician engagement and high-quality patient care.

CHAPTER OUTLINE

- Role of Management in Governance
- Role of Board of Directors in Governance
- Role of Clinicians in Governance
- Governance Structure and Processes

INTRODUCTION

Health services managers do not run health care organizations (HCOs) alone. Healthcare **governance** is the term that describes how these groups collaborate to make important decisions for an HCO. Governance establishes the structures and processes that prevent individuals or factions from wresting control and making unilateral decisions that impact the whole organization (Moyo, 2021). In a hospital or health system, the major groups that share power through governance include board of directors, CEO and management team, medical staff, nursing staff, and patients. During prosperous times, the give-and-take among these powerful groups enables necessary attention to critical strategic and operational issues. In troubled times, however, power struggles imperil effective governance and undermine HCO success by dissatisfying physicians, distressing the board, angering nurses, alienating patients, and leaving the management team—the CEO in particular—seeking employment opportunities elsewhere.

FIGURE 7.1 Health care organization governance model.

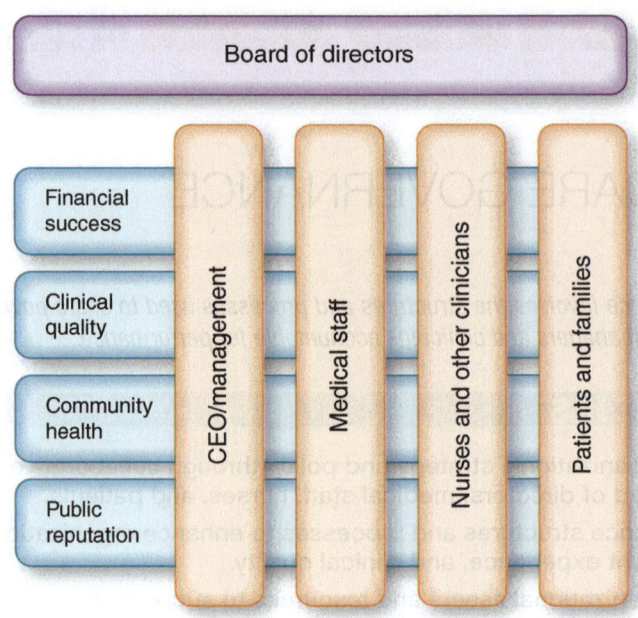

In addition to sharing power, good healthcare governance balances several priorities. As isexplained in this chapter, governance structures and processes are responsible for ensuring that financial success, clinical quality, community health, and a favorable public reputation can all be accomplished simultaneously. However, each of the power groups holds varying levels of interest in each of the priorities. As these groups compete to obtain resources, good governance enables powerful groups to respect the perspectives of others, share decision-making, and hold each other accountable for performance. Figure 7.1 illustrates the various groups and priorities involved in governance.

This chapter reviews the roles that health services managers, boards of directors, nurses, clinicians, and patients play in HCO governance and how these groups work together to achieve common goals. As is explained, the board of directors is the highest authority in the governance structure but relies on the CEO and their management team to turn strategy into action. The medical staff is legally authorized to set clinical policy but shares governance responsibilities with nurses and other clinicians. Finally, some health services managers rely on patients to play roles in governance, creating new opportunities for HCOs to become more responsive to their needs, preferences, and values.

ROLE OF MANAGEMENT IN GOVERNANCE

Relationship Between the Board and the CEO

Successful CEOs form strong working relationships with members of the **board of directors**. Board members, also called **trustees**, are elected to jointly guide the direction of the HCO (Kovner, 1990). The board of directors has the collective authority to make the final decisions. As a group, the board serves as the CEO's boss (Tyler & Biggs, 2001). As such, the CEO-board relationship has the potential to generate conflict, especially if the CEO resents deferring to people with less healthcare management knowledge. Nevertheless, the CEO is hired to faithfully implement the board's directives, whether they agree with their orders or not.

> **△ KEY IDEA**
>
> The board of directors has the collective authority to make the final decisions and act as the CEO's boss.

Agency theory explains the dynamics of CEO-board relationships. In agency theory, the principals of a firm (i.e., board of directors) hire independent agents (i.e., CEO and other executives) to run the organization on their behalf. While management is supposed to act in accordance with the interests of the organization, disputes can arise. The incentive for the CEO to make self-interested decisions is called the agency problem (Ross, 1973). To prevent agency problems, governing boards align the CEO's compensation with the HCO's performance, including profitability, quality of care, and community health (Collum et al., 2014). Ideally, well-written employment contracts create financially prosperous HCOs, which translates into salary increases and other rewards for health services managers (Karpoff, 2021).

Building supportive relationships with board members takes work and constant attention. Successful CEOs work diligently on board relations efforts, including the following (Biggs, 2011; Brown, 2014; Moyo, 2021; Sonnenfeld, 2002; Tyler & Biggs, 2001):

- *Establish boundaries:* Emphasize the management role as distinctive from the board's responsibility for governance.
- *Cultivate relationships:* Meet informally with board members outside of the boardroom and between board meetings. Trust in the CEO prevents board members from developing back channels to health services managers who report to the CEO.
- *Communicate with candor and listen for insights:* Speak with candor, transparency, and clarity and listen to board members' opinions.
- *Share critical issues:* Never surprise the board with bad news. Hidden negative information can be perceived as deception.
- *Seek regular feedback:* Regularly request informal feedback, allowing the board to provide any criticism in private (and praise in public).
- *Defuse harmful conflict:* Promote healthy conflict, build trust, and enable better decision-making.
- *Avoid political maneuvering:* Manipulating board members can erode a CEO's credibility. A prudent CEO avoids pitting one faction against another.

> **CAREER BOX 7.1: Managing Upward**
>
> Managing your boss, like the CEO-board relationship, takes collaborative problem-solving, a willingness to speak honestly, and an acknowledgment that your boss makes the final decisions. To influence your boss, it helps to frame your ideas in terms of what they want to achieve. Your boss is interested in accomplishing their goals, not necessarily yours. To understand what your boss wants, engage with them regularly to learn about their concerns, goals, priorities, and professional aspirations. Successful proposals solve issues that are important to them. Of course, your boss may disagree with you, which is fine. If you discuss your perspective in a respectful, productive way, you can maintain trust and continue in a collaborative working relationship. Your next proposal just might get approved.

Support the Board of Directors

To promote effective governance, CEOs and other executive health services managers provide board members with social and material support (Brown, 2014). Health services managers encourage the board to fulfill their governance responsibilities in a variety of ways, including the following (Brown, 2014; Collum et al., 2014; De Regge & Eeckloo, 2020; Tyler & Biggs, 2001):

- *Promote the higher purpose*: When the board believes that their role is important and consistent with their values, they are more likely to participate in governance activities.
- *Provide healthcare context*: HCO governance can be challenging for members who work outside the healthcare industry. Management should avoid jargon and simplify information to avoid overwhelming board members.
- *Encourage recruitment of competent board members*: Boards are responsible for recruiting new members, but the CEO can recommend capable people for consideration.
- *Control board size*: Most experts advise keeping board membership large enough to ensure representation on all committees but small enough that everyone can contribute meaningfully.
- *Provide training*: Boards who feel more competent in their abilities are more likely to successfully guide their HCOs.
- *Collaborate on agenda setting*: The CEO should ask the board chair and other members to suggest meeting agenda items that they think are important.
- *Cultivate trust*: If the board members respect one another, they develop trust, which creates a sense of **psychological safety** needed for expressing opinions without fear of negative consequences.
- *Consider compensating board members*: Almost all board members of investor-owned HCOs are paid for their participation. Most nonprofit HCO board members are not compensated or only receive a stipend.

Under the direction of the CEO, an administrative staff member acts as the primary contact for board meeting logistics, such as distributing agenda packets, keeping meeting minutes, and storing board documents. Although HCO board members serve part-time and meet infrequently, meetings are held at least once every other month (De Regge & Eeckloo, 2020). The CEO's staff spends substantial time and resources organizing regular meetings and annual strategic planning retreats. Apart from the usefulness of retreats for strategic planning, gatherings at appealing off-site locations offer enticing incentives for board members.

INFORMATIONAL INTERVIEW 7.1
Board of Directors Member, Community Health Center
Access the informational interview online at http://connect.springerpub.com/content/book/978-0-8261-4807-0/chapter/ch00.

Engage Medical Staff in Governance

According to federal and state law, hospitals must create a distinct governance body called a **medical staff**, which is made up of physicians and potentially other clinical practitioners who are licensed to provide patient care, if allowed by law. All physicians who admit patients to or work in the hospital are a part of the medical staff and are subject to its rules. For example, medical staff members are expected to participate in performance improvement activities and other governance functions as needed. However, many physicians avoid active participation because of the limited time available for administrative responsibilities. As such, health services managers work with physician leaders to recruit medical staff members to volunteer for governance activities, such as special projects or committee assignments. Through engagement in these experiences, physicians learn firsthand about the challenges that HCOs face and develop an appreciation for the management role. This, in turn, builds trust between health services managers and physicians and establishes shared commitment to organizational goals (Oostra, 2016).

> △ **KEY IDEA**
>
> When physicians engage in medical staff governance, they learn firsthand about the challenges that HCOs face and develop an appreciation for the management role.

Include Nurses and Other Clinicians in Governance

Nurses are not afforded the same advantages in hospital governance structures as physicians because nurses are not required by law to participate. Nevertheless, a concept called **shared governance** encourages nurses to influence governance decisions (Hess, 2017). As with physicians on the medical staff, shared governance means that nurses assume the obligation to meet the professional standards of practice of their profession. However, engagement from frontline nurses can prove difficult. Apathy, distractions, and lack of follow-through can undermine even the best intentions to involve nurses in self-governance (Ballard, 2010). Therefore, it is important to sustain nurses' involvement in shared governance through the constant attention from health services managers and nurse leaders. More importantly, health services managers should avoid using shared governance as a way to manage nurses but as a demonstration of respect for professional autonomy and a dedication to inclusive governance.

> △ **KEY IDEA**
>
> Shared governance is not a way to manage nurses but a demonstration of respect for professional autonomy and a dedication to inclusive governance.

Shared governance is not a threat to management authority. Instead, when managers share decision-making authority with nurses, they are empowered to influence issues that impact patient care (Porter-O'Grady, 2017). Health services managers who support shared governance among nurses and other clinicians create formal communication processes to express concerns with management (Moreno et al., 2018). Instead of suppressing frustrations, shared governance persuades frontline nurses to identify challenges and propose solutions related to professional practice and clinical quality. Through shared governance practices, health services managers not only enhance quality of care but also contribute to the overall success of the HCO.

ROLE OF BOARDS OF DIRECTORS IN GOVERNANCE

Set the Strategic Direction

The board possesses the ultimate responsibility for setting the HCO's strategic direction. The board reviews detailed strategic plans developed by the CEO and executive management team (Moseley, 2018). If the strategic plan is sound and consistent with the HCO's mission, vision, and values, then the board will vote to approve it. If not, the management team will revise their strategic recommendations based on the board's feedback. Once approved, the CEO and the management team must implement the strategy and deliver results.

Oversee Management and Clinicians

The board selects, evaluates, and compensates the CEO based on annual appraisals that compare the CEO's performance against established goals for the HCO (Biggs, 2011). If successful, the board financially rewards the CEO with bonuses or merit-based raises. In instances where HCO performance does not meet expectations, the board provides the CEO guidance and support on how to improve future performance. When the CEO blunders or commits ethical lapses, the board may fire the CEO (or force them to resign). More frequently, CEO employment separations occur when the board and CEO disagree about the strategic direction of the HCO. Being fired due to conflict with the board happens to even the most competent executives and usually does not severely damage a health services management's career (Gamble, 2014). In fact, other healthcare executives will sympathize with fired CEOs, realizing that CEO-board relationships can be especially challenging.

INFORMATIONAL INTERVIEW 7.2
Manager, Corporate Governance
Access the informational interview online at http://connect.springerpub.com/content/book/978-0-8261-4807-0/chapter/ch00.

The HCO board also oversees the management team's performance (Erwin et al., 2019). Boards regularly monitor operational performance metrics, such as market share and patient volume, to ensure that management is meeting established goals. An untrained board member may want to directly fix operational problems but managing HCO operations is not the role of the board (Kovner & Lemak, 2018). Instead, effective boards communicate performance expectations and hold management accountable for missing operational goals.

Boards are also responsible for financial oversight to ensure compliance with laws and regulations. The **Sarbanes-Oxley Act** of 2002 is a federal law designed to prevent fraudulent financial reporting for publicly traded for-profit companies. Nonprofit HCOs may not be directly affected by Sarbanes-Oxley requirements, but many high-performing HCOs implement relevant financial controls described under the law (Griffith, 2009). Nonetheless, all HCO boards select independent firms to audit the financial processes and reports of the HCO, consistent with good governance practice. A **management letter** from the auditors to the board and management reports any existing or potential financial irregularities or items of concern. The management letter is meant to help the HCO's board and management team address any issues or recommendations.

△ KEY IDEA

High-performing boards require health services management teams to provide regular updates about key clinical quality measures, including mortality rates, healthcare-acquired infections, and patient experience scores.

Finally, HCO boards oversee patient safety and health care quality, holding both management and clinicians accountable for clinical performance (Erwin et al., 2019). High-performing boards require health services management teams to provide regular updates about key clinical quality measures, including mortality rates, healthcare-acquired infections, and patient experience scores. When the board closely monitors clinical performance, management is more likely to invest in safe, high-quality clinical practices (Tsai et al., 2015).

> **CAREER BOX 7.2:** Career Board of Directors
>
> Health services managers need career boards of directors, a small group of people who help them navigate career challenges and celebrate successes. Informal in nature, the ideal career board includes people of various professional perspectives, such as a great leader, a technical expert, a sympathetic friend, an experience manager, or a strong writer (Stelter, 2022). Members of your career board of directors can be job specific, such as those working in a certain setting or area of specialization. A career board of directors will ask difficult questions about your career strategy and plans, make introductions to hiring managers, and give needed advice. They can also help with career transitions, such as negotiating a promotion or changing jobs. People will want to serve on your career board because successful people like to help others, just like others helped them when they were in need. The best way to assemble a career board of directors is to simply ask for guidance. Some may decline the request, but others will be happy to serve.

Recruit New Board Members

HCO boards are **self-perpetuating**, meaning that the board is responsible for recruiting new members, usually elected for terms of 3 years and no more than a total of 9 years (Center for Healthcare Governance [CHG], 2009). Board members are typically influential people with records of accomplishment and interest in serving the HCO. While some may be recruited because they are rich, famous, or well connected, the minimum qualifications for board membership are not that lofty. To qualify, potential board members must demonstrate the ability to collaborate with management and clinicians, the initiative to monitor HCO performance, and the desire to advocate for the interests of the HCO and community (Sonnenfeld, 2002). Board members usually possess one or more of the following qualifications (Erwin et al., 2019; Moyo, 2021; Sonnenfeld, 2002):

- Respected community standing
- Volunteer experience
- Business or finance knowledge
- Clinical expertise
- Healthcare background
- Mentorship experience
- Philanthropic capacity or fundraising skills

> △ **KEY IDEA**
>
> **Without diverse perspectives and experience on boards, HCOs will struggle to create diverse, equitable, and inclusive environments in which to care for patients and their families.**

To eliminate health disparities and improve health equity, some HCOs actively recruit a more diverse set of representatives to their boards (Bass, 2020). Achieving diversity in board membership means balancing skills, expertise, perspectives, gender, race, and ethnicity (Moyo, 2021). While HCOs have experienced modest gains in female board members, there has been less success in recruiting racial or ethnic minority representation (Silvera et al., 2023). Without diverse perspectives and experience on boards, HCOs will struggle to create diverse, equitable, and inclusive environments for patients and their families.

> ⚠ **KEY IDEA**
> Without diverse perspectives and experience on boards, HCOs struggle to create diverse, equitable, and inclusive environments for patients and their families.

Ethical Principles of Board Practice

Serving on HCO boards means accepting a position of trust. **Fiduciary** responsibility is the ethical obligation to maintain the trust of the people who they represent. Ethical board service upholds three fiduciary duties (CHG, 2009; Sonnenfeld, 2002):

- *Duty of care:* Board members must make themselves sufficiently informed before making decisions, relying on information, opinions, and reports provided by management. Board members are shielded from personal legal jeopardy as long as they act as any prudent person would in a similar situation
- *Duty of loyalty:* Board members must act in the best interest of the HCO. This includes avoiding **conflicts of interest**, which include using board service for personal gain.
- *Duty of obedience:* Board members must ensure that the HCO complies with applicable laws and regulations and act within the scope of their legal and governance authority.

As part of its ethical responsibilities, some HCO boards take stances on a variety of social and environmental issues, embracing what is known as **corporate social responsibility** (Erwin et al., 2019). For instance, many HCOs focus on increasing the proportion of women and people of color in HCO executive positions (Capozzalo, 2020; Lewis, 2022). Board oversight on these gender and racial equity goals prompts the management team to invest in leadership development programs, executive succession plans, pay equity initiatives, and fair evaluation and promotion practices (Development Dimensions International [DDI], 2021). In addition, environmental concerns have led hospitals to institute sustainable health services delivery practices that aim to reduce carbon emissions and wastefulness (Greenhill & Khalil, 2023). These social and environmental goals are a part of a concept known as the **triple bottom line**, which states that businesses should be committed to measuring not only profits but also its social and environmental impact (Senay et al., 2022). Table 7.1 outlines social and environmental measures that some HCO boards monitor.

TABLE 7.1 Social and Environmental Issues and Measures for Board Monitoring

ISSUE	CATEGORY	MEASURE
Environmental	Waste and pollution	Total annual waste by weight, type, and disposition (e.g., on-site incineration, landfill)
	Energy efficiency	Total annual energy consumed; percentage of grid electricity, percentage of renewable energy
	Climate change	Total annual greenhouse gas emissions per patient
Social	Diversity, equity, and inclusion	Percent of supplies expenses from minority procurement sources
	Safety and well-being	Number of hours and expenses of safety training per employee

Representation of External Stakeholders

Boards also represent external **stakeholders**, the term for groups of people who have interests in the HCO's success (Brown, 2014). For example, government HCO boards represent citizens who contribute funds through taxes. Investor-owned HCO boards represent investors in for-profit companies, who expect increased stock value and/or profits. Not-for-profit HCO boards represent the priorities of religious organizations, foundations, or communities in which the HCOs operate (CHG, 2009). Effective governance ensures that the HCO thrives, or at least survives, to provide health care services to the community (Brown et al., 2018). By federal law, all not-for-profit hospitals and health systems must demonstrate how they provide **community benefit**. Not-for-profit hospitals are exempt from paying taxes to the Internal Revenue Service (IRS) and must explain to the IRS how the HCO invests in community health. Boards hold hospital management teams accountable for justifying its tax-exempt status to the IRS. Some boards create permanent community benefit oversight committees to guide management's community efforts (Prybil & Killian, 2013).

ROLE OF CLINICIANS IN GOVERNANCE

Medical Staff Governance

Regulators and accreditors require hospitals and health systems to create medical staff structures and processes to oversee quality of care and patient safety (Cairns & Matzka, 2014). While typically a physician-only body, federal regulations allow HCOs to appoint other independent licensed practitioners to the medical staff, such as dentists, psychologists, APRNs, midwives, PAs, chiropractors, or podiatrists (Centers for Medicare and Medicaid Services [CMS], 2020). The medical staff influences clinical practice and negotiates resource allocation and capital equipment purchases. Figure 7.2 illustrates the standing committees and subcommittees of the medical staff. Within the governance structure, the medical executive committee includes a chief of staff, department chairs of medical departments (e.g., surgery, medicine, and pediatrics), and chairs of various committees (e.g., quality and safety). The **chief of staff** is viewed as the main physician representative of the medical staff. The **chief medical officer** is a separate position employed by the HCO to serve as a medical advisor to management.

The **medical staff bylaws** are guidelines for physician self-governance and vary by organization and state law but usually include the following (CHG, 2009; Crawford, 2013):

- *The medical executive committee:* Votes on governance processes, structures, rules, and regulations proposed by the subcommittees. If approved, the medical staff then makes recommendations to the board for review and approval.
- *Qualifications for membership:* Membership is typically limited to doctors of allopathy (MD) and doctors of osteopathy (DO), although some states allow HCOs to appoint other types of independent licensed practitioners.
- *Credentialing:* Medical staff administrators review applications for physicians to gain **privileges**, which allow them to practice medicine at the HCO. The credentialing committee makes recommendations to the board, who makes the final determination.
- *Organizational structure:* Defines clinical departments, such as surgery or gastroenterology, and the rules for electing chiefs of the clinical departments
- *Clinical review:* Protects patients from substandard care and abuse through **peer review** of medical practice. Physicians on the medical staff hold one another accountable to the performance standards of their profession. Physicians with similar practices review the work of one another, especially in cases of adverse events, such as patient death.
- *Disciplinary processes:* Defines rules for when a medical staff physician performs below standard or behaves disruptively, including corrective actions, suspensions, and fair hearing rights

FIGURE 7.2 Medical staff organization.

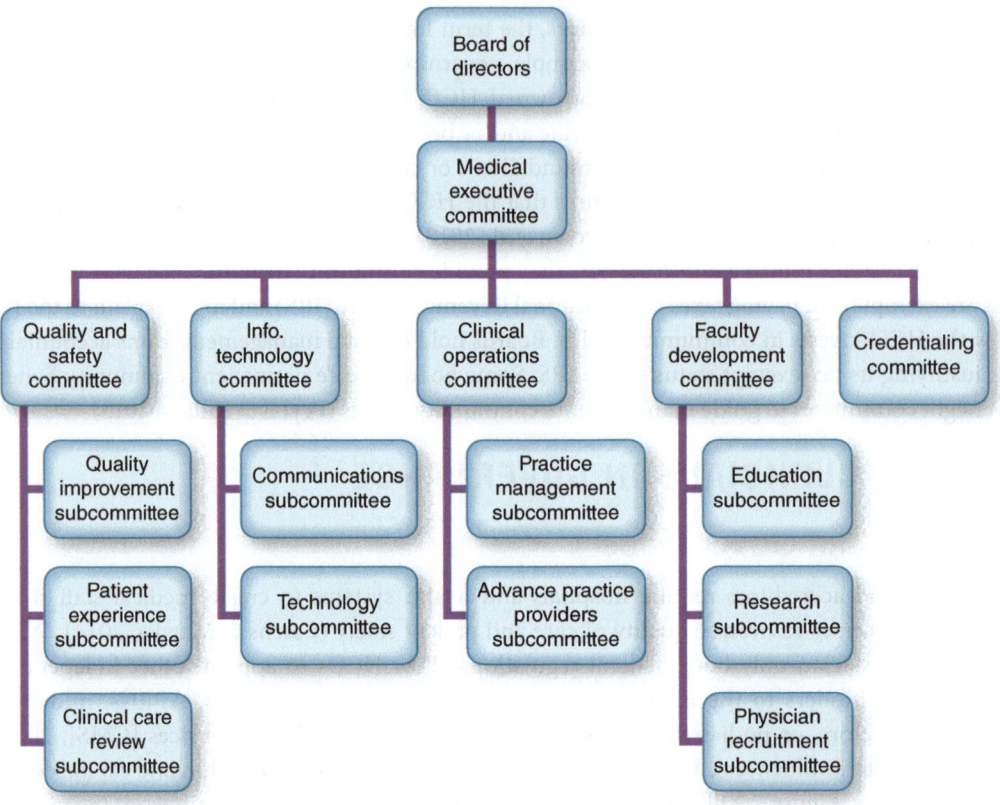

When the medical staff members actively engage in governance practices, HCOs tend to invest in quality initiatives, such as surgical infection prevention programs, that positively impact the quality of care (Bai & Krishnan, 2015; Jiang et al., 2009; Rotar et al., 2016).

Shared Governance Councils

Nurses and other clinicians influence institutional policies through shared governance. Frontline staff nurses and other bedside clinicians are encouraged to participate on shared governance councils to express their professional autonomy and promote best practices in patient care (Hess, 2017). Figure 7.3 illustrates a model for shared governance councils. These interprofessional councils often include the following (Moreno et al., 2018):

- *Coordinating council:* Provides guidance and cross-council communication related to shared governance issues. Members include representatives from each of the patient care departments and clinical professions.
- *Patient care leadership council:* Allocates resources and advocates for frontline clinical staff. Provides accountability and facilitates professional autonomy. Members include the chief nursing officer, administrative directors, directors of nursing, and directors of other clinical professions.
- *Quality and safety council:* Guides continuous quality improvement processes and establishes a fair process of peer review, including examination of incidents. Members include representatives from each of the clinical care departments.

FIGURE 7.3 Shared governance councils.

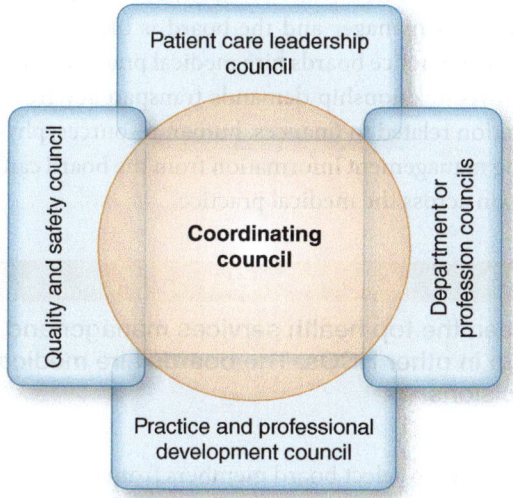

Source: Adapted from Westrope, R. A., Vaughn, L., Bott, M., & Taunton, R. L. (1995). Shared governance from vision to reality. *JONA: The Journal of Nursing Administration, 25*(12), 45–54. https://doi.org/10.1097/00005110-199512000-00008

- *Practice and professional development council*: Promotes professional development; implements new evidence-based clinical practices; and ensures practice of competence, accountability, and responsibility. Identifies needs and makes recommendations regarding products, equipment, and technology that impact patient care
- *Department or profession councils:* Each department/unit or specialty creates councils to review the patient care and share concerns and potential solutions to the coordinating council. Members include representatives from each of the patient care departments (or units) and clinical professions.

Finally, when nurses engage in governance, including governing boards and shared governance councils, they improve nursing practice and patient safety (Carthon et al., 2019; Kutney-Lee et al., 2016). However, nurses rarely serve as members on boards of directors. Even though nurses are the largest clinical profession in HCOs, they make up less than 5% of the board positions (American Hospital Association [AHA], 2022). Increased representation of nurses on boards could improve governance practices because they can provide valuable insights into patient needs and improve management-nurse relations (Kacik, 2023).

Medical Practice and Other Governance Structures

Physicians who collectively own and operate medical practices establish a special form of shared governance, which differs from that of hospitals and health systems in that medical practice board members are comprised of mostly physician owners (CHG, 2015). Ownership structures of medical practices vary widely, where some practices are owned by a small number of physicians who employ other physicians, while others are collectively owned by all the practicing physicians, each of whom have an ownership stake in the practice (Wagner, 2017). Regardless of the ownership arrangements, large medical practices create governance structures and processes to share decision-making among physicians.

Typically, board members of physician-owned medical practice are experts in the practice of medicine but not in the business of healthcare (Wagner, 2017, p. 277). As such, the relationship between the top health services manager and the board is like the CEO-board relationship in other HCOs. Namely, medical practice boards hire medical practice managers to implement their decisions. This boss-employee relationship demands transparency from the practice managers, including sharing information related to finances, human resources, physician performance, and ethical lapses. Withholding management information from the board can result in a decay of trust and ineffective collaboration across the medical practice.

> ⚠ **KEY IDEA**
>
> The relationship between the top health services manager and the board is like the CEO-board relationship in other HCOs. The boards hire medical practice managers to implement their decisions.

Large medical practices tend to select board members from diverse areas of the organization, including different practice locations or from different physician specialties. Such **representational governance** may impede effectiveness if the board members believe their role is to represent the interests of a group rather than the interests of the entire medical practice. To create more effective governance, some medical practices add external members with competencies in business or community relations, as well as physicians from outside the practice. Figure 7.4 illustrates an example medical practice governance structure that applies the representational model.

Another representational governance model includes healthcare business entities called Accountable Care Organizations (ACOs). Established by the Affordable Care Act and regulated by the Centers for Medicaid & Medicare (CMS), ACOs are legal entities made up of a collection of HCOs (i.e., hospitals, physician groups, long-term care) that assume responsibility for the total cost of treating patients and the quality of care provided to their patients. In exchange, the ACO

FIGURE 7.4 Physician practice governance structure.

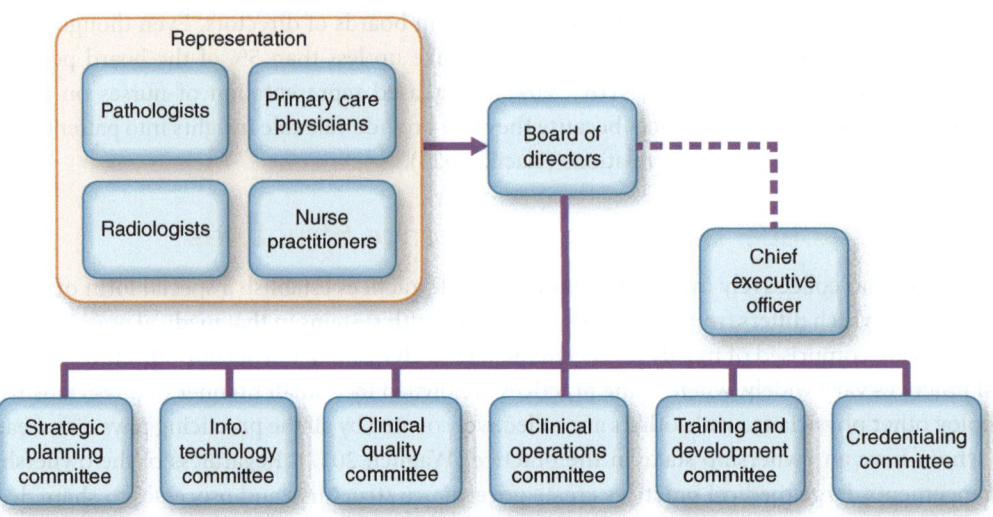

is eligible to receive financial bonuses based on the level of cost reduction, if any. The ACO board must, by law, provide meaningful governance contributions from each of the participating organizations. Representatives from each of the participating ACO groups will serve on the board, including physicians and management. In addition, CMS requires that at least 75% of the governing board be comprised of ACO patients, providing another example of consumer governance.

ROLE OF PATIENTS IN GOVERNANCE

Patient-Centered Governance

Patient-centered care addresses the patient preferences, needs, and values when making all clinical decisions (Institute of Medicine [IOM], 2001). One way HCOs achieve patient-centered care is to include patients in governance structures, an approach called **consumer governance** (Wright, 2013). Patient involvement in governance provides a respectful way to gather feedback from patients about actions that affect them. Consumer governance also increases a community's perception that the HCO wants to build trusting relationships with patients (DeCamp et al., 2021).

In many instances, national and state health policy requires that HCOs participate in consumer governance practices (DeCamp et al., 2019). These governance regulations are intended to improve patient safety and clinical quality, give patients power to influence the strategic direction of the HCO, and promote responsiveness to patient needs. For example, the CMS requires that ACOs and other value-based purchasing programs include patient representatives in governance (Hendrickson, 2019). The federal government requires 51% of community health center boards to be patients (Wright, 2013).

Patient and Family Advisory Councils

The most common way that HCOs involve patients in governance practices is through **Patient and Family Advisory Councils** (PFACs). PFACs are designed to encourage patients and families to collaborate with HCOs to improve the quality, safety, and experience of care. When health services managers actively engage with PFACs, it demonstrates commitment to patient centeredness, quality care, and transparency in decision-making. Effective PFAC consumer governance practices include the following (Center for Health Care Strategies [CHCS], 2019; DeCamp et al., 2021; Jones, 2018; NYHealth Foundation, 2018):

- *Commit HCO resources:* Name a health services manager executive sponsor and provide a staff liaison to assist with scheduling and planning regular meetings.
- *Gain staff and clinician buy-in:* Communicate the rationale and benefits of PFACs throughout the HCO.
- *Define goals and evaluate impact:* Set expectations for performance and measure the impact of PFAC activities.
- *Train and educate:* Offer effective orientation and continuing education opportunities that allow PFAC representatives to influence governance structures and processes.
- *Reflect diversity of communities:* Avoid tokenism. Engage in ongoing recruitment to ensure recruitment of representatives that reflect the communities they serve.
- *Compensate members:* Pay stipends or wages to encourage participation, especially among disadvantaged populations. Provide logistical support, such as childcare, parking, transportation, and lunches.

Community Representation

Effective PFACs represent their communities. As such, ideal PFAC members possess good interpersonal and communications skills so that they can interface with members of the community, a powerful public relations approach for improving the HCO's reputation (Dukhanin et al., 2020). Health services managers establish ways for the community to contact PFAC members, including email, suggestion boxes, town hall gatherings, and open council meetings (DeCamp et al., 2019). During such interactions, patients frequently share their positive and negative health care experiences with PFACs.

However, for PFACs to serve as trustworthy contacts for the community, PFAC membership should reflect the diversity of the communities served (Jones, 2018). Diversity can be defined very broadly, such as a mix of age, gender, race, ethnicity, culture, sexual orientation, financial situation, overall health and disability status, physical and mental ability, and educational background. To recruit PFAC members from diverse backgrounds, health services managers can attend community meetings to develop relationships and ask community leaders, physicians, nurses, and public relations staff for referrals. To make a diverse set of potential PFAC members feel valued, health services managers can make sure language interpreters are at meetings, hold meetings at different times and modalities (i.e., in person or virtual), and make sure their opinions are used to improve the HCO.

GOVERNANCE STRUCTURES AND PROCESSES

Charters and Bylaws

Boards document basic rules for the conduct of governance matters of the HCO (CHG, 2009). A **charter** is a legal document, frequently called the articles of incorporation, that legally creates the HCO and is filed with the secretary of the state. **Governance bylaws** are the board's operating instructions that describe the formal self-governance structure and processes by which the HCO is governed. Bylaws typically include the following:
- Board authority, functions, and responsibilities
- Board membership size and composition
- Recruitment and election of board members
- Performance expectations of board members
- Descriptions of standing committees and the process for creating ad hoc committees
- Written standards of ethical conduct
- Committee membership, including nonboard members with specialized expertise

Bylaws also describe the parliamentary authority, which is the set of procedures for conducting board meetings. A board may develop their own set of rules governing the conduct of meetings, or it may adopt formalized rules, such as *Robert's Rules of Order*, a book that explains the basic steps for **parliamentary procedures** (Robert, 2020). Examples of Robert's Rules procedures include the following:
- A board member makes a **motion** that proposes an action for the consideration of the board (e.g., "I move that we create a special committee to . . .").
- Another board member must second a motion (e.g., "I second it."). Without a second, the motion will die.
- The board debates using formal rules, such as one person being allowed to speak at a time.
- The board votes when two-thirds of the members present agree to end the debate (e.g., say "I call the question.").
- Final vote taken. Those in favor say "aye," and those opposed say "nay."
- **Meeting minutes** are a record of what was done in a meeting (not what was said), including motions and results of votes.

Not all motions in a board meeting need debate. In fact, board meetings are full of routine reports handled using **consent agenda** that allow the board to approve items, such as meeting minutes or committee reports. Consent agenda items must be sent out to board members before the meeting. If requested, a board member can request that an item be pulled out of the consent agenda for discussion and possible rejection.

Committee Membership and Structures

Board bylaws outline the rules for committee formation, member selection, and performance evaluation. Although there is little agreement on the size and composition of the ideal HCO board, the number of people serving on a board is usually proportional to the size of the HCO, ranging from nine to 15 members (De Regge & Eeckloo, 2020; Erwin et al., 2019). In most cases, board members are not employees of the HCO. When HCO boards decide to include CEOs, CFOs, physicians, and nurses, there is a tendency to hold **executive sessions** without managers or clinicians present so that they may discuss particularly sensitive issues related to those parties (Sonnenfeld, 2002).

While the number and type of governance committees vary, shared best practices create commonalities across the healthcare industry (CHG, 2009). All committees report to the board of directors. **Standing committees** are permanent entities whose purposes are defined in the bylaws. **Special committees** (i.e., ad hoc or task committees) are created for specific duties and disbanded upon the completion of the assigned tasks, such as handling a public relations crisis or conducting a search for a new CEO (CHG, 2009). Common standing committees, illustrated in Figure 7.5, include the following (CHG, 2009; Prybil & Killian, 2013):

- *Executive committee:* Meets when urgent matters arise, such as serious high-level workplace matters, and may be empowered to make decisions on the board's behalf in specific circumstances. All directors are invited to participate in executive committee meetings.
- *Strategic planning committee:* Establishes strategic direction (i.e., mission, vision, and values) of the HCO to create competitive advantage and meet the needs of the populations the board is elected to serve
- *Finance and audit committee:* Responsible for financial oversight of the HCO, including allocating capital to operations, reviewing capital expenditures, critically evaluating financing alternatives, and auditing accounting processes
- *Quality and patient safety committee:* Oversees clinical quality, patient safety, and risk management

FIGURE 7.5 Health care organization governance structure.

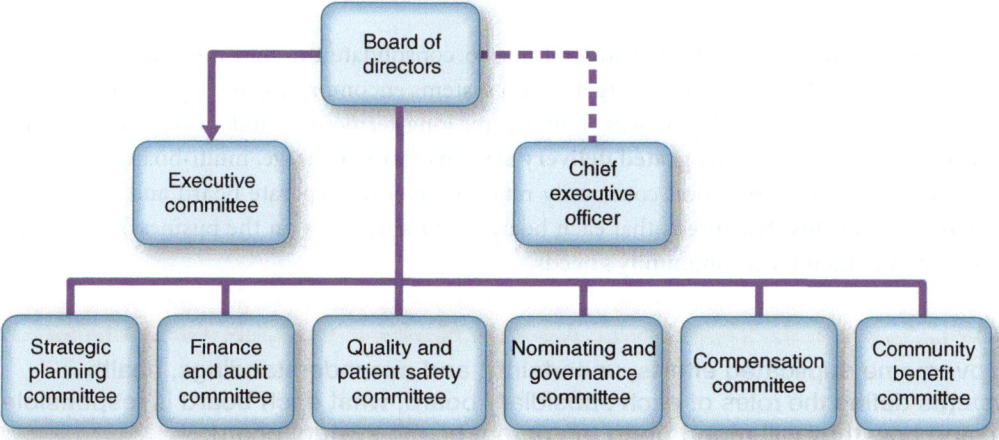

- *Nominating and governance committee:* Oversees recruitment of proposed nominees for election to the board and evaluate board governance practices
- *Compensation committee:* Makes decisions regarding CEO selection, evaluation, and compensation. The IRS recommends hiring an independent third party to compare salaries and bonuses of CEOs at similar HCOs.
- *Community benefit committee:* Although not common, some boards form a committee tasked to ensure that the HCO appropriately provides community benefit to the standards established by IRS regulations.

Governance Policies and Procedures

Boards are responsible for overseeing the HCO's operations, including efforts to ensure compliance with applicable laws and regulations. Through the standing committees, boards approve written **policies and procedures** that set the expectations for certain situations and to describe in step-by-step detail how the HCO should operate. External authorities (e.g., regulators and accreditors) require that HCOs document, implement, and follow policies and procedures. There can be dozens of policies and procedures, each of which are reviewed, revised, and approved by the board on a regular basis. Common policies and procedures cover issues related to conflicts of interest, charity care, executive compensation, selection of external auditors, joint ventures, whistleblower protections, prevention of disruptive behavior, and hiring practices consistent with the Civil Rights Act of 1964 and the Age Discrimination in Employment Act of 1967.

Regulators are government bodies that verify whether a business is working according to laws. The executive branch of the federal government operates dozens of regulators impacting HCOs, including the CMS and the Occupational and Safety and Health Administration (AHA, 2017). State government regulators, such as departments of health, also require specified policies and procedures and conduct regular audits of HCO performance. **Accreditors** also inspect HCOs to determine whether the appropriate policies and procedures are documented and followed. Accreditation is a system of standards deemed essential for health services delivery. Most acute care hospitals opt to become accredited because the CMS requires that hospitals either be accredited or pass state inspections to qualify for payments from Medicare. Most acute care hospitals (about 88%) choose to become accredited by **The Joint Commission** but may choose from among several accrediting bodies (Jha, 2018).

HCOs utilize templates that establish an efficient way for policy and procedure to be written, tracked, and reviewed. Table 7.2 illustrates an example of the typical components of a policy and procedure for conflicts of interest.

Multi-Organization Governance

The healthcare industry is expected to continue to consolidate through mergers, acquisitions, partnerships, or affiliations to create larger health systems encompassing multiple types of HCOs, including hospitals, medical practices, home care, long-term care, and insurance companies (Erwin et al., 2019). These **integrated delivery systems** form one large, multi-board governance structure with each organization commonly retaining its own separate board and committees. The advantage of this structure is that each board maintains focus on the business's unique circumstance and their local community's needs.

△ KEY IDEA

To overcome duplicated efforts, uncertainty, and misunderstandings, health systems define the roles of each subsidiary board, what each board is responsible for, and how they will report up to the parent health system board.

TABLE 7.2 Example Policy and Procedure

HCO POLICY AND PROCEDURE MANUAL			
Subject:	Institutional Conflicts of Interest		
Index title:	Ethics and Compliance		
Policy Number: HCO-EC009	Effective Date: 2/17/22		Revision date: 9/19/24
Purpose:	While relationships with external entities are a part of normal business operations, financial interests must not compromise, or appear to compromise, the objectivity or integrity of the HCO's mission.		
Policy:	Gifts from corporate entities must not influence, or appear to influence, HCO's business decisions or the integrity of patient care. Organizational representatives must not use their positions or influence to gain advancement for themselves, immediate family, or other personal and business associates at the expense of the HCO. The HCO personnel must comply with conflict management plans that are formulated by the board of directors.		
Procedures:	<ul><li>Disclosures of potential or actual conflict of interests must be made by completing the Conflict of Interest Declaration Form.</li><li>Significant external activity involving honoraria, gifts, or other in-kind compensation of more than $5,000 per year must be disclosed.</li><li>Significant external activity related to consulting income, salary (excluding that from the HCO), or other in-kind compensation of more than $5,000 per year must be disclosed.</li><li>The board reviews the details of declared conflicts and determines appropriate actions, according to the conflict management plan.</li><li>Conflicts declared previously do not need to be declared again unless specifics have changed.</li></ul>		
Definitions:	Conflict of interest: Employee's outside activities, personal financial interests, or other personal interests influence, or appear to influence, their ability to make unbiased decisions in their job responsibilities. Conflict management plan: A structured approach to address and resolve conflicts that may arise within the HCO and is used to maintain integrity or objectivity of patient care or the business transactions of the HCO Significant external activity: External engagements providing more than $5,000 in income in a 12-month period or exceed 5% ownership in external entity		
Name and Title:	Pranesh Rima, chief compliance officer		
Signature of Approval:			

HCO, health care organization.

However, when multi-unit boards seek to operate autonomously, it can lead to duplicated efforts, uncertainty, and misunderstandings. To overcome these challenges, health systems define the roles of each subsidiary board, what each board is responsible for, and how they will report up to the parent health system board. The system-level boards establish control and authority over the local boards to direct effective strategic decisions and manage system-wide strategic initiatives and investments (Prybil et al., 2012). Figure 7.6 illustrates the hierarchy of system-level and local boards and the coordination between committees, as represented by the dotted line connections.

FIGURE 7.6 Health system governance structure.

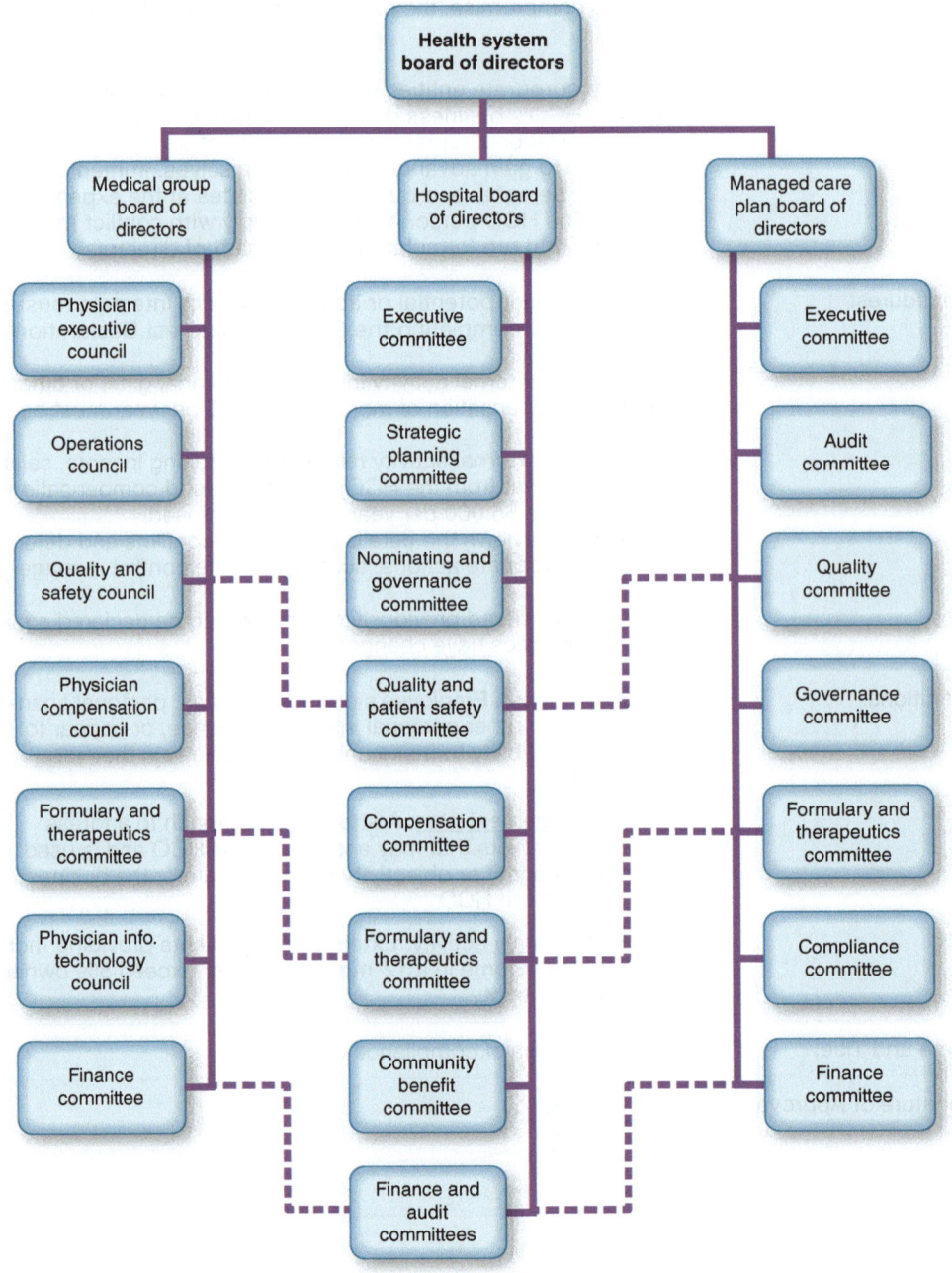

FUTURE DIRECTIONS

Hospitals and physician practice sectors are expected to further consolidate into regional health systems through mergers and acquisitions. These multi-organization structures require significant coordination and collaboration of different boards, each with different missions, visions, and values. Without governance alignment, the health systems will not be able to take advantage of consolidation. Therefore, the future challenge for HCOs will be to design governance structures that balance the interests of boards of directors, management teams, medical staffs, nursing staffs, and patients across multiple communities.

SUMMARY

- Governance is the legal process of sharing power, control, and authority through formal committee structures and decision-making processes.
- Major groups govern hospitals and health systems—the board of directors, CEO and management, medical staff, nurses and other clinicians, and patients—and each have distinctive roles in healthcare governance.
- Boards set strategic direction, recruit new board members, oversee the CEO, and represent the community for which they were elected to represent. Management runs day-to-day operations.
- Board fiduciary responsibilities include duty of care, duty of loyalty, and duty of obedience. Some HCO boards expand their fiduciary responsibilities beyond community health to include social and environmental issues.
- The medical staff is a separate legal entity with responsibilities for oversight of the quality of clinical care and the processes involved with analyzing and improving medical care services.
- Shared governance enables frontline nurses and other bedside clinicians to express their professional autonomy and promote best practices in patient care. Representatives from departments and professions form councils that communicate concerns and potential solutions to management.
- Other types of HCOs, such as physician-owned medical practices and community health centers, form governance structures in which the CEO reports to the board, no matter if the board is constituted with physicians or patients.

KEY TERMS*

*For the full list of key terms, please see the online glossary at **http://connect.springerpub.com/content/book/978-0-8261-4807-0.**

accreditors
agency theory
board of directors
charter
chief of staff
chief medical officer
community benefit
conflicts of interest
consent agenda
consumer governance
corporate social responsibility
duty of care
duty of loyalty

duty of obedience
executive sessions
fiduciary
governance
governance bylaws
integrated delivery systems
The Joint Commission
management letter
medical staff
medical staff bylaws
meeting minutes
motion
parliamentary procedures

patient and family advisory councils
patient-centered care
policies and procedures
privileges
psychological safe
regulators
representational governance
Robert's Rules of Order
Sarbanes-Oxley Act
self-perpetuating
shared governance
special committee
stakeholders
standing committee
triple bottom line
trustees

LEARNING ACTIVITIES

Professional Development and Reflection

1. Boards of directors advise the chief executive officers of HCOs. Reflect on the "board members" who advise you on your career. Where are there gaps in skills or perspectives among your board of directors? What steps with you take to recruit new career board members?
2. Based on best practices for CEO-board relations, create a list of rules for effectively "managing upward" to your boss or other senior executive health services managers.

Discussion Questions

1. Reflect on the potential conflicts that may arise in the relationship between CEOs and boards of directors. How can these conflicts be effectively managed to ensure productive collaboration?
2. Should nurses and other clinicians be given legal authority in the governance structure of hospitals and health systems? Why or why not?
3. Discuss the challenges and benefits of reflecting the diversity of communities in PFAC memberships. How can health services managers avoid tokenism and ensure that PFAC members represent the broad range of demographics within their communities.

RECOMMENDED READING AND MEDIA

Badowski, R., & Gittines, R. (2004). *Managing up: How to forge an effective relationship with those above you*. Currency.

Bass, K. H. (2020, November 10). *Recruiting for a diverse health care board: Practices and processes to better reflect community diversity*. American Hospital Association Trustee Services. https://trustees.aha.org/recruiting-diverse-health-care-board

Ford, E. W. (2022). Creating your personal board of directors. *Journal of Healthcare Management, 67*(5), 303–305. https://doi.org/10.1097/jhm-d-22-00160

Robert, H. M., Evans, W. J., Honemann, D. H., Balch, T. J., Seabold, D. E., & Gerber, S. (2020). *Robert's rules of order, newly revised in brief: Updated to accord with the twelfth edition of the complete manual* (3rd ed.). PublicAffairs.

Stelter, S. (2022, May 9). Want to advance in your career? Build your own board of directors. *Harvard Business Review*. https://hbr.org/2022/05/want-to-advance-in-your-career-build-your-own-board-of-directors

Wagner, S. E. (Host). (2021, September 17). *The board's role in advancing health equity strategies* [Audio podcast]. American Hospital Association Trustee Services. https://trustees.aha.org/podcasts/2021-09-17-boards-role-advancing-health-equity-strategies

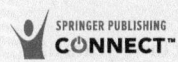

A robust set of instructor resources designed to supplement this text is located at http://connect.springerpub.com/content/book/978-0-8261-4807-0.
Qualifying instructors may request access by emailing textbook@springerpub.com.

REFERENCES

American Hospital Association. (2017). *Federal agencies with regulatory or oversight authority impacting hospitals*. https://www.aha.org/system/files/2018-01/info-regulatory-burden-federal-agencies.pdf

American Hospital Association. (2022). *AHA 2022 national health care governance survey report*. https://trustees.aha.org/aha-2022-national-health-care-governance-survey-report

Bai, G., & Krishnan, R. (2015). Do hospitals without physicians on the board deliver lower quality of care? *American Journal of Medical Quality, 30*(1), 58–65. https://doi.org/10.1177/1062860613516668

Ballard, N. (2010). Factors associated with success and breakdown of shared governance. *The Journal of Nursing Administration, 40*(10), 411–416. https://doi.org/10.1097/nna.0b013e3181f2eb14

Bass, K. H. (2020, November 10). *Recruiting for a diverse health care board: Practices and processes to better reflect community diversity*. American Hospital Association Trustee Services. https://trustees.aha.org/recruiting-diverse-health-care-board

Biggs, E. L. (2011). *Healthcare governance: A guide for effective boards* (2nd ed.). Health Administration Press.

Brown, W. A. (2014). Antecedents to board member engagement in deliberation and decision-making. In C. Cornforth & W. A. Brown (Eds.), *Nonprofit governance: Innovative perspectives and approaches* (pp. 100–116). Routledge.

Brown, A., Dickinson, H., & Kelaher, M. (2018). Governing the quality and safety of healthcare: A conceptual framework. *Social Science & Medicine, 202*, 99–107. https://doi.org/10.1016/j.socscimed.2018.02.020

Cairns, C. S., & Matzka, K. (2014). *Verify and comply: Credentialing and medical staff standards crosswalk*. HCPro Inc.

Capozzalo, G. L. (2020). *Healthcare systems have an imperative to advance gender equity* [blog]. American College of Healthcare Executives. https://www.ache.org/blog/2020/healthcare-systems-have-an-imperative-to-advance-gender-equity

Carthon, J. M. B., Davis, L., Dierkes, A., Hatfield, L., Hedgeland, T., Holland, S., Plover, C., Ballinghoff, J., Del Guidice, M., Sanders, A. M., Visco, F., & Aiken, L. H. (2019). Association of nurse engagement and nurse staffing on patient safety. *Journal of Nursing Care Quality, 34*(1), 40. https://doi.org/10.1097/ncq.0000000000000334

Center for Healthcare Governance. (2009). *The guide to good governance for hospital boards*. American Hospital Association.

Center for Healthcare Governance. (2015). *Governance of physician organizations: An essential step to care integration*. American Hospital Association. https://www.aha.org/resources/2019-05-14-governance-physician-organizations

Center for Health Care Strategies. (2019, December). *Best practices for convening a community advisory board*. https://www.chcs.org/resource/best-practices-for-convening-a-community-advisory-board

Centers for Medicare and Medicaid Services. (2020). State operations manual appendix a - survey protocol, regulations, and interpretive guidelines for hospitals. https://www.cms.gov/Regulations-and-Guidance/Guidance/Manuals/downloads/som107ap_a_hospitals.pdf

Collum, T., Menachemi, N., Kilgore, M., & Weech-Maldonado, R. (2014). Management involvement on the board of directors and hospital financial performance. *Journal of Healthcare Management, 59*(6), 429–445. https://doi.org/10.1097/00115514-201411000-00009

Crawford, T. (2013). *Medical staff bylaws, rules, and regulations: Read before you sign.* [blog]. NEJM CareerCenter. https://resources.nejmcareercenter.org/article/medical-staff-bylaws-rules-and-regulations-read-before-you-sign

De Regge, M., & Eeckloo, K. (2020). Balancing hospital governance: A systematic review of 15 years of empirical research. *Social Science & Medicine, 262*, 113252. https://doi.org/10.1016/j.socscimed.2020.113252

DeCamp, M., Brewer, S. E., & Dukhanin, V. (2021). Patient, public, consumer, and community engagement: From consucrat to representative comment on "the rise of the consucrat". *International Journal of Health Policy and Management, 10*(8), 503–506. https://doi.org/10.34172%2Fijhpm.2020.148

DeCamp, M., Dukhanin, V., Hebert, L. C., Himmelrich, S., Feeser, S., & Berkowitz, S. A. (2019). Patients' views about patient engagement and representation in healthcare governance. *Journal of healthcare management/American College of Healthcare Executives, 64*(5), 332–346. https://doi.org/10.1097/jhm-d-18-00152

Development Dimensions International. (2021). *Leadership transitions report 2021.* https://www.ddiworld.com/research/leadership-transitions-report

Dukhanin, V., Feeser, S., Berkowitz, S. A., & DeCamp, M. (2020). Who represents me? A patient-derived model of patient engagement via patient and family advisory councils (PFACs). *Health Expectations, 23*(1), 148–158. https://doi.org/10.1111/hex.12983

Erwin, C. O., Landry, A. Y., Livingston, A. C., & Dias, A. (2019). Effective governance and hospital boards revisited: Reflections on 25 years of research. *Medical Care Research and Review, 76*(2), 131–166. https://doi.org/10.1177/1077558718754898

Gamble, M. (2014, May 9). The CEO's guide to getting fired. *Becker's Hospital Review.* https://www.beckershospitalreview.com/hospital-management-administration/the-ceo-s-guide-to-getting-fired.html

Greenhill, R. G., & Khalil, M. (2023). Sustainable healthcare depends on good governance practices. *Frontiers of Health Services Management, 39*(3), 5–11. https://doi.org/10.1097/hap.0000000000000163

Griffith, J. R. (2009). Finding the frontier of hospital management. *Journal of Healthcare Management, 54*(1), 57–72. https://doi.org/10.1097/00115514-200901000-00011

Hendrickson, S. W. (2019). Practitioner application: Patient's views about patient engagement and representation in healthcare governance. *Journal of Healthcare Management, 64*(5), 347–348. https://doi.org/10.1097/jhm-d-19-00155

Hess, R. G., Jr. (2017). Professional governance: Another new concept? *JONA: The Journal of Nursing Administration, 47*(1), 1–2. https://doi.org/10.1097/NNA.0000000000000427

Institute of Medicine. (2001). *Crossing the quality chasm: A new health system for the 21st century.* National Academy Press.

Jha, A. K. (2018). Accreditation, quality, and making hospital care better. *JAMA, 320*(23), 2410–2411. https://doi.org/10.1001/jama.2018.18810

Jiang, J. H., Lockee, C., Bass, K., & Fraser, I. (2009). Board oversight of quality: Any differences in process of care and mortality? *Journal of Healthcare Management, 54*(1), 15–29. https://doi.org/10.1097/00115514-200901000-00005

Jones, K. (2018). *Diverse voices matter: Improving diversity in patient and family advisory councils.* Institute for Patient- and Family-Centered Care. https://ipfcc.org/resources/Diverse-Voices-Matter.pdf

Kacik, A. (2023, March 2023). *Nurses on boards could impact hospital governance—If there were enough.* Modern Healthcare. https://www.modernhealthcare.com/esg/nurses-on-boards-hospital-governance-palo-pinto-aha

Karpoff, J. M. (2021). On a stakeholder model of corporate governance. *Financial Management, 50*(2), 321–343. https://doi.org/10.1111/fima.12344

Kovner, A. R. (1990). Improving hospital board effectiveness: An update. *Frontiers of Health Services Management, 6*(3), 3.

Kovner, A. R., & Lemak, C. H. (2018). J. Knickman & B. Elbel (Eds.), In *Health Care Delivery in the United States*. New York: Springer Publishing Company.

Kutney-Lee, A., Germack, H., Hatfield, L., Kelly, M. S., Maguire, M. P., Dierkes, A., Del Guidice, M., & Aiken, L. H. (2016). Nurse engagement in shared governance and patient and nurse outcomes. *JONA: The Journal of Nursing Administration, 46*(11), 605–612. https://doi.org/10.1097/nna.0000000000000412

Lewis. J. A. (2022). *In 2022, we were bold. In 2023, we'll do even more* [blog]. American Hospital Association Institute for Diversity and Health Equity. https://ifdhe.aha.org/news/blog/2022-12-13-2022-we-were-bold-2023-well-do-even-more

Moreno, J. V., Girard, A. S., & Foad, W. (2018). Realigning shared governance with Magnet® and the organization's operating system to achieve clinical excellence. *JONA: The Journal of Nursing Administration, 48*(3), 160–167. https://doi.org/10.1097/nna.0000000000000591

Moseley, G. B. (2018). *Managing Health Care Business Strategy.* (2nd ed.). Jones & Bartlett Learning.

Moyo, D. (2021). *How boards work: And how they can work better in a chaotic world*. Basic Books.

NYHealth Foundation. (2018, June 11). *Strategically advancing patient and family advisory councils in New York State hospitals*. https://nyhealthfoundation.org/wp-content/uploads/2018/06/strategically-advancing-patient-and-family-advisory-councils.pdf

Oostra, R. D. (2016). Physician leadership: A central strategy to transforming healthcare. *Frontiers of Health Services Management, 32*(3), 15–26. https://doi.org/10.1097/01974520-201601000-00003

Porter-O'Grady, T. (2017). A response to the question of professional governance versus shared governance. *JONA: The Journal of Nursing Administration, 47*(2), 69–71. https://doi.org/10.1097/nna.0000000000000439

Prybil, L., & Killian, R. (2013). *Community benefit: Community benefit needs board oversight*. Health Progress. Journal of the Catholic Health Association of the United States. https://www.chausa.org/publications/health-progress/article/july-august-2013/community-benefit---community-benefit-needs-board-oversight

Prybil, L., Levey, S., Killian, R., Fardo, D., Chait, R., Bardach, D. R., & Roach, W. (2012). *Governance in large nonprofit health systems: Current profile and emerging patterns*. Commonwealth Center for Governance Studies, Inc.

Ross, S. A. (1973). The economic theory of agency: The principal's problem. *The American Economic Review, 63*(2), 134–139.

Rotar, A. M., Botje, D., Klazinga, N. S., Lombarts, K. M., Groene, O., Sunol, R., & Plochg, T. (2016). The involvement of medical doctors in hospital governance and implications for quality management: A quick scan in 19 and an in depth study in 7 OECD countries. *BMC Health Services Research, 16*(2), 160. https://doi.org/10.1186/s12913-016-1396-4

Senay, E., Cort, T., Perkison, W., Laestadius, J. G., & Sherman, J. D. (2022). What can hospitals learn from the Coca-Cola company? Health care sustainability reporting. *NEJM Catalyst Innovations in Care Delivery, 3*(3), CAT-21. https://doi.org/10.1056/CAT.21.0362

Silvera, G. A., Erwin, C. O., & Garman, A. N. (2023). A Seat at the table: An examination of hospital governing board diversity, 2011–2021. *Journal of Healthcare Management, 68*(2), 132–142. https://doi.org/10.1097/jhm-d-22-00068

Sonnenfeld, J. A. (2002). What makes great boards great. Harvard business review, 80(9), 106–113.

Stelter, S. (2022, May 9). Want to advance in your career? Build your own board of directors. *Harvard Business Review*. https://hbr.org/2022/05/want-to-advance-in-your-career-build-your-own-board-of-directors

Tsai, T. C., Jha, A. K., Gawande, A. A., Huckman, R. S., Bloom, N., & Sadun, R. (2015). Hospital board and management practices are strongly related to hospital performance on clinical quality metrics. *Health Affairs, 34*(8), 1304–1311. https://doi.org/10.1377/hlthaff.2014.1282

Tyler, J. L., & Biggs, E. L. (2001). Practical governance: CEO performance appraisal. *Trustee: The Journal for Hospital Governing Boards, 54*(5), 18–18.

Wagner, S. L. (2017). *Fundamentals of medical practice management.* Health Administration Press.

Wright, B. (2013). Who governs federally qualified health centers? *Journal of Health Politics, Policy and Law, 38*(1), 27–55. https://doi.org/10.1215/03616878-1898794

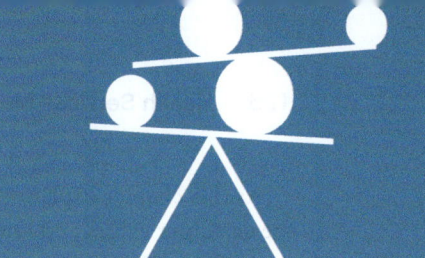

CHAPTER 8

HEALTHCARE STRATEGY AND MARKETING

Healthcare strategy refers to making choices that position the organization to uniquely provide value to patients, families, clinicians, and communities. Marketing entails designing, delivering, and communicating the value of health services.

COMPETENCIES

- Conduct internal and external assessments to determine strategic opportunities.
- Formulate strategic plans to maximize market opportunities.
- Assess strategic alternatives using evidence.
- Allocate resources to improve the long-term viability of the organization.
- Develop business plans that align with organizational strategy.
- Create operational plans that implement organizational strategy.
- Evaluate legal and regulatory implications of affiliations, mergers, and other strategic alliances.
- Segment and target audiences with marketing and promotional tactics.

CHAPTER OUTLINE

- Strategic Analysis
- Three Levels of Strategy
- Marketing Health Services
- Promotional Mix

INTRODUCTION

Health services managers guide health care organizations (HCOs) in an exceedingly complex and rapidly evolving U.S. healthcare system. Planning for the future requires that health services managers understand the competitive, demographic, financial, political, and regulatory circumstances affecting their HCOs. Health services managers must also understand what makes their HCO better than the competitors. Healthcare **strategy** means making choices that uniquely position the HCO to create value for patients, families, clinicians, and communities in ways competitors cannot (Porter & Lee, 2016).

Some health services managers may be tempted to pursue any appealing opportunity that might increase their HCO's revenue, profits, or prestige. However, agreeing to pursue just any opportunity is a recipe for disaster. Strategically oriented managers decline business opportunities that do not fit with the HCO's capabilities or meet the needs of patients and other stakeholders. As Michael E. Porter (1996, para. 61) wrote, "the essence of strategy is choosing what *not* to do." Successful health services managers learn when to take advantage of opportunities—and when not to—by building competence in healthcare strategy and marketing.

As this chapter explains, **strategic planning** is the management process of determining what the customer values and how the organization delivers services more successfully—more distinctively, more effectively, or more efficiently—than its competitors. This chapter also describes how health services managers align strategy with the operational functions of the HCO, including human resources, clinical operations, finance, and, crucially, health services marketing.

STRATEGIC ANALYSIS

Internal Environmental Assessment

To effectively formulate strategy, health services managers must understand both the internal and external environment of the organization. **Internal environmental assessment** entails the examination of the internal resources of the organization, including human talent, equipment, culture, and operational characteristics. Health services managers can take a variety of approaches to assess the internal environment, but for the sake of simplicity, this chapter only addresses three fundamentals of strategic planning:

- Strategic direction
- Core competencies
- Financial analysis

First, the **strategic direction** serves as the foundation for the organization's strategy and involves stating the mission, vision, and values. The **mission** is the purpose and reason for existence that describes what the organization does and who the organization serves. The mission keeps health services managers focused on meeting the needs of patients, families, the community, and other stakeholders. The **vision** is an aspirational statement of what the HCO wants to become in the future. The vision should be long range (e.g., 3 or 5 years), observable, and challenging to accomplish. Finally, the **values** are the words that define the HCO's basic philosophy, principles, and ideals.

The HCO board of directors is responsible for developing and reviewing these statements in collaboration with the CEO during strategic planning processes. The board and executive health services managers evaluate all strategic alternatives against the established mission, vision, and values. Health services managers at all levels communicate the mission, vision, and values to staff, clinicians, patients, families, and communities.

Another critical part of internal environmental assessment identifying the HCO's **core competencies**, which are the unique combinations of knowledge, processes, and technologies that other competitors do not possess but that customers greatly desire. Ideally, core competencies can be sustained over a long period and are difficult to acquire or develop by competitors. Core competencies are more than the activities that the HCO performs capably, they must make the HCO distinctive in some way.

For example, Kaiser Permanente, the California-headquartered integrated delivery system, possesses many skills, processes, and characteristics that by themselves would not be considered core competencies. Certainly, Kaiser Permanente ably combines team-based care, shared electronic medical records, and standardized clinical protocols intended to reduce costs and improve health care quality. However, over 100 integrated delivery systems in the United States possess these same capabilities (Eickholt, 2019). More distinctively, Kaiser Permanente combines these assets with a unique governance structure in which physicians give up some professional autonomy to health services managers and physician administrators (Chesluk et al., 2017). According

TABLE 8.1 Examples of Mission, Vision, and Values of Health Care Organizations

HCO	MISSION	VISION	VALUES
Mayo Clinic	Inspiring hope and promoting health through integrated clinical practice, education, and research.	Transforming medicine to connect and cure as the global authority in the care of serious or complex diseases.	The needs of the patient come first. Respect, integrity, compassion, healing, teamwork, innovation, excellence, and stewardship
The Johns Hopkins Hospital	To improve the health of our community and the world by setting the standard of excellence in patient care	To lead the world in the diagnosis and treatment of disease and to train tomorrow's great physicians, nurses, and scientists	Excellence and discovery; leadership and integrity; diversity and inclusion; respect and collegiality
Washington Permanente Medical Group	To be the best place to give and receive care	Create world-class health and medical experiences that put our patients at the center of all we do	Innovation, stewardship, collaboration, compassion, excellence, and equity
Select Physical Therapy	Select Physical Therapy is committed to providing an exceptional patient care experience that promotes healing and recovery in a compassionate environment.	To serve our communities as the premier provider of adult rehabilitation care, resulting in the highest level of independence for our patients	We deliver superior quality care in all that we do. We treat others as they would like to be treated. We are results oriented and achieve our objectives. We are team players. We are resourceful in overcoming obstacles.
Northwell Health Physician Partners	Northwell Health Physician Partners provides exceptional, comprehensive, and quality clinical care to patients, families and communities through an integrated approach and with a commitment to exceeding customer expectations.	To be recognized as a world-class leader in the delivery of the highest quality, compassionate, and innovative medical care	As employees of Northwell Health, we uphold our health organization's values. Every role, every person, every moment matters. We put our patients and customers at the center of everything we do, while acting on our core values: caring, excellence, innovation, and integrity.

to Chesluk et al. (2017), the Kaiser Permanente physicians believe that corporate strategies are designed to achieve a shared goal—to improve patient care. Because physicians align with corporate goals, Kaiser Permanente can take advantage of strategies unavailable to other competitors.

> **CAREER BOX 8.1:** Career Core Competencies
>
> Core competencies are unique combinations of capabilities and resources that make the organization different and valuable. You can also use this concept to advance your career by adding a Core Competencies section to your résumé. For each position that you apply, list 10 to 20 skills, knowledge, and experiences that match the words in the job description. In addition to explicitly communicating your value, using the right keywords will help your application pass through the résumé screening technologies. Alternatively, you can combine your core competencies in creative ways to highlight your accomplishments. For example, you could describe your success as the treasurer for a school social club as an example of your strong analytical and interpersonal skills. Also, an internship could serve as an example of how you ambitiously pursued opportunities to humbly learn from more experienced people. A restaurant job could emphasize your ability to make processes more efficient while juggling competing priorities. Combining skills, knowledge, or experiences in creative ways communicates your value to potential employers.

Core competencies can also be viewed as bundles of resources, both tangible and intangible, that deliver value to customers and offer sustainable advantages over competitors (Barney et al., 2011). **Tangible resources** are the physical assets, such as staff, buildings, and technologies, that the HCO uses to provide health services. **Intangible resources** are nonphysical assets, such as brand recognition, intellectual property, ability to innovate, and management skills. Most of the activities conducted in the HCO are indistinguishable by the consumer between different competitors in the healthcare marketplace (Bratucu et al., 2014). Therefore, HCOs tend to have a high proportion of intangible assets serving as core competencies, including brand recognition, clinical protocols and procedures, and organizational culture (Evans et al., 2017). These intangible resources tend to be durable over time and difficult for competitors to imitate.

To identify the most important five or six core competencies of their HCOs, health services managers commonly use two analytical approaches: the SWOT analysis and the value chain analysis. The **SWOT analysis**, which stands for **S**trengths, **W**eaknesses, **O**pportunities, and **T**hreats, is one of the most popular and long-standing methods for conducting an internal analysis (Helms & Nixon, 2010). **Strengths** are internal characteristics that give the organization an advantage over its competitors (Clardy, 2013). **Weaknesses** are the fundamental deficiencies of an organization that inhibit its ability to serve its customers, especially compared to its competitors. One method for identifying strengths and weaknesses is to examine recent events that were considered either triumphs or disappointments, such as negotiating a payment increase from a health insurance company or dealing with electronic medical record failures (Coman & Ronan, 2009).

Another approach to identifying the core competencies of the HCO is called **value chain analysis**, in which health services managers chart the patient care delivery processes (Porter, 2008). By examining the value chain, health services managers can uncover core competencies that prove most valuable to the patient and their families. Figure 8.1 shows Porter's value chain concept from a health services delivery perspective, adapted from Porter (2008) and (Porter and Teisberg, 2006). At the bottom of the chart are the primary activities in the value chain that illustrate the health services delivery processes, through which patients derive value, such as preventing and diagnosing diseases. Core competencies can also be identified from the support activities of the HCO, such as providing superior patient experience during transitions from one health care setting to another.

FIGURE 8.1 Health services value chain analysis.

Support activities	**Organizational infrastructure** Finance, strategic planning, marketing, human resources, facilities, information technology, supply chain, etc.					
	Patient services Registration, scheduling, patient billing, case management, patient experience support, etc.					
	Clinical operations Clinical review, patient safety and quality, medical technologies, credentialing, etc.					
	Clinical support Patient transport, environmental services, nutrition, etc.					
Primary activities	**Monitoring and preventing** • Medical history • Screening • Identifying risks • Prevention	**Diagnosing** • Medical history • Physical exam • Diagnostic testing • Referral and consultation	**Preparing** • Care coordination • Pre-treatment • Patient education	**Intervening** • Treatment procedures • Drug administration	**Recovering and rehab** • Discharging • Rehabbing • Therapy fine-tuning	**Monitoring and managing** • Monitoring and managing conditions

Profit Margin → Patient Value

Source: Adapted from Porter, M. E. (2008). *Competitive advantage: Creating and sustaining superior performance* (2nd ed.). Free Press; Porter, M. E., & Teisberg, E. O. (2006). *Redefining health care: Creating value-based competition on results*. Harvard Business School Press.

Finally, the internal environmental assessment includes financial analyses (Priore, 2021). Without adequate financial resources, HCOs cannot invest in new services, enhance existing services, hire valuable staff, or access capital for growth. Financial ratios describe the financial status of the HCO, which is important to strategic plan formulation and implementation. Financial analyses will be explained in more detail in Chapter 14.

External Environmental Assessment

Health services managers also perform **external environmental assessments** to monitor the health care needs of the community, competitive marketplace, governmental policy, scientific innovations, and social and economic changes. In the SWOT analysis, **opportunities** are the external factors that can help the HCO achieve its strategic vision. Strategic **threats** are those circumstances that could prevent the HCO from achieving success, whether financial, reputational, or otherwise. For example, a threat exists when health insurance companies consolidate in the HCO's market area, resulting in fewer purchasers. This can potentially lead to less revenue or lower profits, as fewer health insurance companies in the market make it difficult for HCOs to negotiate prices.

Figure 8.2 illustrates strengths, weaknesses, opportunities, and threats in a two-by-two matrix. The boxes in the horizontal axis (left to right) are helpful and harmful in achieving the organizational vision. The boxes in the vertical axis (up and down) are internal orientation versus external orientation. In other words, the internal environmental analysis includes only the strengths and weaknesses, while the external environmental assessment includes only the opportunities and threats.

Health services managers should also identify relevant competitors in the market and ask whether they have strengths or weaknesses that would influence their abilities to respond to a particular opportunity or threat, such as the following:

FIGURE 8.2 SWOT analysis 2x2 matrix.

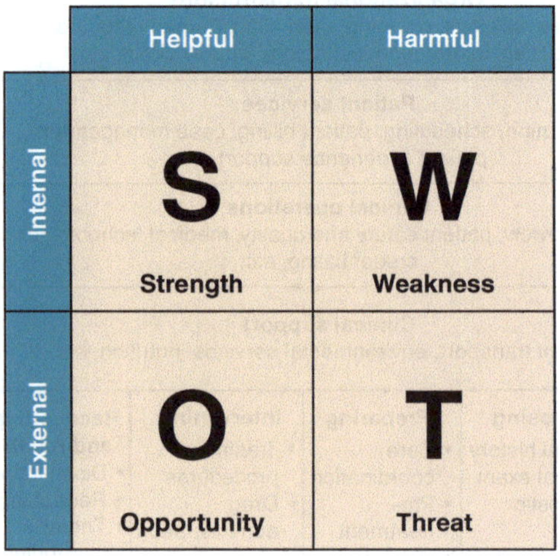

	Helpful	Harmful
Internal	**S** Strength	**W** Weakness
External	**O** Opportunity	**T** Threat

- *Market share:* Do the competitors hold large market shares overall or in certain service lines?
- *Financial assets:* Do competitors have more financial resources? More revenue? More profits?
- *Health insurance contracts:* Do competitors have exclusive contracts with health insurance companies that would prevent patients from choosing their HCO?
- *Size of organization:* Do competitors have more employees, credentialed clinicians, or beds?
- *Service offering:* Do the competitors offer unique services? Are the competitors' services more or less comprehensive?
- *Partnerships:* Are the competitors affiliated with or partnered with other HCOs in the market that may give them an advantage?
- *Reputation:* Do competitors have better brand recognition? What are patients' perceptions of the competitors?
- *Apparent core competencies:* Do the competitors have some key technology, special service, or unique process?

Health services managers also need to understand the competitive dynamics of the external environment. Michael E. Porter (2008) developed a framework for evaluating the intensity of competition in a marketplace, called the **Five Forces model**. The first force—highly influenced by the other forces described in the following—is the overall competitive rivalry of the market. When marketplace competition is intense, the prospects for long-term profitability for the HCO are diminished.

> ⚠ **KEY IDEA**
>
> When marketplace competition is intense, the prospects for long-term profitability for the HCO are diminished.

The intensity of the competitive rivalry can be measured by the concentration of the market. The **Herfindahl–Hirschman Index** (HHI) is calculated by squaring each HCO's market share and then summing the resulting numbers (U.S. Department of Justice, 2018). As the HHI increases, the market becomes more competitive and less profitable. Where there is a single HCO in the market (**monopoly**), the HHI score reaches a maximum of 10,000. Where the market is occupied by a large number of equally sized HCOs, the HHI approaches zero (**perfect competition**). Moderately concentrated markets with HHIs between 1,500 and 2,500 points are called **monopolistic competition**. Where an HHI is greater than 2,500 points, the market is highly concentrated, called an **oligopoly**.

The other four elements of Porter's Five Forces model are the following:

- *Bargaining power of the buyers:* The buyers of health services are typically health insurance companies and government payers (e.g., Medicare), although patients and families also influence these buyer choices. For example, if one health insurance company dominates the marketplace, an HCO's negotiating power is reduced, which decreases the long-term profitability prospects for the market (Geyman, 2022).
- *Bargaining power of the suppliers:* If a market is dominated by a small number of suppliers, then the prices for the supplies increase, making the market less attractive. Supplies include durable medical equipment or pharmaceuticals. Labor is a type of supplier, including nurses and other critical clinical professions. A shortage of clinicians can reduce HCO profitability, which has become a significant issue in the healthcare industry in recent years (Rhodes et al., 2023).
- *Ability of competitors to enter the market:* If there are **barriers to entry**, such as government **certificate of need** laws and regulations that require government permission to build a new facility, then the existing HCOs in that market will enjoy a less intense competitive marketplace.
- *Level of threat of substitution of other services:* Access to close substitutes for services increases the competitiveness of a market. For example, traditional inpatient care can be substituted by technology-enabled home care for a lower price (Baugh et al., 2022).

Because laws and regulations significantly impact healthcare strategy, any well-conceived strategic plan will include an analysis of the current legal and regulatory environment. For example, mergers in a market may require approval from the federal government, namely the Federal Trade Commission (FTC) of the U.S. Department of Justice. According to the **Sherman Antitrust Act,** the federal government can examine the concentration of competition in a market, using HHI scores and other measures, to evaluate whether to give HCOs approval to merge. Other examples of health policies that impact strategy are union-backed laws that restrict the supply of labor, environmental laws that increase operating costs, and regulations that cut Medicare payments.

The final element to consider in the external environmental analysis is the accurate prediction and anticipation of the demand for health services, also called a **community health needs assessment**. The **epidemiological planning model** explains the process of forecasting the health services needs of the community (White & Griffith, 2019). Health services managers use epidemiology, the public health discipline that studies disease in populations, to analyze the number of people contracting the disease or injury (incidence) and how widespread the disease is (prevalence) in a particular community (Ahlbom, 2020). Epidemiological tools can be used to describe the patient **case mix**, which includes the level of severity of the disease (morbidity) and the intensity of care (acuity of care).

Market share data is also needed to accurately predict health service demand for a specific HCO. The market from which the HCO attracts patients is known as the **catchment area**. If there is more than one HCO in the catchment area, patients will have choices about where to seek health services. Therefore, health services managers need to calculate the proportion of the total population that the HCO has historically served for each relevant health service. Most HCOs have sophisticated forecasting models that combine case mix, population estimates, market share, and historical health services utilization data to predict patient demand (Jalalpour et al., 2015).

⚠ KEY IDEA

To calculate health service demand, the forecasting model should recognize that not everyone in the catchment area will get a disease, not everyone who gets the disease will use the service at the same level, and not everyone who needs services will choose the same HCO.

To summarize the epidemiological model, not everyone in the catchment area will get a disease, not everyone who gets the disease will use the service at the same level, and not everyone who needs services will choose the same HCO. For example, assume the expected fertility rate for the catchment area is 56 births per 1,000 population of women ages 15 to 44 per year (National Center for Health Statistics, 2023). A catchment area of 1 million potential mothers would predict 56,000 deliveries annually. A small number of births (1.64%) occur outside the inpatient setting (Lang et al., 2021). Therefore, approximately 55,000 births would be expected. If the hospital typically serves 10% of the maternity care market, then it can expect 5,500 births per year. Similar demand calculations can be made for any number of services.

Competitive Advantage

The results of internal and external environmental analyses can be used to identify and exploit **competitive advantage** over other HCOs in the market area. Competitive advantage is created when the HCO consistently provides greater value to patients in ways that their competitors cannot. To be considered as possessing a competitive advantage, the differences in service or service delivery must create measurable value for patients and health insurance companies. This value comes in the form of reduced costs, improved clinical quality, superior patient experience, or increased access to care.

Competitive advantage is created when the HCO delivers services that are either different from competitors or similar to competitors but are delivered in different ways (Porter, 1996). To make the most of their HCO's competitive advantage, successful health services managers negotiate price increases with payers, price decreases with suppliers, favorable agreement terms with partners and affiliates, outmaneuver competitors, and otherwise preserve their competitive advantage for the future. Differentiated services create sustained profitability, increased market share, and/or reputational excellence through these activities.

 INFORMATIONAL INTERVIEW 8.1
Senior Marketing Coordinator
Access the informational interview online at http://connect.springerpub.com/content/book/978-0-8261-4807-0/chapter/ch00.

In the service differentiation strategy, HCOs offer unique medical services, such as robot surgery, organ transplantation, or burn care, or enjoy superior brand identity. However, in the health services delivery sector, the health services are often indistinguishable from one HCO to the next, at least from the perspectives of patients, families, and health insurance companies (Trinh, 2020). Unless the HCO offers medical care that is otherwise unavailable in the market area, it can be next to impossible to differentiate health services. Therefore, to create competitive advantage, undifferentiated health services must be delivered in ways that are substantially different from their competitors' offerings. There are a variety of approaches to differentiate health services delivery that can create value for patients, including the following (American Hospital Association; 2022, 2023, Permanente Medicine, 2023; Porter, 1996; Stowell & Akerman, 2015; Trinh, 2020):

- *Create unique customer experiences:* Focus on the other aspects of care that patients and families appreciate, such as physician and staff communication styles, attractive and comfortable physical environment, food and beverage options, entertainment, valet parking, and other amenities.
- *Build partnerships with payers:* Collaborate with health insurance companies to develop new ways of pricing health services, such as bundled pricing, pay for performance, or guaranteed health outcomes.
- *Access-based convenience:* Greater access to care through innovative scheduling, telehealth services, retail clinics, or anything making it easier for patients to get care.
- *Collocated, team-based care delivery:* Health services organized around the needs of the patient, instead of the clinicians, can create distinctive value for patients.
- *Connected electronic medical records:* Access to patient medical charts across multiple specialties, healthcare settings, and geographies can create opportunities for improved customer service and coordinated care.
- *Integration of services:* Corporate behemoths, such as CVS Health, Amazon Care, and Walmart, combine health services delivery with technologies and logistical expertise to create competitive advantages that traditional HCOs cannot ignore.

Health services managers can also create competitive advantage through the price of health services. Because patients are represented by third-party payers, such as health insurance companies and governments, HCOs do not usually promote their lower costs publicly. Nevertheless, the low-cost strategy is a viable approach for HCOs to create competitive advantage. Beyond innovative pricing strategies, such as the aforementioned bundled pricing or pay-for-performance contracting, HCOs can create a cost leadership position by vigorously cutting costs and tightly controlling expenses. Lowering costs in healthcare can be challenging, but as a core strategy, it can be effective at creating value for patients and their health insurance companies (Porter & Teisberg, 2006). Creating value leads to competitive advantage, which generates sustained profitability.

△ KEY IDEA

HCOs do not usually promote their lower costs publicly. Nevertheless, the low-cost strategy is a viable approach for HCOs to create competitive advantage.

No matter how HCOs seek to create competitive advantage (e.g., differentiation of service, differentiation of delivery, or cost leadership), successful health services managers intentionally connect the chosen strategy to business operations. If the strategy cannot be executed effectively, then the HCO may be better off not offering the services to patients (Magretta, 2011). Strategic implementation is about accepting the operational limitations of the HCO. This means that HCOs cannot be everything to everyone. In other words, strategic success means making trade-offs between the operational activities that align with strategy and those that may seem like a good idea but do not match the given strategy.

THREE LEVELS OF STRATEGY

Corporate Strategy

Many HCOs are large multiservice operations containing multiple businesses, divisions, and service lines. In many ways, HCOs operate like corporations, irrespective of their nonprofit or for-profit status. Executives at the corporate headquarters drive strategic planning for the entire

HCO. Their role is to link all of the businesses together so that the whole organization is more valuable than the sum of its services and business. Therefore, the strategic planning methods devised for the modern corporation apply to a significant portion of the healthcare sector. Three such approaches include adaptive strategies, portfolio analysis, and product life cycle analysis.

Simply stated, HCOs can either expand, contract, or maintain their current strategic scope. Ginter et al. (2018) call these options **adaptive strategies** because HCOs adapt to the environment. In today's healthcare marketplace, most HCOs are seeking to expand their operations. However, some HCOs face shrinking markets or obsolete services. For example, nearly 30% of all rural hospitals in the United States are at risk of closing because of severe financial problems (Center for Healthcare Quality and Payment Reform, 2023). Rural hospitals are divesting their facilities and liquidating equipment to meet their existing financial obligations. In other instances, HCOs want to maintain their size and reinvest in existing operations in an effort to prepare for future opportunities.

HCOs pursue **expansion strategies** to gain more power in the market (Azzoparde et al., 2022). Expansion is a way to create **economies of scale** (e.g., buying supplies in bulk at reduced prices per unit) or increase negotiating power with health insurance companies. At the corporate level, there are three ways that HCOs expand the size of their organizations: vertical integration, horizontal integration, or diversification. Figure 8.3 illustrates healthcare expansion through vertical and horizontal integration.

FIGURE 8.3 Healthcare expansion: Vertical and horizontal integration.

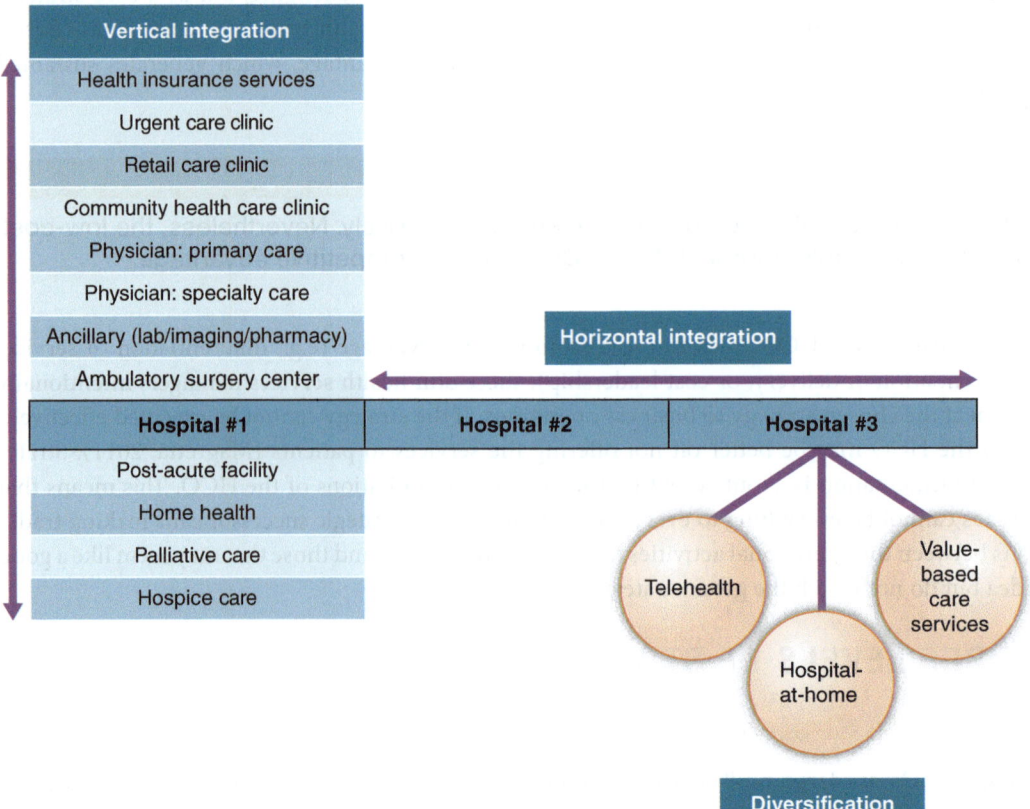

Vertical integration occurs in healthcare when two or more health services delivery settings are combined into one HCO. As shown in Figure 8.3, vertical integration can occur throughout the various healthcare businesses and settings. Most frequently, vertical integration happens when hospitals or health systems employ physicians and/or acquire physician practices to create integrated delivery systems. In recent years, however, large for-profit healthcare corporations have embarked upon a vertical expansion strategy by purchasing other large corporations. For example, the retail pharmacy giant CVS acquired MinuteClinic for $170 million in 2006, pharmacy benefits manager Caremark Rx for $24 billion in 2007, and health insurance company Aetna for $69 billion in 2018 (Harris, 2007; Richman, 2018; St. Paul Business Journal, 2006). Recently, CVS accelerated its vertical integration strategy with the acquisition of home health provider Signify for $8 billion in 2022, the launch of kidney care specialist services at CVS Kidney Care in 2023, and the purchase of primary care clinic operator Oak Street Health for $10.6 billion in 2023 (Goddard, 2022; Landi, 2023; Minemyer, 2022).

Horizontal integration is an expansion strategy in which two or more entities that offer the same services combine to create a larger organization. Figure 8.3 shows the horizontal integration of three hospitals that provide similar acute care services. Horizontal integration can occur through a **merger**, where two similar-sized firms combine to become a separate organization; through acquisition, where one HCO buys another; or through a **strategic alliance**, where a strategic partnership of two independent organizations is formed. **Horizontal expansion** can take place in the same catchment area or by combining two HCOs from different markets. Figure 8.3 also shows how a hospital can expand through **diversification**, which enables HCOs to generate additional revenue through related or unrelated businesses. For example, most health systems in the United States are diversifying inpatient services with telehealth, remote monitoring technologies, and/or value-based care services, according to McKinsey & Company (Azzoparde et al., 2022).

As the size of an HCO grows to include dozens of disparate services or business units, the formation of a corporate-level strategy demands performance evaluations of all services or businesses within the HCO. **Portfolio management** is the process of allocating resources to services or businesses based on their potential for growth and profitability. Health services managers need to manage their portfolio of services and businesses to ensure that the HCO remains viable. Most HCOs purposefully operate service lines that are not profitable but are necessary for the health and well-being of the community. Consequently, executive health services managers seek to maximize the financial performance of the HCO's service portfolio so that more profitable services subsidize the operation of less profitable services that are needed by the community.

The **Boston Consulting Group (BCG) Matrix** is an analytical tool used by corporations to evaluate and balance the portfolios of business and services (Henderson, 1970). The BCG Matrix analyzes business and services along two dimensions: market growth rate and relative market share. As Figure 8.4 illustrates, when a service or business in the HCO's portfolio falls within one of the four boxes, then the BCG matrix gives it a name: stars, question marks, cash cows, and dogs. Each of the four quadrants indicates the level of cash need and cash generation. Depending on which category the service or business falls within the BCG matrix, the health services management executive can take certain actions.

Stars need a lot of cash to buy assets, but they also generate substantial cash. Health services managers pay plenty of attention to stars by investing the maximum number of resources to encourage growth and long-term profitability. **Cash cows** are also coveted by health services managers, but they rarely generate the same investments from managers. Instead, cash cows are "milked" of their cash to fund other services and businesses, especially those that are needed in the community. **Question marks**, however, require plenty of cash, but they generate much less cash flow. They are

FIGURE 8.4 Boston consulting group matrix. https://www.bcg.com/publications/1970/strategy-the-product-portfolio.

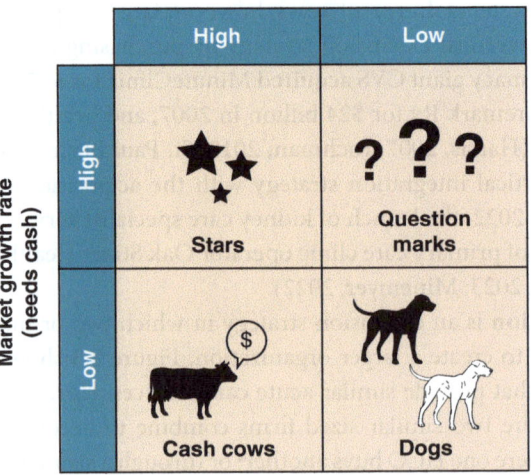

called question marks because it is often uncertain if the service or business will eventually become a star (or a dog). The **dogs** are the worst of the four categories with low relative market share and low growth, so health services managers should consider divesting these services or business units, depending on the health services needs of the community.

△ KEY IDEA

Cash cows are also coveted by health services managers but rarely generate the same investments of resources. Instead, cash cows are "milked" of their cash to fund other services and businesses, especially those that are needed in the community.

Over time, stars may become cash cows, question marks, or dogs. To stabilize the HCO's revenue and profits, health services managers need to predict the decline of services and replace them with others. Theodore Levitt (1965), in his classic article, "Exploit the Life Cycle," suggested that the **life cycle management** approach be used to forecast the rise and decline of products and services. According to this view, there are four stages of a product or service's life cycle, as illustrated in Figure 8.5, each with several developmental stages that present opportunities and constraints:

1. *Market development or introduction:* A new service in a marketplace requires facilities, equipment, and marketing investments by the HCO. The revenues are very low, and the expenses are very high (i.e., profits are low).
2. *Market growth:* Revenues and profit increase, but more competitors will try to enter the business placing pressure on the long-term sustainability of profits.
3. *Market maturity:* The market is saturated with competitors. The growth in revenues starts to decline and profitability decreases as competitors start to compete more on price and less on differentiation. Strong competition requires more marketing efforts to maintain market share.
4. *Market decline:* Both revenues and profits decline.

FIGURE 8.5 Product life cycle.

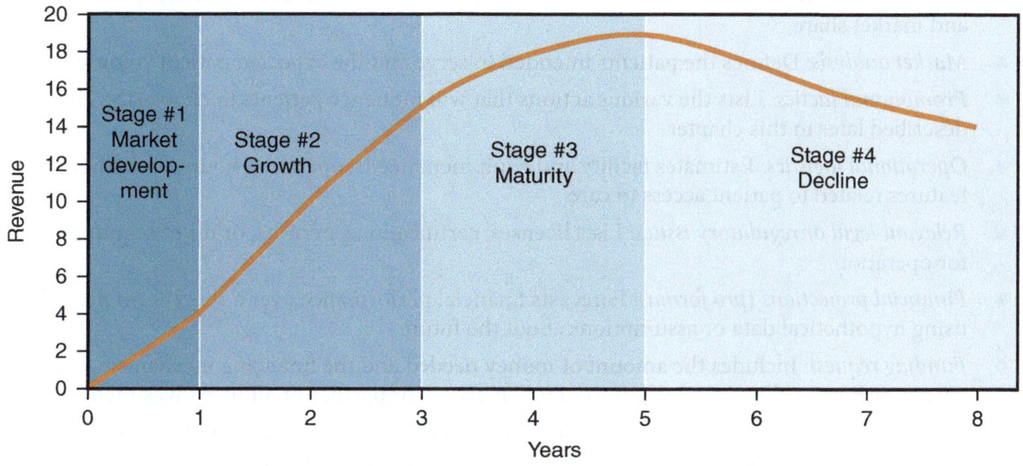

Stage #1 Market development
Stage #2 Growth
Stage #3 Maturity
Stage #4 Decline

Source: Adapted from Levitt, T. (1965). Exploit the product life cycle. *Harvard Business Review*. https://hbr.org/1965/11/exploit-the-product-life-cycle

Life cycle management concepts apply to the healthcare services delivery sector. For example, inpatient revenues are expected to either remain constant or decline due to decreased payments from government payers and health insurance companies, coupled with advances in health care technologies (Gliadkovskaya, 2022). Therefore, inpatient services can be considered either in maturity or decline. Consequently, many health systems are developing new services to replace declining inpatient services. For example, health systems are investing in hospital-at-home services with monitoring technologies. These services are expected to grow rapidly in the next few years, and the investments by HCOs are examples of effective life cycle management.

Business Unit Strategy

A **strategic business unit** is an independently managed, specialized unit, division, or line of business that focuses on a particular service and customer. A corporation, such as a health system, may have many strategic business units, each of which provide distinct services, such as inpatient, outpatient, diagnostics, home health, and insurance services. Within each of these businesses or divisions are multiple service lines, and within these service lines are individual service offerings, often identified by disease classification or procedure type. Within health services, most HCOs hold the same assumptions for how to successfully run a health services delivery business. The common **business model** for HCOs entails preventing, diagnosing, and treating diseases and injuries through highly trained clinicians applying medical knowledge and technologies, and most HCOs are paid by third-party payers, such as the government and health insurance companies.

Strategic planning at the business level must align with and contribute value to the corporate strategy. For new businesses or services to obtain funding from corporate executives, health services managers create proposals called **business plans** that analyze the merits of the opportunity. There are many components of a business plan, including the following:

- *Executive summary:* Briefly (one or two pages) describes the relevant sections found in the business plan
- *Service or business overview:* Describes the new venture and explains how the services will fill a need in the market

- *Staffing:* Defines the management, clinicians, and nonclinical support staff necessary to operate
- *Competitor analysis:* Describes each competitor's services, strengths, weaknesses, positioning, and market share
- *Market analysis:* Defines the patients intended to serve and the expected patient volume
- *Promotional tactics:* Lists the various actions that will influence patients to choose the HCO, as described later in this chapter
- *Operational logistics:* Estimates facility and equipment needs, operating hours, and other features related to patient access to care
- *Relevant legal or regulatory issues:* Lists licenses, certifications, permits, or other requirements for operation
- *Financial projections (pro forma):* Forecasts financial performance over a short-term period using hypothetical data or assumptions about the future
- *Funding request:* Includes the amount of money needed and the financing mechanism, such as corporate budget allocation, access to capital markets, or partner or affiliate investments
- *Performance monitoring:* Defines specific performance measures, targets, and milestones that will be used to evaluate the success of the business plan implementation

Once a business plan is approved, health services managers translate strategic plans into action. The **strategic management** process involves allocating resources, creating operational plans, organizing people, and implementing processes to support new services or businesses. An **operational plan** is a detailed document that outlines the specific actions, activities, and processes necessary to achieve the strategic objectives and goals of an organization. An operational plan guides day-to-day operations within the organization, typically for defined periods, such as a year, and provides direction to staff. Under the guidance and oversight of executives, health services managers monitor the performance of the operational plan and take corrective actions to ensure that strategic objectives are met, if necessary.

Functional Level Strategy

Based on the corporate- and business-level strategy, health services managers allocate resources to the operating functions of the HCO. Functional departments and units include finance, clinical operations, information technology, human resources, and marketing. When strategic decisions are made at the corporate or business level, functional area managers tailor their operations to fit those choices. Without strategic fit, the HCO will blunder in its strategic implementation and weaken any established competitive advantage (Porter, 1996).

△ KEY IDEA
Without strategic fit, the HCO will blunder in its strategic implementation and weaken any established competitive advantage.

For example, an orthopedic ambulatory surgery center (ASC) may choose to serve only elderly patients insured by Medicare, as opposed to the sports injury-focused market preferred by a key competitor. Consequently, successful strategic implementation demands that the ASC purchase orthopedic implant devices that work for disabled elderly patients (i.e., stabilizing joints). If the ASC instead purchased devices more suitable for athletic patients (i.e., flexible joints), then the purchasing function would be acting inconsistently with the overall strategy. To implement a simplified strategy focused on disabled elderly patients, the ASC should purchase less expensive devices that are designed specifically for stabilizing older patients.

> **INFORMATIONAL INTERVIEW 8.2**
> *Director, Business Development and Physician Relations*
> Access the informational interview online at http://connect.springerpub.com/content/book/978-0-8261-4807-0/chapter/ch00.

MARKETING HEALTH SERVICES

Trust and Ethics in Health Services Marketing

While all business functions contribute to the development and execution of HCO strategies, the marketing department plays an especially significant role. Health services **marketing** is the function responsible for developing strategies for distribution, pricing, and promoting health services to patients. Health services managers who specialize in the marketing function develop clear and compelling brand identities for HCOs, build long-term relationships with patients and clinicians, and enhance employee engagement and patients' overall care experience (Lee, 2021).

Fundamental marketing practices are common to all businesses, but unique characteristics of the healthcare sector significantly shape health services marketing, including the following (Berry & Bendapudi, 2007; Brownlee et al., 2017):

- The expertise and reputation of clinicians play an important role in the decision-making process of patients. Therefore, health services managers often focus on marketing to clinicians to encourage referral of patients to services.
- Third-party payers, such as health insurance companies, bear most of the costs of health services, making patients unaware of prices.
- Intense federal and state regulations of health services add complexity and risk to the HCO marketing function.
- Most money in healthcare is spent on services that people need but do not want.
- Patients are often sick, under stress, and lack medical knowledge, which makes them feel more uncertain, anxious, emotional, and demanding than other types of consumers.
- Obtaining more services will not necessarily produce better health outcomes for patients. Promoting unnecessary health services may harm patients and HCOs.

Because health services are unique, health services managers must market the HCO in ways that engender trust and confidence from patients, clinicians, communities, potential employees, and other stakeholders. Trust plays a significant role in shaping patients' perceptions, influencing their decision-making process and impacting their overall satisfaction with the chosen HCO. Patients want to feel confident in HCOs and the clinicians responsible for their care. Therefore, health services managers should ensure that marketing approaches maintain trust of patients, not undermine it.

> **△ KEY IDEA**
> Patients want to feel confident in HCOs and the clinicians who will be responsible for their care. Therefore, health services managers should ensure that marketing approaches maintain trust of patients, not undermine it.

While the professional associations for health services management, such as the American College of Healthcare Executives (ACHE) and Medical Group Management Association (MGMA) do not have specific guidelines for marketing health services, its members are expected to adhere to ethical standards in their professional conduct. Some medical societies, such as the American Medical Association (AMA), provide specific guidelines for the ethical marketing of health services. The following are some health services marketing ethical guidelines to follow (ACHE, 2022; AMA, 2019; Medical Group Management Association-American College of Medical Practice Executives, 2015):

- Avoid deceptive, aggressive, and high-pressure marketing tactics. Claims that imply that clinicians offer unique health services are typically considered deceptive because it is unlikely that any clinician provides truly exclusive services.
- Avoid making false or misleading claims about the benefits, effectiveness, or outcomes of health services. Marketing messages and materials should provide information that assists patients in making informed decisions.
- Avoid disclosing sensitive personal health information.
- Avoid using fear-based tactics or exaggerating the severity of health conditions to influence patients' decisions that exploit patients' vulnerabilities, fears, or emotions.
- Avoid discrimination, stereotypes, or any form of bias that may marginalize certain populations. Marketing tactics should be culturally sensitive, inclusive, and respectful of the diversity of patients' backgrounds, beliefs, and values.

Market Segmentation and Targeting

Health services managers are responsible for attracting the right patients, convincing them to choose the HCO over their competitors, and earning long-lasting loyalty (Gunawardane, 2020). To analyze which audience to market to, health services managers engage in a two-step analytical process: segmentation and targeting. **Segmentation** divides the market of potential customers into homogenous groups of prospective buyers. **Targeting** involves selecting the best segment or segments of potential customers for whom the marketing efforts will be most successful.

Market segments are created based on relevant characteristics, such as demographics (e.g., age, gender, location), psychographics (e.g., lifestyle, interests, values), behavior (e.g., purchasing habits, online activity), or other specific criteria. Within each segment, the patients will be similar in terms of the chosen characteristics. By understanding what influences patient behaviors and decision-making processes, health services managers can predict how each segment of patients may respond to certain marketing tactics.

△ KEY IDEA
By understanding what influences patient behaviors and decision-making processes, health services managers can predict how each segment of patients may respond to certain marketing tactics.

There is no single way to segment a market, but the desired result is to distinguish the groups of patients who will buy the health services from those who will not. Examples of characteristics used to create market segments include the following:

- *Geographics:* The catchment area from which an HCO attracts patients is defined by zip code; census tract; counties; or urban, suburban, or rural categorizations. HCOs use Geographic Information System (GIS) software to create maps of current or prospective patient homes by distance from the HCO.
- *Payer types:* Health insurance coverage, including commercial, **Medicare, Medicaid,** and uninsured, impacts access to care and purchasing behaviors.

- *Psychographics:* This refers to what people want and why they act in certain ways, including their values, lifestyle, perceptions, motivations, and attitudes.
- *Sociodemographics:* Attributes such as age, generation, race, ethnicity, income, and others are important to consider.
- *Health needs and disease states:* Diagnoses and health service utilization patterns that predict health services demand can be accessed from electronic medical records.

Psychographics and health needs are the most important factors in influencing health services purchasing behaviors, which can be gathered from patient surveys. Woodside et al. (1988), Deloitte Center for Health Solutions (2012), and Liu and Chen (2009) used survey data to segment the health services market by a variety of characteristics, as summarized in Table 8.2.

Once the segments of the market are defined, health services managers need to choose which market segments to target with marketing campaigns (Gunawardane, 2020). Health services managers create customized marketing content and/or deliver personalized service experiences that cater to the specific motivations and needs of a **target audience**. Wise choices of target

TABLE 8.2 Examples of Health Services Market Segmentation

SEGMENT NAME	PATIENT SEGMENT DESCRIPTION	PROPORTION OF MARKET
"Preference segmentation of health care services" by Woodside et al. (1988)		
Old-fashioneds	Retirees or disabled; want hospital with same religious affiliation; want hospital close to home	8%
Value conscious	Want lower prices; want best doctors in area	39%
Affluents	High income, high education; want hospital to act as wellness center, not just a place for sick care; want a hospital with a caring reputation	25%
Professional want-it-alls	High income, high education (similar to affluents); 70% of the segment want all the preferences (e.g., close to home, reputation for caring, best doctors, best nurses, best equipment, best reputation for emergency care)	27%
Total:		100%
"Using data mining to segment health care markets from patients' preference perspectives" by Liu and Chen (2009)		
Performance driven	Lower education levels; more retired people; interested in efficienct, compassionate, and responsive care	51%
Reputation driven	Most with high school education; clinical reputation of hospital most important	27%
Empowerment driven	Higher proportion of college degrees and private insurance; desire for more information; want more involvement in medical decisions	22%
Total:		100%

TABLE 8.2 Examples of Health Services Market Segmentation (*continued*)

SEGMENT NAME	PATIENT SEGMENT DESCRIPTION	PROPORTION OF MARKET
"How do consumers navigate the healthcare frontier?" by Read and Korenda (2018)		
Bystanders	Wants convenience and low costs; complacent; tech reluctant; resistant to change providers; oldest segment; most likely to be in poor health	14%
Trailblazers	Tech savvy; self-directed, engaged in wellness; willing to share tracked health data; healthiest and youngest segment	16%
Prospectors	Rely on recommendations from providers & friends/family; willing to use technology	30%
Homesteaders	Wants convenience; reserved, cautious traditionalists; least likely to share health data	40%
	Total:	100%

Source: Liu, S. S., & Chen, J. (2009). Using data mining to segment healthcare markets from patients' preference perspectives. *International Journal of Health Care Quality Assurance, 22*(2), 117–134. https://doi.org/10.1108/09526860910944610; Read, L., & Korenda, L. (2018, October 29). *How do consumers navigate the health care frontier?* Deloitte Insights. https://www2.deloitte.com/us/en/insights/industry/health-care/healthcare-consumer-patient-segmentation.html; Woodside, A. G., Nielsen, R. L., Walters, F., & Muller, G. D. (1988). Preference segmentation of health care services: The old-fashioneds, value conscious, affluents, and professional want-it-alls. *Journal of Health Care Marketing, 8*(2), 14–24.

audiences will increase the chances of attracting patients to the HCO's services. Since marketing budgets are limited, health services managers select the target audience that will yield the biggest results.

Marketing Mix (Four Ps of Marketing)

The **marketing mix** is the set of actions used to promote a brand, product, or service in the market. Also known as the "**Four Ps**," the concepts of product, pricing, placement, and promotion can be used by health services managers to build comprehensive marketing campaigns. Effective health services marketing entails more than just promotional tactics; it also encompasses other essential elements within the marketing mix: product, pricing, and placement. Using the full marketing mix enables campaigns to communicate the unique value offered by the HCO and take advantage of the competitive advantages identified in the strategic plan.

> ⚠ **KEY IDEA**
>
> Effective health services marketing entails more than just promotional tactics; it also encompasses other essential elements within the marketing mix: product, pricing, and placement.

In the health services marketing mix, the **product** encompasses the range of medical treatments, procedures, consultations, diagnostics, and therapies offered to patients. Defining the product means describing the key features of the health services (e.g., cleanliness and comfort of patient rooms, state-of-the-art facilities, access to top clinicians, or the functionality of the telehealth platform) and benefits provided to patients (e.g., reduced fear, time saved, or improved health outcomes). Effective marketing campaigns highlight the features and benefits of the service, known as **value proposition**. Marketing campaigns that communicate the value proposition to a target audience will attract patients and reinforce competitive advantage.

Pricing in the health services marketing mix involves setting prices for various services. Because health services are mostly paid for through **third-party payers**, the pricing element of the marketing mix is complicated. In general, the listed price of health services is not what is paid by the patient. Therefore, price reductions, coupons, or rebates for health services are not usually used as marketing tactics. However, HCOs commonly use pricing strategies when negotiating prices for their services with health insurance companies.

CAREER BOX 8.2: Four Ps of Job Searches

The marketing mix's Four Ps can be used to market yourself to potential employers (Pelzel, 2021). First, the product is the value you bring to an organization. Describe yourself in terms of the needs of the organization and what sets you apart from other potential applicants. Next, price what the potential employer would give you in exchange for your services. Price may include more than just salary, so identify other things you value, such as opportunities for career progression, work-life balance, commute time, and professional fulfillment. To attain a higher price for your contributions, you may need to invest in yourself. Consider how credentials or new skills will increase your value to potential employers. Next, promotions are the actions that create interest in you as a potential employee, such as résumés (brochures), LinkedIn with testimonials (product reviews), and cover letters (press releases). Finally, placement may be the most crucial element to marketing yourself to potential employees. Career advancement is about who you know, so put yourself in positions where prospective employers can evaluate your value, such as by attending professional events or volunteering with community organizations.

Placement means how products or services are distributed in the marketplace. For health services to be distributed, they must be made accessible to patients. There are a variety of access points for health services, depending on the type of HCO. For example, a patient who needs acute care can access services through the physician's office, the emergency department, or via direct admission to an inpatient facility. Health services managers market health services by developing **marketing channels** through which patients can access services, such as physician-hospital partnerships, social media interactions, or exclusive contracts with health insurance companies. Developing new marketing channels is a primary reason HCOs engage in vertical integration strategies, such as building urgent care clinics or purchasing physician medical practices.

Finally, **promotion** of health services includes the methods of communication and advertising used to attract patients to HCOs. The promotional strategy depends on the chosen target audience, such as the patient, family, or physician. Promotions enhance brand awareness, distribute information about specific services, convey health campaigns, and ultimately influence patients to select an HCO.

INFORMATIONAL INTERVIEW 8.3

Executive Director, Strategic Planning

Access the informational interview online at http://connect.springerpub.com/content/book/978-0-8261-4807-0/chapter/ch00.

PROMOTIONAL MIX

Branding, Advertising, and Public Relations

The promotional mix of health services marketing refers to the methods used by HCOs to promote services, such as branding, advertising, and public relations. Healthcare **branding** refers to creating and managing a unique identity that creates economic value for the HCO. A compelling brand identity includes attractive logos, typography, and visual elements that represent the HCO's values and character. Creating a recognizable brand requires consistent application of the brand identity in print materials, signage, websites, social media profiles, and educational content. A strong brand is a valuable tool for health services managers to achieve the following HCO goals (Agency for Healthcare Research and Quality [AHRQ], 2020; Khosravizadeh et al., 2017; Read et al., 2021; Sciulli & Missien, 2015):

- *Trust, credibility, and loyalty:* Building strong reputation among patients, clinicians, and the community is critical to branding.
- *Competitive positioning:* Reinforce value proposition and competitive advantage for the HCO or specific services.
- *Consumer awareness:* Improves knowledge of medical specialists ability to treat special diseases and the benefits of health services.
- *Create more positive experience:* The brand includes cleanliness of the HCO; the convenience of appointment scheduling; and helpful, courteous, and respectful office staff.
- *Employee recruitment:* Increase people's intention to pursue job opportunities.
- *Confirm medical decision:* Brand supports physicians' decisions about treatments.
- *Improves perceived clinical quality:* Brand reinforces patients' positive perceptions of treatment quality.

Advertising, a form of paid promotion, takes the form of mass communication that is channeled through different media platforms, such as billboards, newspapers, radio, television, mailings, the internet, social media, and bus station benches. Although spending on pharmaceutical advertising overshadows that of health services by nearly ten to one, the growth in health services advertising has increased much more in recent decades (Schwartz & Woloshin, 2019). Since the American Hospital Association and the AMA lifted bans on HCO advertising in the 1980s, health services advertising has grown rapidly (Strach, 2004). Historically, most of the money for health service advertising has been spent on television. However, internet and mobile spending have become the second largest advertising category over the last decade.

> **CAREER BOX 8.3: Cover Letter as a Press Release**
>
> Press releases and cover letters have a lot in common. While press releases remain invaluable marketing tools for HCOs to build a credible brand, reporters have become inundated with press releases. The same can be said of recruiters, who are besieged by online applications. To generate publicity or land a job interview, write press releases or cover letters like a storyteller. Instead of just listing the who, when, what, where, and why, effective press releases pitch stories so that reporters do not have to work too hard to imagine why their audience would be interested in the HCO. Compelling cover letters focus on story elements, such as the hero (you), desire (the job, career aspirations), conflict (the main problem the company is seeking an employee to solve), and transformation (how desires will be realized, or conflict resolved). By creating a compelling story, the hiring manager or recruiter can easily realize why you fit the position.

For many decades, the **public relations** function has been the dominant method by which HCOs have communicated with the public, favored by its low costs and high credibility (Elrod & Fortenberry, 2020a). The public relations staff within the marketing department works with media contacts to pitch stories that enhance the public's perception and reputation of the HCO. The main functions of the public relations staff include the following:

- *Press releases:* Press releases are written and distributed to the news media to tell stories about the HCO. To attract attention, press releases must be compelling to the media outlet and their potential viewers/readers.
- *Prepare for interviews:* Marketing staff train clinicians, executives, and others to serve as spokespeople for the HCO.
- *Social media:* Social media platforms and other online channels are used to share information, engage with the public, monitor online conversations, address patient concerns, and manage the HCO's online reputation.
- *Community relations:* HCOs can collaborate with nonprofit organizations, local leaders, and other health services providers to demonstrate their commitment to the well-being of the community.
- *Patient education programs:* Marketing creates and distributes educational materials, organizes health fairs and events, and promotes health-related information.

Negative attention detracts from the reputation of the HCO. When natural disasters, bad press, social media backlash, or employee whistleblowing happen, the marketing function provides accurate and timely information to minimize potential damage to the HCO's reputation. A well-conceived **crisis communications plan** that outlines roles, responsibilities, and protocols for addressing potential crises enables health services managers to react faster than those HCOs without such preparations (Alotaibi, 2019).

Internal Marketing

Internal marketing includes the activities that promote a positive work environment and foster engagement among clinicians and other staff (Asiamah et al., 2018). Internal marketing includes sharing important information, team building activities, recognition and rewards programs, and efforts that seek employee feedback, encourage participation, and provide collaborative decision-making opportunities. Internal marketing initiatives often emphasize the importance of treating patients with respect, empathy, and attentiveness, which has been found to improve employee satisfaction and increase employee retention rates (Kukreja, 2017; Rahman & Pribadi, 2022).

When internal marketing creates engaged HCO staff and clinicians, patients report better experiences with care (Fortenberry & McGoldrick, 2016). **Patient experience** is a multifaceted concept that can be defined as the patient's subjective and objective assessments of care related to communication, responsiveness, and environment compared to their expectations for services (Wolf et al., 2014). While patient experience is an **intangible standard** (i.e., a benchmark that cannot be easily quantified), the Centers for Medicare & Medicaid Services (CMS) measures patient experience through surveys, called the Consumer Assessment of Healthcare Providers and Systems (CAHPS; CMS, 2023). The surveys measure key aspects of patient care, such as communication and coordination of healthcare needs, but these services do not ask whether patients were satisfied with their treatment or the amenities of the HCO.

HCOs want to improve patient experience for a variety of reasons, such as the following (Anhang Price et al., 2014; Quigley et al., 2021; Richter & Muhlestein, 2017):

- *Obtain financial bonuses:* Scores on CAHPS patient experience surveys impact payment levels from the CMS.

- *Motivate clinicians:* Most clinicians want meaningful, impactful experiences with patients that positively impact their health.
- *Improve word-of-mouth marketing:* Positive experiences motivate patients to recommend the HCO to others.
- *Increase intent to return to HCO:* Patient experience ratings of nursing and physician care are associated with higher intent to return for services.
- *Improve clinical outcomes:* Higher patient experience scores are related to better adherence to treatments, improved patient safety, and better survival rates.

Marketing to Clinicians

HCOs generate patient referrals by engaging clinicians through marketing campaigns, including advertising, educational luncheons, informative blog posts, articles, webinars, online advertising, email marketing campaigns, and social media. However, the most effective form of clinician marketing is the use of salespeople (Elrod & Fortenberry, 2020b). While significantly more expensive than advertising or public relations, personal selling can be valuable in situations where face-to-face, interactive dialogue is required. For example, hospitals and large specialist physician practices employ physician relations representatives to promote the benefits of admitting patients to their hospital. These representatives also resolve any customer service issues, aiming to facilitate future patient referrals from physicians.

Physicians strongly influence patient decisions about health services and HCOs. If a physician prefers to admit patients to one hospital over another, then patients will typically agree to be admitted to that hospital instead of switching to another physician. **Switching costs** refer to the expenses, efforts, or barriers associated with changing from one service provider to another. Patients often develop trust with their clinicians, so switching providers may result in emotional costs, including anxiety, uncertainty, and concerns. Switching providers also involves onerous logistical barriers, such as obtaining patient records or scheduling appointments.

However, health services managers need to be aware of the legal constraints involved with engaging in clinician marketing (Satiani et al., 2020). Named after the sponsor of the bills, U.S. Representative Pete Stark of California, **Stark laws** prohibit physicians or immediate family members who have a financial relationship with an HCO from making Medicare referrals to those entities, except in certain situations. While physician self-referral laws do not apply to all health services, certain services are exempt, such as clinical laboratory services or occupational health. Like Stark laws, the federal Anti-kickback Statute was established to prevent financial abuse of the healthcare system. **Kickbacks** in healthcare are any financial reward (i.e., bribe or rebate) given in exchange for patient referrals. For example, physician landlords cannot offer kickbacks disguised as low-cost rent to induce referrals from other physicians. The law provides certain **safe harbor regulations** that define payment and business practices that are not considered kickbacks. A basic rule of safe harbor regulations is that financial transactions between potential referring parties should be conducted at fair market value.

FUTURE DIRECTIONS

Competition is intensifying as HCOs consolidate and patients become more discerning consumers, thus demanding that HCOs improve the unacceptable value of health services. Health services managers are accountable for the long-term viability of the HCO, but success is far from assured. The largest 10 hospital systems control a quarter of the inpatient market, and the health insurance industry has consolidated to the point where nearly three quarters of all metropolitan areas are considered highly competitive markets (Waddill, 2021). These large payer and provider corporations battle each other for dominance in contract negotiations, creating a zero-sum game where one party collects profits at the expense of the other. These system-level battles create no real value for patients or communities (Porter & Tiesberg, 2006).

However, the emerging healthcare conglomerates created by vertical consolidations may diminish the importance of negotiations between health systems and insurance companies. When health insurers consolidate with health service providers to create "payviders," profits cannot be secured at the bargaining table (Goldberg & Nash, 2021). Instead, these large, vertically integrated HCOs may be forced to capture profits along the health services delivery value chain, which could lead to health system improvements that benefit patients.

SUMMARY

- To effectively formulate strategy, health services managers must understand both the internal and external environment of the organization.
- Based on the directional strategy (i.e., mission, vision, and values) and core competencies identified in the environmental assessments, health services managers make strategic choices designed to create a competitive advantage.
- Healthcare strategy takes place at three levels: corporate, business, and function. Executives at the corporate level drive strategic planning for the entire HCO and align businesses and service lines with that strategy. Functional departments, such as finance, human resources, and marketing, align their operations with corporate and business strategy.
- Business plans are proposals that describe which businesses or services may have the highest potential for success. Operational plans guide the implementation of strategic plans.
- Health services marketing is the function responsible for distribution, pricing, and promoting health services. Health services marketing needs to be appropriate in tone, message, and method, according to ethical guidelines.
- Effective and efficient health services marketing largely depends on the ideal segmentation of the market. The right selection of target audiences will improve the performance of marketing campaigns.
- The health services marketing promotional mix includes branding, advertising, public relations, internal marketing, and clinician marketing.

END-OF-CHAPTER RESOURCES

KEY TERMS*

*For the full list of key terms, please see the online glossary at **http://connect.springerpub.com/content/book/978-0-8261-4807-0.**

adaptive strategies
barriers to entry
Boston Consulting Group (BCG) matrix
branding
business model
business plan
cash cows

catchment area
certificate of need
case mix
community health needs assessment
core competencies
crisis communications plan
dogs

economies of scale
environmental assessment
epidemiological planning model
expansion strategies
Five Forces model
Four Ps
Herfindahl-Hirschman Index
horizontal expansion
intangible resources
intangible standard
internal marketing
kickbacks
life cycle management
marketing
marketing channels
marketing mix
market share
merger
mission
monopoly
monopolistic competition
oligopoly
operational plan
opportunities
patient experience
perfect competition
portfolio management
placement
pricing
product
promotion
question marks
safe harbor regulations
segmentation
Sherman Antitrust Act
Stark laws
stars
strategy
strategic alliance
strategic business unit
strategic direction
strategic management
strategic planning
strengths
SWOT analysis
switching costs
tangible resources
target audience
targeting
values
third-party payers
threats
value proposition
vertical integration
vision
weaknesses

LEARNING ACTIVITIES

Professional Development and Reflection

1. Create a list of your strengths that will facilitate your future career success. To generate ideas, examine academic program competencies, course objectives, performance assessments (school and work), strength surveys, and input from trusted advisors. Also, ask yourself: What do I enjoy doing? What comes easily to me that others find difficult? What if I were to enhance my current skills?

2. Choose at least three (3) potential target healthcare settings, such as inpatient, physician practice, hospice, managed care, consulting, and others. Locate the website of at least one representative organization within each of these settings and describe how each of their missions, visions, and values are consistent with yours. Write reflections about whether you would fit in these organizations and why.

Discussion Questions

1. Discuss the challenges faced by rural HCOs that may lead to shrinking markets or obsolete services. How can these HCOs adapt their strategies to remain financially viable and prepare for future opportunities?

2. Reflect on the challenge of managing service lines that may not be profitable but are necessary for the community's health and well-being. How do health services managers seek to maximize the financial performance of an HCO's service portfolio?
3. What makes marketing health services different from marketing other types of consumer products and services? How do you suggest that health services marketers maintain the trust of patients and their families?

RECOMMENDED READING AND MEDIA

Barnett, B. (2015). *The strategic career: Let business principles guide you.* Stanford Business Books.

Dafny, L. S., & Lee, T. H. (2016). Health care needs real competition. *Harvard Business Review.* https://hbr.org/2016/12/health-care-needs-real-competition

Martin, R. (2022, June 29). *A Plan Is Not a Strategy* [YouTube]. Harvard Business Review. https://www.youtube.com/watch?v=iuYlGRnC7J8.

McKeown, G. (2014). *Essentialism: The disciplined pursuit of less.* Currency.

Porter, M. E. (1996). What is strategy? *Harvard Business Review.* https://hbr.org/1996/11/what-is-strategy

Porter, M. E., & Lee, T. H. (2015). Why strategy matters now. *New England Journal of Medicine, 372*(18), 1681–1684.

Porter, M. E., & Lee, T. H. (2016). The strategy that will fix healthcare. *Harvard Business Review.* https://hbr.org/2013/10/the-strategy-that-will-fix-health-care

Yankelovich, D., & Meer, D. (2006). Rediscovering market segmentation. *Harvard Business Review.* https://hbr.org/2006/02/rediscovering-market-segmentation

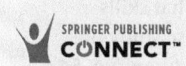

A robust set of instructor resources designed to supplement this text is located at http://connect.springerpub.com/content/book/978-0-8261-4807-0.
Qualifying instructors may request access by emailing textbook@springerpub.com.

REFERENCES

Agency for Healthcare Research and Quality. (2020, September). *CAHPS clinician and group survey 3.0 measures.* https://www.ahrq.gov/cahps/surveys-guidance/cg/about/survey-measures.html

Ahlbom, A. (2020). Epidemiology is about disease in populations. *European Journal of Epidemiology, 35*(12), 1111–1113. https://doi.org/10.1007/s10654-020-00701-9

Alotaibi, M. M. (2019). The Role of Public Relations in Informing a Crisis Plan for the Texas Health Presbyterian Hospital and the Broward Health Medical Center in Florida. *Mass Communication Research, 52*(52), 39–94. https://doi.org/10.21608/jsb.2019.42833

American College of Healthcare Executives. (2022, December 5). *Code of ethics.* https://www.ache.org/about-ache/our-story/our-commitments/ethics/ache-code-of-ethics

American Hospital Association. (2022). *Why 2022 will be a year of disruptor differentiation.* https://www.aha.org/aha-center-health-innovation-market-scan/2022-01-11-why-2022-will-be-year-disruptor-differentiation

American Hospital Association. (2023). *Retail clinics target chronic diseases.* https://www.aha.org/aha-center-health-innovation-market-scan/2023-05-30-retail-clinics-target-chronic-diseases

American Medical Association. (2019, December 15). *Truth in advertising.* https://www.ama-assn.org/delivering-care/patient-support-advocacy/truth-advertising

Anhang Price, R., Elliott, M. N., Zaslavsky, A. M., Hays, R. D., Lehrman, W. G., Rybowski, L., Edgman-Levitan, S., & Cleary, P. D. (2014). Examining the role of patient experience surveys in measuring health care quality. *Medical Care Research and Review, 71*(5), 522–554. https://doi.org/10.1177/1077558714541480

Asiamah, N., Opuni, F. F., & Mensah, H. K. (2018). The nexus between internal marketing in hospitals and organizational commitment: Incorporating the mediation roles of key job characteristics. *International Journal of Healthcare Management, 11*(4), 1–15. https://doi.org/10.1080/20479700.2018.1551951

Azzoparde, J., Malani, R., Rao, N., & Singhal, S. (2022, November 15). *U.S. health systems: Diversify to thrive*. McKinsey & Company, Inc. https://www.mckinsey.com/industries/healthcare/our-insights/us-health-systems-diversify-to-thrive

Barney, J. B., Ketchen Jr., D. J., & Wright, M. (2011). The future of resource-based theory: Revitalization or decline? *Journal of Management, 37*(5), 1299–1315. https://doi.org/10.1177/0149206310391805

Baugh, C. W., Dorner, S. C., Levine, D. M., Handley, N. R., & Mooney, K. H. (2022). Acute home-based care for patients with cancer to avoid, substitute, and follow emergency department visits: A conceptual framework using Porter's Five Forces. *Emergency Cancer Care, 1*(1), 1–10. https://doi.org/10.1186/s44201-022-00008-3

Berry, L. L., & Bendapudi, N. (2007). Health care: A fertile field for service research. *Journal of Service Research, 10*(2), 111–122. https://doi.org/10.1177/1094670507306682

Bratucu, R., Gheorghe, I. R., Purcarea, R. M., Gheorghe, C. M., Velea, O. P., & Purcarea, V. L. (2014). Cause and effect: The linkage between the health information seeking behavior and the online environment: A review. *Journal of Medicine and Life, 7*(3), 310.

Brownlee, S., Chalkidou, K., Doust, J., Elshaug, A. G., Glasziou, P., Heath, I., Nagpal, S., Saini, V., Srivastava, D., Chalmers, K., & Korenstein, D. (2017). Evidence for overuse of medical services around the world. *The Lancet, 390*(10090), 156–168. https://doi.org/10.1016/S0140-6736(16)32585-5

Center for Healthcare Quality and Payment Reform. (2023). *Rural hospitals at risk of closing*. https://ruralhospitals.chqpr.org/downloads/Rural_Hospitals_at_Risk_of_Closing.pdf

Centers for Medicare and Medicaid Services. (2023, January 25). *Consumer Assessment of Healthcare Providers & Systems (CAHPS)*. https://www.cms.gov/research-statistics-data-and-systems/research/cahps

Chesluk, B., Tollen, L., Lewis, J., DuPont, S., & Klau, M. H. (2017). Physicians' voices: What skills and supports are needed for effective practice in an integrated delivery system?: A case study of Kaiser Permanente. *INQUIRY: The Journal of health care organization, provision, and financing, 54*, 0046958017711760. https://doi.org/10.1177/0046958017711760

Clardy, A. (2013). Strengths vs. strong position: Rethinking the nature of SWOT analysis. *Modern Management Science & Engineering, 1*(1), 100–122. https://doi.org/10.22158/mmse.v1i1.54

Coman, A., & Ronan, B. (2009). Focused SWOT: Diagnosing critical strengths and weaknesses. *International Journal of Production Research, 47*(20), 5677–5699. https://doi.org/10.1080/00207540802146130

Deloitte Center for Health Solutions. (2012). *The U.S. health care market: A strategic view of consumer segmentation*. https://www2.deloitte.com/content/dam/Deloitte/us/Documents/life-sciences-health-care/us-lshc-health-care-market-consumer-segmentation.pdf

Elrod, J. K., & Fortenberry, J. L. (2020a). Public relations in health and medicine: Using publicity and other unpaid promotional methods to engage audiences. *BMC Health Services Research, 20*(1), 821. https://doi.org/10.1186/s12913-020-05602-x

Elrod, J. K., & Fortenberry, J. L. (2020b). Personal selling in health and medicine: Using sales agents to engage audiences. *BMC Health Services Research, 20*(1), 819. https://doi.org/10.1186/s12913-020-05600-z

Eickholt, L. (2019). Why many integrated delivery systems have not enhanced consumer value, and what's next. *NEJM Catalyst Innovations in Care Delivery, 1*(1). https://doi.org/10.1056/CAT.19.1086

Evans, J. M., Brown, A., & Baker, G. R. (2017). Organizational knowledge and capabilities in healthcare: Deconstructing and integrating diverse perspectives. *SAGE Open Medicine, 5*, 2050312117712655. https://doi.org/10.1177/2050312117712655

Fortenberry, J. L., & McGoldrick, P. J. (2016). Internal marketing: A pathway for healthcare facilities to improve the patient experience. *International Journal of Healthcare Management, 9*(1), 28–33. https://doi.org/10.1179/2047971915Y.0000000014

Geyman, J. (2022). Health Insurance in the United States: Failure of Private and Multi-Payer Financing. In A. I. Tavares (Ed.). *Health Insurance*. IntechOpen.

Ginter, P. M., Duncan, W. J., & Swayne, L. E. (2018). *Strategic management of health care organizations* (8th ed.). John Wiley & Sons, Inc.

Gliadkovskaya, A. (2022, March 17). *Moody's: Shift away from inpatient care will continue to shrink hospital margins*. Fierce Healthcare. https://www.fiercehealthcare.com/providers/moodys-report-shifting-care-trends-will-continue-shrink-hospital-margins

Goddard, R. (2022, September 14). *Healthcare vertical integration: Back to the future*. Lumeris. https://www.lumeris.com/healthcare-vertical-integration-back-to-the-future

Goldberg, Z. N., & Nash, D. B. (2021). The payvider: An evolving model. *Population Health Management, 24*(5), 528–530. https://doi.org/10.1089/pop.2021.0164

Gunawardane, G. (2020). *Modern health care marketing*. World Scientific.

Harris, P. (2007, March 16). *CVS finally wins Caremark for $24 billion*. Reuters. https://www.reuters.com/article/us-caremark-cvs/cvs-finally-wins-caremark-for-24-bln-idUSWEN549420070316

Helms, M. M., & Nixon, J. (2010). Exploring SWOT analysis–where are we now? A review of academic research from the last decade. *Journal of Strategy and Management, 3*(3), 215–251. https://doi.org/10.1108/17554251011064837

Henderson, B. (1970). *The Product Portfolio*. Boston Consulting Group. https://www.bcg.com/publications/1970/strategy-the-product-portfolio

Jalalpour, M., Gel, Y., & Levin, S. (2015). Forecasting demand for health services: Development of a publicly available toolbox. *Operations Research for Health Care, 5*, 1–9. https://doi.org/10.1016/j.orhc.2015.03.001

Khosravizadeh, O., Vatankhah, S., & Maleki, M. (2017). A systematic review of medical service branding: Essential approach to hospital sector. *Annals of Tropical Medicine & Public Health, 10*(5), 1137–1146. https://doi.org/10.4103/ATMPH.ATMPH_328_17

Kotter, P. (1994). *Marketing management* (8th ed.). Prentice Hall.

Kukreja, J. (2017). Internal marketing: A prelude or an outcome of Employee Motivation? *BVIMSR's Journal of Management Research, 9*(1), 54.

Landi, H. (2023, May 2). *CVS closes $10.6B acquisition of Oak Street Health to expand primary care footprint*. Fierce Healthcare. https://www.fiercehealthcare.com/providers/cvs-closes-106b-acquisition-oak-street-health-expand-primary-care-footprint

Lang, G., Farnell IV, E. A., & Quinlan, J. D. (2021). Out-of-hospital birth. *American Family Physician, 103*(11), 672–679.

Lee, C. (2021). Patient loyalty to health services: The role of communication skills and cognitive trust. *International Journal of Healthcare Management, 14*(4), 1254–1264. https://doi.org/10.1080/20479700.2020.1756111

Levitt, T. (1965). Exploit the product life cycle. *Harvard Business Review*. https://hbr.org/1965/11/exploit-the-product-life-cycle

Liu, S. S., & Chen, J. (2009). Using data mining to segment healthcare markets from patients' preference perspectives. *International Journal of Health Care Quality Assurance, 22*(2), 117–134. https://doi.org/10.1108/09526860910944610

Magretta, J. (2011, December 15). Jim Collins, meet Michael Porter. *Harvard Business Review*. https://hbr.org/2011/12/jim-collins-meet-michael-porte

Medical Group Management Association-American College of Medical Practice Executives. (2015, September 29). *Code of ethics*. https://www.mgma.com/MGMA/media/files/about/Code-of-Ethics-Approved.pdf

Minemyer, P. (2022, March 25). *How CVS Kidney Care is thinking about personalized care for patients*. Fierce Healthcare. https://www.fiercehealthcare.com/retail/how-cvs-kidney-care-thinking-about-personalized-care-patients

National Center for Health Statistics. (2023, May 17). *Births and natality*. Centers for Disease Control and Prevention. https://www.cdc.gov/nchs/fastats/births.htm

Permanente Medicine. (2023, April 10). *Driving health care innovation in 10 steps*. https://permanente.org/medical-excellence/driving-healthcare-innovation-in-10-steps

Pelzel, K. (2021, December 11). Marketing Yourself Using the 4 Ps and Cs [Blog post]. Upskilling. https://medium.com/upskilling/marketing-yourself-using-the-4-ps-and-cs-a6e930e37628

Porter, M. E. (1996). What is strategy? *Harvard Business Review*. https://hbr.org/1996/11/what-is-strategy

Porter, M. E. (2008). *Competitive advantage: Creating and sustaining superior performance* (2nd ed.). Free Press.

Porter, M. E., & Lee, T. H. (2016). The strategy that will fix healthcare. *Harvard Business Review*. https://hbr.org/2013/10/the-strategy-that-will-fix-health-care

Porter, M. E., & Teisberg, E. O. (2006). *Redefining health care: Creating value-based competition on results*. Harvard Business School Press.

Priore, R. J. (2021). *Improving financial and operations performance: A healthcare leader's guide*. Springer Publishing Company.

Quigley, D. D., Reynolds, K., Dellva, S., & Price, R. A. (2021). Examining the business case for patient experience: A systematic review. *Journal of Healthcare Management, 66*(3), 200–224. https://doi.org/10.1097/JHM-D-20-00207

Rahman, A. N., & Pribadi, F. (2022). Effective marketing strategies in health services: Systematic literature review. *Expert Journal of Marketing, 10*(2), 73–84.

Read, L., Korenda, L., & Nelson, H. (2021, August 5). *Rebuilding trust in health care: What do consumers want—and need—organizations to do?* Deloitte Insights. https://www2.deloitte.com/us/en/insights/industry/health-care/trust-in-health-care-system.html

Rhodes, J. H., Santos, T., & Young, G. (2023). The early impact of the covid-19 pandemic on hospital finances. *Journal of Healthcare Management, 68*(1), 38–55. https://doi.org/10.1097/JHM-D-22-00037

Richman, E. (2018, November 28). *CVS closes $69B acquisition of Aetna in a 'transformative moment' for the industry*. Fierce Healthcare. https://www.fiercehealthcare.com/payer/cvs-closes-69-billion-acquisition-aetna

Richter, J. P., & Muhlestein, D. B. (2017). Patient experience and hospital profitability. *Health Care Management Review, 42*(3), 247–257. https://doi.org/10.1097/HMR.0000000000000105

Satiani, B., Zigrang, T. A., & Bailey-Wheaton, J. L. (2020). Proposed stark regulations: Small step in the right direction. *Physician Leadership Journal, 7*(3), 30.

Schwartz, L. M., & Woloshin, S. (2019). Medical marketing in the United States, 1997–2016. *JAMA, 321*(1), 80–96. https://doi.org/10.1001/jama.2018.19320

Sciulli, L. M., & Missien, T. L. (2015). Hospital service-line positioning and brand image: Influences on service quality, patient satisfaction, and desired performance. *Innovative Marketing, 11*(2), 20–29.

St. Paul Business Journal. (2006, July 13). *CVS to buy MinuteClinic*. https://www.bizjournals.com/twincities/stories/2006/07/10/daily30.html

Stowell, C., & Akerman, C. (2015, September 17). Better value in health care requires focusing on outcomes. *Harvard Business Review*. https://hbr.org/2015/09/better-value-in-health-care-requires-focusing-on-outcomes

Strach, L. (2004). Hospital advertising in the beginning: Marketplace dynamics and the lifting of the ban. *Essays in Economic & Business History, 22*, 229–239.

Trinh, H. Q. (2020). Strategic management in local hospital markets: Service duplication or service differentiation. *BMC Health Services Research, 20*(1), 880. https://doi.org/10.1186/s12913-020-05728-y

U.S. Department of Justice. (2018, July 31). *Herfindahl–Hirschman Index*. https://www.justice.gov/atr/herfindahl-hirschman-index

Waddill, K. (2021, September 29). *Health Insurance Industry Consolidation Grew from 2014 to 2020*. Health Payer Intelligence. https://healthpayerintelligence.com/news/health-insurance-industry-consolidation-grew-from-2014-to-202

White, K. R., & Griffith, J. R. (2019). Marketing and strategy. In *The Well-Managed Healthcare Organization* (9th ed., pp. 471–506). Health Administration Press.

Wolf, J. A., Niederhauser, V., Marshburn, D., & LaVela, S. L. (2014). Defining patient experience. *Patient Experience Journal, 1*(1), 7–19. https://doi.org/10.35680/2372-0247.1004

Woodside, A. G., Nielsen, R. L., Walters, F., & Muller, G. D. (1988). Preference segmentation of health care services: The old-fashioneds, value conscious, affluents, and professional want-it-alls. *Journal of Health Care Marketing, 8*(2), 14–24.

CHAPTER 9

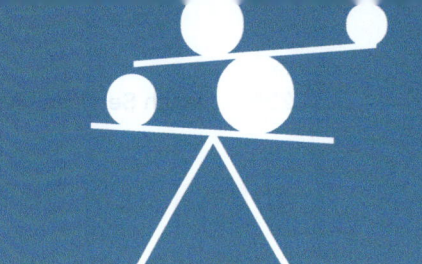

HUMAN RESOURCE MANAGEMENT

Human resource management involves recruiting and hiring people who fit the job and organization, paying them, training them, evaluating them, rewarding them, and retaining them so that the organization can succeed.

COMPETENCIES

- Manage hiring processes including recruitment, screening, selection, and on-boarding.
- Develop competitive compensation and benefits structures.
- Comply with human resources laws and regulations.
- Build staffing models and workload forecasts.
- Develop effective physician and employee retention programs.
- Design staff training, development, and engagement programs.
- Create evaluations systems to assess employee performance.
- Align human resource practices with organizational strategy.
- Manage staff within collective bargaining rules.
- Maintain succession and replacement plans for employees.
- Assure safety and well-being of employees.

CHAPTER OUTLINE

- Human Resources and Early Careerists
- Human Resources Business Partners and Health Services Managers
- Strategic Human Resources and Healthcare Executives

INTRODUCTION

Human resource management plays a critical function in the health care organization (HCO), and yet, many business leaders once considered human resources (HR) as merely a clerical function (Drucker, 1954). Despite this dim view, healthcare HR professionals have increasingly become operational partners and strategic collaborators with health services managers. Without competent HR management to support the health services manager, the challenges—staffing shortages, retention problems, low morale, burnout, patient harm, and legal liability—would be much more difficult to solve.

HR management is a popular career specialization for health services managers. Early career positions in HR focus on day-to-day tactical tasks, but with experience and ambition, HR specialists can rise through the ranks to executive roles. This chapter, however, examines the value that HR professionals provide to health services managers throughout their career stages.

HUMAN RESOURCES AND EARLY CAREERISTS

Administrative Functions of Human Resources

Many early career health services managers first encounter HR practices when they go through the hiring process themselves. From the perspective of the early careerist applicant, HR professionals manage a series of administrative processes (applications, interviews, job offers, and others). At this stage, HR can seem like an impediment—not an ally—to career advancement. This is understandable, given the frustrations typically associated with submitting online job applications. However, HR processes are not designed to assist applicants per se but to create efficient and effective employment systems that support hiring managers.

Job Analysis

HR professionals offer valuable, time-saving human capital management services. For example, when a health services manager requires new staff, HR specialists will help to formally define the position, an HR management practice called **job analysis**. This systematic process documents the roles, responsibilities, work tasks, credentials, and capabilities needed to perform the job. Based on the job analysis, the HR analyst collaborates with the hiring manager to create a **position description**, which documents the following elements (Chmiel et al., 2017; Society for Human Resource Management [SHRM], 2015):

- *Job identification:* Identifies the title, department, supervisor, classification, and date written or last reviewed
- *Position control number:* Assigned by HR and tied to a job classification system that tracks vacancies, assists with staffing and budgeting, and controls the creation of new jobs in a centralized system
- *Salary grade/level/family:* A grouping of compensation levels or pay ranges by similar job type, including minimum and maximum pay bands
- *Summary/objective:* A statement of the purpose and essential functions of the job
- *Competency profile:* The knowledge, skills, and attitudes required of the worker to be effective in the position
- *Essential duties:* The basic functions of the job that must be performed, with or without **reasonable accommodations** made for individuals with disabilities
- *Required/preferred credentials or job experience:* Includes mandatory or optional education and experience levels based on job-related requirements and laws
- *Supervisory responsibilities:* The number of employees and level of oversight required
- *Legal information:* Federal or state regulations, such as the Americans with Disabilities Act and U.S. **Equal Employment Opportunity Commission (EEOC)**, as appropriate

Job seekers entering the health services management profession should be aware that most early career position descriptions will appear highly repetitive and rather boring. This perception is due more to the poorly written position descriptions than a reflection of the actual work (Parker et al., 2019a). Hiring managers and their HR department collaborators tend to write position descriptions that are overly prescriptive and task focused, which can make jobs seem tedious and unattractive to outside applicants. Many early career health services manager roles feature variety in day-to-day activities and somewhat independent decision-making (Bonica & Hartman, 2018). To avoid discouraging ambitious early career health services managers, HR specialists and hiring managers would be better served to highlight the variety of tasks, relative autonomy, and the overall purpose of the work (Parker et al., 2019b). Well-described position descriptions are probably the exception, so early career health services managers should further investigate whether the job is more interesting than the position description makes it sound.

> ### △ KEY IDEA
> Well-described position descriptions are probably the exception, so early career health services managers should further investigate whether the job is more interesting than the position description makes it sound.

Job Applications

Position descriptions for open jobs are usually posted to the career sections of HCO websites, where individuals can submit applications directly into a tracking system. A software automatically scans applications and résumés for keywords related to the position description, and only the résumés that contain the specific language used in the position description will ever be reviewed by an actual person. Once prescreened, the number of applicants may be reduced from a hundred to fewer than 20 who are minimally qualified and a potential good fit for the company (Burnison, 2018).

In any case, hiring managers often circumvent the applicant screening rules for people that they know. HR recruiters often run two separate processes—one for candidates who only submit through the website and one for applicants referred by the hiring manager or other employees. This means that the job may be filled by someone who the hiring manager knows even before other candidates are considered (Adler, 2016). Therefore, successful early career health services managers use their professional contacts to gain introductions to hiring managers.

Recruiting

Recruiters are specialized HR professionals who are responsible for connecting the HCO to potential employees best suited for the position. In addition to sifting through job applications, recruiters hold career fairs and other hiring events with community partners and universities to find well-qualified candidates. Recruiters conduct interviews and assessments to confirm that the candidate's background, goals, personality, and skills fit the position description and work environment. Due to a shortage of many types of healthcare caregivers and other team members, recruiters often have dozens of open positions that they are responsible for filling (Leavy-Detrick, 2012). Table 9.1 describes the different recruiting challenges associated with recruiting various healthcare human capital.

FIGURE 9.1 Employee hiring process.

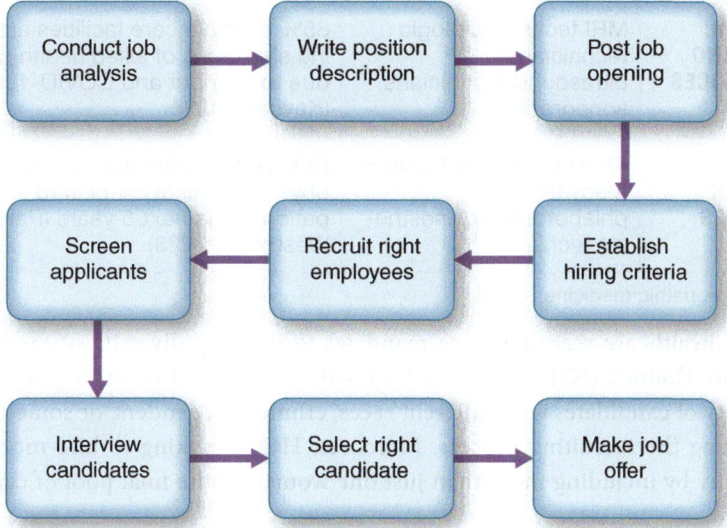

TABLE 9.1 Recruiting Challenges Associated With Recruiting Healthcare Human Capital

ROLE CATEGORY	TYPES	NEEDS AND CHALLENGES
ADMINISTRATIVE SUPPORT JOBS	Front desk specialists, maintenance technicians	Replacing healthcare billers takes months due to jobs asking for longer hours and increased focus on productivity (Akasa, 2021); 88% of physician practices are having difficulties recruiting front-of-office staff (Medical Economics, 2021).
HEALTH SERVICES MANAGERS	Various specialists, coordinators, analysts, managers, directors, executives	Job demand for health services managers is expected to increase faster than other occupations (BLS, 2022).
REGISTERED NURSES	Bedside and nonbedside nursing roles	Limited capacity for associate's and bachelor's prepared nursing programs (Apen, 2021); increased demand means challenges for nurse staffing (Buerhaus, 2021)
NURSE PRACTITIONERS	Specialty types of nurse practitioners, such as primary care, nurse anesthetists, and nurse midwives	Some state laws limit ability of nurse practitioners to practice independently from physicians (Cimiotti, 2019).
OTHER NURSES	Licensed practical nurses, certified nursing assistants	Lack of academic programs and lower pay reduce worker supply (Gingerelli, & Mulhern, 2021).
PHYSICIANS	MD (allopathic) and DO (osteopathic)	Physician shortages of between 37,800 and 124,000 physicians by 2034 are caused by high cost of training and people leaving the profession due to burnout (IHS Markit, 2021).
SUPPORT SERVICES	Environmental services, patient transport, food delivery, facilities technicians	Staffing shortages caused by the COVID-19 pandemic, retiring staff, and poor workforce planning (Burmahl, 2022)
ALLIED HEALTH: DIAGNOSTIC AND IMAGING SERVICES	MRI techs, radiologic technicians, ultrasound technicians, sonographers	85% of healthcare facilities are experiencing shortages of allied health professionals due to burnout and COVID-19 pandemic (Kayser, 2022).
OTHER ALLIED HEALTH PROFESSIONALS	Medical assistants, pharmacy techs phlebotomists, anesthesia techs	Difficult to recruit due to low pay and physical labor, 21% plan to leave occupation in the next 5 years (Paiewonsky & Westhead, 2023)

DO, doctor of osteopathic medicine.

In addition, healthcare recruiters face mandates to improve diversity of candidates (Nashville Health Care Council [NHCC], 2022). HCOs that embrace diversity, equity, and inclusion identify a variety of candidates with different races, ethnicities, genders, or some other category of identity during the recruiting process. Moreover, HCOs looking to hire more women can improve diversity by including more than just one woman in the final pool of candidates. One study found that if a four-person candidate pool had only one woman, then the likelihood that she would be hired was virtually zero (Johnson et al., 2016). Slim chances were also found in situations where there was only one person from an underrepresented racial or ethnic group among the candidate pool.

>
> ## INFORMATIONAL INTERVIEW 9.1
> *Human Resources Coordinator*
> Access the informational interview online at http://connect.springerpub.com/content/book/978-0-8261-4807-0/chapter/ch00.

Interviewing

If an applicant makes it through the screening process, an HR recruiter will coordinate first round interviews, either virtually or in person. HR professionals train hiring managers and other staff on how to comply with employment laws and improve the effectiveness of interviews. Anti-discrimination laws and regulations prohibit interviewers from asking a variety of personal questions about national origin, age, marital status, religion, disabilities, and criminal record. Creating objective hiring criteria based on job analyses and position descriptions is the best way to avoid non-compliance with employment laws.

In addition, HR specialists often collaborate with hiring managers to develop **structured interview** questions based on the job analysis and position description. By asking each candidate the same set of job-relevant questions in the same order, the interviewers can evaluate interviewee responses more validly and reliably (Levashina et al., 2014). In some organizations, even rapport-building questions (e.g., "How are you doing today?") are standardized to remove any extraneous information not related to job performance. Structured interviews, when implemented correctly, can reduce bias in the interview process. For example, the **halo effect** is a cognitive bias that leads recruiters or hiring managers to form a positive impression of a candidate based on irrelevant characteristics, such as how they look or whether they belonged to the same fraternity.

The most popular types of structured interview questions are behavioral and situational (Levashina et al., 2014). **Situational interview** questions ask applicants how they might react to hypothetical workplace situations. Common situational questions start with "What would you do if" and commonly relate to interpersonal skills and time management. **Behavioral interview** questions predict future behaviors by asking about an interviewee's past experiences. These kinds of questions usually begin with "Describe a time when you" and address the candidate's ability to deal with adversity, use good judgment, or handle conflict. The difference between the two types is that situational interview questions are hypothetical, while behavioral questions are based on actual events.

Early career health services managers can prepare for these types of interview questions in similar ways. A commonly used format for these types of questions is called the STAR technique, an acronym that reflects a step-by-step approach to answering interview questions. As shown in Figure 9.2, interviewees state the situation, the task they were responsible for, the action they took, and the result of that action (Development Dimensions International, Inc. [DDI], 2023). The best answers to behavioral questions are specific and pertain to work, school, or volunteer experiences. If the example involves a team, the actions should relate to the part the interviewee played in achieving the result.

FIGURE 9.2 STAR interview response technique.

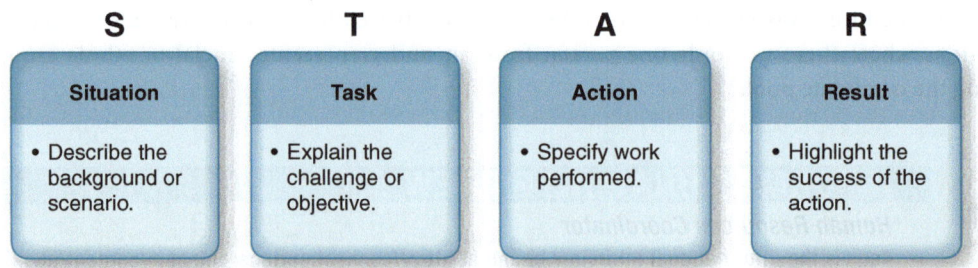

Source: Adapted from STAR Method by Development Dimensions International, Inc. https://www.ddiworld.com/solutions/behavioral-interviewing/star-method

Selection

Prior to making job offers, many HCOs use **selection tools** that evaluate candidates against predetermined selection criteria. Some HCOs conduct preemployment screening assessments to give hiring managers a chance to evaluate candidates based on skill, which can reduce bias and increase diversity (Sans, 2019). For health services managers, examples of assessments include critical thinking tests, case study analyses, or software aptitude proficiency tests (e.g., Microsoft Excel® simulations). Another way to ensure that offers are made to the best candidate is by conducting **realistic job previews**, where HR professionals arrange structured observations or meetings between applicants and hiring manager and staff. Equipped with both positive and negative information about the job, the job previews allow both organization and job applicant to make informed choices about whether the person is a good fit for the position (Baur et al., 2014).

> ⚠ **KEY IDEA**
>
> Preemployment screening assessments, such as critical thinking tests, case study analyses, or software aptitude proficiency tests, give hiring managers a chance to evaluate candidates based on skill, which can reduce bias and increase diversity.

Once candidates are interviewed (often multiple times) and vetted, the HR professional will help the hiring manager decide which candidate to hire. The hiring manager makes the final selection of candidates based on predetermined criteria. A **person-job fit** is determined by how the candidate's competencies match the specific requirements listed in the position description. A **person-organization fit** is concerned with how the candidate matches the values, culture, and vision of the organization. Hiring managers can consider both person-job and person-organization fit simultaneously to determine the preferred candidate, but person-job fit is a stronger predictor of success than person-organization fit (Kristof-Brown et al., 2005). Once the final decision is made, the HR professional will then extend an employment offer, either verbally or in writing. If the candidate is determined to be a good fit for the organization, most HCOs will administer drug screens, physical exams, background checks, credential reviews, and verify prior employment before extending job offers.

Compensation and Benefits

When the HR recruiter makes an employment offer, the early career health services manager should ask for all the details of the compensation package and request a reasonable amount of time to consider the offer (i.e., 2 to 3 days, sometimes up to a week). Each position falls within a

salary band that defines the acceptable salary range, even if the published compensation amount is only a single number. HR uses these salary bands—confidential within the HCO—to control workforce costs and to keep the compensation levels of similar positions in the organization equitable. Salary bands are determined by an HCOs **compensation philosophy** that guides how HCOs pay employees, including decisions about who to compensate, what amount, and for which accomplishments. A well-defined compensation philosophy ensures that salaries, bonuses, and benefits are equitable among employees of the HCO and in-line with compensation packages of competitors in the marketplace.

Pay equity means that employees receive equal pay for equal work regardless of gender, race, or other protected characteristics. Health services managers work with HR to monitor HCO compensation data for new and existing employees and to continuously communicate compensation decisions to employees, ensuring transparency and fairness in compensation packages. To promote pay equity, some states and cities require that employers share the salary bands with candidates, which has been found to reduce pay discrepancies between men and women and minorities (National Women's Law Center [NWLC], 2023). Nevertheless, candidates can research salary ranges at similar organizations in the region to determine where to start negotiations. Most healthcare recruiters expect that job candidates will negotiate their salaries (Birt, 2023). Once the compensation is agreed upon, the HR recruiter will send an official offer letter for signature by the candidate.

Once employed by the HCO, salary and benefit administration becomes the responsibility of HR specialists. Some benefits packages are mandated by law, while some vary depending on the level of the employee. Benefits can vary by HCO, which use these packages as a way to differentiate themselves when competing for employees. Common benefits at HCOs include the following:

- *Health insurance:* U.S. companies pay an average annual cost of $7,954, and an individual employee is responsible for $1,327 each year (Claxton et al., 2022).
- *Flexible spending account*: It is a special account with pretax money that can be used to pay for certain medical expenses; dental care and vision care; and dependent care, such as preschool, summer camp, and day care.
- *Qualified retirement plan*: It is an employer-sponsored, tax-deductible retirement plan that meets the federal tax code requirements.

CAREER BOX 9.1: Negotiating First Positions in Health Services Management

Before any job offer, investigate salary ranges for the type of positions you seek and be ready with salary expectations and probable ranges of offers. Once the job has been offered, the recruiter will likely ask—in writing or on the telephone—how much salary will be required to accept the position. Instead of answering this question directly, convey gratitude for the offer, excitement for the position, and desire for fair wage for the position. Then, ask the recruited what the pay range for the position is. They might not answer this question, or they might offer something on the lower end of the pay band. In either case, you should ask for pay that is close to the top of the expected salary range. For example, if the likely salary is between $55,000 and $65,000, ask for something closer to $65,000. This reasonable offer moves the negotiations to the higher end without provoking negative reactions from the recruiter or hiring manager (Maaravi & Segal, 2022). Do not worry if the offer is met with silence; recruiters use this technique to get candidates to agree to a lower amount. If the offer is below expectations, the pause in negotiations may lead to an increased offer (Curhan et al., 2021). Once a final offer is made, it is always okay to ask for 2 to 3 days to consider a job offer.

- ***Defined contribution plan:*** It is a retirement plan, such as the 401(k), to which the employer matches an employee's investment up to a certain amount. Upon retirement, the employee can withdraw the money and the accrued interest at a reduced tax rate.
- ***Short-term disability insurance:*** It provides a percentage of pre-disability wages when an employee is unable to work for extended time due to an illness or injury.
- *Paid time off (PTO):* The average PTO depends on years of service with the HCO and includes vacation, sick time, and holidays.
- *Paid parental leave:* The United States does not have national standards, but top hospitals offer an average of 7.8 weeks of paid parental leave per year. The annual mean paid parental leave among economically similar nations is 18.6 weeks (Lu et al., 2021).
- *Tuition reimbursement:* To encourage career growth and improve employee retention, many large HCOs offer educational assistance, and $5,250 of the benefit each year is tax-free for the organization (Internal Revenue Service [IRS], 2023).

Onboarding

HR specialists administer onboarding (i.e., orientation) programs designed to ensure that new employees are as comfortable and productive as possible when they start their new jobs. This includes plenty of paperwork that will be entered into the human resources information system (HRIS). The HRIS is used for recordkeeping, payroll processes, benefits administration, PTO tracking, and performance evaluation rating from which a variety of reports can be generated.

However, onboarding is far more than filling out forms. Onboarding also teaches new employees about the culture of the HCO. This may include explaining workplace policies to employees, such as dress codes or anti-harassment rules, or individualized content, such as job shadowing with a manager and training on job-related computer systems (Hegwer, 2019). Onboarding may also involve team-building exercises that support diversity, equity, and inclusion, as well as trainings that cover the HCO's mission, patient safety standards, patient experience, and employee health and wellness. Long after the initial onboarding, high-performing HCOs will provide on-the-job training for new employees to increase employee retention (Klein et al., 2015).

HUMAN RESOURCES BUSINESS PARTNERS AND HEALTH SERVICES MANAGERS

Human Resources Business Partners

Human resources business partners (HRBPs) are HR experts teamed with health services managers to help them achieve their goals (Ramlall & Melton, 2019). As a partner, HRBPs enable health services managers to act as managers for the employees who report to them. When HR problems occur, HRBPs accept partial responsibility—along with their health services management partners—for solving them. Ideally, HRBPs attend business meetings where the problems are identified and remain as the dedicated HR point of contact until the employee issues are resolved (McCracken, 2017).

As health services managers advance in their careers, they can rely on HR professionals to support their people management practices. While not responsible for managing people—which is the job of managers—HRBPs use their expertise with HR functions and familiarity with the business to act as internal employee champions, trusted business advisors, and creative problem solvers (Storey et al., 2019).

> **INFORMATIONAL INTERVIEW 9.2**
> *Senior Human Resources Business Partner*
> Access the informational interview online at http://connect.springerpub.com/content/book/978-0-8261-4807-0/chapter/ch00.

Employee Relations

An effective HRBP empowers health services managers to make day-to-day workforce decisions and handle interpersonal conflict or employee grievance issues on their own. The HR department is responsible for the development, maintenance, and communication of policies and procedures. These documents provide health services managers with step-by-step guidance on how to solve problems within their business units. Moreover, when health services managers follow guidance of their HRBP, they can avoid costly litigation. Some HR organizational policies and procedures that are important for managing people include the following (Rothwell et al., 2012; Showalter, 2020):

- *Grievance*: A formal complaint filed when an employee is dissatisfied with the financial, social, physical, and emotional aspects of their workplace. In unionized HCOs, grievances are filed when there is a violation of the collective bargaining agreement. HR professionals coordinate investigations and resolutions of grievances.
- *Hostile environment*: Unwelcomed sexual advances, requests for sexual favors, and other verbal or physical harassment of a sexual nature. HR has the responsibility for investigating the issue or identifying a neutral third-party investigator.
- *Mediation*: It is a process required by The Joint Commission accreditation standards where an impartial third-party attempts to resolve disputes and conflicts to avoid escalation into grievances or legal action.
- *Credentialing*: It is a legal requirement in which HCOs verify that a provider is licensed to provide medical services.
- *Negligent hiring*: Legal liability occurs when HCOs engage in negligent hiring in the credentialing review and the clinician harms a patient or another employee.
- *Progressive discipline systems*: It is a method of discipline using graduated steps for addressing employee misconduct or performance issues, increasing in severity from counseling to verbal warnings, written warnings, demotion, suspension, and termination.
- *Performance Improvement Plans (PIPs)*: For employees who need to improve performance, PIPs document job performance goals, identify skill gaps, and set clear expectations for future conduct.
- *Retaliatory discharge*: It is a term used to refer to an employer terminating an employee for something other than work performance reasons, such as filing a complaint about a manager or coworker.

> **△ KEY IDEA**
> Effective HRBPs empower health services managers to handle employee issues on their own.

Human Resources Laws and Regulations

The HRBPs assist health services managers with following laws and regulations related to hiring, paying, and managing people. It would be a mistake, however, to think that the primary role of HR professionals is to keep health services managers out of legal trouble (McCracken, 2017). Ignorance of laws and regulations is not an excuse for noncompliance. Although HR professionals can act as consultants on human capital issues, health services managers are responsible for understanding and following labor laws and regulations, including the following (Rothwell et al., 2012; Showalter, 2020):

- *Age Discrimination in Employment Act of 1967*: Protects applicants and employees 40 years of age and older from discrimination based on age in hiring, promotion, termination, compensation, or other terms of employment
- *Civil Rights Act of 1964*: Established the regulatory body, EEOC, prohibiting discrimination based on race, color, religion, sex, national origin, disability, or age in hiring, promoting, firing, pay, and other terms of employment. It is unlawful to sexually harass anyone at work.
- *Employee Retirement Income Security Act of 1974 (ERISA):* Sets minimum standards for retirement and health plans
- *Equal Pay Act of 1963:* Requires that men and women in the same workplace be given equal pay for equal work, as enforced by the EEOC
- *Fair Labor Standards Act*: Establishes minimum wage and overtime pay standards. Nonexempt employees must be paid at least the federal minimum wage and any overtime must be paid at one and a half times the regular rate of pay over 40 hours per week. Exempt employees are executive, administration, and professional employees who are paid a salary, so overtime regulations do not apply.
- *Family and Medical Leave Act (FMLA)*: Entitles employees to take unpaid, job-protected leave for specified family and medical reasons with continuation of group health insurance coverage. Example reasons include care for a newborn, care for adopted child, or serious health condition of the employee or their family member.
- *Health Insurance Portability and Accountability Act (HIPAA):*Enables employees to continue health insurance coverage after they leave an employer without discriminating against preexisting health conditions (i.e., portability). Privacy and security rules assure confidentiality of health information and protect patients from data breaches.
- **Americans with Disabilities Act** *(ADA):* Ensures that qualified individuals with disabilities have equal rights in employment and have reasonable accommodations for their work environment
- *Occupational Safety and Health Act (OSHA):* Establishes guidelines to help employers create a safe and sanitary working environment, including safety training, reporting, and anti-retaliation protections for employees who report unsafe working conditions
- *Workers' compensation*: State laws require disability pay for employees who are injured on the job.

△ KEY IDEA

Ignorance of laws and regulations is not an excuse for noncompliance. Although HR professionals can act as consultants on human capital issues, health services managers are responsible for understanding and following labor laws and regulations.

Fortunately, health services managers and HR managers are not the only parties who work to assure compliance with HR laws and regulations. In HCOs, the compliance department is responsible for communicating laws and regulations and addressing violations (Showalter, 2020). Historically, the relationship between compliance and HR departments has been reactive, joining together to address a particular legal predicament (Grimm, 2018). Increasingly, though, the collaboration between departments has evolved to proactively avoid legal problems through training programs, hotlines, and compliance audits (Rosen & Thiel, 2022). Successful HR compliance programs support health services managers by providing consistent compliance messaging, reviewing disciplinary actions, and conducting HR-related investigations.

Efforts to prevent HR compliance violations can sometimes be unsuccessful. **Disparate impact**, sometimes referred to as unintentional discrimination, occurs when HR practices appear to be impartial but result in a disproportionate impact on a protected group. For example, artificial intelligence (AI) tools automate the résumé screening process but have been found to cause unfair exclusion of women and underrepresented groups (Ore & Sposato, 2022). One study found that Black and Asian applicants were more than twice as likely to get interviews if they removed elements from their résumés that revealed their race or ethnicity (Kang et al., 2016). Even though AI creates the impression of objectivity, these computer programs are created by humans, who may unintentionally introduce bias into the process to the disadvantage of some applicants. However, HCOs can take a variety of tactics to reduce systematic exclusion of applicants based on racial or ethnic factors, such as revising screening software, removing identifying factors in résumés, and conducting training for HR professionals and hiring managers alike (Gerdeman, 2017; Li, 2020).

Staffing

Day-to-day staffing of employees, including clinicians and support services, is the responsibility of health services managers. Critical to the financial health of the HCO, staffing levels of clinicians are related to patient care outcomes (Aiken et al., 2017). A variety of approaches to staffing can be used, but common methodologies include the following (Griffiths et al., 2020):

- *Fixed:* Determined by clinician hours per patient day or clinician-to-patient ratio, depending on the acuity of the patient care units. For example, an intensive care unit with sicker patients would have a lower patient-to-nurse staffing ratio than a general medical-surgical unit.
- *Acuity based:* Based on a comprehensive assessment of the illness severity of patients and the intensity of care that patients require
- *Skill mix:* Staffing based on number of clinicians, their educational preparation, and their experience working in a clinical setting. For example, on a 12-hour day shift, a care unit could schedule either seven RNs and one LPN or six RNs and two LPNs.
- *Flexible:* Staffing that dynamically responds to changing numbers of patients by employing clinicians with flexible unit assignments (i.e., "float nurses") who are required to work in any unit where needed
- *Capacity*: Staffing based on the predicted number of patients, depending on time-of-day, day-of-week, and seasonal patterns

When the current number of employees or their skill sets are insufficient to accomplish future staffing demands, HCOs may turn to **contingent staffing**, which is the use of temporary employees, part-time employees, independent contractors, and consultants to fill staffing needs. Caution for this approach is necessary, especially when used to fill persistent staffing gaps. **Travel nurses**, a type of contingent staff, can be a very expensive approach to long-term nursing shortages, as their wages can be one and a half to three times higher than permanent nurse wages (Robertson, 2022; Stromstad, 2022).

Workload Forecasting

Staffing schedules are typically based on **workload forecasts**, which involve predicting the number of patients, severity of illness, intensity of care, and provider skill mix required to care for the patients (Tarpey, 2017). Health services managers determine how many clinicians of each skill type should be recruited, hired, and staffed in the department based on the overall annual budget of the department. AIe and machine learning software can use staffing mix and minimum staffing levels to predict the workload forecasts based on prior period patient volumes and severity (The Health Management Academy [HMA], 2023). A staffing matrix, shown in Figure 9.3, indicates the skill mix required to care for a predicted range of patients per day in an acute care unit of a hospital. Effective HRBPs help avoid conflict by advocating for staffing needs with HR executives acting as liaison with other HR departments. In some instances, staff can be better distributed throughout the HCO to increase productivity and create safe staffing levels.

In 2021 workforce challenges displaced financial challenges as the top issue facing healthcare executives (Gooch, 2023). Ninety percent of the CEOs ranked shortages of RNs as the biggest staffing need, followed by shortages of technicians (83%) and burnout among nonphysician staff (80%). A poll found that about 30% of health care workers considered leaving their profession in 2021 (Wan, 2021). This dissatisfaction leads to high employee **turnover rates**, measured as the percentage of workers who leave an organization and are replaced by new employees over a certain time. HRBPs work with health services managers to retain employees. **Retention** efforts, such as creating career growth opportunities, showing appreciation, encouraging self-care, and improving communication with management, are less expensive than hiring replacement employees.

FIGURE 9.3 Nurse staffing matrix for acute care unit.

Patient census	Time	Charge nurse	Register nurse	Certified nurse assistant	Unit assistant (UC)	Total staff
5–6	0700–1930	1	1	1		3
	1900–0730	1	1	1		3
	0700–1530				1	1
	1500–2300				1	1
	Hours worked	24	24	24	16	88

Patient census	Time	Charge nurse	Register nurse	Certified nurse assistant	Unit assistant (UC)	Total staff
7–10	0700–1930	1	2	2		5
	1900–0730	1	2	2		5
	0700–1530				1	1
	1500–2300				1	1
	Hours worked	24	48	48	16	136

Patient census	Time	Charge nurse	Register nurse	Certified nurse assistant	Unit assistant (UC)	Total staff
11–15	0700–1930	1	3	3		7
	1900–0730	1	3	3		7
	0700–1530				1	1
	1500–2300				1	1
	Hours worked	24	72	72	16	184

Performance Evaluations

A **performance evaluation** is a formal process in which a manager assesses the job performance of an employee. Almost all HCOs conduct performance evaluations annually, and many conduct them more often, such as 2 weeks after starting a job and then every 4 or 6 months thereafter (Murphy, 2020). HRBPs work with health services managers to administer performance reviews according to the HCO's policies and practices. Performance evaluations are used for promotions and pay increases. However, not all employees seek to be promoted from the frontlines to supervisor, manager, or executive role. A **career ladder** is one way for clinicians to advance in their careers without losing direct patient contact. Through professional development and education, clinicians can increase their pay and gain more autonomy and responsibility in the practice setting.

Focusing on career growth helps the HCO avoid the concept of the **Peter principle**, in which an employee is promoted based on their performance in the current role rather than on abilities relevant to the position that they are promoted to. For example, clinicians who excel at the bedside may not succeed in management roles, so when promoted, they become ineffective managers. The Peter principle states that high-performing employees are promoted to higher levels of the organizational hierarchy until they reach the point where they can no longer perform well (Peter & Hull, 2011). Once they have risen to the level of incompetence, they stay in that job to the detriment of the organization and employee.

Training and Organizational Development

Health services managers are responsible for making sure that their employees obtain the necessary skills to complete their work effectively. HCOs often centralize training and organizational development functions and deliver mandatory HCO-wide training and development programs, such as patient safety, employee wellness, and harassment prevention. When health services managers have specific needs, HRBPs collaborate with health services managers to develop and deliver training and development programs.

CAREER BOX 9.2: Excelling at Performance Self-Assessments

HCOs commonly require employees to complete annual performance selfassessments, which are unofficial supplements to a manager's official review (Grote, 2011). Even though self-assessments can provide valuable reminders to the manager about strong performance, many people are particularly bad promoting their successes. Acting too humbly is unlikely to advance your career. To excel at performance self-assessments, take the following actions:

- *Track your wins:* Keep a journal of individual and team-based accomplishments, both large and small. If you want to ask for more training, support, or resources, record missed goals and opportunities for improvement.
- *Ask your peers and colleagues:* Others may have insights about your work. Your exceptional performance may not be obvious to you.
- *Review your job description:* Describe your performance relative to the official job responsibilities. Make sure you are doing what you were hired to do.
- *Address the performance standards directly:* Explain how you met or exceeded the criteria that you are being measured against. Give examples.
- *Focus on growth:* State career growth or professional goals you hope to achieve. Request resources to help you accomplish those goals.
- *Ask for the raise or promotion:* Research the pay range for similar positions and request the upper part of that range. If you are ready for a promotion, say so in writing.

There are two categories of education that the HR department provides to HCO employees—functional training and organizational development. **Functional training** focuses on the short-term development of job-related skills and knowledge, whereas **organizational development** is concerned with the long-term growth of the employees through conceptual and general knowledge. Training is intended to increase productivity and improve performance; development seeks to increase employee retention and enhance competitive advantage. Table 9.2 lists examples of functional training and organizational development programs in HCOs.

HR departments ensure that employees develop the needed competencies through effective **training designs** that create training and organizational development programs with sequenced content, detailed schedules, and evaluation plans. Training design frameworks clarify training problems, define instructional objectives, incorporate adult learning principles, and identify effective teaching methods (Carliner, 2015).

HR professionals also develop coaching and mentorship programs to support health services managers and their employees. **Coaching** is the short-term, goal-oriented process in which a coach helps their client set goals and develop plans for improving work performance. For example, coaches can help health services managers with leadership skills, people management, communication skills, or work–life balance. **Mentoring** programs are frequently operated by HR departments to connect high-potential employees with more senior employees to build long-term, mutually beneficial relationships. The more knowledgeable mentor guides and advises their mentee on career-related decisions based on their experiences.

Successful HCOs provide training and development programs focused on compliance with EEOC laws and regulations; cultural competency; and diversity, equity, and inclusion (Upadhyay et al., 2022). Increasingly, HR training and development programs are taking extra steps to address interpersonal and systemic bias within HCOs (Cox, 2022). Health services managers can partner with HR training professionals to create environments in which underrepresented groups can voice their experiences with discrimination and everyone can share their perspectives on diversity, equity, and inclusion. By understanding the experiences of diverse groups of employees—not exclusively but especially those from underrepresented populations—health services managers and HR professionals can create more diversity, equity, and inclusion training programs.

TABLE 9.2 Functional Training and Organizational Development Programs in Health Care Oganizations

FUNCTIONAL TRAINING	ORGANIZATIONAL DEVELOPMENT
Work skills, such as effective use of electronic medical records	Leadership development
Knowledge of laws, regulations, and accreditation standards	Change management strategies
Continuous quality improvement methodologies	Job enrichment or job design
Interpersonal skills	Health and well-being awareness and tactics
Cultural competency and implicit bias	Career laddering for clinicians
Harassment awareness and prevention	Health systems knowledge

> **⚠ KEY IDEA**
>
> Health services managers can partner with HR training professionals to create environments in which underrepresented groups can voice their experiences with discrimination and everyone can share their perspectives on diversity, equity, and inclusion.

Employee Safety and Well-Being

Health services managers are also responsible for assuring the health, well-being, and safety of employees. Hospitals are almost twice as hazardous as the average workplace (Occupational Safety and Health Administration [OSHA], 2020). OSHA and The Joint Commission have regulatory and accreditation provisions that encourage workplace safety, including the following (Joint Commission Resources, 2020):

- *Workplace wellness programs:* Offer free health screenings and provide staff support centers, healthy lifestyle classes, peer support groups, and psychological and spiritual resources.
- *Health and safety training*: Provide training to improve patient handling and reduce workplace hazards, such as bullying and work-related fatigue.
- *Violence prevention:* Create programs that prevent and mitigate verbal and nonverbal threats and intervene in all forms of violence, bullying, and aggression.
- *Safe patient handling programs:* Train staff to reduce and prevent the risk of musculoskeletal injuries as a result of improper patient handling and movement.
- *Fall prevention training:* Carry out measures to prevent slips, trips, falls, and other common causes of injury among health care workers.
- *Hazardous chemicals and blood-borne pathogens training:* Create appropriate measures to protect employees from illness and injury due to hazardous chemicals and blood-borne pathogens.

STRATEGIC HUMAN RESOURCES AND HEALTHCARE EXECUTIVES

Strategic Human Resources Management

At the executive level, the HR function links the workforce to the strategy of the HCO. **Strategic human resource management** (SHRM) is the process of aligning HR strategies and tactics with the organization's overall strategy. SHRM represents a shift from HR as an administrative function to a full strategic partner with equal input into decision-making. The HR department creates value for health services management executives by understanding the composition and skills of the workforce needed to position the HCO for competitive advantage. SHRM is, in many ways, a revolutionary concept that not all HCO executives have embraced (Fried & Fottler, 2015). Nevertheless, HR professionals advocate for SHRM as an effective way to help HCOs achieve business goals by aligning workforce strategies and tactics with overall HCO strategies.

> **INFORMATIONAL INTERVIEW 9.3**
>
> *Vice President, Human Resources*
> Access the informational interview online at http://connect.springerpub.com/content/book/978-0-8261-4807-0/chapter/ch00.

Workforce Planning

SHRM connects HR management activities to business strategy. More than ever before, healthcare HR is utilizing data to plan future human capital needs. Data include population-level demographics, public health trends, and community-specific healthcare utilization. Workforce analytics seeks to predict staffing levels to meet patient demand and to make decisions about HCO strategy. Several distinct steps need to be taken in health services workforce planning:

- *Demand forecasting:* Review future business plans and create workload forecasts based on the prior period's patient volumes, severity, and employee skill mix.
- *Supply analysis:* Analyze the current labor supply and skills.
- *Gap analysis:* Examine the differences in the workforce supply and demand forecasts.
- *Solution:* Meet strategic needs by increasing efficiency, improving productivity, recruiting, training and development, contingent staffing, outsourcing, and changing compensation and benefits structures.

Moreover, HR collects data throughout the employment processes, using onboarding surveys, engagement surveys, and exit interviews, all of which are combined to model workforce solutions. Along with electronic health records and population-level data, these HR data are combined in AI and machine learning applications to predict staffing needs, recommend staffing models, and support HR workforce planning decisions (HMA, 2023).

Unions and Collective Bargaining

Health services management executives, in collaboration with senior HR managers, design and are responsible for labor relations. The National Labor Relations Act gives workers the right to form unions that can negotiate with HCO management for better pay and safer working conditions. This negotiation process is known as **collective bargaining**. Some states have "right-to-work" laws that guarantee that no individual can be forced to join a union. Nevertheless, 20% of RNs and 10% of LPNs belong to a union, compared to a national average of 13% across other professions (Bureau for Labor Statistics [BLS], 2022). Unions offer employees job security, but if a strike is held to protest unfair labor practices, then all members must stop working without pay or benefits.

If an HCO has a unionized workforce, then health services managers and HR executives will be responsible for negotiating with the **bargaining unit**, which is the group of employees represented by a union. Unions can negotiate numerous matters, but there are certain **mandatory bargaining issues**, such as wages; hours of work; pensions; bonuses; insurance; grievance procedures; safety practices; seniority; and procedures for discharge, layoffs, and discipline (National Labor Relations Board [NLRB], 1997). Negotiations determine the extent to which health services management executives can implement HCO policy without approval from the union, called the **management rights clause**. This union contract language generally states that managers can direct employees, evaluate performance, discipline and discharge for just cause, and establish standards of performance for employees, just as long as their action falls within the scope of a bargained-for management rights. Management and unions may also negotiate alternative dispute resolution procedures that allow the parties to resolve issues through **arbitration**, a service in which a neutral party helps settle differences outside the court system.

The lack of dignity and respect—not wages and benefits—are what motivate employees to unionize (Morse, 2015). Health services managers can avoid unionization by assuring safe working conditions, respectful treatment of employees, and responsiveness to criticisms of management. If employees elect to form a union, then HCO executives can expect to work with the union for the long term, as decertification of a union is rare.

> **△ KEY IDEA**
> The lack of dignity and respect—not wages and benefits—are what motivate employees to unionize.

Physician Recruitment and Retention

Demand for physician services will likely outpace the supply due to the aging population and innovations in treatment, making the shortage of physicians worse over the next 10 years, especially in many rural areas (Zhang et al., 2020). Succeeding in this competitive landscape depends on investments in physician recruitment and retention programs (Fried & Fottler, 2015). HCOs hire specialized teams, such as physician recruiters, recruiting firms, and physician liaisons, and build attractive compensation and benefits packages to recruit and retain physicians.

Health services managers coordinate with marketing staff to highlight the positive aspects of the HCOs community physician candidates. Compelling marketing materials underscore organizational values, highlight community features, and assist in attracting and recruiting physicians who will fit the culture, whether it is an urban, suburban, or rural setting. Recruiting materials and pitches should also consider community assets that meet the specific needs and interests of physician recruits, which may include assisting with a spouse's job search or information about local schools. Vacation time, flexible on-call schedules, work-life balance, and other benefits may attract and retain the right physicians. Generous signing bonuses, income guarantees, or loans for repaying medical school debt in exchange for staying with the HCO are also common approaches to physician recruitment and retention. Other physician recruitment and retention incentives include reward and recognition systems, innovation teams, and wellness programs.

Succession Planning

High-level HR professionals also support HCO executives with succession planning, which is the process by which high-performing employees are identified to fill top-level positions when needed. Current and potential future vacancies and employee readiness can be tracked using **replacement charts**, a tool commonly used in succession planning for executives. Health services managers identify high-potential employees in the HCO and work with HR professionals to evaluate their readiness to ascend to the next level of responsibility. A succession plan can help foster employee commitment because it demonstrates to employees that the organization supports their development and internal growth (SHRM, 2017). Figure 9.4 shows an example replacement chart.

Organizational Culture

Health services management executives are responsible for creating organizational cultures that enhance competitive advantage and improve patient outcomes. SHRM practices facilitate organizational culture improvement, including the following:

- Conducting organizational climate surveys to identify opportunities to enhance the work environment
- Creating policies that define what the organization considers proper workplace behavior, including bullying or incivility prohibitions

FIGURE 9.4 Personnel replacement chart.

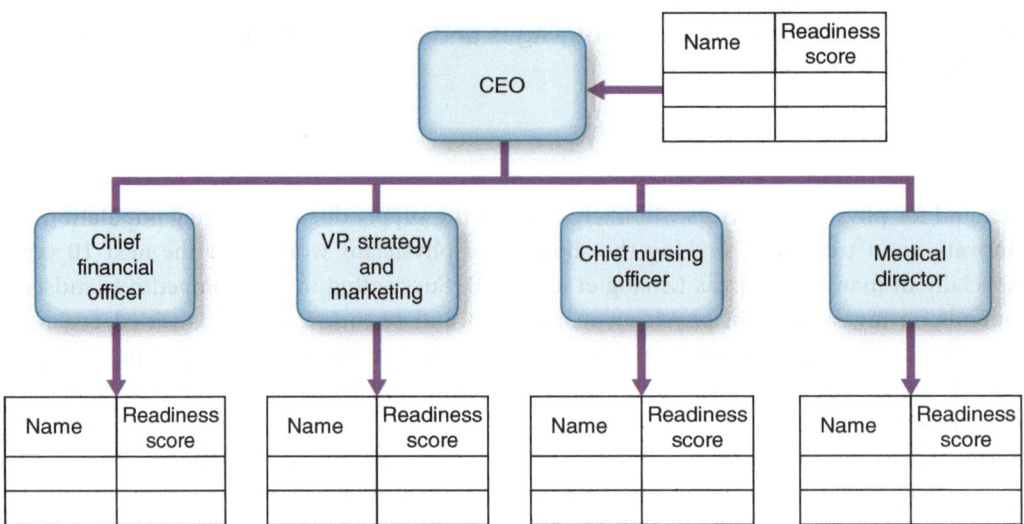

- Developing education and development programs designed to enhance culture, such as cultural competence training
- Encouraging employees to observe, report, and fix errors or problems that place patient, visitor, or staff safety in jeopardy
- Devising performance evaluation programs that set clear expectations, encourage valuable feedback, and hold employees accountable for upholding HCO values

Moreover, improved employee **engagement** can help health services managers and HR professionals create cultures that embrace diversity, equity, and inclusion principles. Engagement is the emotional and intellectual commitment toward a person's work and the organization, resulting in improved employee satisfaction, decreased turnover, and increased productivity (Saks, 2006). When climate surveys reveal employee perceptions of exclusion, SHRM practices can engage team members as a way to promote inclusivity, such as providing team members with a process to voice their concerns, forming and funding inclusivity councils, and celebrating employee differences (Gurchiek, 2018). Through purposeful SHRM practices, engagement can lead to increased diversity, equity, and inclusion (Battle, 2022).

FUTURE DIRECTIONS

After decades of being perceived as a necessary administrative cost, HR professionals have emerged as strategic partners to health services managers. Strategic HR is an innovative, future-oriented function intended to solve business problems through workforce expertise. However, the full capabilities of the HR function have not been universally adopted across the healthcare industry. Staffing shortages, already severe, will become even more challenging for HCOs, and the remaining staff will be asked to do more with less, causing stress, burnout, and unsafe patient care. To respond to tomorrow's healthcare workforce challenges, health services managers will need to maximize the expertise of the HR function to rethink hiring practices, redesign work, train a new kind of workforce, and enhance the well-being of people who care for others.

SUMMARY

- The HR department supports health services managers in recruiting, hiring, onboarding, and training employees.
- HR professionals ensure that hiring managers comply with antidiscrimination laws and regulations, such as asking personal questions about national origin, age, marital status, religion, disabilities, and criminal record.
- HR recruiters negotiate with job candidates within each position's predetermined salary band. Wise job seekers research salary ranges for positions at similar organizations.
- HRBPs assist with employee relations, legal and regulatory compliance, and performance evaluations.
- Effective workforce planning and workload forecasting can help reduce the need for expensive contingent staff.
- Centralized HR professionals deliver mandatory HCO-wide training and development programs. Coaching and mentorship help health services managers manage themselves and their careers so that they can effectively manage others.
- Health services managers and HR professionals collaborate to identify high-potential employees, evaluate their readiness for promotion, and develop succession plans and replacement charts to assure business continuity when employees leave their positions.
- Strategic HR management is the process of aligning HR strategies and tactics with the organization's overall strategy to meet HCO business objectives.

END-OF-CHAPTER RESOURCES

KEY TERMS*

*For the full list of key terms, please see the online glossary at **http://connect.springerpub.com/content/book/978-0-8261-4807-0**.

Age Discrimination in Employment Act
Americans with Disabilities Act
arbitration
bargaining unit
behavioral interviews
career ladder
Civil Rights Act
coaching
collective bargaining
compensation philosophy
contingent staffing
credentialing
defined contribution plan
disparate impact
engagement
Equal Employment Opportunity Commission
Fair Labor Standards Act

Family and Medical Leave Act
flexible spending account
functional training
grievance
halo effect
Health Insurance Portability and Accountability Act (HIPAA)
hostile environment
human resources business partner
management rights clause
mandatory bargaining issues
mediation
mentoring
negligent hiring
Occupational Safety and Health (OSH) Act
organizational development
pay equity

performance improvement plans
person–job fit
person–organization fit
Peter principle
progressive discipline system
qualified retirement plan
realistic job preview
reasonable accommodation
replacement charts
retaliatory discharge
retention
salary band
selection tools
sexual harassment
short-term disability insurance
situational interview
strategic human resources management
structured interview
training design
travel nurses
turnover rate
workers compensation
workload forecasts

LEARNING ACTIVITIES

Professional Development and Reflection

1. Write a performance self-evaluation for a position that you have recently held using a combination of unstructured and rating scale methods. Assesses your job performance using a rating scale for the qualities required for the job, such as reliability, dependability, and leadership. Be sure to list your achievements, goals, opportunities for improvement. Depending on your corporate culture and your boss's needs, you might consider developing a PowerPoint presentation to share.
2. Identify a position description in an online job posting for which you are at least somewhat qualified. Write or edit your résumé using keywords and phrases from the position description that will pass the prescreening stage of application review.

Discussion Questions

1. Reflect on how the chapter describes the early careerist's interactions with human resources during the hiring process. Based on your experiences, do you agree with this perception? Do you think human resources functions are facilitators or impediments to early career advancement?
2. Discuss the concept of disparate impact in human resources practices. Do you think automated résumé screening using AI is ethical? How can AI tools inadvertently introduce bias, and what impact does this have on applicants, especially from underrepresented groups?
3. Discuss the inclusivity practices of the human resources function in HCOs, such as providing a process for voicing concerns, forming inclusivity councils, and celebrating employee differences. How can these practices contribute to a more inclusive organizational culture?

RECOMMENDED READING AND MEDIA

Burnison, G. (2018). *Lose the résumé: Land the job*. John Wiley & Sons, Inc.

Cox, G. (2022). *Leading inclusion: Drive change your employees can see and feel*. Page Two.

Friedman, L. H., & Kovner, A. R. (2018). *101 careers in healthcare management* (2nd ed.). Springer Publishing Company.

Jotform. (2022, February 9). *How to conduct a performance appraisal* [Video]. YouTube. https://www.youtube.com/watch?v=6RcYCS-W4ow

Rosen, M., & Thiel, D. [ProviderTrust]. (2022, February 24). Bridging the compliance & HR gap: Drive operational efficiency in a shifting regulatory world [Video]. YouTube. https://www.youtube.com/watch?v=ymIAhKUxVxI

Sutton, R. I. (2010). *The no asshole rule: Building a civilized workplace and surviving one that isn't*. Business Plus.

Tinline, G., & Cooper, C. (2016). *The outstanding middle manager: How to be a healthy, happy, high-performing mid-level manager*. Kogan Page.

Wilkinson, B. (2021). *The diversity gap: Where good intentions meet true cultural change*. HarperCollins Leadership.

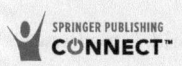

A robust set of instructor resources designed to supplement this text is located at http://connect.springerpub.com/content/book/978-0-8261-4807-0. Qualifying instructors may request access by emailing textbook@springerpub.com.

REFERENCES

Adler, L. (2016). *New survey reveals 85% of all jobs are filled via networking*. LinkedIn.com https://www.linkedin.com/pulse/new-survey-reveals-85-all-jobs-filled-via-networking-lou-adler

Aiken, L. H., Cimiotti, J. P., & Lake, E. T. (2017). Association of nurse work environment and safety climate on patient mortality: A cross-sectional study. *International Journal of Nursing Studies, 74*, 155–161. https://doi.org/10.1016/j.ijnurstu.2017.06.004

Akasa. (2021, January 26). *Recruitment costs, long hiring timelines negatively impact healthcare finance teams*. https://akasa.com/press/staffing-challenges-within-the-healthcare-revenue-cycle

Apen, L. V., Rosenblum, R., Solvason, N., & Chan, G. K. (2021). Nursing academic leadership: An urgent workforce shortage in nursing education. *Nursing Education Perspectives, 42*(5), 304–309. https://doi.org/10.1097/01.nep.0000000000000851

Battle, B. (2022). DEI in the healthcare workforce: Advancing equity systemwide to improve service, care, and innovation. *Journal of Healthcare Management, 67*(4), 230–233. https://doi.org/10.1097/jhm-d-22-00105

Baur, J. E., Buckley, M. R., Bagdasarov, Z., & Dharmasiri, A. S. (2014). A historical approach to realistic job previews: An exploration into their origins, evolution, and recommendations for the future. *Journal of Management History, 20*(2), 200–223.

Birt, J., Herrity, J., & Esparza, E. (2023, March 3). *How to negotiate your salary during economic uncertainty*. Indeed Career Coaches. https://www.indeed.com/career-advice/pay-salary/salary-negotiation-economic-uncertainty

Bonica, M. J., & Hartman, C. (2018). Managing up and followership: Competencies for first-year health administrators. *Journal of Health Administration Education, 35*(3), 327–352.

Buerhaus, P. I. (2021). Current nursing shortages could have long-lasting consequences: Time to change our present course. *Nursing Economics, 39*(5), 247–250.

Bureau for Labor Statistics. (2021). *Occupational outlook handbook: Medical and health services managers*. U.S. Department of Labor. https://www.bls.gov/ooh/management/medical-and-health-services-managers.htm

Bureau for Labor Statistics. (2022). *Union members - 2022*. U.S. Department of Labor. https://www.bls.gov/news.release/pdf/union2.pdf

Burmahl, B. (2022, March 17). *Worker shortages hit health care facilities teams*. Health Facilities Management. https://www.hfmmagazine.com/articles/4406-worker-shortages-hit-health-care-facilities-teams

Burnison, G. (2018). *Lose the résumé: Land the job.* John Wiley & Sons, Inc.

Carliner, S. (2015). *Training design basics.* Association for Talent Development Press.

Chmiel, N., Fraccaroli, F., & Sverke, M. (2017). An Introduction to work and organizational psychology: An international perspective (3rd ed.). Wiley-Blackwell.

Cimiotti, J. P., Li, Y., Sloane, D. M., Barnes, H., Brom, H. M., & Aiken, L. H. (2019). Regulation of the nurse practitioner workforce: Implications for care across settings. *Journal of Nursing Regulation, 10*(2), 31–37. https://doi.org/10.1016/s2155-8256(19)30113-9

Claxton, G., Rae, M., Damico, A., Wager, E., Young, G., & Whitmore, H. (2022). Health benefits in 2022: Premiums remain steady, many employers report limited provider networks for behavioral health. *Health Affairs, 41*(11), 1670–1680. https://doi.org/10.1377/hlthaff.2022.01139

Cox, G. (2022). *Leading inclusion: Drive change your employees can see and feel.* Page Two.

Curhan, J. R., Overbeck, J. R., Cho, Y., Zhang, T., & Yang, Y. (2021). Silence is golden: Extended silence, deliberative mindset, and value creation in negotiation. *Journal of Applied Psychology, 107*(1), 78–94. https://psycnet.apa.org/doi/10.1037/apl0000877

Development Dimensions International, Inc. (2023). *What's the STAR method?* DDI World. https://www.ddiworld.com/solutions/behavioral-interviewing/star-method

Drucker, P. (1954). *The Practice of Management.* Harper & Row, Publishers, Inc.

Fried, B. J., & Fottler, M. D. (2015). *Human resources in healthcare: Managing for success* (4th ed.). Health Administration Press.

Gerdeman, D. (2017, May 17). *Minorities who 'Whiten' Job Résumés get more interviews.* Harvard Business School Working Knowledge. https://hbswk.hbs.edu/item/minorities-who-whiten-job-résumés-get-more-interviews

Gingerelli, A., & Mulhern, W. (2021, April 12). *The future of the certified nursing assistant workforce in Massachusetts.* Project on Workforce. https://www.pw.hks.harvard.edu/post/the-future-of-the-cna

Gooch, K. (2023, February 13). The No. 1 problem keeping hospital CEOs up at night. Becker's *Hospital Review.* https://www.beckershospitalreview.com/hospital-management-administration/the-no-1-problem-keeping-hospital-ceos-up-at-night.html

Griffiths, P., Saville, C., Ball, J., Jones, J., Pattison, N., Monks, T., & Safer Nursing Care Study Group. (2020). Nursing workload, nurse staffing methodologies and tools: A systematic scoping review and discussion. *International Journal of Nursing Studies, 103*, 103487. https://doi.org/10.1016/j.ijnurstu.2019.103487

Grimm, D. A. (2018). Compliance: An ounce of prevention is worth a pound of cure. *Frontiers of Health Services Management, 34*(4), 32–41. https://doi.org/10.1097/hap.0000000000000035

Grote, D. (2011). *How to be good at performance appraisals.* Harvard Business Review Press.

Gurchiek, K. (2018, March 19). *6 steps for building an inclusive workplace.* SHRM. https://www.shrm.org/hr-today/news/hr-magazine/0418/pages/6-steps-for-building-an-inclusive-workplace.aspx

Hegwer, L. R. (2019). Retaining your most valued resource. *Healthcare Executive, 34*(1), 20–28.

IHS Markit. (2021). *The complexities of physician supply and demand: Projections from 2019 to 2034.* Association of American Medical Colleges.

Internal Revenue Service. (2023). *Employer's tax guide to fringe benefits.* U.S. Department of Treasury Internal Revenue Service. https://www.irs.gov/pub/irs-pdf/p15b.pdf

Johnson, S. K., Hekman, D. R., & Chan, E. T. (2016, April 26). If there's only one woman in your candidate pool, there's statistically no chance she'll be hired. *Harvard Business Review.* https://hbr.org/2016/04/if-theres-only-one-woman-in-your-candidate-pool-theres-statistically-no-chance-shell-be-hired

Joint Commission Resources. (2022). *OSHA alliance resources.* https://www.jcrinc.com/about-us/osha-alliance/osha-alliance-resources

Kang, S. K., DeCelles, K. A., Tilcsik, A., & Jun, S. (2016). Whitened résumés: Race and self-presentation in the labor market. *Administrative Science Quarterly, 61*(3), 469–502. https://doi.org/10.1177/0001839216639577

Kayser, A. (2022, October 20). 85% of health facilities short on allied health workers. *Becker's Hospital Review*. https://www.beckershospitalreview.com/workforce/85-of-health-facilities-short-on-allied-health-workers.html

Klein, H. J., Polin, B., & Leigh Sutton, K. (2015). Specific onboarding practices for the socialization of new employees. *International Journal of Selection and Assessment, 23*(3), 263–283. https://doi.org/10.1111/ijsa.12113

Kristof-Brown, A. L., Zimmerman, R. D., & Johnson, E. C. (2005). Consequences of individuals' fit at work: A meta-analysis of person–job, person–organization, person–group, and person–supervisor fit. *Personnel Psychology, 58*(2), 281–342. https://doi.org/10.1111/j.1744-6570.2005.00672.x

Leavy-Detrick, D. (2012, March). *Behind the scenes in HR: What's taking so long to hear back?* http://aspyresolutions.com/2012/03/behind-the-scenes-hr/

Levashina, J., Hartwell, C. J., Morgeson, F. P., & Campion, M. A. (2014). The structured employment interview: Narrative and quantitative review of the research literature. *Personnel Psychology, 67*(1), 241–293. https://doi.org/10.1111/peps.12052

Li, M. (2020, October 26). To build less-biased AI, hire a more-diverse team. *Harvard Business Review*. https://hbr.org/2020/10/to-build-less-biased-ai-hire-a-more-diverse-team

Lu, D. J., King, B., Sandler, H. M., Tarbell, N. J., Kamrava, M., & Atkins, K. M. (2021). Paid parental leave policies among US news & world report 2020–2021 best hospitals and best hospitals for cancer. *JAMA Network Open, 4*(5), e218518. https://doi.org/10.1001/jamanetworkopen.2021.8518

Maaravi, Y., & Segal, S. (2022). Reconsider what your MBA negotiation course taught you: The possible adverse effects of high salary requests. *Journal of Vocational Behavior, 139*, 103803. https://doi.org/10.1016/j.jvb.2022.103803

McCracken, M., O'Kane, P., Brown, T. C., & McCrory, M. (2017). Human resource business partner lifecycle model: Exploring how the relationship between HRBPs and their line manager partners evolves. *Human Resource Management Journal, 27*(1), 58–74. https://doi.org/10.1111/1748-8583.12125

Medical Economics. (2021, December 31). *Top challenges of 2022, No. 1: Hiring and retaining staff*. Medical Economics Journal. https://www.medicaleconomics.com/view/top-challenges-of-2022-no-1-hiring-and-retaining-staff

Morse, S. (2015, July 9). As unions grow, healthcare execs need to know how to handle them. *Healthcare Finance*. https://www.healthcarefinancenews.com/news/unions-grow-healthcare-execs-need-know-how-handle-them

Murphy, K. R. (2020). Performance evaluation will not die, but it should. *Human Resource Management Journal, 30*(1), 13–31. https://doi.org/10.1111/1748-8583.12259

Nashville Health Care Council. (May 01, 2022). *How healthcare leaders can support DEI initiatives and improve health equity*. Modern Healthcare. https://www.modernhealthcare.com/ethics/how-healthcare-leaders-can-support-dei-initiatives-and-improve-health-equity

National Labor Relations Board. (1997). *Basic guide to the national labor relations act*. https://www.nlrb.gov/sites/default/files/attachments/basic-page/node-3024/basicguide.pdf

National Women's Law Center. (2023, January). Salary range transparency reduces gender wage gaps. National Women's Law Center Fact Sheet. https://nwlc.org/wp-content/uploads/2022/09/Salary-Transparency-FS-1.13.23.pdf

Occupational Safety and Health Administration. (2020). *Worker safety in hospitals*. https://www.osha.gov/hospitals

Ore, O., & Sposato, M. (2022). Opportunities and risks of artificial intelligence in recruitment and selection. *International Journal of Organizational Analysis, 30*(6), 1771–1782. https://doi.org/10.1108/IJOA-07-2020-2291

Paiewonsky, A., & Westhead, M. (2023, January 30). *The state of the clinical workforce*. The Advisory Board. https://www.advisory.com/topics/health-care-workforce/2023/01/state-of-the-clinical-workforce

Parker, S. K., Andrei, D. M., & Van den Broeck, A. (2019a). Poor work design begets poor work design: Capacity and willingness antecedents of individual work design behavior. *Journal of Applied Psychology, 104*(7), 907–928. https://psycnet.apa.org/doi/10.1037/apl0000383

Parker, S. K., Andrei, D. M., & Van den Broeck, A. (2019b, June 12). *Why managers design jobs to be more boring than they need to be.* SHRM. https://www.shrm.org/resourcesandtools/hr-topics/organizational-and-employee-development/pages/why-managers-design-jobs-to-be-more-boring-than-they-need-to-be.aspx

Peter, L. J., & Hull, R. (2011). *The Peter principle: Why things always go wrong.* Harper Business.

Ramlall, S., & Melton, B. (2019). The role and priorities of the human resource management function: Perspectives of HR professionals, line managers, and senior executives. *International Journal of Human Resource Studies, 9*(2), 9–27. https://doi.org/10.5296/ijhrs.v9i2.14492

Robertson, M. (2022, December 15). Average nurse pay vs. travel nurse pay for all 50 states. *Becker's Hospital Review.* https://www.beckershospitalreview.com/compensation-issues/travel-nurse-vs-rn-pay-gap-for-all-50-states.html

Rothwell, W. J., Prescott, R. K., Lindholm, J., Yarrish, K. K., Zaballero, A. G., & Benscoter, G. M. (2012). *The encyclopedia of human resource management.* Pfeiffer.

Saks, A. M. (2006). Antecedents and consequences of employee engagement. *Journal of Managerial Psychology, 21*(7), 600–619. https:/doi.org/10.1108/02683940610690169

Sans, N. (2019, Dec 5). 10 recruiter strategies to improve diversity and inclusion in hiring. *Forbes.* https://www.forbes.com/sites/forbesbusinesscouncil/2019/12/05/10-recruiter-strategies-to-improve-diversity-and-inclusion-in-hiring

Showalter, J. S. (2020). *The law of healthcare administration* (9th ed.). Health Administration Press.

Society for Human Resource Management. (2015). *How to develop a job description. How-To Guides.* https://www.shrm.org/resourcesandtools/tools-and-samples/how-to-guides/pages/developajobdescription.aspx

Society for Human Resource Management. (2017). *Society for Human Resource Management (SHRM) resources & tools: Practicing the discipline of workforce planning.* https://www.shrm.org/resourcesandtools/tools-and-samples/toolkits/pages/practicingworkforceplanning.aspx

Storey, J., Ulrich, D., & Wright, P. M. (2019). *Strategic human resource management: A research overview.* Routledge.

Stromstad, D. (2022). Moving past business as usual to meet future hospital staffing needs. *Frontiers of Health Services Management, 38*(4), 4–8. https://doi.org/10.1097/hap.0000000000000143

Tarpey, R. J. (2017). Human interaction management impact on hospital labor planning. *Muma Business Review, 1*(11), 125–139. https://doi.org/10.28945/3847

The Health Management Academy. (2023, March 15). *Survey by the health management academy reveals accelerating use of AI to overcome workforce challenges* [Press release]. https://www.businesswire.com/news/home/20230314005243/en/Survey-by-The-Health-Management-Academy-Reveals-Accelerating-Use-of-AI-to-Overcome-Workforce-Challenges

Upadhyay, S., Weech-Maldonado, R., & Opoku-Agyeman, W. (2022). Hospital cultural competency leadership and training is associated with better financial performance. *Journal of Healthcare Management, 67*(3), 149–161. https://doi.org/10.1097/jhm-d-20-00351

Wan, William. (2021, April 22). Burned out by the pandemic, 3 in 10 health-care workers consider leaving the profession. *Washington Post.* https://www.washingtonpost.com/health/2021/04/22/health-workers-covid-quit/

Zhang, X., Lin, D., Pforsich, H., & Lin, V. W. (2020). Physician workforce in the United States of America: Forecasting nationwide shortages. *Human Resources for Health, 18*(1), 8. https://doi.org/10.1186/s12960-020-0448-3

CHAPTER 10

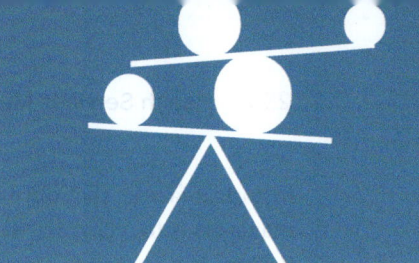

ORGANIZATIONAL DESIGN

Organizational design is the process of defining work, arranging people according to responsibilities, assigning decision-making authority, and coordinating work among staff.

COMPETENCIES

- Apply organizational design concepts to improve performance.
- Assess advantages and disadvantages of various organizational designs.
- Utilize formal and informal decision-making structures to accomplish goals.
- Integrate clinical professionals and nonclinical staff with goals of the organization.
- Build effective collaborations across the continuum of care.
- Understand how organizational structure impacts patient care and experience.
- Establish and coordinate external supplier services.
- Examine interdependence, integration, and competition of external organizations.

CHAPTER OUTLINE

- Defining the Work
- Assigning the Work
- Coordinating the Work
- Expanding the Organization
- Extending the Organization

INTRODUCTION

Organizational design is the process of arranging people according to their work responsibilities, delegating decision-making authority, establishing workflows, and coordinating work among and within the units of the organization. Managers ask questions about the structure of work. What needs to get done? How do we divide up the work? Who reports to whom? Who makes decisions? Answering to these questions is organizational design. Managers define the work, assign tasks to the right people, and coordinate the work among units and teams. Health services managers design roles and relationships with the goal of improved organizational performance.

Organizational design can be forward-looking, thoughtful, methodical, and theory based. In this way, organizational design is consistent with the classical managerial theory of the manager who plans, organizes, directs, coordinates, and controls people and processes (Fayol, 1916). However, designing organizational structures from the beginning rarely happens in healthcare. Health services managers often inherit existing organizational structures that have evolved from vague historical factors that once addressed patient needs. Therefore, the challenge for health services managers is to recognize when circumstances require new ways of thinking about organizational design. Health services managers must constantly consider restructuring the organization to meet the current patient needs and to respond to the external competitive environment.

This chapterdescribes how health services managers (1) divide tasks among different workers, (2) organize people to get the work done, and (3) coordinate the work among people and across the organization. This chapter also reviews organizational structures of larger and more complex health care organizations (HCOs).

DEFINING THE WORK

Standardized Work

When designing the organizational structure, health services managers must first define what needs to get accomplished to achieve shared goals. Breaking up the work into discrete, repeatable tasks and subtasks is called **standardized work**. The work standardization concept was first articulated by the "father of scientific management," Frederick W. Taylor, who famously conducted time-and-motion studies in the early 20th century (Kanigel, 2005). Taylorism focused on dividing up tasks to create the most efficient process possible, a management innovation that was later applied to manufacturing in Henry Ford's automobile assembly line (Ford & Crowther, 1926). Later, Taylorism was criticized for how dividing up work into smaller, less meaningful tasks could sap people of their motivation (Huang et al., 2013).

Standard Operating Procedures

Standard operating procedures (SOPs), also known as policies and procedures (P&Ps), functional protocols, best practices, work instructions, or checklists, serve to document standardized work practices. The SOPs are written to set clear expectations for nonclinical and clinical operational functions. Nonclinical SOPs include hiring new employees, purchasing supplies, billing insurance companies, maintenance of facilities, and the like. In addition to nonclinical SOPs, patient care functions also require SOPs, sometimes called functional protocols (White & Griffith, 2019). SOPs are used to secure consistency in staff performance, eliminate errors, and avoid confusion about assigned tasks.

> △ **KEY IDEA**
>
> **SOPs are used to secure consistency in staff performance, eliminate errors, and avoid confusion about assigned tasks.**

Certain health care-related processes are routine and repetitive and warrant standardization (Rousseau, 2020). For example, the World Health Organization (WHO) developed a 19-item Surgical Safety Checklist that outlines the mandatory steps in preparing a patient for surgery (WHO, 2008). The checklists are explicit reminders to clinicians to complete the minimum necessary tasks—the standardized work practices—before surgery, such as the patient confirming their identity, surgical site, procedure, and consent (Gawande, 2009). Health services managers work in partnership with the surgical team to develop and adopt the checklist and implement the process as best practice.

In collaboration with nurses, health services managers define SOPs related to nursing processes. Once such SOP includes purposeful hourly rounding at set intervals can improve patient safety (Ryan et al., 2019). Nurses on the patient care unit should use professional judgment regarding how to follow the SOPs in place, depending on each patient's circumstances (Cleveland Clinic, 2018). For instance, if a patient is sleeping, a nurse could simply check on the patient instead of conducting a detailed health assessment.

> △ **KEY IDEA**
>
> A nurse on the patient care unit should be empowered to use professional judgment about how to follow the SOPs, depending on the patient's circumstances.

Health services managers also create SOPs to standardize the work of less routine practices, such as disaster preparation and response. For example, mass casualty emergencies can overwhelm ill-prepared trauma centers. To prevent the mistakes and misunderstandings that can occur under stressful situations, health services managers work to define logistical procedures in advance. Such mass casualty SOPs include designing an intensive care unit overflow space, mobilizing blood banks, and adopting shortened patient registration forms (Einav, et al., 2014; Gates, et al., 2014; Sánchez, & Sánchez, 2020). These tasks are put in place by health services managers before the mass casualty event so that well-trained clinicians can respond effectively (Gawande, 2013).

Clinical Protocols

Health services managers also collaborate with clinical professionals to define tasks associated with direct patient care (Begun et al., 2011). For example, the health services manager can provide resources (e.g., time, money, training, or support staff) for clinicians to develop and document standard clinical procedures. These science-based rules are known as a variety of names, such as clinical protocols, standards of practice, integrated care pathways, clinical practice guidelines, patient management protocols, or interdisciplinary plans of care (Campbell et al., 1998; Field & Lohr, 1990; White & Griffith, 2019). Healthcare is not a one-size-fits-all endeavor. Therefore, clinicians are authorized to depart from clinical protocols when patient circumstances dictate (White & Griffith, 2019). Table 10.1 lists the terms used for different clinical and nonclinical types of standardized work documentation.

TABLE 10.1 Terms Used for Different Types of Standardized Work Documentation

NONCLINICAL	CLINICAL
Best practices	Clinical practice guidelines
Checklists	Clinical protocols
Policies and procedures	Interdisciplinary plans of care
Functional protocols	Integrated care pathways
Standard operating procedures	Patient management protocols
Work instructions	Standards of practice

ASSIGNING THE WORK

Division of Labor

The idea of creating collections of specialized teams of workers has been around since the 18th century and is commonly used today (Smith, 2002). According to classical organization design theory, efficiencies are created when workers are organized by their areas of expertise and directed by a top manager. When a manager assigns a set of tasks to a separate person or group of persons, it is called **division of labor**. The assignment of collections of similar tasks to one individual or position creates areas of expertise, such as finance, marketing, or operations, called **specialization**. In organizational theory, the process of organizing task assignments to groups of people by specialization is called **departmentalization** (Galbraith, 1977).

Departmentalization creates a **functional structure**, which can be illustrated in an **organizational chart** that shows the links between and among top managers, **middle management**, and staff. Figure 10.1 shows the executive team for a fictional hospital with the board of directors at the top of the organization. The functional organizational structure creates a pyramid shape, with one boss at the top and many workers at the bottom. The hierarchical layout denotes the **chain of command**, with each worker lower on the chart reporting to a single person higher up on the chart. Separate organizational charts can be created for each of the functional areas, such as finance, operations, and clinical support services.

Authority and Responsibility

Organizational charts reflect two important concepts—authority and responsibility. **Authority** refers to the ability to compel workers to act, while **responsibility** means accepting accountability for a work commitment. The assignment of responsibility by a person with authority is called

FIGURE 10.1 Functional organizational chart.

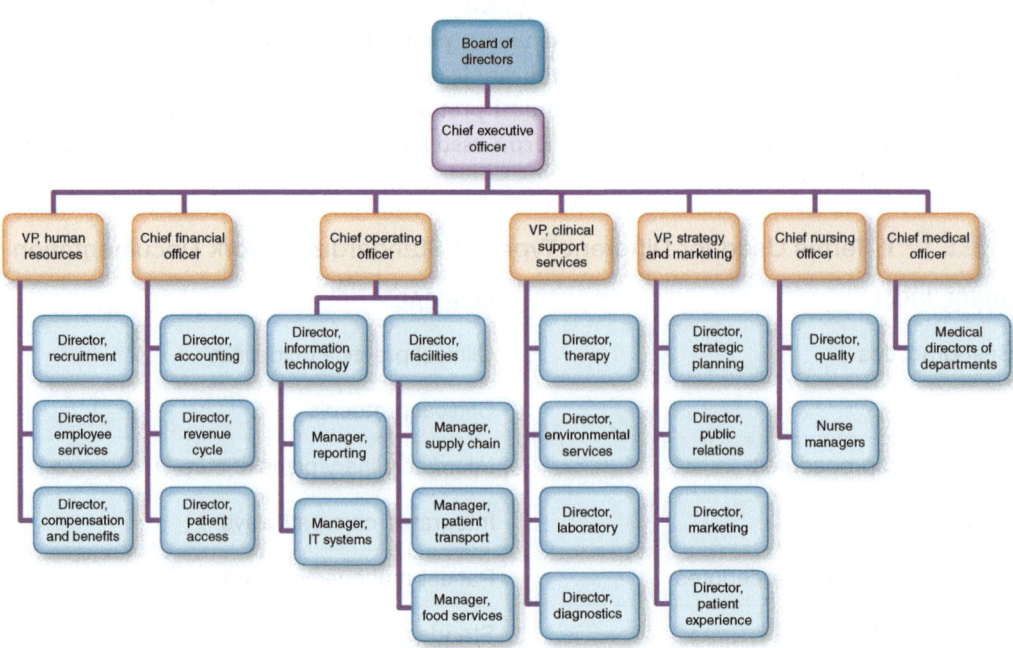

delegation. As shown in Figure 10.1, the board of directors has the ultimate authority and delegates operational authority and responsibility to the CEO. Among the managers, the CEO has the most authority and responsibility. In the functional organization, the CEO then delegates responsibility and authority to different parts of the organization, according to their functional expertise. The boss delegates responsibilities down the line of authority, and the individual accepts responsibility for the work. This top-down delegation of authority and responsibility is called the **line of authority** or **chain of command**.

> △ **KEY IDEA**
>
> The board of directors has the ultimate authority and delegates operational authority and responsibility to the CEO.

Organizational design specifies how, where, and by whom authority is given for decisions (Fredrickson, 1986). Highly prescribed roles and responsibility tend to lead to formalized rules and procedures for completing tasks and making decisions (Baker et al., 1999). The delegating manager defines the decision-making processes. This includes telling the employee to "decide, but ask before acting" or "act, then tell the result." For example, the CEO delegates responsibility to the CFO for financial matters. The CEO and CFO meet on a regular basis to review performance according to the established goals. In certain instances, the CEO will authorize the CFO to make decisions and act; for important financial matters, the CEO may insist on making the decisions. This same process occurs down the hierarchy, with the CFO delegating responsibility for accounting tasks to the director of accounting and so on.

In functional organizational design, only recognized experts with authority and responsibility can make decisions about how to perform certain tasks, a term called **functional authority**. Highly formalized decision-making processes discourage managers outside of the functional department from making decisions for which they do not have authority. For example, the human resources department is ultimately responsible for hiring employees in an HCO. Even though the health services manager may be responsible for the budget and strategic execution of a particular business, they may not be able to hire employees without human resources decision-making oversight. Ideally, managers collaborate with human resources specialists to perform certain tasks (e.g., hire employees) and make decisions about how to accomplish goals (e.g., set salary levels).

> **CAREER BOX 10.1: Responsibility and Authority in Entry-Level Jobs**
>
> Health services management careers do not start in the management ranks but rather in lower level positions with job titles like representative, specialist, coordinator, project manager, or analyst. Early careerists usually perform basic administrative tasks typical of entry-level positions in other industries, such as documenting, processing, tracking, retrieving, and assisting. Even at lower positions in the hierarchy, health services managers can be responsible for independent decision-making under stressful conditions. Successful early careerists are willing to accept responsibility for tasks without authority to make decisions or delegate work. Entry-level jobs undeniably prepare career-minded administrators to take on more responsibility and to make the right decisions without direct oversight from people with higher levels of authority.

Figure 10.1 shows that seven senior managers report to the CEO. The vice president of human resources only has three direct reports, and the vice president of clinical support services has four direct reports. While only fictional, the illustration presents the ratio of workers for each manager, a concept called **span of control**. When bosses need to closely monitor their workers, a narrow span of control is ideal. When there are multiple levels of management in the hierarchy and managers have a narrow span of control, it is called a **tall organizational structure**. Figure 10.2 shows three layers of management (director, manager, and supervisor) and one level of worker (staff). In this representation, the director has two direct reports, each manager has three direct reports, and each supervisor has three subordinates. Decisions get made more slowly in tall organizations because they need to make their way through "proper channels" to gain approval (Drucker, 1954).

When workers require less oversight from their boss, a wide span of control is ideal. A wide span of control is seen in a **flat organizational structure** where there are fewer layers of management. This organizational structure is used when managers have less time for direct oversight, thus empowering the staff to take on responsibility for tasks, work independently, and solve problems collaboratively. As shown in Figure 10.3, bosses have many direct reports. In the flat structure, decisions can be made quickly. However, wide spans of control can overwhelm supervisors, and subordinates may feel ignored by their supervisor. Many HCOs design a flat organization where physician managers in HCOs possess wide spans of control because of their substantial professional independence (Mintzberg, 1981).

FIGURE 10.2 Tall organizational structure.

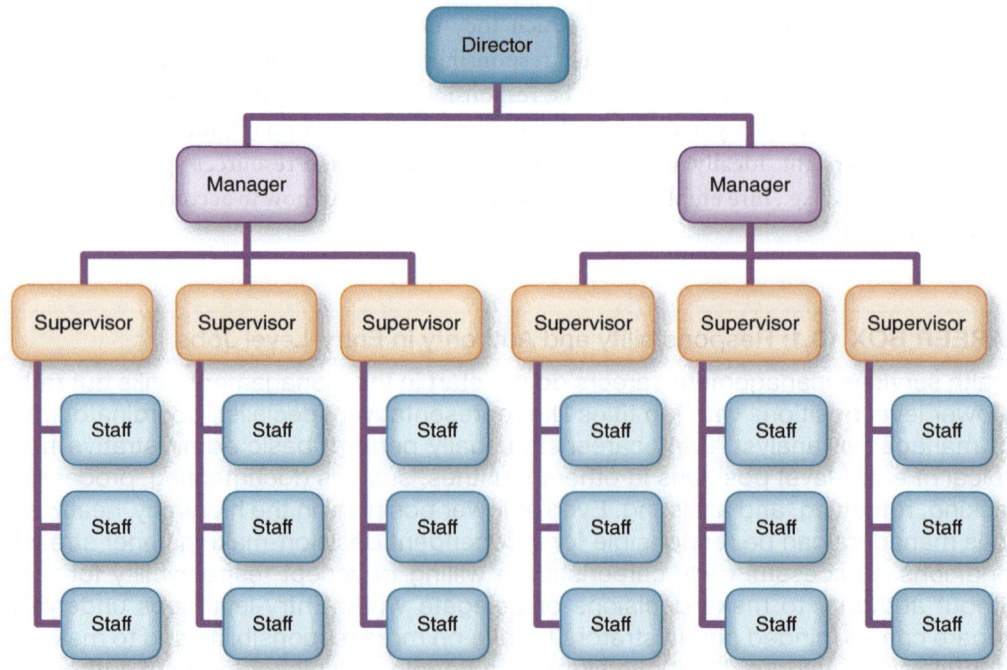

FIGURE 10.3 Flat organization.

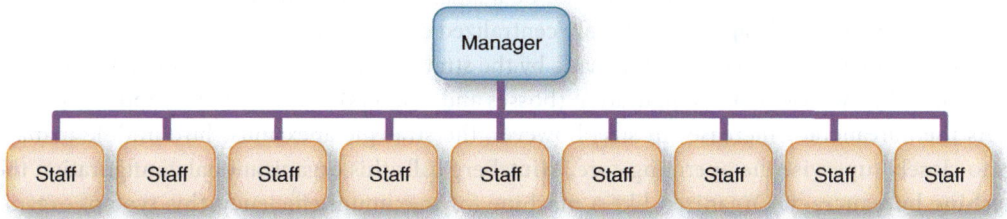

The Professional Bureaucracy

The term **bureaucracy** was first used by 20th-century sociologist and political economist Max Weber (1947) to describe an organization that is arranged in a hierarchal fashion with formal lines of authority and responsibility. Most bureaucracies give bosses the authority to assign responsibilities to workers who report to them. Healthcare is different, though. The frontline workers of healthcare—doctors, nurses, pharmacists, respiratory therapists, physical therapists, and others—are more likely to follow their profession's rules and state laws than any directive issued by health services managers. Therefore, health services delivery is a special kind of bureaucracy called a **professional bureaucracy** (Mintzberg, 1981).

To understand what makes the structure of the HCO unique, it is helpful to first understand the basics of theorist Henry Mintzberg's organizational framework (Mintzberg, 1983). As depicted in Figure 10.4, there are five basic parts:

- Strategic apex (e.g., senior managers and the board of directors)
- Middle management (e.g., managers between the CEO and workers)
- Technostructure (e.g., strategy planners and quality improvement specialists)
- Support staff (e.g., human resources and compliance)
- Operating core (e.g., frontline workers)

FIGURE 10.4 Mintzberg's organizational framework.

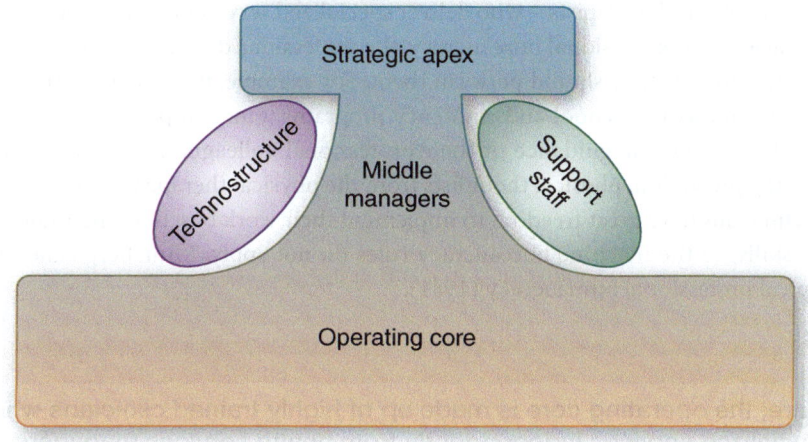

Source: Adapted from Mintzberg, H. (1981). *Organization design: Fashion or fit?* Harvard Business Press.

Mintzberg uses these five basic parts to describe a variety of archetypal organizational structures. For example, the simple structure can be a small entrepreneurial company where senior managers of the **strategic apex** exert highly centralized control over frontline staff of the **operating core**. In other words, decisions are made by the strategic apex and implemented by the operating core. This two-element configuration (bosses and workers) is swift, nimble, and innovative.

As the bureaucracy increases in size, however, the strategic apex must hire middle managers to closely supervise the operating core. Mintzberg calls this organizational configuration the **machine bureaucracy**. Organized like a machine for maximum efficiency, this type of organizational structure evolved from the industrial revolution when manufacturers demanded that low-skilled workers perform repetitive tasks. In machine bureaucracy, various layers of managers are needed to standardize and control the work that is delegated in a top-down manner through the ranks of middle managers (i.e., the tall organizational structure). The machine bureaucracy tends to respond slowly to change, giving the term "bureaucracy" a negative connotation today.

INFORMATIONAL INTERVIEW 10.1
Integration Project Manager
Access the informational interview online at http://connect.springerpub.com/content/book/978-0-8261-4807-0/chapter/ch00.

As an organization grows even more, the strategic apex adds more specialized workers, called the technostructure and support staff, to further support the operating structure. The **technostructure** includes technical experts who plan and control the work of the operating core, such as human resources, information technology, compliance, accounting, strategic planning, and quality management. The technostructure does not generate any revenue but only formalizes the work of the operating core by creating standardized processes. The **support staff** provides indirect services, such as customer service, patient registration, facility maintenance, patient transportation, environmental services, supply chain, and food services. In Figure 10.4, the technostructure and support staff elements are placed outside the operating core because they do not provide direct services to customers.

In healthcare, the operating core is made up of highly trained clinicians—physicians, nurses, pharmacists, and physical therapists—who deliver specialized services independently from health services managers. In a professional bureaucracy, the professions determine what tasks clinicians should perform and how they should perform them. For example, physicians learn how to practice medicine from medical school and residency programs. Once in practice, they follow state medical board rules and the guidance of their professional colleagues. Nurses follow guidance from the nursing profession, physical therapists from the physical therapist profession, and so on. In practice, clinicians have great freedom to implement their work based on their knowledge and professional skills, so the machine bureaucracy rules do not apply. Mintzberg called healthcare the prototypical professional bureaucracy (1981).

△ KEY IDEA

In healthcare, the operating core is made up of highly trained clinicians who deliver specialized services independently from health services managers. In a professional bureaucracy, the professions determine what tasks clinicians should perform and how they should perform them.

> **CAREER BOX 10.2:** Staff and Line Positions
>
> From an organizational design perspective, positions of health services management can be categorized as line or staff positions. In Mintzberg's (1981) terminology, health services manager staff positions are jobs in the technostructure and administrative support staff. These specialized jobs are responsible for extensive work processes that support frontline clinical professionals. In common business terms, jobs in both technostructure and support staff structures are just called **staff positions** (Burns et al., 2019). Staff position functions include human resources, finance, business planning and development, supply chain management, marketing, strategic planning, and patient experience. Job promotions in staff positions can include supervisor, manager, director, vice president, and so on.
>
> In contrast, some health services management jobs are called **line positions.** In Mintzberg's organizational model, line positions are the middle managers who oversee the operating core and are responsible for the financial profits (or losses) of the business unit. Early careerists often start in staff positions (e.g., analyst) and can be promoted to a line position with additional authority running smaller businesses, such as hospital departments, medical specialty physician office (i.e., surgery, pathology, or pediatrics), or medical clinics, and other organizational units (e.g., home health). Examples of mid-career line position titles include administrator, practice manager, service line manager, program manager, or operations manager. Jobs of this kind can also be promoted to directors, vice presidents, and so on.

Physicians often retain organizational autonomy over hospital administrators, in addition to professional autonomy. Only a minority of physicians (about 40% in 2020) are employed directly by a hospital (American Medical Association, 2021). In the case of independent medical practices, the physicians themselves are the owners, and health services managers are hired to run their business while they practice medicine. Even though managers have organizational authority and responsibility, their initiatives may fail because physicians ignore, resist, or reject their decisions. The best way to integrate physicians into the decision-making structures of HCOs has been a challenge for many decades (Starr, 1982).

Dyad Models of Authority and Responsibility

To improve physician integration with organizational goals and improve operations, HCOs' health services managers increasingly include physicians in authority structures. When the organization creates a **dyad model**, the operations executive and physician executive share authority and responsibility for organizational decision-making and performance. This arrangement is very common in medical group practices and increasingly common in hospitals (Comstock, 2019; Trandel, 2015). Through dyad partnerships, health services managers expand their awareness of day-to-day medical practice issues, and physician leaders gain insight into operational issues. The dyad model of shared authority and responsibility can occur throughout the hierarchy of the organization, from the executive level to the department or unit level.

At the executive level, dyad partners report to a board of directors or the group of physician owners, who hold the responsibility for dividing tasks between the executive manager and the executive physician (Yates, 2021). Health services managers are typically responsible for operations, finance, human resources, supply chain, facilities, and performance management; physician managers are responsible for clinical standards of practice, clinical quality, provider productivity, and referring provider relations. Both the physician and manager share responsibility and authority for strategy and overall performance (Zismer et al., 2010). Table 10.2 presents the division of labor in a management-clinician executive dyad model.

The dyad model divides the responsibilities and maximizes the authority of business managers and clinical managers. Unfortunately, shared responsibility and authority can lead to potential conflicts in decision-making processes (Yates, 2021). Nonetheless, due to the complexity of healthcare and the need to gain physician buy-in for effective operational implementation, the dyad partnership can be viewed as a necessary structure to achieve organizational goals (Young, 2017).

Alternatives to the Functional Structure

While functional organizational design is most common in healthcare, there are various alternatives. Consider Stanford Health Care Cancer Center's streamlined patient registration function design (Dapelo-Garcia, 2015). Originally, Stanford Health Care organized outpatient cancer services in the functional organizational design. Patients who received multiple oncology services on the same day had to register for each service, such as chemotherapy infusion, laboratory testing, and a physician visit, all of which had different scheduling and billing requirements. To improve the patient experience, Stanford Health Care streamlined the organizational design to allow patients to register, pay, and schedule multiple services through a single point of contact.

Another modification to the functional structure is called **adhocracy**. The term ad hoc literally means "to this" but translates as something like "for this specific purpose." Mintzberg (1981) used the term adhocracy to describe the type of organizational unit created when the bureaucratic structure would be too slow or inflexible. Under the authority of the senior managers, ad hoc project teams—also called performance improvement teams, tiger teams, self-directed teams, or task forces—are charged with fixing a specific problem with a creative solution (Dunn, 2021; White & Griffith, 2019; McBeth et al., 2021). Ad hoc project teams are comprised of a variety of experts throughout the organization, including project managers and implementation experts, and are ideally provided budgets and clear goals (Waterman, 1990).

TABLE 10.2 Division of Labor in a Dyad Model of Authority and Responsibility

MANAGEMENT EXECUTIVE	DYAD	CLINICIAN EXECUTIVE
Financial management	Mission, vision, values	Clinical quality
Human resources management	Clinical, patient service, and business goal setting	Physician recruiting
Competition and market share	Organizational culture	Clinical supply chain (e.g., surgical and devices)
Community relations	Overall clinical and business performance	Clinical protocol development and implementation
Promotion of evidence-based management practices	Organizational design	Promotion of evidence-based medicine practices

For example, the Mayo Clinic in Rochester, Minnesota, created a task force to solve the personal protective equipment (PPE) shortage during the COVID-19 pandemic (Francis, 2020). The team was comprised of supply chain specialists, engineering experts, and clinical advisors tasked with sourcing a critical supply of surgical masks, respirators, gowns, welder-style face shields, glasses, and goggles. The structure of the PPE task force enabled more informal, agile decision-making processes. The PPE task force quickly developed pandemic-related protocols, redesigned distribution processes, and identified supply sources to significantly increase the availability of PPE.

COORDINATING THE WORK

Coordinating Health Services

When creating organizational structures, health services managers create "systems of coordinated action" to accomplish organizational goals (Chandler, 1962; March & Simon, 1993, p. 2). How managers achieve coordination (who works on what and how they go about it) determines the structure of the organization (Mintzberg, 1981). Effective coordination of administrative roles and health professions across functional structures can enhance HCO performance. Ineffective coordination can lead to inefficiencies, conflict, and patient harm.

INFORMATIONAL INTERVIEW 10.2
Vice President, Service Lines
Access the informational interview online at http://connect.springerpub.com/content/book/978-0-8261-4807-0/chapter/ch00.

A variety of approaches to coordination can occur in a large HCO, depending on the type of work. For minimally complex administrative work, health services managers can give directives to workers and closely supervise their performance, though healthcare rarely features that kind of work. More common in the HCO, health services managers need to standardize administrative tasks, such as patient check-in procedures, patient scheduling rules, and billing processes. As the tasks get more complex, additional layers of management and specialists are added to coordinate the work within and among units. Health services managers also coordinate the actions of the support staff who assist clinical professionals. This includes managers supporting clinical performance through recruiting and hiring clinical support personnel and administrative support functions, such as patient registration and billing.

Clarifying Health Services Roles

Health services managers clarify clinical and nonclinical roles and responsibilities in HCOs. Due to the ever-changing nature of healthcare, tasks assigned to a particular role can unofficially transfer from one person to another. Sometimes, role expansion means effective use of worker capabilities that are appropriate to the circumstance and consistent with the organizational goals (Hoff, 2019). Other times, however, tasks migrate from one role to another without justification, often leading to misalignment and ineffectiveness.

Health services managers assess the extent to which all roles support organizational goals (Pruitt et al., 2018). For example, the patient navigator position has been created in many HCOs to support patients as they obtain care from different parts of the health system. These nonclinical navigators—also known as liaisons or care guides—can be beneficial in many contexts. Cleveland Clinic previously had patient navigators who helped with nonclinical tasks that made clinicians' jobs of caring for patients easier (Merlino, 2015). However, navigators were often given unnecessary tasks that did not meaningfully improve patients' experiences, according to their systematic study. The Cleveland Clinic health services managers discontinued that navigator program because it did not help reach their patient experience improvement goals.

When ambiguous and overlapping, job roles can cause conflict among workers. For example, APRNs and physicians often disagree about the expanding clinical responsibilities of APRNs. Despite changes in some state laws that permit APRNs to conduct some patient care tasks without physician oversight, APRNs are sometimes prevented from performing essential patient care procedures unless under medical doctor supervision (Kleinpell et al., 2022). Scope of practice expansion can lead to contentious discussions among clinician groups, as each profession cherishes its autonomy. Such interprofessional conflict requires health services managers to bring the clinical professionals together to identify the capabilities of each role, coordinate tasks accordingly, and mediate disagreements across clinical professions about roles, resolving any lingering disagreements (Begun et al., 2011).

> ### △ KEY IDEA
> When roles are ambiguous and overlapping, conflict among workers can occur. It is the job of the health services managers to mediate disagreements across clinical professions about roles and to resolve any lingering disagreements.

Coordinating Processes and Structures

In hospitals and outpatient physician practices, clinical services are typically organized around physician specialty (surgery, endocrinology, and others). When a patient needs treatment for a condition that requires many different specialists, the patient is often forced to travel from one doctor to the next, repeating their medical history and symptoms, sometimes with their printed medical records in hand. This functional organizational design in healthcare leads to what is known as "fragmentation." **Fragmented care** refers to when services are obtained across many providers, making coordination difficult and causing many problems, such as wasted time, repeated tests, confused patients, misaligned resources, and medical errors (Stange, 2009).

To solve fragmentation, health services managers attempt to improve coordination between different organizational units. For example, patient discharges from the hospital are fraught with process missteps and miscommunications. Poorly executed discharges can result in admissions again soon after patients leave the hospital. Also, when there are delays in sending patients home from the hospital, patients cannot be admitted, and crowding occurs in the emergency department (Franklin et al., 2020).

Some health services managers have created new organizational designs that accelerate discharge processes. Managers at WellStar Kennestone Regional Medical Center in Georgia created a new care unit called a "discharge lounge" (Franklin et al., 2020). Staffed with registered nurses, a care coordinator, and a pharmacy team member, the discharge lounge allows patients to wait for transportation, prescriptions, durable medical equipment, or other needs without occupying a hospital bed. Nurses repeat discharge instructions, care coordinators confirm follow-up appointments and arrange transportation, and pharmacy team members ensure prescription delivery. In addition to improving patient throughput, WellStar Kennestone decreased inpatient readmissions following the implementation of the discharge lounge.

Outpatient care also serves more as a collection of different medical specialties than a fully integrated cooperative system of care. To solve this kind of fragmentation, some health services managers design organizational structures where all relevant providers occupy one physical space, forming a patient-oriented facility of clustered clinical experts. For example, a specialized diabetes outpatient treatment and education center features a multidisciplinary team of endocrinologists, ophthalmologists, certified diabetes educators, nutrition specialists, nurse practitioners, laboratory testing specialists, physician assistants, and pharmacists. Patients at diabetes centers receive their integrated diabetes care under one roof. This organizational design better coordinates care and results in improved health outcomes and reduced total costs (Bratcher & Bello, 2011).

EXPANDING THE ORGANIZATION

Divisionalized Organizations

The organizational design concepts presented so far have applied to a single organizational entity, such as the hospital or physician practice. However, more complex businesses offering multiple products or services may create **divisionalized** forms of the functional organizational structure. These divisions are businesses coordinated by a common administrative corporate headquarters. In healthcare, divisions typically focus on specific service or customer types, such as hospitals, ambulatory surgery centers, urgent care centers, skilled nursing facilities, home health services, and medical groups, or by geography, such as regions of the marketplace.

In the divisionalized form, health systems designate managers with authority and responsibility for each specific operating unit. That means each division runs as a separate business with its own hierarchical structure (CEO, CFO, and others), as described in Figure 10.1. Each unit in the health system is led by a senior manager who is responsible for a separate budget, performance results, and profits. Mintzberg (1981) called these divisional bosses the middle line managers, as distinguished from the strategic apex managers at the corporate headquarters.

Divisional managers oversee their respective divisions but must report to their bosses at the corporate headquarters. Though many decisions are left up to division managers, the corporate headquarters still formally retains the right to make some decisions, a distinction called **reserved powers**. Executives higher up in the corporate organization hold authority over all division managers' decisions, and depending on the relationship between them, an informal review takes place on decisions (Baker et al., 1999). That means divisional managers who make questionable choices can see their decisions overturned by their corporate bosses. Even if unfavorable decisions are made and implemented by divisions, poor performance can result in decision reversal (and firing of the divisional manager).

Centralized and Decentralized Organizations

Despite having authority over all decisions—explicitly or implicitly—the top corporate managers rarely wield total control over division managers. Therefore, top managers at the corporate office establish organizational structures that maintain control over the divisional managers. Multi-organizational structure relationships between corporate headquarters and the divisions range from relatively independent to highly dependent.

The most independent form of a division is called a **strategic business unit,** where a unique business implements a different type of strategy than that of the corporate business. In healthcare, an example of a strategic business unit might be a real estate division that leases office space and manages properties. On the other hand, a **decentralized** organization is when division managers follow the corporate strategy but independently make decisions depending on local circumstances. The performance of division managers is tracked by corporate headquarters on a regular basis (e.g., quarterly) to decide if they agree with certain important decisions made by division managers. The corporate headquarters reserves the right to retract certain decisions, as necessary.

Top managers at the corporate level may prefer to maintain more control over divisions by reserving decision-making power and standardizing functions at a central location (Mintzberg, 1981). In the **centralized** organizational structure, higher level managers make the decisions, including about which operational functions to control. A common scenario for centralized structures in healthcare occurs in multi-hospital systems that has a corporate headquarters and separate local hospitals. These health systems emerged in the late 1980s to mid-1990s to create efficiencies in purchasing and power in negotiations with payers (Heeringa et al., 2020). For example, Hospital Corporation of America (HCA) Healthcare, an investor-owned multi-hospital health system with locations throughout the world, centralizes many functions, such as the supply chain (i.e., purchasing and distributing supplies) and revenue cycle (i.e., payer contracting and billing) within separate corporate divisions (HCA Healthcare, 2023).

In the simple reporting structure, everyone reports to only one boss or **unity of command**, guaranteeing that workers will not be taking orders from different people. However, some divisionalized organizations establish **matrix structures**, a kind of hybrid decision-making configuration where divisional employees report to more than one boss—one from corporate and one from division. In large medical group practices, for example, a practice manager can report to both the managing physician at the local office and the chief operating officer (COO) at the headquarters. In a multi-hospital health system, the local hospital's vice president of finance can report to both the local hospital's CEO and the CFO of the corporate headquarters. While preferred by top managers at the corporate office because they can maintain consistent standards across divisions, the matrix reporting structures can create problems of unclear or duplicate instructions from multiple bosses. To address this issue, health services managers document the responsibilities of employees who have multiple supervisors to help assess the workload of the employee, prioritize tasks, and assure accountability.

Service Line Structures

While the functional organizational structure is an efficient way to organize people, managers must devote significant time to coordinating the work among the units as well. Healthcare viewed across various types of services or places of care is called the **continuum of care**. For example, the continuum of care for pregnancy care might include reproductive health care, prenatal care, childbirth care, and postnatal care. A patient can also move through the continuum of care settings. From this perspective, the continuum of care can include outpatient primary care, diagnostics, outpatient specialist care, inpatient acute care, post-acute rehabilitation, home care, and long-term care. Even for services as common as pregnancy care, health services managers must work diligently to coordinate health services delivery across the fragmented continuum of care.

INFORMATIONAL INTERVIEW 10.3

Chief Transformation and Service Line Officer

Access the informational interview online at http://connect.springerpub.com/content/book/978-0-8261-4807-0/chapter/ch00.

U.S. healthcare policy makers are attempting to remedy problems associated with the fragmented continuum of care. Health care payers, such as Medicare, are moving away from paying HCOs for the volume of services they provide and, instead, are choosing to pay based on high-quality care for less expense through new value-based purchasing schemes. Value-based purchasing represents a significant shift in financing policy that requires HCOs to reorganize around **service line** organizational structures that group patients with similar medical needs together, sometimes called a **center of excellence** (Louis et al., 2019). Service lines centralize the work and resources for addressing a particular medical condition at a single physical site (Elrod & Fortenberry, 2017). The service line structure creates services for patients with a common diagnosis using synchronized care processes, common management teams, and aligned incentives.

Using orthopedic services as an example, Medicare pays a single fee (a lump sum of money) for an entire hip replacement episode of care—from diagnostics to surgery to physical rehabilitation—to encourage coordinated services across the continuum of care (CMS, 2021). Before the move to value-based purchasing, HCOs would separate hospital-based orthopedics care from the ambulatory care center and the rehabilitation center. Individuals with hip joint problems would seek care from a surgeon first without the benefit of alleviating pain through rehabilitation. From the surgery department's perspective, hip replacement surgery may represent good business and effective patient care. However, from the patient's perspective, rehab might have been enough care to fix the problem without the risk of surgery. From Medicare's perspective, hip surgery would be viewed as a waste of money. As such, Medicare no longer pays a different fee for the hospital and the outpatient surgery center. Instead, Medicare pays one fee and leaves it to the hospital to determine the best setting for care.

Banner Health, a multi-hospital system based in Phoenix, Arizona, restructured their organization across many regions and services to account for value-based payment models (Fine & Kuhlenbeck, 2021). The corporate managers combined multiple functional organizations, including the hospital, ambulatory surgery centers, outpatient rehabilitation, post-acute care, and other orthopedic-related settings (Lutz et al., 2021). This new orthopedic service line aligned finances, tracked performance metrics, and placed responsibility and authority for profit and loss of the service line under one divisional manager. Figure 10.5 describes this service line structure across the orthopedics continuum of care.

FIGURE 10.5 Service line organizational structure.

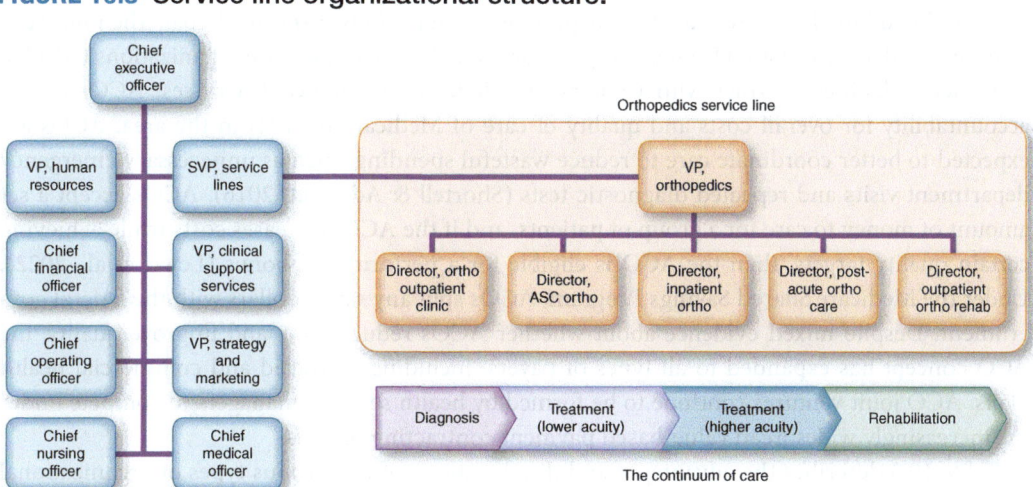

> **△ KEY IDEA**
> All types of payers are moving toward value-based payments to incentivize HCOs to control spending, optimize care coordination, and improve quality. HCOs are responding with service line organizational structures.

Coordinated Divisional Structures

Healthcare payment reforms and competitive pressures have motivated the establishment of other forms of coordinated **divisional structures**, such as integrated delivery systems and accountable care organizations (Lewis et al., 2022). When many different divisions across the continuum of care are highly connected, the health systems are known as **integrated delivery systems**. As with service line structures, the drive to create integrated delivery systems is the response to competitive pressures with other HCOs, as well as the need for improved negotiating power with insurance companies and the push for improved coordination of care imposed by value-based payments (Lewis et al., 2022; Shortell et al., 1996).

Integrated delivery systems are structured to promote coordination between various hospitals, medical groups, skilled nursing care, and health plans with a corporate headquarters at the top. Top managers of these very large multidivisional healthcare corporations use various mechanisms to integrate the organizations, including governance structures, strategic planning, ownership ties, contractual relationships, information and communication technologies, common SOPs, and centralized administrative functions (Heeringa et al., 2020). The most tightly integrated delivery systems combine financing (i.e., health plans), inpatient services, physician groups, and a collaborative network of providers, such as post-acute care providers and behavioral health. Top corporate managers coordinate the performance of both provider side (hospitals and clinics) and payer side (health plans) to reduce overall costs and increase financial stability for the entire integrated delivery system (Walberer, 2017).

In addition, the Patient Protection and Affordable Care Act of 2010 (ACA) created a new value-based payment arrangement, called the Medicare Shared Savings Program, to encourage HCOs to better coordinate care (Huang et al., 2023). Participating organizations create formal partnerships between hospitals, physicians, long-term care, and other providers that deliver services across the continuum of care. Medicare requires HCOs to create a type of business arrangement called a **joint venture** that has common ownership, official governance and management structures, and combined resources for the purpose of accomplishing a specified goal. The joint ventures in the Medicare Shared Savings Program are called accountable care organizations (ACOs).

Under a distinct contract with Centers for Medicare & Medicaid Services, ACOs accept accountability for overall costs and quality of care of Medicare patients in the area. ACOs are expected to better coordinate care to reduce wasteful spending, such as unnecessary emergency department visits and repeated diagnostic tests (Shortell & Addicott, 2016). ACOs accept a set amount of money to care for a group of patients, and if the ACO decreases costs while achieving certain quality targets, then the ACO is eligible for a performance bonus (Lewis et al., 2022). Under the Medicare Shared Savings Program, ACOs split any saved dollars with the federal government. Despite mixed evidence about whether ACOs reduce costs and improve quality, the ACO concept has expanded to all types of payers, including Medicaid and commercial health plans. ACO joint ventures continue to be formed by health services managers to compete under the increasingly widespread value-based payment contracting models.

Table 10.3 describes the advantages and disadvantages of the various types of organizational structures discussed in this chapter.

TABLE 10.3 Advantages and Disadvantages of Types of Organizational Structures

STRUCTURE	ADVANTAGES	DISADVANTAGES
Functional	Efficiency, productivity, accountability, and clarity of roles and responsibilities	Fragmentation, poor communication, difficult coordination across units, lack of overall organizational perspective
Divisionalized	Diversity of products and services; enables geographic growth	Duplication of functions among headquarters and divisions
Matrixed	Alignment across organizational units	Reporting confusion, unclear roles, lack of accountability
Centralized	Clear authority for decision-making, standardization of tasks	Slow and inflexible decision-making
Decentralized	Responsive to local environment	Conflicting perspectives among divisions, inefficient functions
Dyad model	Divides responsibilities based on strengths and expertise of coleaders; integrates clinical perspective in organizational decisions	Slows decision-making process with potential conflict and lengthy deliberations
Service line	Improves coordination across continuum of care; aligns with value-based payment incentives	Requires authority sharing across medical specialties and settings
Joint venture	Gain access to expertise; share risks and costs	Difficult to mix differing cultures and management styles

EXTENDING THE ORGANIZATION

Organizational Affiliations and Alliances

HCOs can create other types of partnerships that are designed to improve coordination among organizational structures. **Affiliations** and **alliances**, terms often used interchangeably, operate through voluntary collaboration rather than hierarchical control, and each entity maintains its own governance structure and financial independence (Alexander et al., 2015). Affiliation and alliance relationships can expand the capabilities and meet specific business needs but allow each HCO to remain independent business entities. Nevertheless, these structures can be effective at extending the coordination of the work outside the organization.

For example, care transitions—the movement of a patient from one setting of care to another—can be a challenging organizational design problem for health services managers to solve. Patient discharges from the hospital to post-acute care services (skilled nursing, home health, rehabilitation, and others) are particularly fraught with delays and mistakes. While health services managers sometimes develop these post-acute care businesses as a corporate division, they often prefer to establish affiliate relationships (Hogan et al., 2019). If a hospital is affiliated with a post-acute care organization, they may be able to solve the discharge coordination problems without spending additional money.

Outsourcing to Suppliers

Health services managers can also **outsource**, an alternative form of organizational design in which managers purchase work from outside firms. Typically, outsourcing occurs when the work does not require a high degree of coordination between entities. Health services managers outsource to external organizations because these organizations have specialized expertise that makes it less expensive than operating the service in-house. A variety of services are commonly outsourced in healthcare, including information technology, housekeeping/environmental services, laundry, food and concessions, patient transport, laboratory operation, and medical facilities management (Berry et al., 2021). If health services managers can maintain oversight of the outsourced services, then they can realize reduced costs and improved quality for their organization.

> **△ KEY IDEA**
>
> **If health services managers can maintain oversight of the outsourced services, then they can realize reduced costs and improved quality for their organization.**

To outsource services, health services managers follow similar steps as the design of the internal organization; they define the work, contract the work, and coordinate the work. Work is typically defined in a request for proposal (RFP), which documents the requirements for formal bids from external suppliers. Once qualified third parties have responded to the RFP, health services managers use standard criteria to evaluate potential suppliers, set contract terms, establish performance expectations, and manage vendor relationships (O'Connor, 2015). The full cost of outsourcing should be considered when deciding to contract with external suppliers, including costs associated with maintaining vendor relationships and coordinating the services with internal operations.

For example, health services managers usually outsource some portion of supply chain systems. The healthcare supply chain is a complex system of purchasing, receiving, controlling, distributing, and paying for all supplies and equipment (O'Connor, 2015). HCOs commonly outsource at least some of the supply chain to **group purchasing organizations** (GPOs), which act as cooperatives of many HCOs that negotiate and purchase supplies at discounted rates from manufacturers and distributors (Burns, 2022). For example, instead of purchasing directly from a medical device company, the HCO would rely on the outsourced services from the GPO to manage the procurement process, including evaluation of the product quality and negotiation of the contract terms. Outsourcing to GPOs can substantially reduce costs and improve the quality of supplies acquired by the HCO.

However, the cost savings benefits of outsourcing may not always outweigh the loss of control over the work. Health services managers may prefer to contract with external management companies who are responsible for recruiting, hiring, and managing emergency department physicians. When health services managers outsource clinical care, they risk losing control over clinical quality and may jeopardize the HCO's reputation, due to weakened employee morale and lack of confidence in management decisions (Berry et al., 2021).

Cooperation Among Competitors

Health services managers also cooperate with managers of competing HCOs to improve internal operations and coordination of patient care processes. Relationships between competitors can be structured as informal memoranda of understanding to unincorporated joint ventures (formal, though not legally binding). For example, ICU beds are scarce in many communities, so groups of competing hospitals create a central coordinating team who impartially assigns transfer patients to the hospital with available ICU beds (Newton, 2015). When health services managers successfully extend the organizational structure to collaborating competitors, the HCO can improve patient care and operational effectiveness.

FUTURE DIRECTIONS

Rapid adoption of virtual technologies during the COVID-19 pandemic will likely change how HCOs organize their workforces and health care delivery structures. For healthcare workers who do not provide direct patient care, working remotely has become normal practice. As a result, HCOs will need to determine how teams coordinate, solve problems, and make decisions when they are not physically in the same room. In addition, the growth of telehealth services for patient care, education, and monitoring will reshape how HCOs organize health services teams. It is likely that innovative HCOs will reinvent the health care workflow to solve the problem of patient care fragmentation with the integration of telehealth technologies and in-person care. Nevertheless, HCOs are likely to make substantial changes in how the work is defined, coordinated, and structured in response to virtual technologies in the near-term future.

SUMMARY

- Health services managers divide the work for clinical and nonclinical operational functions of HCOs into discrete, repeatable tasks that are documented to set clear expectations for the performance.
- Health services managers assign the work to people and organizational units for better decision-making and coordinated workflows. The division of labor creates areas of specialization. Dividing tasks by specialization into departments creates a functional organizational structure.
- Individuals higher up in the chain of command have the authority to assign responsibility for certain tasks to a person lower in the chain of command. When assigned by their authorized manager, workers accept responsibility for tasks related to their area of specialization.
- Health services managers often operate with responsibility but with limited authority over clinicians on the frontlines. Decisions on how to care for patients are made by clinicians with the guidance from their professional organizations, not by health services managers.
- To meet organizational goals, health services managers hire specialized administrative support staff who implement extensive work processes that support frontline clinical professionals.
- Health services managers coordinate work among and between staff and departments, including clarifying roles and responsibilities among workers.
- As organizations become more complex, health services managers create divisions that operate as separate businesses run by authorized senior managers who are responsible for distinct budgets, performance results, and profits.

END-OF-CHAPTER RESOURCES

KEY TERMS*

*For the full list of key terms, please see the online glossary at **http://connect.springerpub.com/content/book/978-0-8261-4807-0.**

adhocracy
affiliation
alliances
authority
bureaucracy
chain of command
continuum of care
center of excellence
centralized
decentralized
delegation
departmentalization
division of labor
divisional structure
divisionalized
dyad model
flat organizational structure
fragmented care
functional authority
functional structure
group purchasing organizations
integrated delivery systems
joint venture
line position

line of authority
machine bureaucracy
matrix structure
middle management
operating core
organizational chart
organizational design
outsource
outsourcing
professional bureaucracy
reserved powers
responsibility
service line
span of control
specialization
staff position
standardized work
standard operating procedure
strategic apex
strategic business unit
support staff
tall organizational structure
technostructure
unity of command

LEARNING ACTIVITIES

Professional Development and Reflection

1. Reflect on the ideal job. What are the authority, responsibility, span of control, and decision-making processes of the position? For example, reflect on the level of authority and responsibility desired in the ideal job. Would an "act, then inform your boss of the result" decision-making process be preferred? Would frequent interaction with your boss (narrow span of control) be preferred? Which of these elements would have to change for you to leave the job for another?

2. Mintzberg described five basic parts of organizations. In HCOs, the operating core consists of clinicians. Imagine that you had three similar job opportunities in three different parts of the organization: middle management, support structure, and technostructure. Another way to describe health services management positions within the organizational structure is staff or line positions (see Career Box 10.2). A staff position can be located in the support structure or the technostructure. A line position is considered middle management. Which part of the organization would you prefer for your next job? Why? Does your preference align with your overall career goals?

Discussion Questions

1. The desire to improve the effectiveness and efficiency of healthcare has resulted in consistent efforts to implement standardized processes in HCOs. However, some clinicians resist the efforts to standardize their work, instead preferring to improvise when faced with unexpected and unpredictable events that are inevitable in many health services delivery settings, such as emergency care. Do you think clinicians are justified in resisting efforts to standardize their work? Why or why not?
2. Reflect on the professional bureaucracy concept in HCOs. What role do physicians play in a professional bureaucracy, and how does it impact health services delivery? How does the professional bureaucracy impact the health services management role?

RECOMMENDED READING AND MEDIA

Bard, M., & Nugent M. (2011). *Accountable care organizations: Your guide to strategy, design, and implementation*. Health Administration Press.

Belasen, A. T. (2019) *Dyad leadership and clinical integration: Driving change, aligning strategies*. Health Administration Press.

Bolman, L. G., & Deal, T. E. (2021). *Reframing organizations: Artistry, choice, and leadership* (7th ed.). Jossey-Bass.

Burns, L. R. (2022). *The healthcare value chain: Demystifying the role of GPOs and PBMs*. Palgrave Macmillan.

Christensen, C. M., Grossman, J. H., & Hwang J. (2017). *The innovator's prescription: A disruptive solution for health care*. McGraw-Hill Education.

Clayton, M. (2022). Henry Mintzberg's 4 plus 2 Organizational Types. [video]. YouTube. https://www.youtube.com/watch?v=JmvYcskjh3E

Cleveland Clinic Nurses – Purposeful Hourly Rounding. [video]. YouTube. https://www.youtube.com/watch?v=Ue1bYNR9ysc

Dunn, R. (2015). *Dunn & Haimann's Healthcare Management* (10th ed.). Health Administration Press.

Gawande, A. (2009). *The checklist manifesto: How to get things right*. Metropolitan Books.

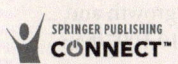

A robust set of instructor resources designed to supplement this text is located at http://connect.springerpub.com/content/book/978-0-8261-4807-0. Qualifying instructors may request access by emailing textbook@springerpub.com.

REFERENCES

Alexander, J. A., Heardl, L. R., & Shi, Y. (2015). Assessing organizational change in multisector community health alliances. *Health Services Research, 50*(1), 98–116. https://doi.org/10.1111%2F1475-6773.12216

American Medical Association. (2021). *AMA analysis shows most physicians work outside of private practice*. https://www.ama-assn.org/press-center/press-releases/ama-analysis-shows-most-physicians-work-outside-private-practice

Baker, G., Gibbons, R., & Murphy, K. J. (1999). Informal authority in organizations. *Journal of Law, Economics, and Organization, 15*(1), 56–73. https://doi.org/10.1093/jleo/15.1.56

Begun, J. W., White, K. R., & Mosser, G. (2011). Interprofessional care teams: The role of the healthcare administrator. *Journal of Interprofessional Care, 25*(2), 119–123. https://doi.org/10.3109/13561820.2010.504135

Berry, L. L., Letchuman, S., Ramani, N., & Barach, P. (2021, November). The high stakes of outsourcing in health care. In *Mayo Clinic Proceedings* (Vol. 96, No. 11, pp. 2879–2890). Elsevier.

Burns, L. R. (2022). *The healthcare value chain: Demystifying the role of GPOs and PBMs*. Palgrave Macmillan.

Burns, L. R., Bradley, E. H., & Weiner, J. (2019). *Shortell and Kaluzny's health care management organization design & behavior*. Cengage Learning.

Bratcher, C. R., & Bello, E. (2011). Traditional or centralized models of diabetes care: The multidisciplinary diabetes team approach. *The Journal of Family Practice, 60*(11 Suppl), S6–11.

Campbell, H., Hotchkiss, R., Bradshaw, N., & Porteous, M. (1998). Integrated care pathways. *BMJ, 316*(7125), 133–137. https://doi.org/10.1136/bmj.316.7125.133

Centers for Medicare and Medicaid Services. [CMS]. (2021, April 29). *Comprehensive Care for Joint Replacement Model*. https://www.cms.gov/priorities/innovation/innovation-models/cjr.

Chandler, A. (1962). *Strategy and Structure: Chapters in the history of industrial enterprise*. Doubleday.

Cleveland Clinic. (2018, May 24). *Finding the way to purposeful hourly rounding*. https://consultqd.clevelandclinic.org/finding-the-way-to-purposeful-hourly-rounding/

Comstock, N. H. (2019, October 31). *Better together: Most healthcare leaders report using a dyad leadership model*. Medical Group Management Association. https://www.mgma.com/data/data-stories/better-together-most-healthcare-leaders-report-us

Dapelo-Garcia, A. (2015). Stanford Health Care creates universal registration: Stanford Health Care developed a seamless, single-point-of-contact registration process for patients receiving multiple services at its cancer center. *Revenue Cycle Strategist, 12*(8), 5–7.

Drucker, P. (1954). *The practice of management*. Harper & Row, Publishers, Inc.

Dunn, R. (2021). *Dunn and Haimann's healthcare management* (11th ed.). Health Administration Press.

Elrod, J. K., & Fortenberry, J. L. (2017). Centers of excellence in healthcare institutions: What they are and how to assemble them. *BMC Health Services Research, 17*(1), 15–24. https://doi.org/10.1186/s12913-017-2340-y

Einav, S., Hick, J. L., Hanfling, D., Erstad, B. L., Toner, E. S., Branson, R. D., ... & Task Force for Mass Critical Care. (2014). Surge capacity logistics: care of the critically ill and injured during pandemics and disasters: CHEST consensus statement. *Chest, 146*(4), e17S–e43S.

Fayol, H. (1916). General principles of management. *Classics of Organization Theory, 2*(15), 57–69.

Field, M. J., & Lohr, K. N. (Eds.). (1990). *Clinical practice guidelines: Directions for a new program*. Committee to Advise the Public Health Service on Clinical Practice Guidelines. Institute of Medicine, U.S. Department of Health and Human Services. https://doi.org/10.17226/1626

Fine, P. S., & Kuhlenbeck, K. (2021). Implementing a new service line model to support growth and serve patients. *Frontiers of Health Services Management, 37*(3), 4–13. https://doi.org/10.1097/hap.0000000000000104

Ford, H., & Crowther, S. (1926). *Today and tomorrow*. Doubleday, Page & Co.

Francis, J. R. (2020). COVID-19: Implications for supply chain management. *Frontiers of Health Services Management, 37*(1), 33–38. https://doi.org/10.1097/hap.0000000000000092

Franklin, B. J., Vakili, S., Huckman, R. S., Hosein, S., Falk, N., Cheng, K., Murray, M., Harris, S., Morris, C. A., & Goralnick, E. (2020). The inpatient discharge lounge as a potential mechanism to mitigate emergency department boarding and crowding. *Annals of Emergency Medicine, 75*(6), 704–714. https://doi.org/10.1016/j.annemergmed.2019.12.002

Fredrickson, J. W. (1986). The strategic decision process and organizational structure. *Academy of Management Review, 11*(2), 280–297. https://doi.org/10.2307/258460

Galbraith, J. R. (1977). *Organization design*. Addison-Wesley Publishing Company, Reading, MA.

Gates, J. D., Arabian, S., Biddinger, P., Blansfield, J., Burke, P., Chung, S., ... & Yaffe, M. B. (2014). The initial response to the Boston marathon bombing: lessons learned to prepare for the next disaster. *Annals of Surgery, 260*(6), 960–966.

Gawande, A. (2009). *The checklist manifesto: How to get things right*. Metropolitan Books.

Gawande, A. (2013, April 17). Why Boston's Hospitals Were Ready. *The New Yorker*. https://www.newyorker.com/news/news-desk/why-bostons-hospitals-were-ready

HCA Healthcare. (2023). *Who we are: Doing business with HCA healthcare*. https://hcahealthcare.com/about/doing-business-with-hca.dot

Heeringa, J., Mutti, A., Furukawa, M. F., Lechner, A., Maurer, K. A., & Rich, E. (2020). Horizontal and vertical integration of health care providers: A framework for understanding various provider organizational structures. *International Journal of Integrated Care, 20*(1), 2. https://doi.org/10.5334%2Fijic.4635

Hoff, T. (2019). Activities and sensemaking associated with frontline role expansion in primary care settings. *Journal of Healthcare Management, 64*(5), 315–329. https://doi.org/10.1097/jhm-d-18-00187

Hogan, T. H., Lemak, C. H., Hearld, L. R., Sen, B. P., Wheeler, J. R., & Menachemi, N. (2019). Market and organizational factors associated with hospital vertical integration into sub-acute care. *Health Care Management Review, 44*(2), 137–147. https://doi.org/10.1097/hmr.0000000000000199

Huang, H., Zhu, X., Ullrich, F., MacKinney, A. C., & Mueller, K. (2023). The impact of Medicare shared savings program participation on hospital financial performance: An event-study analysis. *Health Services Research, 58*(1), 116–127. https://doi.org/10.1111%2F1475-6773.14085

Huang, K. P., Tung, J., Lo, S. C., & Chou, M. J. (2013). A review and critical analysis of the principles of scientific management. *International Journal of Organizational Innovation (Online), 5*(4), 78.

Kanigel, R. (2005). *The one best way: Frederick Winslow Taylor and the enigma of efficiency*. MIT Press.

Kleinpell, R., Myers, C. R., Likes, W., & Schorn, M. N. (2022). Breaking down institutional barriers to advanced practice registered nurse practice. *Nursing Administration Quarterly, 46*(2), 137–143. https://doi.org/10.1097/naq.0000000000000518

Lewis, C., Abrams, M. K., Seervai, S., Horstman, C., & Blumenthal, D. (2022, April 28). *The impact of the Payment and Delivery System Reforms of the Affordable Care Act*. The Commonwealth Fund. https://www.commonwealthfund.org/publications/2022/apr/impact-payment-and-delivery-system-reforms-affordable-care-act

Louis, C. J., Clark, J. R., Gray, B., Brannon, D., & Parker, V. (2019). Service line structure and decision-maker attention in three health systems: Implications for patient-centered care. *Health Care Management Review, 44*(1), 41–56. https://doi.org/10.1097/hmr.0000000000000172

Lutz, J. A., Zalucki, P. M., & Finarelli, M. (2021). Service lines: Working toward a value-based future. *Frontiers of Health Services Management, 37*(3), 14–28. https://doi.org/10.1097/hap.0000000000000105

March, J. G., & Simon, H. A. (1993). Introduction to the second edition. In J. G. March & H. A. Simon (Eds.). *Organizations* (2nd ed., pp. 1–19). Wiley.

McBeth, B., Karanas, Y., Nguyen, P., Kurani, S., & Bhimani, M. (2021). Improving communication between hospital administrations and healthcare providers during COVID-19: Experience from a large public hospital system in Northern California. *Journal of Communication in Healthcare, 14*(4), 274–282. https://doi.org/10.1080/17538068.2021.1975250

Merlino, J. (2015). *Service fanatics: How to build superior patient experience the Cleveland Clinic way*. McGraw-Hill.

Mintzberg, H. (1981). *Organization design: Fashion or fit?* Harvard Business Press.

Mintzberg, H. (1983). *Structure in fives: Designing effective organizations*. Prentice-Hall.

Newton, S. M., & Fralic, M. (2015). Interhospital transfer center model: Components, themes, and design elements. *Air Medical Journal, 34*(4), 207–212. https://doi.org/10.1016/j.amj.2015.03.008

O'Connor, C. J. (2015). *Healthcare supply chain at the intersection of cost, quality, and outcomes: The essential guide*. Nexera/Greater New York Hospital Association.

Pruitt, Z., Taylor, P., & Bryant, K. B. (2018). A managed care organization's call center-based social support role. *The American Journal of Accountable Care, 6*, e16–e22.

Rousseau, D. M. (2020). The realist rationality of evidence-based management. *Academy of Management Learning & Education, 19*(3), 415–424. http://doi.org/10.5465/amle.2020.0050

Ryan, L., Jackson, D., Woods, C., & Usher, K. (2019). Intentional rounding – An integrative literature review. *Journal of Advanced Nursing, 75*(6), 1151–1161. https://doi.org/10.1111/jan.13897

Sánchez, C. E., & Sánchez, L. D. (2020). Case study: emergency department response to the Boston marathon bombing. *Operational and medical management of explosive and blast incidents*, 363–367.

Shortell, S. M., & Addicott, R. (2016). A new lens on innovations in health care: Forms and functions. In E. Ferlie, K. Montgomery, & A. R. Pedersen (Eds.), *The Oxford handbook of healthcare management*. Oxford University Press.

Shortell, S. M., Gillies, R. R., & Anderson, D. A. (1996). *Remaking healthcare in America* (2nd ed.). Jossey-Bass.

Smith, A. (2002). *The wealth of nations*. Oxford, England: Bibliomania.com Ltd. [Web.] https://lccn.loc.gov/2002564559

Stange, K. C. (2009). The problem of fragmentation and the need for integrative solutions. *The Annals of Family Medicine, 7*(2), 100–103. https://doi.org/10.1370%2Fafm.971

Starr, P. (1982). *The social transformation of American medicine: The rise of a sovereign profession and the making of a vast industry*. Basic Books.

Trandel, E. (2015). *Advocating for dyad leadership at your organization? Use our slides*. https://www.advisory.com/research/physician-executivecouncil/prescription-for-change/2015/03/dyad-leadership-slides

Walberer, P. (2017). The Geisinger model. In A. Schmid & S. Singh (Eds.), *Crossing borders - Innovation in the U.S. health care system*, P.C.O.-Verlag.

Waterman, R. H. (1990). *Adhocracy: The power to change*. Whittle Direct Books

Weber, M. (1947). *Theory of social and economic organization*. Translated by A. M. Henderson & T. Parsons. The Free Press.

White, K. R., & Griffith, J. R. (2019). Foundations of clinical excellence. In *The well-managed healthcare organization* (9th ed., pp. 337–366). Health Administration Press.

White, K. R., and J. R. Griffith. 2019. "Foundations of well-managed healthcare organizations." In *The well-managed healthcare organization* (9th ed., pp. 3–33). Chicago: Health Administration Press.

World Health Organization. (2008). *Implementation manual: WHO surgical safety checklist (first ed.)*. https://apps.who.int/iris/handle/10665/70046

Yates, M. A. (2021). *An exploration of Dyad leadership in private practice within the United States* [Doctoral dissertation, The University of Mississippi Medical Center].

Young, R. (2017, January 30). *It takes two: Can Dyad leadership provide a durable pathway in healthcare's brave new world?* Innovate Healthcare Cardiology Business.

Zismer, D. K., Brueggemann, J., & James, M. (2010). Examining the "dyad" as a management model in integrated health systems. *Physician Exec, 36*(1), 14–19.

CHAPTER 11

PERFORMANCE MANAGEMENT

Performance management includes the processes of setting organizational goals and connecting them to operational initiatives and individual achievement.

COMPETENCIES

- Translate organizational strategy into actionable and measurable goals.
- Define, measure, and monitor indicators of performance.
- Compare performance against benchmarks to identify opportunities for improvement.
- Hold self and others accountable for achievement.
- Report performance metrics to accrediting agencies and other external stakeholders.
- Balance financial achievement with other perspectives, including innovation; clinical quality; population health; employee wellness; and diversity, equity, and inclusion.
- Operationalize measures of effectiveness, efficiency, and productivity.
- Monitor performance of functional areas of health care organizations, including marketing, supply chain, human resources, and clinical quality.
- Connect organizational goals to individual performance.
- Recognize the effects of rewards and penalties in health care organizations.

CHAPTER OUTLINE

- Accountability to Stakeholders
- Strategic Performance
- Performance Management Process
- Goal Setting
- Executing, Monitoring, and Learning
- Individual Performance

INTRODUCTION

Successful health services managers possess an **achievement orientation**, a drive to accomplish goals and outperform competitors (National Center for Healthcare Leadership [NCHL], 2018). When health services managers discover that performance measures have fallen below expectations, they accept accountability and motivate themselves and others to improve. Even when performance is deemed successful, high-achieving health services managers set more challenging goals to encourage the health care organization (HCO) to become more efficient; effective; productive; and valued by patients, families, communities, and payers.

As is described in this chapter, a health services manager's drive to succeed can be harnessed into a system of practices called performance management. **Performance management** involves the activities of setting goals, focusing the organization on the highest priority actions, monitoring and evaluating performance, holding individuals and teams accountable, and improving performance through organizational learning. This chapter explains how effective managers translate complex strategies into high-level, long-term strategic objectives and collaborate with individuals at various levels of the organization to set precise, actionable, and objective performance goals. This chapter also describes the competencies associated with performance measurement, monitoring, and evaluation of individuals and business operations (Otley, 1999).

ACCOUNTABILITY TO STAKEHOLDERS

Stakeholder View of Performance

Various healthcare stakeholders, such as boards of directors, regulators, payers, and accreditors, rigorously monitor the performance of clinical and business operations of HCOs. Successful health services managers incorporate these stakeholder's perspectives into the HCO's performance management systems and report the results to stakeholders at regular intervals (Kfuri et al., 2021). Failure to meet certain performance standards can result in significant patient, organizational, and professional consequences. **Accountability** means the practice of being held answerable for achieving expected standards (McGrath & Whitty, 2018). Successful health services managers hold themselves and others accountable for achievement and allocate resources to improve clinical and operational performance.

> △ **KEY IDEA**
> **Failure to meet certain performance standards can result in significant patient, organizational, and professional consequences.**

Boards of Directors

The board of directors is the stakeholder group that monitors the overall performance of the HCO and the CEO. The board of directors regularly monitors high-level strategic performance objectives to ensure that managers are achieving agreed-upon goals (Erwin et al., 2019). If successful, the board will reward the management team with bonuses or merit-based raises. In instances where performance does not meet expectations, effective boards will hold managers, especially the CEO, accountable for missing performance targets. Sometimes, the board will force the CEO to resign or dismiss them from their executive position for poor performance. More likely, however, the board will expect that managers invest in performance improvement practices and demand progress toward success.

HCO boards of directors also oversee clinical performance. During regular board meetings, health services management teams provide updates about key clinical quality measures, such as healthcare-acquired infections, patient experience scores, and various forms of **mortality** (i.e., death) and **morbidity** (i.e., illness) rates. When clinical performance does not meet or exceed standards, health services managers are responsible for allocating resources designed to improve clinical quality (Tsai et al., 2015). When significant patient safety events are caused by clinician negligence, boards may revoke the ability for those clinicians to practice at the HCO (Erwin et al., 2019).

Regulators

Healthcare **regulators** are the various government authorities who are responsible for monitoring and enforcing laws, rules, and regulations designed to protect the public's health and safety. The federal agency, Centers for Medicare & Medicaid Services (CMS), requires HCOs to collect and submit a variety of performance reports. With these data, the CMS publishes the Hospital Compare website that displays performance rankings so that potential patients can compare the quality of care between HCOs (Glance et al., 2020). State and local public health agencies also require HCOs to report performance measures, such as healthcare-associated infections and patient falls (Metcalfe et al., 2018).

CAREER BOX 11.1: Career Stakeholders

Stakeholder identification and prioritization theory is a framework for organizations to make more informed decisions and build positive relationships with stakeholders who can contribute to their long-term success (Serna et al., 2022). Career stakeholders refer to individuals, groups, or entities that are likely to be affected by your choices or anyone in a position to influence the outcomes of your career decisions. The following groups are some of the stakeholders who may impact your career:

- *Family members:* Provide support and connections to mentors, employers, or industry contacts. The desire to balance career goals with family considerations can influence decisions.
- *Professors and mentors:* Teach knowledge and skills, offer valuable insights, help navigate challenges, and provide networking opportunities.
- *Colleges and universities:* Provide education and career counseling services. Their reputation is linked to career achievements of graduates.
- *Current bosses:* Recognize areas for improvement and provide opportunities for skill development and training. Understands strengths and assigns challenging projects to expand capabilities.
- *Colleagues and peers:* Provide collaboration, knowledge sharing, skill development, and networking opportunities.
- *Customers, clients, or patient*s: Contribute feedback and recommendations based on achievement.
- *Professional associations:* Deliver workshops and conferences that enhance competencies. Offer networking opportunities, career fairs, and resources for job seekers.

By identifying and prioritizing the interests of key stakeholders, you can build stronger relationships and make better career decisions.

Payers

HCOs also submit performance results to health care **payers**, including Medicare, Medicaid, commercial health insurance companies, and large corporate entities who self-insure their employees. The National Committee for Quality Assurance (NCQA) is responsible for developing performance measures within their **Healthcare Effectiveness Data and Information Set (HEDIS)**, a standard measure set used by health insurance companies use to evaluate the performance of HCOs. NCQA updates this HEDIS measurement set each year through workgroup discussions among management and clinical experts from HCOs and health insurance companies (NCQA, 2023). Payers also hold HCOs accountable for performance through contracts that seek to improve quality of care and decrease costs, called **pay for performance** or **value-based purchasing** (Powers et al., 2017).

Accreditors

Accreditors also collect performance data to hold HCOs accountable for performance and to motivate continuous improvement (Kfuri et al., 2021). The CMS requires that HCOs maintain accreditation as a condition for serving Medicare beneficiaries, which makes accreditation a veritable necessity. **The Joint Commission** is the most widely recognized accrediting organization in the United States for hospitals, home care organizations, nursing homes, rehabilitation centers, and behavioral health organizations. The Joint Commission collects and publicly reports core measures on HCO performance as a part of their certification and accreditation programs (Leape, 2021). Other accrediting organizations include Utilization Review Accreditation Commission (URAC) and Accreditation Association for Ambulatory Health Care (AAAHC). Health services manager create programs designed to reduce the risks of noncompliance, such as unexpected instances of death or serious physical or psychological injury, known as **sentinel events** or **never events**. A failure by an HCO to provide a prudent standard of care is known as **negligence**, which is a form of noncompliance. Events of noncompliance such as these can lead to significant legal and financial penalties for HCOs and even a loss of accreditation.

INFORMATIONAL INTERVIEW 11.1

Manager, Patient Experience
Access the informational interview online at http://connect.springerpub.com/content/book/978-0-8261-4807-0/chapter/ch00.

Awards and Recognitions

Health services managers also engage in performance management practices so that their HCOs can be recognized for outstanding performance (Beaudin-Seiler & Fogarty, 2016). The **Malcolm Baldrige National Quality Award** recognizes organizations for high achievement. The American Nurses Credentialing Center's (ANCC's) **Magnet Recognition** and **Pathway to Excellence** programs provide performance management framework for monitoring and improving the nursing practice environment (ANCC, 2017). These certification programs recognize HCOs for quality patient care and professional nursing practices and have been found to improve hospital financial performance (Karim et al., 2018).

△ KEY IDEA

Health services managers also engage in performance management practices so that their HCOs can be recognized for outstanding performance.

Ranking Organizations

Nongovernmental performance **ranking organizations**, such as U.S. News and World Report, Fortune/Merative Top Hospitals and Health Systems, Consumer Reports, Healthgrades, and the Leapfrog Group, publish scores and rankings on HCOs. To derive their rankings, a number of performance measures, including mortality, patient safety measures, and the expert opinions of physicians, are combined into composite scores (Thomas Craig et al., 2020). A **composite score** is a single variable that represents a combination of weighted measures to summarize overall performance.

Many health services managers pay close attention to the performance criteria of ranking organizations, as public rankings influence where patients seek care. HCO marketing campaigns often tout success in one or more of these rankings. However, these ranking organizations and their methodologies are criticized for causing HCOs to align their strategic focus on improving their rankings, instead of caring for patients (Plott et al., 2021; Svrluga, 2023). Nevertheless, ranking organizations influence how funds are allocated by health services managers due to the importance rankings have on HCO prestige and patient care revenues.

STRATEGIC PERFORMANCE

Benchmarking

Health services managers track hundreds of performance measures and compare them to average performance metrics of the best-performing HCOs. **Benchmarking** is the systematic approach of comparing performance to successful HCOs, identifying gaps between the HCO and the best performers, and implementing new actions intended to improve performance (Ellis, 2006). The actions that are most likely to improve performance are known as **best practices**. Benchmarking can be used to set goals or to motivate adoption of best practices when their HCO's performance lags behind similar types of HCOs.

Strategic Scorecard

While high-performing HCOs diligently track hundreds of performance benchmarks, reacting to all of them can distract from achievement of overall strategic goals. Health services managers who monitor too many performance goals will become bogged down in operational issues unrelated to long-term strategies. Successful health services managers commit to strategic choices and monitor only a smaller number of strategic objectives that are most critical to those strategies (Doerr, 2018; White & Griffith, 2019). As Stephen R. Covey (1989) wrote in his influential book, *The 7 Habits of Highly Effective People*, "The main thing is to keep the main thing the main thing."

> △ **KEY IDEA**
>
> **Health services managers who monitor too many performance goals will become bogged down in operational and tactical issues unrelated to long-term, high-level strategies.**

To maintain focus on key drivers of performance, some HCOs adopt a strategic performance management framework created by Kaplan and Norton (1996), called the **balanced scorecard** approach, which offers two main advantages. First, the balanced scorecard forces managers to reduce complexity of the strategic planning and execution process by focusing managers on the most critical measures of performance (Kaplan & Norton, 2007). Second, the balanced scorecard offsets the tendency of businesses to focus solely on financial goals, such as profit, market share, return-on-investment, or revenue growth. Whereas traditional performance measurement systems focus only on the financial perspective, the balanced scorecard approach "balances" many different perspectives so that that the organization does not excel at one performance perspective at the expense of another.

According to Kaplan and Norton (1992), the balanced scorecard creates a framework that views the business from four important perspectives: financial, internal business processes, learning and growth, and customers, as reflected in Table 11.1 (Gurd & Gao, 2007; Kaplan & Norton, 2007).

TABLE 11.1 Four Perspectives of Kaplan and Norton's Balanced Scorecard

PERSPECTIVE	DEFINITION	KEY QUESTION	HEALTHCARE PERFORMANCE AREAS
FINANCIAL	The efficient and effective use of resources	How do we appear to stakeholders?	Profit, supply costs, market share, labor productivity, fundraising
INTERNAL BUSINESS PROCESSES	Processes or business systems most critical to reducing costs, enhancing products and services, or improving productivity	What must we excel at?	Patient throughput, cost per discharge, length of stay, resource utilization, supply chain processes
INNOVATION AND LEARNING	Learning is more than training; it seeks innovation.	How will we sustain our ability to improve?	Employee development, new market penetration, scientific development
CUSTOMER	Creating value for customers, including patients and referring physicians	How do customers see us?	Patient satisfaction, physician satisfaction

Healthcare Perspectives

According to Kaplan and Norton (2001), organizations may alter the four perspectives of their original balanced scorecard framework to reflect the values of the HCO but should maintain the overall simplicity of their approach. Health services delivery features perspectives uncommon in other industries, such as life-and-death decisions, high-stress work, and the incentive to address diversity, equity, and inclusion that are essential to serving patients. Table 11.2 shows some of the common perspectives chosen by HCOs when implementing the balanced scorecard approach (Amer et al., 2022; Gurd & Gao, 2007; Hadden et al., 2022; Lantz, 2019).

PERFORMANCE MANAGEMENT PROCESS

Strategic Scorecard

A strategic scorecard approach aligns strategy to organizational and individual performance. Figure 11.1 illustrates the performance management cycle steps. The remaining content of this chapter will discuss performance management cycle, which includes the following steps:

1. Set strategic, organization-wide, long-term, high-level objectives.
2. Communicate strategic objectives to multiple levels of organization.
3. Link strategic objectives to operationalized performance goals (i.e., measures, metrics, or key performance indicators).
4. Create short-term initiatives, projects, or actions designed to achieve goals.
5. Monitor performance metrics to track progress toward objectives.
6. Reward or improve performance of individuals based on performance.
7. Collect feedback and incorporate learning into strategic planning.

TABLE 11.2 Balanced Scorecard Perspectives Common to Health Care Organizations

PERSPECTIVE	DEFINITION	KEY QUESTION	PERFORMANCE AREAS
CLINICAL QUALITY	The degree to which clinical services meet established standards, evidence-based guidelines, and best practices	Is the healthcare being provided safe, effective, efficient, patient centered, timely, and equitable?	Mortality, morbidity, patient safety, access to care, health outcomes, health care processes
POPULATION HEALTH	Distribution of health-related risks and outcomes in a population	How healthy is the community?	Social and economic needs, health behaviors, health services utilization, disease burden
EMPLOYEE WELL-BEING	Physical, mental, and emotional health of employees	How satisfied, healthy, and engaged are employees in the workplace?	Job satisfaction, employee engagement, employee retention
SOCIAL RESPONSIBILITY	Impacts on society, community, and environment	How can the HCO act responsibly toward the environment, communities, and society?	Environmental impact, support for community organizations, health disparities by race, ethnicity, gender, and/or socioeconomic status
DIVERSITY, EQUITY, AND INCLUSION	Diverse and inclusive environment where all individuals, regardless of their backgrounds, identities, and experiences, achieve optimal health and feel valued, respected, and empowered	How can we promote diversity, equity, and inclusion within our HCO?	Cultural competency, workplace equity, supplier diversity

HCO, health care organization.

FIGURE 11.1 Performance management cycle.

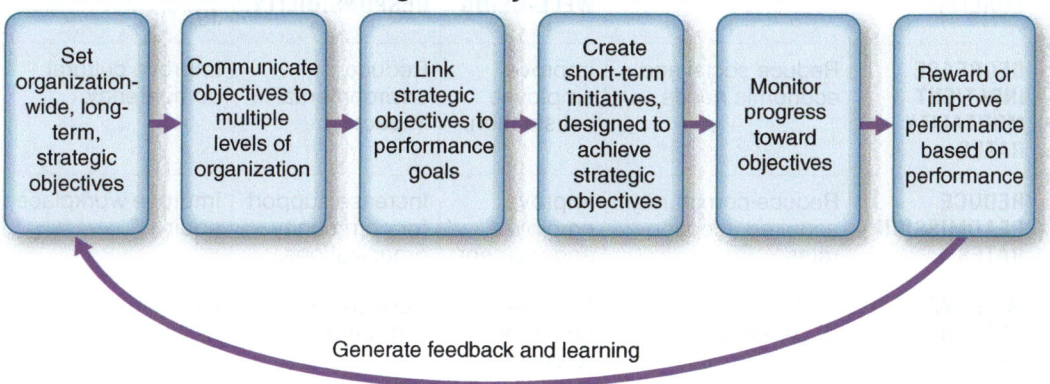

Set Strategic Objectives

Effective performance management begins with defining strategic priorities, a management function described in Chapter 8. Within each strategic perspective of the balanced scorecard, health services managers choose a limited number of strategic objectives (Kaplan & Norton, 1996). **Strategic objectives** are organization-wide, high-level goals that express what the board of directors and health services management executives want to accomplish in the long term (i.e., more than 1 year). Table 11.3 lists healthcare-related examples of strategic objectives within the four perspectives of Kaplan and Norton's balanced scorecard.

Health services managers also select strategic objectives that match the HCO's more expansive strategic perspectives, such as clinical quality; population health; employee well-being; social responsibility; and diversity, equity, inclusion, and justice. Table 11.4 lists examples of strategic objectives within these healthcare-related perspectives.

TABLE 11.3 Healthcare-Related Strategic Objectives Within the Four Perspectives of the Balanced Scorecard

FINANCIAL	INTERNAL BUSINESS PROCESSES	INNOVATION AND LEARNING	CUSTOMER
INCREASE PROFITS	Increase patient throughput.	Enhance employee development.	Improve patient satisfaction.
REDUCE OPERATING COST	Decrease cost per discharge.	Improve employee training.	Improve clinician satisfaction.
INCREASE LABOR PRODUCTIVITY	Decrease length of stay.	Enter new health services markets.	Decrease patient complaints.
INCREASE MARKET SHARE	Decrease resource utilization.	Increase scientific development.	Improve communication with patients.
INCREASE FUNDRAISING	Improve supply chain processes.	Increase investment in technology.	Improve communication with clinicians.

TABLE 11.4 Strategic Objectives Within Common Healthcare Balanced Scorecard Perspectives

CLINICAL QUALITY	POPULATION HEALTH	EMPLOYEE WELL-BEING	SOCIAL RESPONSIBILITY	DIVERSITY, EQUITY, INCLUSION, AND JUSTICE
DECREASE INPATIENT MORTALITY RATES	Reduce social and economic needs.	Improve employee satisfaction.	Reduce environmental impact.	Improve cultural competency.
REDUCE READMISSION RATES	Reduce community-acquired infection rates.	Improve employee engagement.	Increase support for community organizations.	Improve workplace equity.
IMPROVE PATIENT SAFETY	Reduce chronic disease burden.	Increase employee retention.	Reduce health disparities.	Increase supplier diversity.

Communicate Strategic Objectives

Once long-term strategic objectives are set, health services managers clearly communicate the high-level strategic objectives throughout the various levels of the HCO. Kaplan and Norton (2007) refer to the process of communicating strategic goals throughout the various levels of the organization as **cascading**. Cascading strategic objectives involves communicating the overarching goals from the top corporate level down to the divisional, business unit, departmental, and individual levels, making sure that everyone is working toward the same overarching objectives. Cascading ensures that each level's objectives match the corporate strategic objectives. However, it does not simply mean making the HCO aware of the strategic objectives, nor does it mean that the executive managers mandate goals. To create accountability and to motivate actions, cascading requires that health services managers involve frontline employees in the performance management processes.

GOAL SETTING

Link Strategic Objectives to Goals

Effective performance management requires that various levels of the organization—divisions, business units, functional areas, departments, teams, and individuals—translate the strategic objectives into relevant, measurable, and actionable terms. This collaborative process is known as **goal setting** (Ogbeiwi, 2021). The goal-setting process is more successful when employees set their personal goals. When goals are meaningful to people, performance management systems can act as a catalyst to inspire effective action (Latham & Locke, 2007). If individuals do not believe in the goals or in their ability to accomplish them, then they can become discouraged. Therefore, effective health services managers empower people to control the goal-setting processes that impact their work (Bandura, 1997).

> **INFORMATIONAL INTERVIEW 11.2**
> *Chief Executive Officer, Academic Medical Center Physician Practice*
> Access the informational interview online at http://connect.springerpub.com/content/book/978-0-8261-4807-0/chapter/ch00.

In addition, goals set at the various levels of the organization do not depend on the next higher level setting their goal first. As long as the goals are relevant, meaningful, and aligned with the corporate strategic objectives, the goal setting process can occur simultaneously at each organizational level (Grote, 2011). For example, individuals can set goals and measures that do not match the department's goals, as long as they are strategically appropriate and match the person's job responsibilities.

> ⚠ **KEY IDEA**
>
> As long as the goals are relevant, meaningful, and aligned with the corporate strategic goals, the goal setting process can occur simultaneously at each organizational level.

The most prominent framework for setting measurable and actionable goals is known as the SMART framework. Developed by George T. Doran (1981), the SMART framework is an acronym that stands for **S**pecific, **M**easurable, **A**ssignable, **R**ealistic, and **T**ime bound. Doran's easy-to-remember

FIGURE 11.2 SMART goal framework.

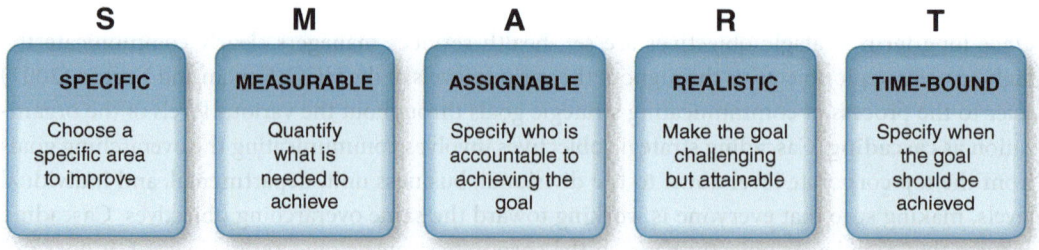

Source: Adapted from Doran, G. T. (1981). There's a S.M.A.R.T. way to write management's goals and objectives. *Management Review, 70(11)*, 35–36.

mnemonic indicates the minimum components necessary for operationalizing strategic objectives into measures. Figure 11.2 illustrates the SMART goal framework. Using this mnemonic can be useful for effectively defining performance measures. Effective goal setting requires the following criteria:

- *Specific:* Goals should apply to the areas for which the business unit or functional area can control.
- *Measurable:* Abstract performance concepts must be stated using variables that can be used to objectively monitor and compare performance.
- *Assignable:* Whether self-selected or determined by a team, a person or team should be responsible and accountable for the goal.
- *Realistic:* An achievement orientation leads to creation of challenging but achievable goals. Ambitious targets drive breakthrough results; benchmarks are good starting points.
- *Time bound:* Performance management systems occur on a regular cadence. Regular milestones (e.g., weekly, monthly, quarterly, and annually) should be agreed upon by everyone.

Goals must be stated in precise terms so that they can be compared accurately to external benchmarks, established expectations, or performance over time. **Operationalization** is the process of turning abstract performance concepts into measurable observations. Managers use a number of words to describe operationalized performance, such as **goal**, aim, **metric, statistic, key performance indicator** (KPI), outcome, or target. Some scholars and practitioners parse their meanings, but there is no agreement on which words to use within performance management systems (Ogbeiwi, 2021). Kaplan and Norton (2007) use the word "**measure**" to describe the operationalized strategic objectives. No matter which term is used, the main point is to translate performance concepts in quantifiable and actionable terms.

Common Healthcare Goals

All goals in business performance management systems are intended to improve effectiveness or efficiency. **Effectiveness** measures the degree to which goals are achieved, and **efficiency** refers to producing the most results for a given amount of resources. Efficiency and effectiveness are distinct abstract concepts, not strategic objectives or measures. The meanings of efficiency and effectiveness can be differentiated through a simple nurse staffing example. Health services managers seek to avoid overstaffing (inefficient) or understaffing (ineffective) in nurse staffing, measured using the **patient-to-nurse ratio** (number of patients per full-time nurse). An efficient but not effective nurse staffing model would staff too few **full-time equivalent** (FTE) nurses to care for patients, which would be less expensive (efficient) but dangerous for the patients (ineffective). An effective but inefficient HCO might staff too many nurse FTEs, which might produce excellent health outcomes (effective) but would cost the HCO too much money (inefficient). Ideally, the patient-to-nurse ratio would be both effective and efficient.

Effectiveness is commonly measured by decreasing patient mortality, a strategic objective within the clinical quality perspective. Mortality can be operationalized as the proportion of individuals who were treated in a hospital and died within 30 days of being admitted to the hospital, including deaths occurring during a stay and those after discharge but within 30 days (30-day hospital mortality rate). Mortality is usually statistically adjusted so that fair comparisons can be made between HCOs that care for patients with different characteristics. **Risk adjustment** accounts for different factors that can influence health outcomes, such as age, gender, medical procedures, and diagnoses present on admission. A predictive statistical model (i.e., logistic regression analysis) estimates the expected mortality rate for each HCO based on the identified patient risk factors (Dalton et al., 2013).

Table 11.5 lists clinical quality strategic objectives and operationalized performance measures commonly used by health services managers (Brar, 2019; Centers for Medicare and Medicaid, 2022; Emanuel et al., 2017).

TABLE 11.5 Examples of Healthcare Measures Within the Clinical Quality Perspective

STRATEGIC OBJECTIVE	MEASURE	OPERATIONALIZED DEFINITION
DECREASE MORTALITY RATES	Risk-adjusted 30-day hospital mortality rate	Percentage of patients who die within 30 days of being admitted to the hospital, including deaths occurring during stay and those after discharge but within 30 days, risk-adjusted for patient-level factors
DECREASE MORBIDITY RATES	Case mix index	MS-DRG weight for each discharge and dividing that by the total number of Medicare and Medicaid discharges in a given month and year
REDUCE READMISSION RATES	30-day hospital-wide all-cause readmission rates	The number of readmissions within the 30-day period divided by the total number of patients discharged from the hospital after their initial admission (for any diagnosis)
IMPROVE PATIENT SAFETY	Serious medication errors	Patient death or serious disability associated with a medication error (e.g., error involving the wrong drug, wrong dose, wrong patient, wrong time, wrong rate, wrong preparation, or wrong route of administration)
IMPROVE INFECTION CONTROL	Surgical site infections	Evidence of infection within 30 days of surgery, identified through International Classification of Diseases or Current Procedural Terminology codes
REDUCE WAIT TIMES	ED wait times	Time patients spend waiting to be seen by a clinician in the emergency department, measured from check-in to clinician assessment

MS-DRG, Medicare Severity Diagnosis Related Group.

Productivity is a performance concept that is defined as the ratio of outputs (a form of effectiveness) relative to the number of inputs (a form of efficiency). In healthcare, productivity measures the number of medical treatments, procedures, consultations, diagnostics, and therapies offered to patients relative to the costs related to those activities. **Labor productivity**, another common performance concept in HCOs, is the effective and efficient use of human resources (Priore, 2021). Labor productivity is one of the most important metrics that health services managers monitor and optimize (Berger, 2005). Improving labor productivity can be accomplished in two basic ways: increase the number of outputs (e.g., number of patients treated) or decrease labor inputs (e.g., hours worked by nurses). For example, productivity can be boosted by making it easier for clinicians to treat more patients (i.e., increased effectiveness). Health services managers can implement artificial intelligence systems to reduce the amount of paperwork clinicians need to complete. Alternatively, health services managers may increase productivity by restricting the amount of overtime expenses paid to staff (i.e., increased efficiency). Sometimes staff need to work overtime, such as when treating a patient in an emergency, but most overtime hours can be avoided, which can reduce extra expense. Table 11.6 lists examples of labor productivity measures commonly used by health services managers (Berger, 2005; Priore, 2021).

As described in Table 11.5, health services managers commonly use **relative value units** (RVUs) to measure clinician productivity (American Medical Association, 2023). Medicare publishes standardized work RVUs based on an estimated amount of time and effort that clinicians spend treating patients for services and procedures. For example, 99214 is the Current Procedural Terminology (CPT) code for an outpatient visit for the evaluation and management (checkup) of an established patient that takes approximately 30 to 39 minutes. In 2023, Medicare assigned 1.92 work RVUs to the 99214 CPT code. A clinician who completed 15 well-checks in one day would

TABLE 11.6 Examples of Common Healthcare Measures of Labor Productivity

STRATEGIC OBJECTIVE	EXAMPLE MEASURE	OPERATIONALIZED DEFINITION
INCREASE LABOR PRODUCTIVITY	Labor expense per adjusted discharge	Total labor expenses divided by discharges, adjusted by CMI for a specified period of time
	Outpatient visits per provider	Number of patient visits divided by the number of clinician FTEs for a specified period of time
	Patient-to-nurse ratio	Total sum of patients receiving care in a specific unit, department, or HCO divided by the total number of nurse FTEs providing care in the same unit, department, or HCO for a specified period of time
	Nursing hours per patient day	Total sum of productive nursing hours (excludes paid time off for illness, vacation, or continuing education) divided by the total number of patient days times 24, for a specified period of time
	Relative value units per provider	Total sum of RVUs, a standardized measure of value and effort associated with specific medical services, divided by the number of clinicians for a specified period of time

CMI, case mix index; FTE, full-time equivalent; HCO, health care organization; RVU, relative value unit.

produce 28.8 work RVUs. Health services managers can use the RVUs to calculate a clinician's productivity compared to others. A clinician's proportion of the HCOs productivity is determined by calculating each provider's total work RVUs divided by the HCO's total work RVUs for a specified period of time. Because Medicare assigns higher RVUs for procedures than for preventive services, health services managers should only compare productivity of similar types of clinicians.

The tendency for health services managers to focus on productivity can be traced to how the U.S. healthcare system pays HCOs. The majority of health services are paid on a fee-for-service basis, meaning that HCOs are paid based on the volume of care provided by clinicians. When more health services are delivered, HCOs generate more revenue and, potentially, profits. As a result, health services managers seek to boost the volume of services provided through increased productivity. Health insurance companies want to control costs by attempting to limit the amount of health services provided by HCOs through a process known as **utilization review**. HCOs spend a significant amount of resources securing permission from health insurance companies to treat patients for certain procedures, called **pre-authorization**. During utilization review, the health insurance companies evaluate the treatment and medical circumstance to determine **medical necessity**, a legal term that means health insurance companies retain the power over HCOs regarding what services can be delivered to patients (Monahan & Schwarcz, 2021).

> △ **KEY IDEA**
>
> An obsession with clinician productivity can be especially problematic in health services management. Clinicians often resent attempts by health services managers to press for more productivity by working faster, longer, or harder.

An obsession with clinician productivity can be especially problematic in health services management. Clinicians often resent attempts by health services managers to press for more productivity by working faster, longer, or harder (Moffatt et al., 2014). Treating clinicians like machines will only serve to sap their motivation and lead to their dissatisfaction or burnout. Instead, successful health services managers focus on making the processes related to patient care more efficient and effective, thus boosting productivity.

Nevertheless, health services managers commonly use volume as an internal measure of performance. For example, hospital **adjusted patient days** (APDs) measures patient activity and health care utilization within a hospital over a specific period. APDs are operationalized as sum of inpatient patient days divided by the ratio of inpatient revenues and outpatient and ancillary revenues. When health services managers monitor APDs, staffing, resource allocation, bed capacity, and financial budgeting can be managed more effectively and efficiently. By comparing APDs over time or against healthcare benchmarks, health services managers can assess HCO performance and identify areas for improvement.

Efficiency is measured by health services managers in many ways (Berger, 2005). A common operational efficiency measure example is **bed occupancy rate**, which measures the percentage of hospital beds that are occupied by patients over a specific period (e.g., day, week, month, quarter, year). Low occupancy rates suggest inefficient use of resources (i.e., beds), and excessively high rates indicate the need to increase the capacity (i.e., number of beds). Table 11.7 lists performance metrics commonly used by health services managers to measure efficiency (Berger, 2005; Burlea-Schiopoiu & Ferhati, 2021; Khalifa & Khalid, 2015).

TABLE 11.7 Examples of Healthcare Measures of Operational Efficiency

STRATEGIC OBJECTIVE	MEASURE	OPERATIONALIZED DEFINITION
REDUCE COSTS	Expenses per inpatient day	Total annual costs for HCO divided by the number of patient days per year
INCREASE RESOURCE UTILIZATION	Clinic appointment utilization	Percentage of available appointment slots that are utilized by patients
IMPROVE OPERATIONAL EFFICIENCY	Operating room turnaround time	Time elapsed between the prior patient exiting the operating room and the next patient entering the operating room
IMPROVE OPERATIONAL EFFICIENCY	Average length of stay	Total number of days of patients stayed in the hospital divided by the number of discharges during a specific period
IMPROVE OPERATIONAL EFFICIENCY	Total asset turnover ratio	Total revenue per dollar of total assets divided by the average value of total assets for the period of time
SUPPLY CHAIN EFFICIENCY	Supply cost per unit of service	Total expense of supplies divided by the number of units of service
SUPPLY CHAIN EFFICIENCY	Inventory turnover	Total revenue divided by the total expenses associated with supply inventory

Define Targets

The final step in the balanced scorecard goal-setting process is to set challenging yet attainable targets for each of the performance measures. According to Kaplan and Norton (2007), **targets** are the quantifiable values for each of the measures that are intended to be achieved in the short term. These targets should be monitored on a weekly, monthly, and/or quarterly basis. Table 11.8 describes examples of health services performance measures with defined targets.

EXECUTING, MONITORING, AND LEARNING

Creating Short-Term Initiatives

After goals and targets are set, health services managers create short-term initiatives that are designed to achieve the strategic objectives. Implementation of strategic initiatives is the most difficult and important phase of performance management (Hadden et al., 2022). Effective health services managers integrate their budgeting processes with strategic planning so that allocated resources support the strategic initiatives (Kaplan & Norton, 2007). Strategic success depends on effectively allocating the necessary resources to achieve performance targets. Figure 11.3 illustrates Kaplan and Norton's balanced scorecard that a division executive would complete for their business unit.

A health services executive responsible for the home health division of a health system would produce something similar to the balanced scorecard described in Table 11.9 (Berger, 2005; Groene et al., 2009; Gurd & Gao, 2007). In this example, the home health division seeks to promote the health system's strategic objectives (increase profitability, enter new health services markets,

TABLE 11.8 Examples of Health Services Performance Measures With Targets

STRATEGIC OBJECTIVE	EXAMPLE MEASURE	OPERATIONALIZED DEFINITION	TARGET
IMPROVE PATIENT SAFETY	Serious medication errors	Patient death or serious disability associated with a medication error (e.g., error involving the wrong drug, wrong dose, wrong patient, wrong time, wrong rate, wrong preparation, or wrong route of administration)	Reduce serious medication errors by 40%
IMPROVE INFECTION CONTROL	Surgical site infections	Evidence of infection within 30 days of surgery, identified through International Classification of Diseases or Current Procedural Terminology codes	Reduce surgical site infections by 50%
IMPROVE CHRONIC DISEASE MANAGEMENT	Adherence to statin medication for individuals with coronary artery disease	Percentage of patients with coronary artery disease who had at least two prescriptions filled for statins and had a proportion of days covered of at least 0.8 for statins during 12 consecutive months	Adherence to statin medication for individuals with coronary artery disease greater than 60%
REDUCE WAIT TIMES	ED wait times	Median time patients spend waiting to be seen by a clinician in the ED, measured from check-in to clinician assessment	Median ED wait time less than 20 minutes
IMPROVE PRIMARY CARE APPOINTMENT SCHEDULING	Third next available appointment	Number of days a patient has to wait to get third next available primary care appointment; first and second available appointments may reflect openings created by patients cancelling appointments	TNAA less than 2 days
INCREASE PATIENT VOLUME	Inpatient average daily census	Total number of patient days in hospital, excluding newborns, divided by the number of days in the period	ACD greater than 266

ADC, average daily census; TNAA, third next available appointment.

increase satisfaction of patients, and improve patient throughput) by implementing an innovative, technology-supported hospital-at-home program. The table demonstrates how the health services executive would define measures, targets, and initiatives for each strategic objective.

As described in Table 11.9, this home health division seeks to achieve the health system's strategic objective to increase profitability. The home health division chose to measure profitability as operating profit margin, which is defined as revenues minus variable costs before paying interest or tax. To achieve the target of an operating profit margin equal to or greater than 15%, the home health division intends to create a hospital-at-home marketing campaign. The health services executive responsible for the home health division would monitor the success of the marketing efforts (e.g., compare results with goals) to ensure that the hospital-at-home campaign has the desired effect on profits. Marketing campaigns could include patient-focused advertising or physician-focused communications. For example, the marketing team could create an internal promotion to the **hospitalists**, physicians who care for patients only in the hospital, to convince them that hospital-at-home services may be medically appropriate for some patients.

FIGURE 11.3 Balance scorecard as a performance management system.

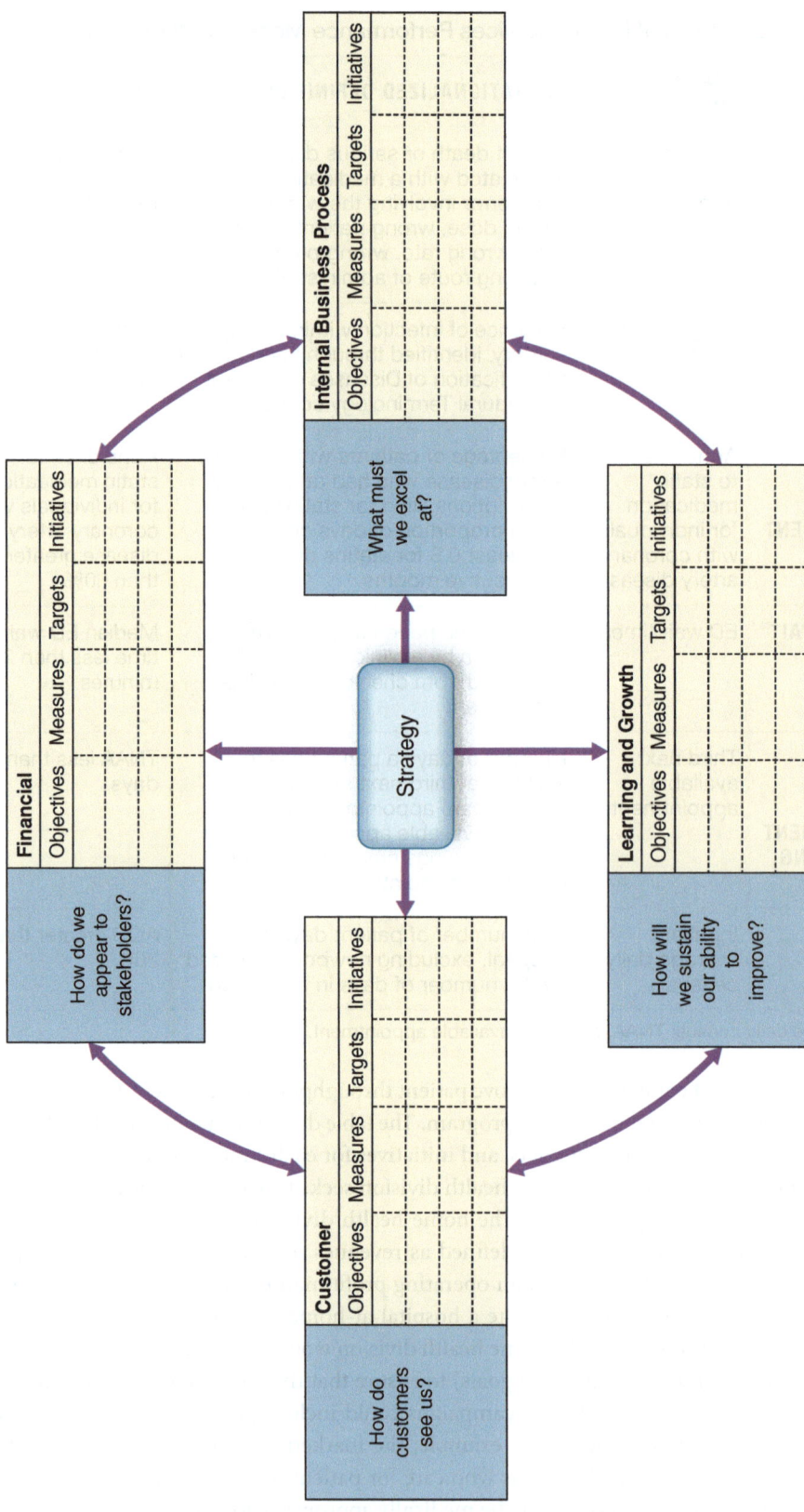

Source: Adapted from Kaplan, R. S., & Norton, D. P. (2007). Using the balanced scorecard as a strategic management system. *Harvard Business Review.* https://hbr.org/2007/07/using-the-balanced-scorecard-as-a-strategic-management-system

TABLE 11.9 Example of a Balanced Scorecard Connecting Strategy to Action in a Home Health Division of a Health System

FINANCIAL	Objective	Increase profitability.
	Measure	Total operating profit margin for home health division
	Target	Increase operating profit margin for home health division to equal to or greater than 15%.
	Initiative	Marketing campaign for hospital-at-home services
LEARNING AND GROWTH	Objective	Enter new health services markets.
	Measure	Total market share of hospital-at-home services
	Target	Increase hospital-at-home market share from 0% to 15%.
	Initiative	Hire clinical liaison to train hospitalists on the hospital-at-home medical evaluation protocol and to promote appropriate referrals of hospital-at-home patients.
CUSTOMER	Objective	Increase satisfaction of patients.
	Measure	NPS
	Target	NPS greater than or equal to 90%.
	Initiative	Institute twice-daily support calls from hospital-at-home clinicians.
INTERNAL BUSINESS PROCESSES	Objective	Improve patient throughput.
	Measure	ALOS
	Target	Reduce ALOS by 10% for inpatient admissions.
	Initiative	Institute nursing midnight rounds with focus on discharging patients to technology-supported hospital-at-home services.

ALOS, average length of stay; NPS, net promoter score.

Also described in Table 11.9, the health system's hospital-at-home program seeks to improve patient satisfaction, an increasingly important outcome for HCOs because payers are linking satisfaction to payments (Stanowski et al., 2015). In health services delivery, patient satisfaction is known as **patient experience** and is measured through the **Consumer Assessment of Healthcare Providers and Systems** (CAHPS) survey, which is created by the federal government and administered by Press Ganey. Different versions of CAHPS measure patient experience issues specific to the particular setting. For example, the hospital version (HCAHPS) measures items such as physician communication and whether the hospital was quiet at night (Agency for Healthcare Research and Quality [AHRQ], 2023). Other survey instruments for patient experience include the CAHPS Clinician & Group Survey (CG-CAHPS), CAHPS Emergency Department Survey (ED CAHPS), CAHPS Home Health Care Survey (HH-CAHPS), and CAHPS Nursing Home Survey (NHCAHPS).

> **CAREER BOX 11.2:** Career Balanced Scorecard
>
> The balanced scorecard approach to performance management can be used for career planning. For one, goal setting provides direction, motivation, and focus for achieving professional success. Perhaps more importantly, the balanced scorecard approach reinforces the idea that career success can mean more than financial success. Some people value extrinsic rewards, such as titles, salary, benefits, and promotions. Others place more importance on intrinsic rewards, such as job security, satisfaction, work-life balance, and congruence with organizational values. Also, the definition of career success varies from person to person and throughout lifetimes (Hildred et al., 2023). Nevertheless, taking a balanced approach to goal setting ensures that people do not excel at one type of career success at the expense of another. For example, someone seeking to improve their work-life balance may set a goal to increase the number of family dinners per week to three or more.

One way to operationalize patient experience is to use the **net promoter score** (NPS), a measure of customer loyalty. CAHPS surveys ask patients to rate their likelihood of recommending the HCO on a scale of 0 to 10. Patients who rate the HCO a 9 or 10 are considered "promoters," those rating 7 or 8 are considered "passives," and individuals answering 0 to 6 are called "detractors." To calculate the NPS, the percentage of "detractors" is subtracted from the percentage of "promoters." In Table 11.9, the customer perspective for the hospital-at-home program describes a patient outreach program where clinicians reach out to patients twice per day with the hopes of identifying issues before they become dissatisfiers, as reflected in the CAHPS survey.

The health system's internal business processes perspective strategic objective in Table 11.9 is improving patient throughput (a measure of efficiency). Patient **throughput** refers to the movement of patients through various stages of care within a hospital, from admission to discharge. Measures of throughput include average length of stay, time spent in the emergency department, bed turnover rate, and outpatient check-in to checkout time. The chosen measure patient throughput in the hospital-at-home example described in Table 11.9 is **average length of stay** (ALOS), defined as the total number of days of patients stayed in the hospital divided by the number of discharges during a specific period. Hospital-at-home programs have been found to reduce inpatient ALOS, but nurses need to make a concerted effort to recognize when patients are eligible for earlier discharge (Leong et al., 2021). In this example, health services managers and nurse managers might institute midnight rounds initiative where nurses identify patients who could benefit from technology-supported hospital-at-home services.

Monitor Performance

Performance management systems require effective monitoring processes to ensure that the HCO is accomplishing its strategic objectives. As a part of the monitoring of performance at the business or functional unit level, health services managers develop and share **operational scorecards** to flag looming problems, modify actions, and/or adjust goals (Doerr, 2018). Operational scorecards help health services managers make better decisions about where to allocate resources—time, people, money—in the day-to-day operations of the HCO (Berger, 2005). Operational scorecards must provide context ("How are we progressing?"), relate to strategic goals ("Are we aligned with our strategy?"), and give feedback on improvement initiatives ("Are we learning and improving?"). As with many elements of performance management, less is more in monitoring and reporting.

△ KEY IDEA

Operational scorecards must provide context ("How are we progressing?"), relate to strategic goals ("Are we aligned with our strategy?"), and give feedback on improvement initiatives ("Are we learning and improving?").

Monitoring performance requires collection of data from a variety of sources. First, electronic medical records contain medical histories, diagnoses, treatments, medications, and test results that can be used to calculate performance measures. Patient surveys collect data on patients' communication with providers, wait times, and overall satisfaction. Also, various HCO systems contain data on hospital operations, such as bed occupancy rates, emergency department wait times, surgical scheduling, supplies, and staff productivity. Human resource data, such as hire dates, compensation, and promotions, can be used to measure workplace equity and other strategic objectives. Finally, HCOs collect vast amounts of financial data from patient revenue collection accounts and vendor management systems. These disparate data sources are collected into a **data warehouse**, which is a centralized repository that stores and organizes various types of data. Management of data is an information technology function called **knowledge management**.

Executive health services managers and frontline employees alike access performance measures collected through HCO information systems. **Dashboards** are interactive, computerized, visual summaries of performance that enable trending, benchmarking, and visualization (Buttigieg et al., 2017). Healthcare managers routinely consult the dashboards to evaluate progress with strategic priorities, allocate resources, and address deficiencies. A variety of business intelligence software vendors, such as IBM, SAP, Tableau, and Qlik, provide platforms for health services managers to create customized dashboards and perform analytics on performance data (El Morr et al., 2019).

While dashboards can be helpful, customization can lead to mistakes in performance data visualization. Dashboards are only valuable for performance management when the data make sense to users. Figure 11.4 shows an example of a basic performance dashboard used in HCOs. Stephen Few (2013), an expert in data visualization, created simple rules for effective, at-a-glance dashboard design, including the following:

- *Simplicity:* Present information in the most straightforward manner possible. Reduce visual clutter by removing unnecessary decorations or excessive labels that can obscure key messages.
- *Parsimony:* Display only the most critical metrics. Allow users to drill down into more detailed information, if necessary.
- *Clarity and precision:* Information should be accurate and easily interpreted by users.
- *Context and comparison:* Performance data should reveal progress relative to set goals, benchmarks, or trends.
- *User centered*: Visualizations should consider the knowledge and abilities of the audience. People with sophisticated understanding of visual data can process more information than those less familiar with measures, graphs, charts, and related concepts.

Feedback and Learning in the Health Care Organization

Health services managers set specific points in time to evaluate metrics relative to the goals of the HCO. Recurring check-in meetings can help managers maintain focus, gather feedback on what is working, and encourage accountability. When performance is lagging, check-in meetings can be best used to focus on root cause analysis, brainstorming, and decision-making, not on discussing the relative merits of the strategic objectives, measures, or initiatives (Perlow, 2017). However,

FIGURE 11.4 Performance dashboard.

Admissions

ED	Other
75%	25%

40 ▲

Revenue

$24 million ▼

Commercial	Other
37%	63%

Readmissions

12% ▲

Medicare	Other
68%	32%

Category	Measure	Actual	Target	% Var
Productivity	FTE	616.5	600	2.2%
	wRVU	87,922	101,923	0.30%
Throughput	ED wait time (min)	25	21	−19%
	Hours to admission	7	6.25	−3.6%
Financial	Operating margin	$4,582,436	$3,200,622	43.2%
	Net patient revenue	$20,371,055	$18,387,786	10.8%
	Total expenses	$16,158,634	$15,579,405	−3.7%

Net promoter score

77.9% ◀ +1.66

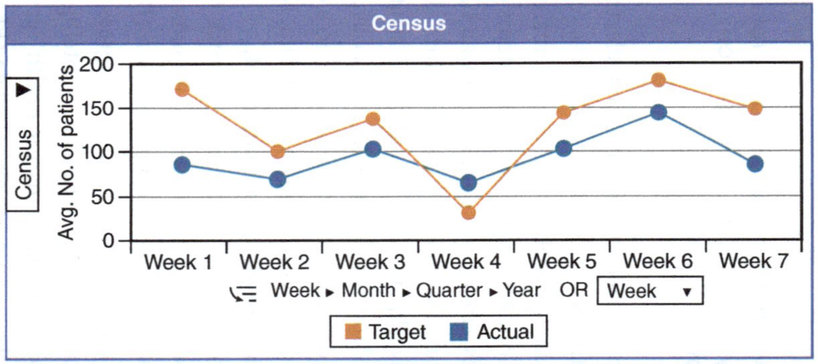

Census

Avg. No. of patients across Week 1–Week 7, with Target and Actual lines.

⛛ Week ▶ Month ▶ Quarter ▶ Year OR Week ▼

■ Target ■ Actual

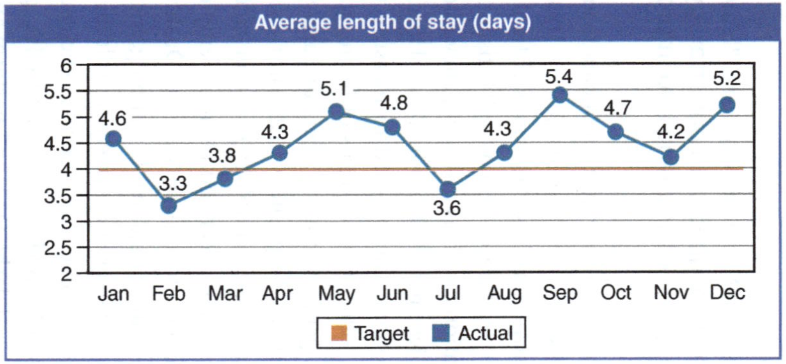

Average length of stay (days)

	Jan	Feb	Mar	Apr	May	Jun	Jul	Aug	Sep	Oct	Nov	Dec
Actual	4.6	4.3	3.8	3.3	5.1	4.8	4.3	3.6	5.4	4.7	4.2	5.2

■ Target ■ Actual

missing goals may require changes in strategy at higher levels of the HCO. When appropriate, the performance results are cascaded back up the organizational hierarchy, creating a feedback loop in the performance management system.

INDIVIDUAL PERFORMANCE

Performance Evaluations

Ultimately, corporate-level performance management systems connect to the individual level. **Performance evaluations** are formal assessments of employees' results compared to their assigned responsibilities. Human resource professionals work with health services managers to administer performance evaluations at least one per year or according to the HCO's policies and practices. Employees must receive **performance standards** in writing and in advance, and standards must be specific, measurable, and realistic. Unfortunately, health services managers may misguidedly give employees poor performance ratings based on ambiguous criteria that are not tied to objective measures of performance or related to their position responsibilities. When there is a gap between the performance standards and how the employee is measured in practice, it is called a **criterion deficiency**. When the goal-setting process is connected to performance evaluations, unconscious bias and accusations of favoritism become less prevalent (Agovino, 2023).

To make performance evaluations fairer, effective health services managers evaluate individual performance based on self-defined goals that are relevant to their job responsibilities (Doheny, 2021). For example, nurses can be evaluated using personal goals set through the balanced scorecard performance management approach (Yang, 2022). Managers responsible for the various nursing departments collaborate with nurse-led workgroups that define personal goal options from which nurses can choose. Health services managers ensure that the measures comply with the SMART framework and align with corporate strategic objectives. Table 11.10 lists options for performance measures for nurses within the four perspectives of Kaplan and Norton's balanced scorecard.

TABLE 11.10 Individual Performance Measures for Nurses Within the Four Perspectives of Kaplan and Norton's Balanced Scorecard

FINANCIAL	INTERNAL BUSINESS PROCESSES	INNOVATION AND LEARNING	CUSTOMER
Medical supplies and drug expiration date management	Punctuality for shifts	Number of preceptor hours for students, as percentage of hours worked	Department-based patient experience score on "nurse communication" domain (HCAHPS)
No medical equipment damaged; actions inconsistent with policy	Proportion of patients discharged by 11 am	Number of training hours, as proportion of total training hours in department	Department-based score on "how to care for yourself at home" patient experience domain (HCAHPS)
Age- and severity-adjusted ALOS	Nursing-related healthcare-associated infections	Participation in quality improvement project	No verified patient complaints

ALOS, average length of stay; HCAHPS, Hospital Consumer Assessment of Healthcare Providers and Systems.

HCOs use various approaches to evaluate employee performances, including the following (Aungsuroch et al., 2021):

- *Unstructured method*: Relies directly on the superior subjective opinion without an objective rating scale. Managers often write essays or short answers to prompts to evaluate employees. To reduce bias, this method is being phased out in HCOs.
- *Rating scale method*: Performance is measured on a numerical (i.e., 1 to 10) or discrete scale (e.g., excellent, very good, good, average, poor) for separate aspects of the position. Most employees will be ranked somewhere in the middle of the scale.
- *Paired comparative method*: An employee's performance is compared to that of every other employee in that department one at a time; then all employees are ranked according to the number of times each person is considered a superior performer in the paired comparisons.
- *Forced distribution*: Ranks employees against one another. Employees are placed along a ranked distribution, such as 20% in the top group of employees, 70% in the middle, and 10% at the bottom.
- *360-degree feedback*: Also known as a **multidimensional appraisal**, it incorporates multiple perspectives from an employee's supervisors, peers, and subordinates to evaluate employee performance.
- *Composite scoring*: Generates a single score of an individual's overall performance by combining multiple measured goals from their performance scorecard. Weighting is used to emphasize the importance of certain measures to create a balanced representation of various factors. Ranked tiers of employees can be created from the composite scores.

In practice, many managers and employees are skeptical of the ability for performance evaluations to fairly link objective measures to individual performance (Murphy, 2020). They sense that measuring performance with numbers misses the true contributions of effective employees (Mackenzie et al., 2019). As the adage goes, "Not everything that matters can be measured, and not everything that can be measured matters." Moreover, some performance evaluation processes are inefficient, convoluted, and biased, making managers and employees distrust the process. With this in mind, some organizations have ended traditional performance appraisals in favor of more rigorous goal-setting sessions (Cappelli & Tavis, 2016). Nonetheless, most organizations will continue to conduct performance evaluations because of their potential to improve performance, usefulness in assigning rewards, and the value of creating legal defensibility for employment separations (Schrøder-Hansen & Hansen, 2023).

Delivering Performance Evaluations

Most health services managers deliver written and verbal performance evaluations at least once a year, although experts advise more frequent conversations about expectations, progress, and development (Doheny, 2021). For top performers, giving feedback on performance is essential to keeping them engaged, focused, and motivated. Top performers want to grow professionally, too, so if there areas in which the employee can improve, effective performance evaluations deliver specific information about their behaviors and focus on what the employee can change in the future to reach their full performance potential (Freedman & Elliot, 2021).

> △ **KEY IDEA**
>
> **Accountability can be misunderstood as punishment, which can lead to shame, cover-ups, and a failure to learn.**

For poor performers, evaluations should communicate the expectations for timely resolution of deficiencies and issue clear warnings about accountability and consequences (Cahill & Sedrak, 2012). However, accountability can be misunderstood as punishment, which can lead to shame, cover-ups, and a failure to learn (Murray et al., 2023). If goals are not met, health services managers can take a variety of approaches to ensure accountability for performance without resorting to blame, including the following (Carucci, 2020; O'Hagan & Persaud, 2009; White & Griffith, 2019):

- *Be open about failure:* Failure is a normal part of the learning process and should be acknowledged and discussed openly.
- *Adjust goals:* Failure to achieve goals may inform the need for goal adjustments. Accountability should not be a one-time occurrence but a process of continuous improvement.
- *Make learning the objective:* Neutralize feelings of shame with a growth mindset. Frame failures positively as opportunities for improvement ("OFIs").
- *Encourage experimentation:* New approaches inherently mean a higher risk of failure. Without experimentation, innovation is impossible. Reassure employees that taking risks will not be punished.
- *Recognize effort:* Celebrate progress toward the goal, even if the desired outcome is not fully achieved.
- *Commit resources and support:* To help them overcome challenges, provide training, mentorship, coaching, or other forms of resources that facilitate performance.
- *Creating plans of action:* Conduct thorough analysis of the root causes and develop follow-up recommendations for improvement.

However, if individuals consistently fail to meet expectations despite support and interventions, appropriate actions must be taken. With a focus on fairness and dignity, health services managers have the option to redeploy underperforming employees to parts of the HCO where they can succeed, implement a performance improvement plans that set clear expectations and consequences, or, as a last resort, separate them from employment at the HCO (Carucci, 2020).

CAREER BOX 11.3: Receiving Performance Evaluations

Most managers and employees dislike the performance evaluation process. For high performers, the negative feedback can seem nitpicky. For poor performers, successes may outweigh shortcomings in their minds (Grote, 2011). Either way, health services managers need to receive criticism professionally (Castrillon, 2022; Nawaz, 2019). The following are best practices for accepting criticism productively:

- *Be polite:* Thank the person for giving feedback. Feeling attacked may trigger an involuntary fight-flight-or-freeze response, so be prepared to be gracious.
- *Process the criticism:* Is the criticism valid? If so, set goals to improve. If the deficiencies are long-standing, it may signal that you are not the right fit for position.
- *Do not take it personally:* Criticism relates to your role, not you as a person.
- *Respond in writing:* If the criticism is unwarranted, prepare a written response with specific examples.
- *Schedule a follow-up:* After a bad performance review, set a meeting with the boss to ask clarifying questions.
- *Rely on trusted advisors:* Seek perspective and advice from people you respect.
- *Maintain well-being:* If feedback is particularly painful, depend on self-care techniques that have helped you through difficult times before.

Performance Incentives

Health services managers design and implement performance incentives to recognize achievement, particularly through compensation, as a way to motivate future action. Performance evaluations are used to create **positive reinforcement** through raises, merit pay, promotions, or other **extrinsic rewards** that recognize performance. However, extrinsic rewards can lead employees to game the performance incentive system. For example, financial bonuses for achieving better patient outcomes can lead to selectively admitting healthier patients (Park et al., 2022). Or if rewards are perceived to be unrelated to performance, then employees will accuse health services managers of giving promotions or merit pay unfairly. **Equity theory** suggests that if employees perceive that their effort does not obtain the same rewards as their peers, they may become demotivated and dissatisfied with their job (Adams, 2005). Alternatively, health services employees can also be motivated by **intrinsic rewards**, such as increased autonomy, additional work challenges, and respect from peers (Kao, 2015). The psychological rewards that employees obtain from doing meaningful work and performing it well can be just as important as financial rewards.

FUTURE DIRECTIONS

In large HCOs, thousands of hours are spent defining strategy, setting goals, budgeting key initiatives, and evaluating employee performance. A year or more can pass between the time that strategic objectives are set to when individuals are evaluated for their performance. Unfortunately, external events—global pandemics, competitive pressures, or economic crises—can render even the most thorough performance management system obsolete. In an uncertain environment, health services managers will need to introduce agility and flexibility into performance management systems to accelerate organizational learning (Short & Mammen, 2020). Future performance management systems will generate real-time performance information, which will require substantial investments into technological infrastructure, business intelligence software, and information technology specialists.

SUMMARY

- Performance management is the activity of setting goals, focusing the organization on the highest priority actions, monitoring and evaluating performance, holding individuals and teams accountable, and improving performance through organizational learning.
- Various healthcare stakeholders, including the board of directors, regulators, accreditors, and ranking organizations, monitor the performance of HCOs to foster accountability and motivate improvements.
- Benchmarking is the systematic approach of comparing performance measures collected from successful HCOs. When health services managers identify disparities between their HCO's metrics and the benchmark, they implement best practices intended to improve outcomes.
- The balanced scorecard is a strategic management system that translates an organization's strategy into a balanced set of performance measures within four perspectives: financial, internal business, learning and growth, and customers.
- The balanced scorecard framework can also be used as a management tool that enables health services managers to align strategy to organizational and individual performance.
- Goal setting is the collaborative process of connecting strategic objectives to individual performance with measures that are specific, measurable, assignable, realistic, and time bound.
- Performance dashboards enable health services managers to evaluate progress using interactive, computerized, visual summaries to determine if strategic implementation is working at various levels of the organization.
- Health services managers conduct performance evaluations based on objective standards that are defined in writing and communicated in advance.

END-OF-CHAPTER RESOURCES

KEY TERMS*

*For the full list of key terms, please see the online glossary at **http://connect.springerpub.com/content/book/978-0-8261-4807-0**.

- 360-degree feedback
- accountability
- achievement orientation
- average length of stay
- balanced scorecard
- bed occupancy rate
- benchmarking
- best practices
- cascading
- composite scores
- Consumer Assessment of Healthcare Providers and Systems (CAHPS)
- criterion deficiency
- dashboards
- data warehouse
- efficiency
- effectiveness
- equity theory
- extrinsic rewards
- forced distribution
- full-time equivalents (FTEs)
- goal
- Health Effectiveness Information Data Set (HEDIS)
- hospitalists
- intrinsic rewards
- key performance indicator
- knowledge management
- labor productivity
- Magnet Recognition
- Malcolm Baldridge National Quality Award
- measure
- metric
- morbidity
- mortality
- multidimensional appraisal
- net promoter score
- never events
- operationalization
- paired comparative method
- patient-to-nurse ratio
- payers
- pay for performance
- performance standards
- positive reinforcement
- pre-authorization
- productivity
- rating scale method
- regulators
- relative value unit (RVU)
- risk adjustment
- statistic
- sentinel event
- strategic objective
- The Joint Commission
- negligence
- throughput
- unstructured method
- utilization review
- value-based purchasing

LEARNING ACTIVITIES

Professional Development and Reflection

1. Identify and prioritize your career stakeholders based on their level of influence, their interest, and the potential impact of your career actions or decisions. Based on your priorities, in what ways will you engage your stakeholders to assist you to build your career? See Career Box 11.1.
2. Develop a career balanced scorecard with objectives that you would like to achieve in 3 to 5 years. What perspectives does your career scorecard include? Define at least

one strategic objective for each perspective. For each strategic objective, create a measure and target. Describe at least one action or initiative for each of your career objectives.

Discussion Questions

1. There is debate about whether HCOs should participate in reporting performance metrics to ranking organizations, as the process can distract from strategic priorities, especially patient care. What are the arguments for and against HCO participation in such rankings?
2. Cascading involves breaking down high-level strategic objectives into specific, actionable goals and targets that are relevant to different organizational levels and meaningful to individuals. Why is flexibility and collaboration important when health services managers cascade strategic objectives throughout the HCO?
3. Among the performance evaluations methods discussed in this chapter, which is the fairest way (or combinations of ways) for an instructor to measure student performance in a course? Why? Which method presents the most risk for unconscious bias by the instructor? Why?

RECOMMENDED READING AND MEDIA

Christensen, C. M. (2017). *How will you measure your life?* Harvard Business Review Press.

Covey, S. R. (1989). *The 7 habits of highly effective people.* Simon & Schuster.

Doerr, J. (2018). *Measure what matters: How Google, Bono, and the Gates Foundation rock the world with OKRs.* Portfolio/Penguin.

Few, S. (2013). *Information dashboard design: Displaying data for at-a-glance monitoring.* Analytics Press.

Freedman, A., & Elliott, P. (2021). *Thrive: The leader's guide to building a high-performance culture.* Lioncrest Publishing.

Grote, D. (2011). *How to be good at performance appraisals: Simple, effective, done right.* Harvard Business Review Press.

Kaplan, R. S., & Norton, D. P. (2001). *The strategy-focused organization: How balanced scorecard companies thrive in the new business environment.* Harvard Business School Press.

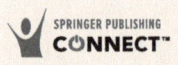

A robust set of instructor resources designed to supplement this text is located at http://connect.springerpub.com/content/book/978-0-8261-4807-0. Qualifying instructors may request access by emailing textbook@springerpub.com.

REFERENCES

Adams, J. S. (2005). Equity theory. In J. B. Miner (Ed.), *Organizational behavior 1: Essential theories of motivation and leadership* (pp. 134–159). M. E. Sharpe.

Agency for Healthcare Research and Quality. (2023). *CAHPS patient experience surveys and guidance.* Agency for Healthcare Research and Quality. https://www.ahrq.gov/cahps/surveys-guidance/index.html

Agovino, T. (2023, March 15). *The performance review problem.* SHRM. https://www.shrm.org/hr-today/news/hr-magazine/spring-2023/pages/the-problem-with-performance-reviews.aspx

Amer, F., Hammoud, S., Khatatbeh, H., Lohner, S., Boncz, I., & Endrei, D. (2022). A systematic review: The dimensions to evaluate health care performance and an implication during the pandemic. *BMC Health Services Research, 22*(1), 621. https://doi.org/10.1186/s12913-022-07863-0

American Medical Association. (2023). *Relative value units*. CPT® International. https://cpt-international.ama-assn.org/relative-value-units

American Nurses Credentialing Center. (2017, October 14). *Organizational programs*. https://www.nursingworld.org/organizational-programs

Aungsuroch, Y., Gunawan, J., & Fisher, M. L. (2021). Performance appraisal. In *Redesigning the nursing and human resource partnership: A model for the new normal era* (pp. 69–79). Springer Singapore.

Bandura, A. (1997). *Self-efficacy: The exercise of control*. W. H. Freeman and Company.

Beaudin-Seiler, B. M., & Fogarty, K. (2016). Quality in healthcare and national quality awards. *American Journal of Accountable Care, 4*(4), 26–32.

Berger, S. (2005). *The power of clinical and financial metrics: Achieving success in your hospital*. Health Administration Press.

Brar, S., Hopkins, M., & Margolius, D. (2019). Time to next available appointment as an access to care metric. *Joint Commission Journal on Quality and Patient Safety, 45*(11), 779–780. https://doi.org/10.1016/j.jcjq.2019.07.007

Burlea-Schiopoiu, A., & Ferhati, K. (2021). The managerial implications of the key performance indicators in healthcare sector: A cluster analysis. *Healthcare, 9*(1), 19. https://doi.org/10.3390/healthcare9010019

Buttigieg, S. C., Pace, A., & Rathert, C. (2017). Hospital performance dashboards: A literature review. *Journal of Health Organization and Management, 31*(3), 385–406. https://doi.org/10.1108/jhom-04-2017-0088

Cahill, T. F., & Sedrak, M. (2012). Leading a multigenerational workforce: Strategies for attracting and retaining millennials. *Frontiers of Health Services Management, 29*(1), 3–15. http://doi.org/10.1097/01974520-201207000-00002

Cappelli, P., & Tavis, A. (2016). The performance management revolution. *Harvard Business Review*. https://hbr.org/2016/10/the-performance-management-revolution

Carucci, R. (2020, November 23). How to actually encourage employee accountability. *Harvard Business Review*. https://hbr.org/2020/11/how-to-actually-encourage-employee-accountability

Castrillon, C. (2022, December 7). 5 steps to deal with a bad performance review. *Forbes*. https://www.forbes.com/sites/carolinecastrillon/2022/12/07/5-steps-to-deal-with-a-bad-performance-review

Centers for Medicare and Medicaid. (2022, April 14). *Quality measures*. https://www.cms.gov/medicare/quality-initiatives-patient-assessment-instruments/qualitymeasures

Covey, S. R. (1989). *The 7 habits of highly effective people*. Simon & Schuster.

Dalton, J. E., Glance, L. G., Mascha, E. J., Ehrlinger, J., Chamoun, N., & Sessler, D. I. (2013). Impact of present-on-admission indicators on risk-adjusted hospital mortality measurement. *Anesthesiology, 118*(6), 1298–1306. https://doi.org/10.1097/aln.0b013e31828e12b3

Doerr, J. (2018). *Measure what matters: How Google, Bono, and the Gates Foundation rock the world with OKRs*. Portfolio/Penguin.

Doheny, K. (2021, January 12). *Annual performance review bows out*. SHRM. https://www.shrm.org/resourcesandtools/hr-topics/people-managers/pages/ditching-the-annual-performance-review-.aspx

Doran, G. T. (1981). There's a S.M.A.R.T. way to write management's goals and objectives. *Management Review, 70*(11), 35–36.

Ellis, J. (2006). All inclusive benchmarking. *Journal of Nursing Management, 14*(5), 377–383. http://doi.org/10.1111/j.1365-2934.2006.00596.x

El Morr, C., & Ali-Hassan, H. (2019). Healthcare, data analytics, and business intelligence: A practical introduction. In *Analytics in healthcare* (pp. 1–13). http://doi.org/10.1007/978-3-030-04506-7_1

Emanuel, E. J., Glickman, A., & Johnson, D. (2017). Measuring the burden of health care costs on US families: The affordability index. *JAMA, 318*(19), 1863–1864. https://doi.org/10.1001/jama.2017.15686

Erwin, C. O., Landry, A. Y., Livingston, A. C., & Dias, A. (2019). Effective governance and hospital boards revisited: Reflections on 25 years of research. *Medical Care Research and Review, 76*(2), 131–166. https://doi.org/10.1177/1077558718754898

Few, S. (2013). *Information dashboard design: Displaying data for at-a-glance monitoring*. Analytics Press.

Freedman, A., & Elliott, P. (2021). *Thrive: The leader's guide to building a high-performance culture*. Lioncrest Publishing.

Glance, L. G., Thirukumaran, C. P., Li, Y., Gao, S., & Dick, A. W. (2020). Improving the accuracy of hospital quality ratings by focusing on the association between volume and outcome: Analysis of using "shrinkage targets" to more accurately classify hospital quality ratings from the Centers for Medicare and Medicaid Services. *Health Affairs, 39*(5), 862–870. http://doi.org/10.1377/hlthaff.2019.00778

Groene, O., Brandt, E., Schmidt, W., & Moeller, J. (2009). The Balanced Scorecard of acute settings: Development process, definition of 20 strategic objectives and implementation. *International Journal for Quality in Health Care, 21*(4), 259–271. https://doi.org/10.1093/intqhc/mzp024

Grote, D. (2011). *How to be good at performance appraisals: Simple, effective, done right*. Harvard Business Review Press.

Gurd, B., & Gao, T. (2007). Lives in the balance: An analysis of the balanced scorecard (BSC) in healthcare organizations. *International Journal of Productivity and Performance Management, 57*(1), 6–21. http://doi.org/10.1108/17410400810841209

Hadden, K., Gardner, S., & Patterson, C. (2022). From strategic planning to strategy impact. *NEJM Catalyst Innovations in Care Delivery, 3*(1). http://doi.org/10.1056/CAT.21.0323

Hildred, K., Piteira, M., Cervai, S., & Pinto, J. C. (2023). Objective and subjective career success: Individual, structural, and behavioral determinants on European hybrid workers. *Frontiers in Psychology, 14*, 1161015. http://doi.org/10.3389/fpsyg.2023.1161015

Kao, A. C. (2015). Driven to care: Aligning external motivators with intrinsic motivation. *Health Services Research, 50*(Suppl 2), 2216–2222. https://doi.org/10.1111%2F1475-6773.12422

Kaplan, R. S., & Norton, D. P. (1992, January-February). The balanced scorecard: Measures that drive performance. *Harvard Business Review*. https://hbr.org/1992/01/the-balanced-scorecard-measures-that-drive-performance-2

Kaplan, R. S., & Norton, D. P. (1996). *The strategy-focused organization: How balanced scorecard companies thrive in the new business environment*. Harvard Business School Press.

Kaplan, R. S., & Norton, D. P. (2007). Using the balanced scorecard as a strategic management system. *Harvard Business Review*. https://hbr.org/2007/07/using-the-balanced-scorecard-as-a-strategic-management-system

Karim, S. A., Pink, G. H., Reiter, K. L., Holmes, G. M., Jones, C. B., & Woodard, E. K. (2018). The effect of the magnet recognition signal on hospital financial performance. *Journal of Healthcare Management, 63*(6), e131–e146. https://doi.org/10.1097/jhm-d-17-00215

Kfuri, A., Davis, N. L., & Giardino, A. P. (2021). External quality improvement: Accreditation, certification, and education. In *Medical quality management: Theory and practice* (pp. 245–281). Springer Publishing Company. http://doi.org/10.1007/978-3-030-48080-6

Khalifa, M., & Khalid, P. (2015). Developing strategic health care key performance indicators: A case study on a tertiary care hospital. *Procedia Computer Science, 63*, 459–466. http://doi.org/10.1016/j.procs.2015.08.368

Lantz, P. M. (2019). The medicalization of population health: Who will stay upstream?. *The Milbank Quarterly, 97*(1), 36–39. https://doi.org/10.1111%2F1468-0009.12363

Latham, G. P., & Locke, E. A. (2007). New developments in and directions for goal-setting research. *European Psychologist, 12*(4), 290–300. http://doi.org/10.1027/1016-9040.12.4.290

Leape, L. L. (2021). *Making healthcare safe: The story of the patient safety movement*. Springer Nature.

Leong, M. Q., Lim, C. W., & Lai, Y. F. (2021). Comparison of Hospital-at-Home models: A systematic review of reviews. *BMJ Open, 11*(1), e043285. https://doi.org/10.1136/bmjopen-2020-043285

Mackenzie, L. N., Wehner, J., & Correll, S. J. (2019, January 11). Why most performance evaluations are biased, and how to fix them. *Harvard Business Review*. https://hbr.org/2019/01/why-most-performance-evaluations-are-biased-and-how-to-fix-them

McGrath, S. K., & Whitty, S. J. (2018). Accountability and responsibility defined. *International Journal of Managing Projects in Business, 11*(3), 687–707. http://doi.org/10.1108/IJMPB-06-2017-0058

Metcalfe, D., Diaz, A. J. R., Olufajo, O. A., Massa, M. S., Ketelaar, N. A., Flottorp, S. A., & Perry, D. C. (2018). Impact of public release of performance data on the behaviour of healthcare consumers and providers. *Cochrane Database of Systematic Reviews,* (9). https://doi.org/10.1002/14651858.cd004538.pub3

Moffatt, F., Martin, P., & Timmons, S. (2014). Constructing notions of healthcare productivity: The call for a new professionalism?. *Sociology of Health & Illness, 36*(5), 686–702. https://doi.org/10.1111/1467-9566.12093

Monahan, A. B., & Schwarcz, D. (2021). Rules of medical necessity. *Iowa Law Review, 107,* 423.

Murray, J. S., Lee, J., Larson, S., Range, A., Scott, D., & Clifford, J. (2023). Requirements for implementing a 'just culture' within healthcare organisations: An integrative review. *BMJ Open Quality, 12*(2), e002237. https://doi.org/10.1136%2Fbmjoq-2022-002237

Murphy, K. R. (2020). Performance evaluation will not die, but it should. *Human Resource Management Journal, 30*(1), 13–31. https://doi.org/10.1111/1748-8583.12259

National Center for Healthcare Leadership. (2018). *Health Leadership Competency Model 3.0.* https://nchl.member365.org/publicFr/store/item/19

National Center for Quality Assurance. (2023, October 26). *HEDIS users group (HUG).* https://www.ncqa.org/hedis/hedis-users-group-hug

Nawaz, S. (2019, April 2). How to take criticism well. *Harvard Business Review.* https://hbr.org/2019/04/how-to-take-criticism-well

Ogbeiwi, O. (2021). General concepts of goals and goal-setting in healthcare: A narrative review. *Journal of Management & Organization, 27*(2), 324–341. http://doi.org/10.1017/jmo.2018.11

O'Hagan, J., & Persaud, D. (2009). Creating a culture of accountability in health care. *The Health Care Manager, 28*(2), 124–133. https://doi.org/10.1097/hcm.0b013e3181a2eb2b

Otley, D. (1999). Performance management: A framework for management control systems research. *Management Accounting Research, 10*(4), 363–382. http://doi.org/10.1006/mare.1999.0115

Park, T. Y., Park, S., & Barry, B. (2022). Incentive effects on ethics. *Academy of Management Annals, 16*(1), 297–333. http://doi.org/10.5465/annals.2020.0251

Perlow, L. A. (2017, July–August). Stop the meeting madness. *Harvard Business Review.* https://hbr.org/2017/07/stop-the-meeting-madness

Plott, C. F., Thornton, R. L., Dankwa-Mullan, I., Punwani, E., Karunakaram, H., Rhee, K., Craig, K. J. T., & Sharfstein, J. M. (2021). *New hospital rankings assess hospitals' contributions to community health with a focus on equity.* Health Affairs Forefront. https://www.healthaffairs.org/content/forefront/new-hospital-rankings-assess-hospitals-contributions-community-health-focus-equity

Powers, B. W., Navathe, A. S., Chaguturu, S. K., Ferris, T. G., & Torchiana, D. F. (2017). Aligning incentives for value: The internal performance framework at Partners HealthCare. *HealthCare, 5*(3), 141–149. https://doi.org/10.1016/j.hjdsi.2016.04.007

Priore, R. J. (2021). *Improving financial and operations performance: A healthcare leader's guide.* Springer Publishing Company.

Schrøder-Hansen, K., & Hansen, A. (2022). Performance management trends: Reflections on the redesigns big companies have been doing lately. *International Journal of Productivity and Performance Management, 72*(5), 1201–1220. http://doi.org/10.1108/IJPPM-07-2021-0391

Serna, L. R., Nakandala, D., & Bowyer, D. (2022). Stakeholder identification and prioritization: The attribute of dependency. *Journal of Business Research, 148,* 444–455. https://doi.org/10.1016/j.jbusres.2022.04.062

Short, J. B., & Mammen, A. (2020). A pandemic application of creative destruction in healthcare. *Frontiers of Health Services Management, 37*(1), 4–9. https://doi.org/10.1097/hap.0000000000000093

Stanowski, A. C., Simpson, K., & White, A. (2015). Pay for performance: Are hospitals becoming more efficient in improving their patient experience?. *Journal of Healthcare Management, 60*(4), 268–284. http://doi.org/10.1097/00115514-201507000-00008

Svrluga, S. (2023, June 26). Penn Medicine quits cooperating with U.S. News hospitals ranking. *Washington Post.* https://www.washingtonpost.com/education/2023/06/26/penn-med-usnews-rankings

Thomas Craig, K. J., McKillop, M. M., Huang, H. T., George, J., Punwani, E. S., & Rhee, K. B. (2020). US hospital performance methodologies: A scoping review to identify opportunities for crossing the quality chasm. *BMC Health Services Research, 20*(1), 1–13. https://doi.org/10.1186/s12913-020-05503-z

Tsai, T. C., Jha, A. K., Gawande, A. A., Huckman, R. S., Bloom, N., & Sadun, R. (2015). Hospital board and management practices are strongly related to hospital performance on clinical quality metrics. *Health Affairs, 34*(8), 1304–1311. https://doi.org/10.1377/hlthaff.2014.1282

White, K. R., & Griffith, J. R. (2019). Foundations of well-managed healthcare organizations. In *The well-managed healthcare organization* (9th ed., pp. 3–33). Health Administration Press.

Yang, G. (2022). The construction of nursing performance evaluation model in community health service center based on the balanced scorecard and hygiene factors. *Nature Scientific Reports, 12*(1), 21793. http://doi.org/10.1038/s41598-022-26334-4

CHAPTER 12

HEALTHCARE QUALITY MANAGEMENT

Healthcare quality management consists of practices designed to deliver high-quality and safe care expected by patients, their families, and their caregivers.

COMPETENCIES

- Elevate quality improvement as a strategic priority for health care organizations.
- Promote organizational cultures that deliver high-quality and safety health care.
- Track, analyze, and report quality measures in compliance with national quality initiatives and accreditation standards.
- Implement risk management programs to provide safe and healthy work environments.
- Analyze business and clinical processes to improve efficiency and effectiveness.
- Prioritize patient experience as vital to patient care and organizational success.
- Apply quality management methodologies and tools to quality improvement initiatives.

CHAPTER OUTLINE

- Healthcare Quality Organization
- Quality and Safety Culture
- Quality Measurement and Improvement
- Quality Management Methodologies

INTRODUCTION

In certain respects, the United States healthcare system is widely admired, especially when clinicians save gravely ill patients with highly technical medical care (Sawyer & McDermott, 2019). And yet, the U.S. healthcare system is the most expensive in the world—nearly twice as much money per person than average—and suffers from frustrations, inefficiencies, and inequities (Shortell et al., 2023). The U.S. healthcare system ranks below other economically prosperous countries in many measures of healthcare system quality, such as lifespan, chronic disease prevalence, and maternal mortality (Schneider et al., 2021). Altogether, Americans do not receive the quality of care one would expect from spending such enormous sums of money.

The Institute of Medicine (IOM) defines **quality of care** as the "degree to which health services for individuals and populations increase the likelihood of desired health outcomes and are consistent with current professional knowledge" (Donaldson et al., 2000, p. 211). While the IOM's definition is widely cited, it is missing a key concept of quality known as **reliability**. Unreliable health services delivery harms patients, confuses processes, and makes high-quality care almost impossible (D'Avena et al., 2020). In addition, just because care is safe, it does not mean that it is high quality. Unreliable health care processes lead to frustrating delays, poor outcomes, and a stressful care environment. To successfully create reliable care, health services managers accept accountability for quality and safety. **Healthcare quality management** is the application of systematic management practices that support the delivery of reliable medical care in health care organizations (HCOs). In this chapter, we describe how health services managers combine fundamental management skills with quality improvement methodologies to build strong organizational cultures capable of solving a variety of healthcare quality challenges.

HEALTHCARE QUALITY ORGANIZATION

Health Services Managers

Most health services managers choose to build their careers in general management roles, running health care businesses of various types. Even in their capacity as general managers, healthcare quality management is a fundamental professional responsibility. For health services managers, their role in healthcare quality management fits the classical conception of management described in Chapter 1 (Fayol, 1916).

- *Planning:* Develop quality improvement plans. Collaborate with clinicians to create quality goals. Select and track quality, safety, and patient experience measures. Allocate resources to quality improvement projects with resources.
- *Organizing:* Organize personnel and other resources to execute improvement activities. Create quality improvement teams with complementary roles in various areas of expertise, such as clinicians, analysts, and others. Delegate authority for implementing solutions.
- *Commanding/directing:* Establish accountability for performance. Give clear instructions for action. Create ongoing training programs.
- *Coordinating:* Facilitate quality improvement collaboration among different teams. Share quality improvement knowledge throughout the organization. Mediate conflict within and among quality improvement teams.
- *Controlling:* Monitor and evaluate performance improvement. Continuously seek ways to improve quality, safety, and patient experience. Track performance against plans through management processes, such as budgeting and performance evaluations.

Some health services managers choose to specialize in healthcare quality management for their careers. Specialized careers in healthcare quality management usually require relevant certifications, such as the Certified Professional in Healthcare Quality (CPHQ) or Lean Sigma expert designations (Indeed Editorial Team, 2023). Specialists can also earn graduate degrees in healthcare quality management. The Commission on Accreditation of Healthcare Management Education (CAHME) accredits graduate programs in quality and safety, such as a Master of Science in Healthcare Quality and Safety, in addition to health administration education programs (CAHME, 2024).

INFORMATIONAL INTERVIEW 12.1

Performance Improvement Coordinator

Access the informational interview online at http://connect.springerpub.com/content/book/978-0-8261-4807-0/chapter/ch00.

Board of Directors

Boards of directors align HCO strategy with quality and safety goals, including mortality rates, medication errors, and patient experience scores (Jalilvand et al., 2024). To help achieve these goals, they approve budgets for quality and safety initiatives that are then implemented by health services managers (Erwin et al., 2019). Boards establish governance committees to review quality and safety goals and mandate performance improvement plans, when necessary (Austin et al., 2017). High-performing HCO boards track quality of care measures with the same level of intensity as financial metrics and hold clinicians and health services managers accountable for performance (Tsai et al., 2015).

Clinicians

Within their respective professions, clinicians hold each other accountable for quality and safety. **Peer review** is the formal HCO process by which physicians examine the medical care practices of each other. Under state law, physicians and other eligible clinicians are governed by medical staff bylaws that establish fair processes for peer reviews, especially in instances of medical errors, patient complaints, or concerns raised by colleagues (Paterick et al., 2020). Peer review committees examine medical records, clinical decisions, and patient outcomes related to the case, and when appropriate, committees offer clinicians constructive criticisms, training recommendations, or suggestions for practice changes. Punitive results of peer reviews can be appealed by clinicians, according to medical staff bylaws.

> **CAREER BOX 12.1: Specialized Certifications**
>
> Professional certifications can demonstrate to hiring managers that you possess specialized skills and requisite knowledge. In healthcare quality management, you can earn a variety of certifications, such as CPHQ and Certified Professional in Patient Safety (CPPS), both offered by the National Association for Healthcare Quality, or Certified Professional in Health Care Risk Management (CPHRM), offered by the American Hospital Association (Pelletier, & Beaudin, 2017). Lean Six Sigma certifications use belts as the designations, such as yellow belt (basic understanding), green belt (small-scale improvement projects), or black belt (large-scale improvement projects). A master black belt certification indicates that a person is a Lean Six Sigma expert who is qualified to lead other belts within an organization.

Quality Improvement Teams

Health services managers commit resources to hire, train, and support multidisciplinary healthcare quality management teams (Rosen et al., 2018). Quality improvement teams in HCOs usually include up to eight people from all areas affected by the proposed improvement (Silver et al., 2016). Healthcare quality improvement specialists, usually professionals with advanced training and certifications, act as facilitators, project managers, and data analysts for many different project teams throughout the HCO (Godfrey et al., 2014). The cross-functional quality improvement teams may include a variety of HCO employee representatives, as described in Table 12.1 (Agency for Healthcare Research and Quality (AHRQ), 2013; Austin et al., 2017; Institute for Healthcare Improvement (IHI), 2024; Silver et al., 2016).

TABLE 12.1 Other Members of Cross-Functional Quality Improvement Teams

ROLE	DESCRIPTION	QUESTIONS ASKED
PROJECT SPONSOR OR CHAMPION	A senior-level health services manager with executive authority who can allocate time and resources to projects and align improvement projects with strategic goals of the organization	What are the highest priority issues? What resources are needed?
TEAM LEAD	An individual who is part of the process that needs to be improved. This person is responsible for managing the quality improvement project and continues to maintain improvements when the project is completed.	What is the problem to be solved? What will fix the issue? How will we sustain improvement?
CLINICAL LEADER	A clinical expert or someone with enough organizational authority to implement quality management interventions consistent with evidence-based recommendations.	What does the patient need? What evidence supports the interventions?
TECHNICAL OR ANALYTICAL EXPERT	Unique knowledge or capability is often required for improvement. The SME can be clinical or nonclinical.	What do the data mean? What are the details involved?
FRONTLINE STAFF	Individuals who have knowledge of the process that is being improved from firsthand experience.	What are the root causes of the problem? What does not work?

SME, subject matter expert.

Risk Management Professionals

In addition to the aforementioned quality improvement team members, most HCOs create units of risk management professionals who are in charge of reporting and addressing serious clinical **adverse events** (Niv & Tal, 2024). Adverse events are preventable physical injuries resulting from medical care, such as patient falls, medication errors, pressure ulcers, or delays in providing necessary medical treatment (AHRQ, 2019b). **Risk management** is the process of proactively identifying, assessing, prioritizing, and mitigating risks in HCOs. Risk management professionals manage risk reduction training, handle malpractice and insurance issues, lead disaster preparedness efforts, and initiate workplace safety initiatives. They are also responsible for developing organizational risk management plans and reviewing outcomes of interventions. HCO risk management professionals are often credentialed with CPHRM (Costello & Huben-Kearney, 2023).

> **△ KEY IDEA**
>
> Risk management professionals manage risk reduction training, handle malpractice and insurance issues, lead disaster preparedness efforts, and lead workplace safety initiatives.

TABLE 12.2 Examples of Administrative and Clinical Support Services Participating on Quality Improvement Teams

ROLE	DESCRIPTION	EXAMPLE PROJECTS
EVS	Clean and sanitize patient rooms, operating rooms, exam rooms, waiting areas, bathrooms, and other areas of the HCO	Fall prevention; room turnover efficiency
PATIENT TRANSPORT	Transport patients between areas of the hospital, such as from their rooms to diagnostic treatment areas	Reduce transport time of patients
FOOD SERVICES	Prepares and delivers meals to patients according to their dietary requirements and medical conditions	Revamp menu to improve nutritional value
SECURITY	Maintains secure environment within the HCO, including visitor management and emergency response	Reduce racial disparities in involuntary sedation in the emergency department
PATIENT FINANCIAL SERVICES	Operates the financial aspects related to patient care, including billing and patient account management	Reduce patient distress associated with medical debt

EVS, environmental services; HCO, health care organization.

Administrative and Clinical Support Services

Clinicians are not the only frontline employees in HCOs responsible for improving healthcare quality and enhancing patient experience. Administrative and clinical support staff of all types also participate on healthcare quality management teams. Table 12.2 provides examples of administrative and clinical support services functions that are included in quality improvement projects (Mantasas, 2021; Southerland et al., 2024; Thom et al., 2023; Wilandh et al., 2024).

Patient and Family Involvement in Quality

When assembling the quality improvement team, health services managers can invite patients and their families to participate in multiple projects (Bombard et al., 2018). Patients, families, and informal caregivers identify problems and make suggestions for improving or redesigning health services delivery. Some patients are provided quality improvement training that helps clarify their responsibilities and expectations for contributions on the teams (Vanstone et al., 2023). More than technical skills, patients are valued for their points of view (Bergerum et al., 2020).

△ KEY IDEA
Patients are valued for their points of view, which helps HCOs improve quality, safety, and patient experiences.

External Quality and Safety Stakeholders

In addition to internal stakeholders, a variety of national organizations set expectations for improving healthcare quality and safety in HCOs. Since at least the early 1980s, various national quality initiatives have pushed health services managers to adopt quality and safety as strategic priorities for their HCOs (Marjoua & Bozic, 2012). Despite some initial resistance from the health services management profession, significant investments in quality and safety programs have been made by HCOs over the decades (Stiles & Mick, 1994).

Several important nongovernmental, not-for-profit organizations establish health care quality and safety standards for the U.S. healthcare sector. For example, **The Joint Commission** seeks to improve quality of care and reduce medical errors through accreditation, auditing more than 250 quality and safety standards in thousands of HCOs nationwide (The Joint Commission, 2024). HCOs that fail to meet these standards can potentially lose federal funding and state licenses to deliver health care services (Ibrahim et al., 2022). The **National Committee for Quality Assurance (NCQA)** is another not-for-profit organization that develops quality measures, sets performance standards, and accredits HCO programs (NCQA, 2023). The **Institute for Healthcare Improvement (IHI)** is a nonprofit organization that focuses on improving healthcare through various initiatives, such as the **Triple Aim** framework that calls for improving patient experience, population health, and reducing costs (Whittington et al, 2015).

The federal government, through the **Centers for Medicare & Medicaid Services (CMS)**, has established numerous national quality initiatives, many of which were introduced since the passage of the Patient Protection and Affordable Care Act of 2010 (CMS, 2023c). CMS runs the national Medicare program that insures 66 million eligible beneficiaries, most of whom are 65 years of age and older (CMS, 2023b). Due to its size and national scope, Medicare quality initiatives greatly impact strategies and operations of HCOs. The following national quality initiatives influence HCO investments in healthcare quality management practices for their HCOs (CMS, 2023c; Hayford & Maeda, 2017):

- *Hospital-Acquired Condition Reduction Program:* Reduces Medicare payments for hospitals with the highest rates of preventable conditions, such as hospital-acquired infections and patient falls
- *Hospital Readmissions Reduction Program (HRRP):* Penalizes hospitals with higher-than-expected readmission rates for certain conditions, such as heart failure, pneumonia, and acute myocardial infarction
- *Medicare Hospital Compare:* The consumer-oriented website allows users to compare hospitals using measures of quality, safety, and patient experience. Hospitals are assigned star ratings based on their performance.
- *Medicare Shared Savings Program (MSSP):* Encourages the formation of accountable care organizations (ACOs), HCOs that share in any cost savings achieved when meeting quality benchmarks
- *Merit-Based Incentive Payment System (MIPS):* Assigns performance scores to eligible physician practices based on reported quality and cost-efficient care measures. MIPS final scores determine positive, neutral, or negative payment adjustments to Medicare Part B physician fees.

QUALITY AND SAFETY CULTURE

Promoting Quality and Safety Culture

Health services managers influence the extent to which HCO cultures embrace the practices associated with high-quality and safe care (Radcliffe et al., 2020). An **organizational culture** comprises the attitudes, norms, and perceptions of employees (Murray et al., 2024). Communication problems, resistance to change, lack of time, and lack of resources all work against creating cultures of quality and safety (Blok et al., 2022). These challenges can be exacerbated by health services managers who act in ways that harm organizational cultures. These negative actions make healthcare quality management practices especially difficult, including the following (Bailey & Madden, 2017):

- *Depriving people of their purpose:* If HCO personnel lack clarity and unity of purpose, then people will not cooperate to improve quality and safety initiatives.
- *Assigning pointless work:* Giving employees unnecessary activities that are not directly related to their core purpose saps their time and energy.
- *Risking employees' physical or emotional harm:* Unnecessary risks, such as being left alone with aggressive patients, undermine quality and safety culture.
- *Overruling professionals' better judgment:* Professionals are guided by expertise and driven by autonomy. Undercutting either will demotivate and frustrate employees.

Instead, health services managers who support organizational culture provide the frontline employees and clinicians with resources to create multidisciplinary performance improvement teams (Begun, White & Mosser, 2011). When unproductive disagreements occur, health services managers encourage quality improvement teams to resolve their differences (Garman et al., 2006).

△ KEY IDEA

Health services managers encourage all employees—especially those at the bedside—to find ways to improve quality and safety and empower people to make quality and safety a part of their work responsibilities.

Empowering Self-Reliance and Responsibility

Frontline clinicians and staff are most likely to discover quality and safety issues in their daily workflows. Health services managers encourage all employees—especially those at the bedside—to find ways to improve quality and safety and empower people to make quality and safety a part of their work responsibilities (AHRQ, 2019a). Empowering actions include the following (American Medical Association [AMA], 2019; Berwick et al., 2017; Desveaux, & Ivers, 2024; Kunnen et al., 2023):

- *Reinforce purpose:* Link safety and quality improvement to meaningfulness of people's roles in the HCO. Consistently communicate organizational mission, vision, and values.
- *Empower improvement:* Assign responsibility to frontline staff for identifying needed change and initiating quality and safety improvement projects.
- *Encourage action:* The people who experience quality and safety problems should be encouraged to fix it when and where it occurs.
- *Destigmatize failure:* Improvement initiatives may not work the first time. Celebrate unsuccessful projects as opportunities to learn.
- *Get rid of stupid stuff:* Ask people to nominate any process they think is poorly designed, unnecessary, or prone to errors. Find opportunities to cut unproductive work. Fully examine processes and remove unnecessary steps.

Health services managers should be open to improving processes, even the ones that they once implemented or supported. This requires health services managers to downplay organizational hierarchy in favor of improving quality and safety in their HCOs. Just because health services managers have authority over a department, they may not be the person with greatest knowledge of a situation that needs improvement. Deference to clinicians, whether entry-level patient care technicians or highly esteemed physicians, is necessary for effective healthcare quality management. In other words, health services managers need to possess enough humility to listen when frontline employees recommend better and safer ways of working.

> ⚠ **KEY IDEA**
>
> **Health services managers need to possess enough humility to listen when frontline employees recommend better and safer ways of working.**

A Just Culture

Patient quality and safety problems can rarely be blamed on people; errors are usually the result of bad systems. As healthcare safety expert Lucian Leape said, "People are not bad when they make errors, . . . [b]ut there may be bad systems, and those systems cause the errors" (Medical Mistakes, 1999, p. 70). This means that punishing people for system failure will not improve quality and safety. In fact, HCOs that blame and punish people for errors create cultures of fear, which makes quality improvement impossible (Boysen, 2013). This does not mean that actions associated with impairment, incompetence, or maliciousness should be excused; accountability is a critical component of a just culture (Wachter, 2013). Blaming employees just delays quality improvement interventions that would prevent errors in the future (Adelman, 2019).

> **CAREER BOX 12.2:** A Purposeful Career
>
> Health services management careers can be stressful, and those who succeed learn to cope with adversity and recover quickly from setbacks. One way to increase your career resilience is to foster a sense of career purpose (Kolaski & Taylor, 2019). When you are able to create meaning from work, you are less likely to experience fatigue, insomnia, illness, and depression related to your career. Many successful health services managers view their work as personally meaningful and as serving a greater purpose, which helps them to maintain optimism in the face of challenges. Meaning in health services management careers, such as helping patients, can be nurtured as defense against career burnout (Bailey & Madden, 2017).

Instead of blaming people, health services managers instill what quality and safety experts call a **just culture**, in which people are unafraid to escalate problems or concerns (Walsh, 2019). Health services managers can establish processes for employees to report **near misses**, which are when mistakes or adverse events are caught before they happened, either by chance or intervention. In a just culture, systems for reporting near misses create opportunities for people to express opinions freely and learn from each other, without fear of blame or retaliation (Shah, 2021). When near misses are reported, risk managers and quality improvement teams can investigate the root causes and implement interventions that avoid those errors in the future (Cochrane et al., 2017).

> **INFORMATIONAL INTERVIEW 12.2**
> *Performance Program Manager*
> Access the informational interview online at http://connect.springerpub.com/content/book/978-0-8261-4807-0/chapter/ch00.

QUALITY MEASUREMENT AND IMPROVEMENT

Quality Measurement

For healthcare quality to be improved, it must be measured. However, quality is a conceptual term that can mean different things to different people. Quality needs to be quantified through empirically precise definitions so they can be calculated objectively. For example, mortality measures whether a patient lived or died, which is objective and measurable. However, to be useful as a quality measure, the specific parameters need to be established, such as which particular group of patients (e.g., inpatient admissions), the time period for assessment (e.g., during hospital stay and within 30 days of discharge), and the measurement period (e.g., annually from January through December). By providing clear definitions, health services managers can track whether quality improvement interventions are successful.

Avedis Donabedian created the first conceptual framework for measuring health care quality in the 1960s that is still used today (Donabedian, 1966). Donabedian's contribution to healthcare quality measurement was a shift away from solely focusing on health outcomes, such as mortality and morbidity, to concentrate on the processes and structures of health services delivery (Donabedian, 1966). Within three domains, hundreds of measures have been adopted by HCOs for quality improvement and accountability applications. Table 12.3 provides examples of measures within Donabedian's healthcare quality measurement domains (AHRQ, 2019b).

Measurement is necessary but not sufficient for quality improvement; healthcare quality management practices must include interventions. The following sections present patient safety, workplace safety, access to care, and patient experience measures and examples of interventions designed to improve them.

Patient Safety

Patient safety is a quality management category that concentrates on mitigating the risk of harm to patients due to accidental injury. To deliver safe care, health services managers and clinicians

TABLE 12.3 Donabedian's Healthcare Quality Measurement Domains

DOMAIN	SUMMARY	DEFINITION	EXAMPLE MEASURES
STRUCTURE	How care is organized	Settings, qualifications, and administrative systems of care	Nurse-to-patient ratio; percent of staff trained on self-disclosure of adverse events
PROCESS	What is done to the patient	Clinical actions performed to maintain or improve patient health	Percentage of patients with asthma prescribed controller medications; Percentage waiting more than 2 days for sick visit appointments
OUTCOMES	What happens to the patient	Impact of health services delivery on the health status, well-being, and satisfaction of patients or populations	30-day mortality rate; ADL

ADL, activities of daily living.

create operational processes that minimize the likelihood of errors and maximize the likelihood of catching them when they happen. Patient safety improvement initiatives have made significant progress in some areas, such as reduced adverse drug events and healthcare-acquired infections (Eldridge et al., 2022). However, patients in the United States still experience preventable safety events. Studies show that for every 100 patients admitted to a hospital, one patient experiences at least one preventable severe or fatal adverse event (Bates et al., 2023; Panagioti et al., 2019). According to the report published by the IOM in 2000, at least 44,000 annual deaths could be attributed to preventable medical errors (IOM, 2000). Despite making health care safer, the risk of death associated with health care services is still too high (Shortell et al, 2023). In 2016, as many people died from medical errors as from diabetes, a disease that causes the seventh highest number of deaths in the United States (Centers for Disease Control [CDC], 2017; Sunshine et al., 2019).

Table 12.4 provides example patient safety measures and interventions (AHRQ, 2019c; CMS, 2023a; Marshall et al., 2022; Meese et al., 2022; Olson et al., 2018).

A systematic approach used to identify and prioritize potential patient safety errors is called the **failure mode and effects analysis (FMEA)** (Liu et al., 2020). FMEA involves analyzing each potential error, determining its likelihood of occurrence, severity of impact, and detectability. The best way to conduct an FMEA is to assemble a team with knowledge about the process, how

TABLE 12.4 Example Patient Safety Measures and Interventions

MEASURE	DEFINITION	EXAMPLE INTERVENTIONS
ADE	Unintended and harmful events associated with medications	Implement electronic prescribing systems with built-in clinical decision support tools
CAUTI	An infection specifically associated with urinary catheterization that patients acquire while receiving medical treatment within an HCO	Proper hand hygiene and sterile technique during catheter insertion
PATIENT FALLS	Number of admissions (patients) who experience a fall	Bed alarms that alert personnel when patients at risk for falls attempt to leave their beds without assistance
SSI	Percentage of adult patients who had an SSI; an adverse surgical outcome, which is often a preventable cause of harm	Prophylactic intravenous antibiotics
UDES	Missed opportunities for earlier diagnosis, lack of timely diagnosis that is likely to have a positive effect on a patient's health for conditions prone to diagnostic error, such as sepsis or colorectal cancer	Artificial intelligence supported differential diagnosis generators
VIOLENCE AGAINST NURSES	Rates of reported assaults against nurses	Strict visitation policies

ADE, adverse drug event; CAUTI, catheter-associated urinary tract infection; HCO, health care organization; SSI, surgical site infection; UDEs, undesirable diagnostic events.

FIGURE 12.1 FMEA for patient falls.

FAILURE MODE AND EFFECTS ANALYSIS

Process name: _____ Responsibility: _____
Team names: _____
FMEA number: _____
FMEA date: _____ Revised date: _____

Process function	Potential failure mode	Potential effect(s) of failure	Severity (1–10)	Potential causes	Occurance (1–10)	Current process controls	Detect (1–10)	Risk priority number	Recommended action(s)
The highest value process step?	In what ways might the process potentially fail?	What is the effect of each failure mode?		How can the failure occur?		What are the existing controls to prevent failure?	How well can you detect cause or failure mode?	SEV×OCC×DET	What are the actions?
Fall risk precaution measures	Insufficient measures	Patient fall	7	Missed bracelets for high risk	7	Check upon admission	3	147	Confirm fall risk status upon shift changes
[Add additional processes here.]									

FMEA, failure mode and effects analysis.

the process fails, and the effects of those failures. The team evaluates each potential failure mode and assigns a value-based occurrence, severity, and detectability. Then, the values of occurrence, severity, and detectability are multiplied together to calculate a risk priority number for each potential failure. Based on the calculated risk priority numbers, the team prioritizes each potential failure mode for action. An FMEA aids HCOs to proactively identify and mitigate potential risks before they occur, thus improving reliability, safety, and overall performance. Figure 12.1 illustrates an FMEA for a potential failure associated with patient falls (Majed et al., 2024).

Workplace Safety

Health services managers, along with risk management specialists, are responsible for improving workplace safety. Unfortunately, in many HCOs, violence against nurses is all too common. Nearly a third of registered nurses report experiencing violence "occasionally" or "frequently" while at work, most events occuring in psychiatric units and emergency departments (Press Ganey, 2024). According to the Emergency Nurses Association (ENA), more than half of surveyed nurses said they had been physically or verbally assaulted or faced threats of violence in the last 30 days (ENA, 2024). Violence and mistreatment from patients, families, and visitors force even the most dedicated nurses to consider leaving their profession, especially when workplace safety concerns are ignored or ineffectively addressed by managers (National Nurses United, 2018).

△ KEY IDEA

Beyond the moral obligation to protect nurses from harm, health services managers are responsible for ensuring that nurses feel safe enough to care for patients.

Beyond the moral obligation to protect nurses from harm, health services managers are responsible for ensuring that nurses feel safe enough to care for patients. After experiencing workplace violence, employees suffer from psychological trauma and a variety of physical and mental health conditions that significantly decrease productivity (Meese et al., 2024). To prevent workplace violence, effective health services managers provide organizational support through the following recommended actions (Meese et al., 2022; Wirth et al. 2021):

- *Create stringent visitor policies:* Set rules that clearly communicate zero tolerance for violence and mistreatment of caregivers by patients and visitors.
- *Screen for at-risk patients or visitors:* Systematically identify patients and visitors who are at high risk for violence.
- *Upgrade security:* Install alarm systems, surveillance cameras, and controls on access to clinical areas.
- *Avoid supply and staff shortages:* Failure to plan for increases in patient volumes, acuity, and intensity creates delays in patient care that can become dangerous in high-stress areas.
- *Train clinicians:* Provide classroom-based training sessions that teach de-escalation and/or self-defense techniques.

Access to Care

One of the primary goals of quality improvement is to increase **access to care**, especially for patients with financial, social, or logistical barriers. Measures of access to care include affordability measures, such as the proportion of patients who were unable to pay their medical bills (Schneider, Shah, Doty, Tikkanen, Fields, & Williams, 2021). Access to care is also assessed through various measures of **timeliness of care**, which measures how quickly patients can obtain information, make appointments, and obtain urgent care after hours. To improve timeliness of care, quality improvement initiatives often aim to improve patient **throughput**, which is the term for the rate at which patients move through a health services delivery care system, including registration, assessment, admission, diagnosis, treatment, and discharge.

Table 12.5 describes example access to care measures and interventions (AHRQ, 2022; Cohen et al., 2024; Rathlev et al., 2020; Zhang, 2022).

Patient Experience

HCOs fail to provide high-quality customer experiences seen in other economic sectors (Poku et al., 2017). **Patient experience** is defined as the "sum of all interactions, shaped by an organization's culture, that influence patient perceptions across the continuum of care" (Wolf, Niederhauser, Marshburn & LaVela, 2021; The Beryl Institute, 2024). Patient experience measurement does not consider clinical outcomes but only whether a patient's expectations about their health services experiences were met. Another concept related to patient satisfaction is **patient-centeredness**, defined as understanding healthcare quality from patients' perspectives and making sure that patients have choices in all circumstances (Berwick, 2009).

△ KEY IDEA
Patient experience measurement does not consider clinical outcomes but only whether a patient's expectations about their health services experiences were met.

TABLE 12.5 Example Access to Care-Related Measures and Interventions

MEASURE	DEFINITION	EXAMPLE INTERVENTIONS
BED TURNOVER RATE	Number of patient discharges divided by the total number of beds over a specific period	Improve inpatient discharge processes
CANCER TREATMENT DELAY	Time from diagnosis to first treatment (chemotherapy, surgery, or radiation)	Create multidisciplinary teams; patient navigation services
OPERATING ROOM TURNOVER TIME	Time between wheels-out of previous patient to wheels-in of the next patient; "patient out to patient in"	Overlapping anesthesia process with other processes continuing in the operating room
PATIENTS LEFT EMERGENCY DEPARTMENT WITHOUT BEING SEEN	Patients who are triaged and register for care but subsequently leave without medical evaluation	More frequent updates on wait time; immediate temporary treatments
TIMELINESS OF GETTING APPOINTMENTS FOR CARE	Percentage of patients who sometimes or never got an appointment for routine care as soon as needed	Flexible scheduling options, including evening and weekend appointments
WAITING TIME	Number of visits in which patients waited to see a physician for 1 hour or more	Avoid overbooking and ensure sufficient time for each patient encounter

Patient experience is generally measured in the United States through standardized survey instruments known as the **Consumer Assessment of Healthcare Providers and Systems (CAHPS)** (AHRQ, 2017). CAHPS (pronounced "caps") surveys evaluate various aspects of patient experiences, and results are publicly available through the Medicare Hospital Compare website, which motivates HCOs to improve patient experience (Padilla, 2017). There are 11 different types of CAHPS surveys, each focused on a different care setting or provider category, such as hospitals, home health, or hemodialysis centers (CMS, 2024). The hospital version of the survey (HCAHPS) includes 29 Likert-style items about a patient's recent hospital stay, including six composite measures, two individual items, and two global items. Each of the six composite measures is constructed from multiple survey questions. Examples of HCAHPS items are listed in Table 12.6 (CMS, 2021).

Health services managers use the CAHPS survey item, "willingness to recommend the hospital," to develop a patient experience measure called the **net promoter score**. Typically, net promoter scores are derived from 10-point scales that range from 1 ("not at all likely") to 10 ("extremely likely"). However, the CAHPS surveys score the willingness to recommend the hospital on a 4-point scale, with response choices of definitely yes, probably yes, probably no, and definitely no. To calculate a net promoter score using the CAHPS survey, respondents answering "definitely yes" are categorized as **promoters**, those answering "probably no" or "probably yes" are **passives**, and "definitely no" are **detractors**. Based on the survey results, the percentage of respondents in each category are calculated. For example, if 100 people were surveyed and 50 answered

TABLE 12.6 Example Items of Consumer Assessment of Healthcare Providers and Systems Surveys

MEASURE	MEASURE TYPE	EXAMPLE SURVEY ITEM
COMMUNICATION WITH DOCTORS	Composite	During this hospital stay, how often did doctors explain things in a way you could understand?
COMMUNICATION WITH NURSES	Composite	During this hospital stay, how often did nurses listen carefully to you?
RESPONSIVENESS OF OFFICE OR HOSPITAL STAFF	Composite	During this hospital stay, after you pressed the call button, how often did you get help as soon as you wanted it?
COMMUNICATION ABOUT MEDICINES	Composite	Before giving you any new medicine, how often did hospital staff tell you what the medicine was for?
DISCHARGE INFORMATION	Composite	During this hospital stay, did doctors, nurses or other hospital staff talk with you about whether you would have the help you needed when you left the hospital?
CARE TRANSITION	Composite	When I left the hospital, I had a good understanding of the things I was responsible for in managing my health.
CLEANLINESS OF HOSPITAL ENVIRONMENT	Individual	During this hospital stay, how often were your room and bathroom kept clean?
QUIETNESS OF HOSPITAL ENVIRONMENT	Individual	During this hospital stay, how often was the area around your room quiet at night?
HOSPITAL RATING	Global	Using any number from 0 to 10, where 0 is the worst hospital possible and 10 is the best hospital possible, what number would you use to rate this hospital during your stay?
WILLINGNESS TO RECOMMEND THE HOSPITAL	Global	Would you recommend this hospital to your friends and family?

"definitely yes," 30 answered "probably no" or "probably yes," and 20 answered "definitely no," then the categories would be calculated as follows:

- *Promoters*: 50% (50 out of 100)
- *Passives*: 30% (30 out of 100)
- *Detractors*: 20% (20 out of 100)

Then, the percentage of detractors are subtracted from the percentage of promoters (50% - 20% = 30%). In this example, the net promoter score is 30%. A positive net promoter score indicates that the HCO has more promoters than detractors. Net promoter scores should be used with caution, however, as comparing services lines or patient populations can be misleading due to the differences in illness acuity and prognosis (Adams et al., 2022). Nevertheless, net promoter scores can be used as a starting point to identify services that require improvement and as baseline for improvements achieved over time.

QUALITY MANAGEMENT METHODOLOGIES

Methodologies and Philosophies

Continuous quality improvement means constant learning through incremental changes to specific problems that have been identified by frontline employees (Radcliffe et al., 2020). Continuous quality improvement approaches are not intended to solve high-level organizational change (Dellifraine et al., 2010; Guo & Hariharan, 2012). More extensive whole-system improvements require different forms of problem-solving, as described in Chapter 2 (Potthoff et al., 2020; Radcliffe et al., 2020). In contrast, continuous quality improvement methodologies are the ideal approach for small-scale projects (Rubenstein et al., 2014).

Lean

The **Lean** quality improvement approach was created from the Toyota manufacturing system developed in Japan in the 1950s and 1960s (Womack & Jones, 1996). Adopted by healthcare in the early 2000s, Lean methodologies have been shown to eliminate inefficiencies in health care processes (Toussaint & Berry, 2013). Despite the benefits of Lean, many healthcare leaders doubted whether manufacturing methods would work in patient care (Laffel & Blumenthal, 1989). Eventually, HCOs recognized the benefits of systematic healthcare quality management methodologies. After ThedaCare of Appleton, Wisconsin, implemented Lean, the total cost of care for inpatient services were reduced by 25% while improving patient satisfaction (Toussaint & Berry, 2013). Virginia Mason Medical Center's application of Lean was so successful that it created the Virginia Mason Institute to train other HCOs on their "Virginia Mason Production System" (Bohl & Kaplan, 2020).

Lean is a philosophy—a way of thinking—that helps organizations make continuous quality improvements. Lean warrants a more detailed instruction, but for the purposes of this chapter,

> **CAREER BOX 12.3:** The Career Ecosystem
>
> Many early career health services managers believe that they want to become hospital CEOs. With this end in mind, careers are viewed as ladders that need to be climbed to the ultimate positions of authority as hospital CEOs. However, the ladder is an inappropriate metaphor for health services management careers. Most career paths are not straight but more dynamic and evolving. A better metaphor for careers is the ecosystem, which is made up of a diverse number of specialized roles, all interacting with one another to collaborate, share resources, and coexist within a complex system (Lancaster et al., 2018). Within the health service management profession, a variety of people fulfill specific niches in the ecosystem that match their goals, talents, and limitations.
>
> You may eventually become a CEO, of course, but you can also build an outstanding career in countless positions that satisfy your desire to contribute at a high level (Pruitt, 2024). Moreover, balancing noncareer priorities, such as child-rearing or physical fitness, is just as important as their careers to most people. So, the interplay between career and personal life should be considered in your conception of career success. As in a dynamic ecosystem, the balance between career and homelife changes over time, just as career environments evolve over time. By adopting the ecosystem conceptual model for your career, you will be able to envision many options for success that account for your growth and the unpredictable changes to your life and the health services environment.

there are a few important concepts that health services managers can adopt in their practice, including the following (Imai, 1986; Womack, 2001; Womack & Jones, 1996):

- *Reduce waste:* Called "muda" in Japanese, waste includes the inefficiencies that consume resources, such as people, time, equipment, space, and money, but do not create value for patients. Lean recognizes eight types of waste, including inventory, motion, waiting, overprocessing, overproduction, transportation, defects, and underutilization of employee skills.
- *Gemba walk:* Gemba means "actual place" in Japanese. Conducting a Gemba walk means visiting the area where the work takes place. A Gemba walk is not a surprise inspection; rather, it is a technique for engaging staff to ask lots of questions and focus on improving processes.
- *Kaizen event:* Kaizen means "change for the better" or "continuous improvement" in Japanese. A kaizen event is collaborative workshop where the quality improvement team (see Table 12.1) analyzes current processes and redesigns health services delivery. A typical kaizen event lasts 4 or 5 days.

Lean approaches continuous quality improvement projects using a simple cycle, called **Plan-Do-Study-Act (PDSA)**. Using the PDSA cycle, quality improvement teams engage in objective measurement and goal setting, rapidly test small-scale projects, and learn from experimentation until the full potential of improvement can be expanded on a larger scale (Knudsen et al., 2019). These are the four steps of the PDSA cycle (Toussaint & Berry, 2013):

1. *Plan:* Define the intervention. Identify measures of success. Develop a plan to test the proposed quality improvement intervention. Make predictions of why the project will improve measures of success.
2. *Do:* Carry out the intervention, collect data, and note observations.
3. *Study:* Study the data to determine if the intervention achieved the measured goal.
4. *Act:* Determine what modifications should be made to the test, if any. Adjust interventions for the next cycle. If it was successful, expand to a larger scale test or fully implement the intervention.

INFORMATIONAL INTERVIEW 12.3

Chief Executive Officer, The Quality Coaching Co.
Access the informational interview online at http://connect.springerpub.com/content/book/978-0-8261-4807-0/chapter/ch00.

For example, Mayo Clinic Hospital in Rochester, Minnesota, used multiple PDSA cycles to improve the timeliness and efficiency of discharge in the NICU (Kaemingk et al., 2022). The quality improvement team identified 31 different causes of the delays and inefficiencies in the discharge process. From these details, the team created a **Pareto chart**, a type of root cause analysis. Health services managers use Pareto charts to identify which causes should be prioritized, addressing the most common root cause first, then the next most common, and so on. According to the Mayo Clinic analysis, the most frequent cause of delays was that the family members/caregivers were not available when the child was ready to be discharged.

Figure 12.2 illustrates a Pareto chart of discharge delays in the Mayo Clinic NICU. The Pareto chart is a combination of the bar and line chart. The axis on the left side of the Pareto chart is count of the occurrences of discharge delays arranged by category in descending order, with largest number occurrences shown on the far left, then the next most frequently occurring instances. The Pareto chart also includes a secondary axis on the right side that measures the cumulative percentage of each category. As illustrated, the first category is 21% of the total, the second category is 20% of the total, and the third category is 20% of the total, for a cumulative percentage of 61%. The cumulative percentage increases with each successive category until it reaches 100%.

FIGURE 12.2 Example Pareto chart for delays in patient care.

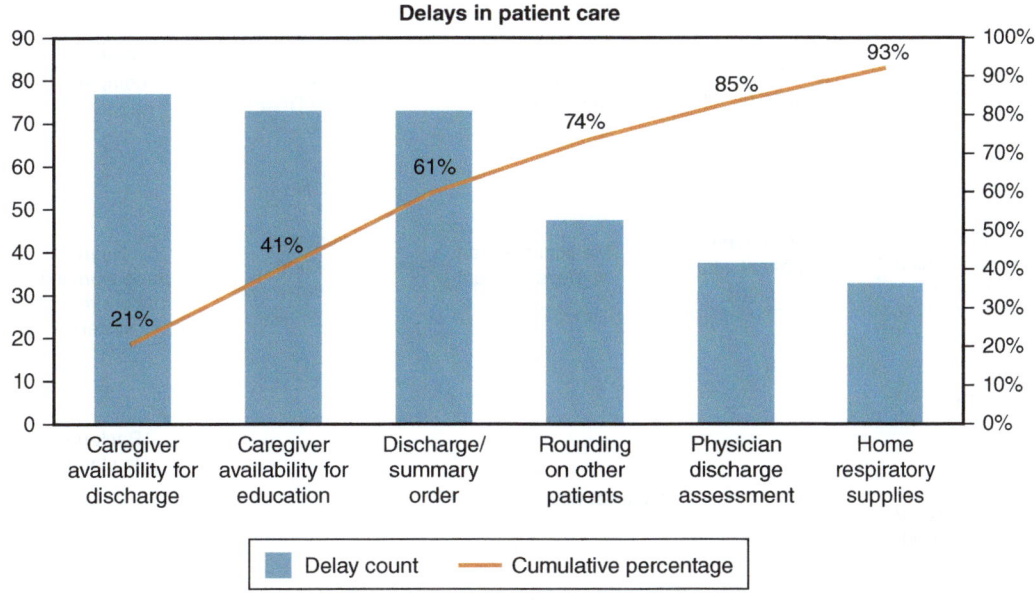

Source: Adapted from Kaemingk, B. D., Hobbs, C. A., Streeton, A. C., Morgan, K., Schuning, V. S., Melhouse, J. K., & Fang, J. L. (2022). Improving the timeliness and efficiency of discharge from the NICU. *Pediatrics, 149*(5), e2021052759.

The Mayo Clinic NICU's first PDSA cycle, which lasted 2 weeks, established a goal of discharging at least 50% of the patients by 11:00 a.m. (Kaemingk et al., 2022). Families were informed of the discharge time by clinical staff and through signs in the NICU patient rooms and common areas. When the 11:00 a.m. discharge goal was missed, the nurse responsible for the discharge sent an email to the team explaining the delay. Five subsequent PDSA cycles were implemented to achieve the discharge goal, and solutions included creating a discharge checklist and prioritized rounding on discharging patients. After completing six PDSA cycles, the percentage of patients discharged from the NICU before 11:00 a.m. improved from 9.4% to 52.4%, with no change in patient satisfaction.

For HCOs struggling with long wait times, medication errors, and the ever-increasing complexities of care, Lean can be used to streamline steps, remove bottlenecks, or make patient care or business processes more reliable (Rotter et al., 2018). **Process improvement** is the proactive, ongoing practice of optimizing inefficient or unreliable processes that produce ineffective results. To identify process inefficiencies in a process, health services managers create **process maps**, also called **flowcharts**, to graphically represent the sequence of steps in a process. Figure 12.3 illustrates a process flow for a patient rooming process for an outpatient clinic. While more details can be incorporated, the following symbols are widely recognized for process mapping:

- *Rounded rectangle:* Marks the start and end of the process
- *Rectangle:* Indicates a specific action or task within the process
- *Arrow connector:* Indicates the sequence of actions or decisions in the process
- *Diamond:* Signifies a point in the process where a yes-no question is posed and answered, leading to different paths depending on the decision outcome
- *Rectangle with a curved bottom:* Represents a document or report
- *Cylinder:* Represents a data file or database

FIGURE 12.3 Process flow of patient rooming process.

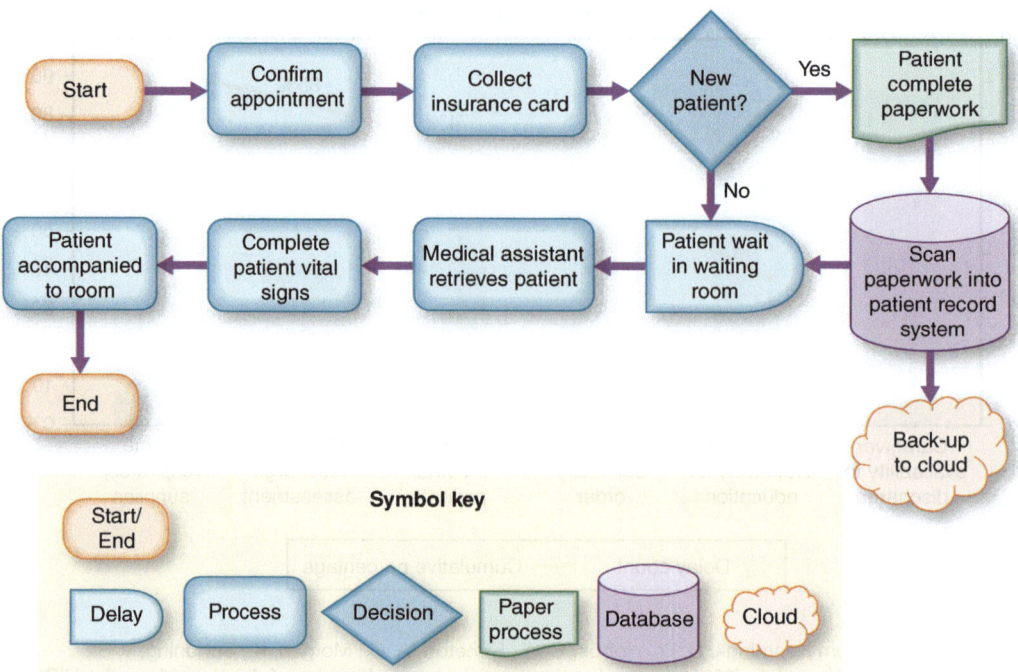

- *Half oval:* Shows a delay or waiting period in a process
- *Cloud:* Processes associated with cloud computing technology

Figure 12.4 illustrates a special type of process map called a **swim lane diagram**. In a swim lane diagram, different functions are assigned lanes, and their associated process steps are placed within their respective lanes to illustrate the sequence of steps involved in the process. After creating a swim lane diagram, redundant steps can be identified and eliminated.

FIGURE 12.4 Swim lane diagram for urgent care visit.

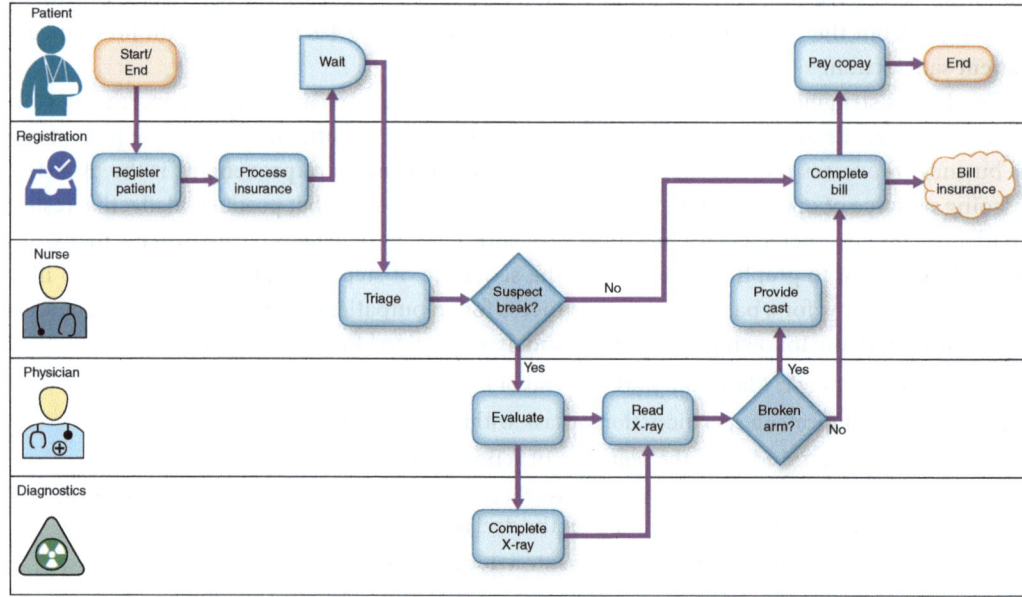

Six Sigma

Six Sigma is another continuous quality improvement methodology borrowed by HCOs from manufacturing. The main focus of Six Sigma is to eliminate defects, errors, or mistakes, often caused by variation in processes (Antony et al., 2018). The name Six Sigma comes from the Greek letter sigma that also represents the statistical measure for variation. **Statistical variation** is defined as the extent to which measurements deviate from the average value, often measured as standard deviation. Under the bell-shaped curve of the standard distribution, the space beyond six standard deviations (six sigma) represents 0.00034% of the outputs for the process. As such, the Six Sigma approach seeks to produce no more than 3.4 defects per million opportunities, or a perfect process 99.99966% of the time.

Table 12.7 provides a closer examination of variation in health services delivery compared to other real-world examples, adapted from Pruitt et al. (2020).

TABLE 12.7 Six Sigma Performance Levels for Health Care and Other Examples

EXAMPLE	RATE	SIGMA LEVEL	EVIDENCE
GLOBAL AIRPLANE FATALITIES	22 fatalities per one million flights	5 to 6 sigma	Worldwide airplane Accident Review from 2002 to 2011 (United Kingdom Civil Aviation Authority, 2013)
ANESTHESIA MORTALITY	25 per million hospital surgical discharges	5 to 6 sigma	Due to due to improvements in anesthesia techniques, monitoring systems, and safety protocols, anesthesia mortality is now rare (Schiff & Wagner, 2016).
U.S. MOTOR VEHICLE FATALITIES	125 per 1 million vehicle miles	5 to 6 sigma	Motor vehicle-related deaths, including pedestrians and cyclists killed by cars (Gorzelany, 2017)
DEFECTS IN MANUFACTURING FOR MOST U.S. COMPANIES	66,807 to 6,210 per million	3 to 4 sigma	The average defects per million opportunities for most manufacturing companies (Thawani, 2004).
MISDIAGNOSIS OF CEREBROVASCULAR EVENTS (STROKE)	71,000 per million strokes	3 to 4 sigma	Strokes happen to approximately 795,000 people in the United States each year (Benjamin et al., 2019). At initial emergency department presentation, roughly 9% patients are misdiagnosed (Tarnutzer et al., 2017).
PREVENTABLE ADVERSE DRUG EVENTS (MEDICATION ERRORS)	112,000 per million inpatient admissions	2 to 3 sigma	According to multisite study, medication errors occurred in 11.2 per 100 admissions (Hug et al., 2010).
MISDIAGNOSIS OF MYOCARDIAL INFARCTIONS (HEART ATTACKS)	182,000 per million heart attacks	2 to 3 sigma	Misdiagnoses of heart attacks occur 18.2% of the time in emergency departments, according one study (Wildi et al., 2015).
INAPPROPRIATE ANTIBIOTIC PRESCRIPTION	182,700 per million cold-related office visits	2 to 3 sigma	Of the over 29 million office-based visits for viral diagnoses, 18.27% were prescribed antibiotics (Imanpour et al., 2017).

Source: Adapted from Pruitt, Z., Smith, C. S., & Pérez-Ruberté, E. (2020). Healthcare quality management: A case study approach. New York: Springer Publishing Company LLC.

FIGURE 12.5 Nurse to patient ratio control chart.

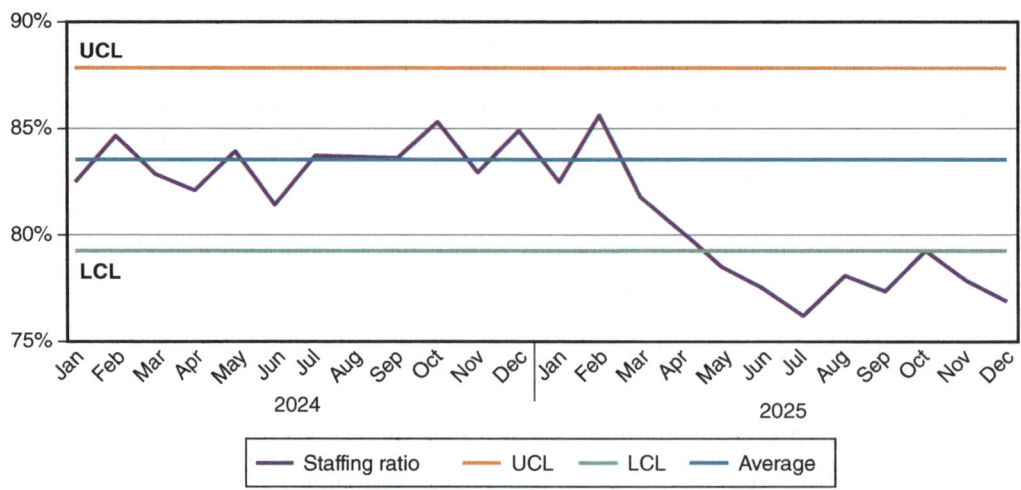

Every process contains some variation, but too much means that the process needs improvement. A **control chart** shows whether a process is performing within normal variation (Woodall, Adams, & Benneyan, 2012). There are two types of variation: common cause variation and special cause variation. **Common cause variation** is the expected variation in the process. When variation exceeds the statistical limits, it indicates **special cause variation**. Figure 12.5 provides an example of a control chart illustrating the variation in nurse-to-patient staffing ratios. The middle line is the mean; the upper and lower lines represent the limits of common cause variation. Values above or below indicate special cause variation. Common cause variation should be ignored as a normal phenomenon; special cause variation should be investigated and eliminated.

Six Sigma also deploys a structured framework for continuous quality improvement, helping organizations to systematically identify, analyze, and address problems in their processes. The Six Sigma methodology is called **DMAIC**, which stands for **Define, Measure, Analyze, Improve, and Control,** and is pronounced "dee-may-ic" (Antony et al., 2018). For example, Johns Hopkins Healthcare System sought to increase the frequency of hemoglobin A1C (A1C) measurement in patients admitted to the hospital who had a history of diabetes (Khan et al., 2023). The quality improvement team included an endocrinology physician, pharmacist, information technology nurse, hospitalist physician, health services manager, and an expert in Six Sigma methodology. Table 12.8 describes each of the DMAIC steps using the Johns Hopkins initiative designed to comply with protocols for hemoglobin A1C blood testing.

Following multiple DMAIC quality improvement cycles, the Johns Hopkins Healthcare System increased A1C testing from 61.2% to 74.5% following the interventions.

High-Reliability Health Care Organizations

While Lean and Six Sigma are different quality improvement methodologies, healthcare quality management practitioners often use the combined phrase "Lean Six Sigma." The combination of the terms reflects the usefulness of both methodologies when used together. In fact, The Joint Commission recommends that HCOs blend principles from Lean (improving flow; eliminates waste), Six Sigma (reducing variability), and formal change management practices to create high-reliability organizations (Cochrane et al., 2017; Veazie et al., 2022). (Change management principles are reviewed in Chapter 4.) **High-reliability organizations** are those that "operate in

TABLE 12.8 Define, Measure, Analyze, Improve and Control Example

STEP	DEFINITION	EXAMPLE
DEFINE	Project goals and deliverables are defined, along with the problem statement and key metrics.	Increase the frequency of A1C testing for diabetic patients who met criteria.
MEASURE	Data are collected to understand the current state of the process.	Percentage of diabetic patients with A1C test sent to inpatient laboratory
ANALYZE	Identify root causes of problems or inefficiencies in the process.	Discovered that laboratory policy only allowed A1C analysis a few times per week, leading to delays in physicians getting the results, which made physicians less likely to request the test. A fishbone diagram illustrated 13 other causes of infrequent A1C testing.
IMPROVE	Potential solutions to address the root causes identified in the analysis phase are developed and implemented.	Implemented four interventions to increase the frequency of A1C testing: new A1C laboratory testing policies, training with medical staff on A1C protocol, and two changes related to the electronic medical record system
CONTROL	Changes are monitored over time and ensure that the improvements are maintained.	The quality improvement team regularly produced control charts that displayed the percentage of A1C tests before and after the deployment of the interventions.

complex, high-hazard domains for extended periods without serious accidents or catastrophic failures" (AHRQ, 2019b). Like Lean and Six Sigma, the concept of high-reliability organizations was borrowed from other industries, such as commercial airlines, where organizations demonstrated exceptional safety records.

△ KEY IDEA

While standardization of workflows to reduce variation is valuable, high-reliability organizations recognize that complexity requires careful evaluation of the entire system of processes for potential threats to quality and safety.

The Joint Commission expects that HCOs apply high-reliability organization principles to consistently provide safe, effective, and high-quality care by making three major organizational commitments (Chassin & Loeb, 2011):

- *Commit to zero patient harm:* Board and executives must measure healthcare quality and safety and hold the organization accountable for performance. Make quality and safety top priorities in strategic decision-making.
- *Create an organizational culture of quality and safety:* Build trust, eliminate blame, encourage employees to report issues, and invest resources to improve.
- *Adopt and deploy quality improvement methodologies:* Use the best available approaches, including Lean and Six Sigma tools and approaches.

In high-reliability organizations, health services managers resist the temptation to oversimplify work processes. While standardization of workflows is valuable, high-reliability organizations recognize that complexity requires careful evaluation of the entire system of processes for potential threats to quality and safety (Chassin & Loeb, 2011). Acknowledging complexity of health services delivery requires that people possess preoccupation with failure. Threats to patient safety can emerge at any time, so constant vigilance is mandatory in high-reliability organizations (AHRQ, 2019b).

FUTURE DIRECTIONS

Patient safety, employee safety, access to care, and patient experience remain top priorities for healthcare quality management practice, but health services managers are increasingly monitoring the environmental impacts of HCOs. Health services delivery systems are responsible for approximately 8.5% of emission in the United States (Eckelman et al., 2020). Pollution and the resultant climate change pose major risks to community health which make environmental sustainability a prerequisite for delivering high-quality health care (Lee & Lee, 2022). Future healthcare quality management practices will include environmental sustainability because high-quality healthcare cannot be delivered when the communities in which HCOs operate lack safe and clean environments (Putnis & Neilson, 2022).

To ensure that HCOs are operating in environmentally sustainable ways, health services managers will increasingly incorporate eco-friendly practices, such as reducing nonrenewable energy consumption, medical waste, and water usage. Like other quality management initiatives, health services managers will allocate resources for training employees and conducting environmental sustainability improvement projects (Aboueid et al., 2023). Only through constant, incremental quality improvements can HCOs reduce their environmental impact and develop environmentally sustainable practices that are consistent with organizational mission and values.

SUMMARY

- Because health services delivery processes are not reliable, health services managers actively identify opportunities to make care safer or higher quality, create collaborative teams to implement changes, and measure the impact of those changes on patient care.
- Boards of directors incorporate quality and safety goals into strategic plans and hold managers and clinicians accountable for performance. A variety of healthcare quality improvement team members are responsible for implementing quality and safety initiatives, including quality experts, risk managers, clinical leaders, and a variety of frontline clinicians and administrative staff.
- Health services managers are responsible for influencing the extent to which HCO cultures embrace the health care quality management practices.
- Health services managers can empower people to make quality and safety a part of their work responsibilities and to report quality and safety improvement opportunities. Health services managers encourage the development of just cultures, an organizational environment characterized by open dialogue without fear of blame for mistakes.
- Hundreds of measures are adopted to track quality, safety, and patient experience improvement. Quality of care can be achieved through reliable processes and medical services delivered according to current professional knowledge.
- Continuous quality improvement is a mindset of constant learning through implementation of small-scale projects designed to achieve incremental changes. A variety of quality improvement methodologies can be adopted in HCOs, including Lean, Six Sigma, and high-reliability organization practices.

END-OF-CHAPTER RESOURCES

KEY TERMS*

*For the full list of key terms, please see the online glossary at **http://connect.springerpub.com/content/book/978-0-8261-4807-0.**

access to care
adverse events
Consumer Assessment of Healthcare Providers and Systems (CAHPS)
Centers for Medicare & Medicaid Services (CMS)
common cause variation
continuous quality improvement
detractors
Define, Measure, Analyze, Improve, and Control (DMAIC)
failure mode and effects analysis (FMEA)
Gemba walk
healthcare quality management
high-reliability organizations
Hospital-Acquired Condition Reduction Program
Hospital Readmissions Reduction Program (HRRP)
Institute for Healthcare Improvement (IHI)
just culture
kaizen event
Lean
Medicare Hospital Compare
Medicare Shared Savings Program (MSSP)
Merit-Based Incentive Payment System (MIPS)
National Committee for Quality Assurance (NCQA)
near misses
outcomes
Pareto chart
patient-centeredness
passives
patient experience
patient safety
peer review
Plan-Do-Study-Act (PDSA)
process
process improvement
promoters
quality of care
reliability
risk management
Six Sigma
special cause variation
statistical variation
structure
The Joint Commission
throughput
timeliness of care
Triple Aim
waste

LEARNING ACTIVITIES

Professional Development and Reflection

1. Identify and define measures of career success. Using external signs of recognition, including titles and salary levels, can make success easy to track. However, broader definitions of success can lead to more personally fulfilling careers. Think of other objective measures of success that align with your values, such as working on interesting projects, overcoming challenges, being recognized as an expert, developing valuable working relationships, helping people, or establishing a secure career.
2. Continuous quality improvement practices can be applied to careers. Based on the career success metrics described earlier, develop interventions designed to achieve your goals. Follow the PDSA or DMAIC cycles described in this chapter to overcome barriers to career success.

Discussion Questions

1. What are some potential drawbacks or limitations of specializing in healthcare quality management compared to pursuing a general management career within HCOs? What are the benefits of specialized health services management careers?
2. How can health services managers effectively balance the competing demands of quality improvement initiatives with financial performance? Are these goals mutually exclusive? Why or why not?
3. What strategies can health services managers implement to create an environment where employees feel comfortable reporting near misses and adverse events without fear of retribution?
4. Consider Lean (i.e., PDSA cycle) or Six Sigma (i.e., DMAIC). Which continuous quality improvement methodology is preferred in healthcare settings? Why?

RECOMMENDED READING AND MEDIA

Black, J. R., Miller, D., & Sensel, J. (2016). *The Toyota way to healthcare excellence: Increase efficiency and improve quality with lean*. Health Administration Press.

Byrnes, J., & Teman, S. (2018). *The safety playbook: A healthcare leader's guide to building a high-reliability organization*. Health Administration Press

Caffrey, M. (2017, November 3). *Catching up with Don Berwick: Where quality improvement is going, and how young people are leading the way*. American Journal of Managed Care. https://www.ajmc.com/view/catching-up-with-don-berwick-where-quality-improvement-is-going-and-how-young-people-are-leading-the-way

Christensen, C. M. (2017). *How will you measure your life?*. Harvard business review press.

Kaemingk, B. D., Hobbs, C. A., Streeton, A. C., Morgan, K., Schuning, V. S., Melhouse, J. K., & Fang, J. L. (2022). Improving the Timeliness and Efficiency of Discharge from the NICU. *Pediatrics, 149*(5), e2021052759.

Pruitt, Z., Smith, C. S., & Pérez-Ruberté, E. (2020). *Healthcare quality management: A case study approach*. Springer Publishing Company.

Vedantamy, S. (Host). (2018, August 27). *You 2.0: Check yourself*. [Audio podcast episode]. https://www.npr.org/transcripts/642310810.

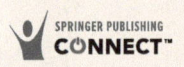

A robust set of instructor resources designed to supplement this text is located at http://connect.springerpub.com/content/book/978-0-8261-4807-0.
Qualifying instructors may request access by emailing textbook@springerpub.com.

REFERENCES

Aboueid, S., Beyene, M., & Nur, T. (2023, November). Barriers and enablers to implementing environmentally sustainable practices in healthcare: A scoping review and proposed roadmap. In *Healthcare management forum* (Vol. 36, No. 6, pp. 405–413). SAGE Publications.

Adams, C., Walpola, R., Schembri, A. M., & Harrison, R. (2022). The ultimate question? Evaluating the use of Net Promoter Score in healthcare: A systematic review. *Health Expectations, 25*(5), 2328–2339. https://doi.org/10.1111/hex.13577

Adelman, J. (2019). High-reliability healthcare: Building safer systems through just culture and technology. *Journal of Healthcare Management, 64*(3), 137–141. https://doi.org/10.1097/jhm-d-19-00069

Agency for Healthcare Research and Quality. (2013). Module 14. Creating Quality Improvement Teams and QI Plans. *Practice facilitation handbook*. https://www.ahrq.gov/sites/default/files/publications/files/practicefacilitationhandbook.pdf

Agency for Healthcare Research and Quality. (2017). *What is patient experience?*. https://www.ahrq.gov/cahps/about-cahps/patient-experience/index.html

Agency for Healthcare Research and Quality. (2019a). *Adverse events, near misses, and errors*. Patient Safety Network. https://psnet.ahrq.gov/primer/adverse-events-near-misses-and-errors

Agency for Healthcare Research and Quality. (2019b). *High reliability*. https://psnet.ahrq.gov/primer/high-reliability

Agency for Healthcare Research and Quality. (2019c). *Measurement of patient safety*. Patient Safety Network. https://psnet.ahrq.gov/primer/measurement-patient-safety

Agency for Healthcare Research and Quality. (2022, October). *2022 national healthcare quality and disparities report measure specifications*. https://www.ahrq.gov/sites/default/files/wysiwyg/research/findings/nhqrdr/2022qdr-measurespecs.pdf

American Medical Association. (2019, December 19). *Getting rid of stupid stuff: Reduce the unnecessary daily burdens for clinicians*. https://edhub.ama-assn.org/steps-forward/module/2757858

Antony, J., Palsuk, P., Gupta, S., Mishra, D., & Barach, P. (2018). Six Sigma in healthcare: A systematic review of the literature. *International Journal of Quality & Reliability Management, 35*(5), 1075–1092.

Austin, J. M., Demski, R., Callender, T., Lee, K. K., Hoffman, A., Allen, L., Radke, D. A., Kim, Y., Werthman, R. J., Peterson, R. R., & Pronovost, P. J. (2017). From board to bedside: How the application of financial structures to safety and quality can drive accountability in a large health care system. *The Joint Commission Journal on Quality and Patient Safety, 43*(4), 166–175. https://doi.org/10.1016/j.jcjq.2017.01.001

Bailey, C., & Madden, A. (2017). Time reclaimed: Temporality and the experience of meaningful work. *Work, Employment, & Society, 31*, 3–18. http://doi.org/10.1177/0950017015604100

Bates, D. W., Levine, D. M., Salmasian, H., Syrowatka, A., Shahian, D. M., Lipsitz, S., Zebrowski, J. P., Myers, L. C., Logan, M. S., Roy, C. G., Iannaccone, C., Frits, M. L., Volk, L. A.,Dulgarian, S., Amato, M. G., Edrees, H. H., Sato, L., Folcarelli, P., Einbinder, J. S., . . . Mort, E. (2023). The safety of inpatient health care. *New England Journal of Medicine, 388*(2), 142–153. https://doi.org/10.1056/nejmsa2206117

Begun, J. W., White, K. R., & Mosser, G. (2011). Interprofessional care teams: The role of the healthcare administrator. *Journal of Interprofessional Care. 25*(2), 119–123.

Benjamin, E. J., Muntner, P., Alonso, A., Bittencourt, M. S., Callaway, C. W., Carson, A., Chamberlain, Chang, A. R., Cheng, S., Das, S. R., Delling, F. N., Djousse, L., Elkind, M. S. V.,Ferguson, J. F., Fornage, M., Jordan, L. C., Khan, S. S., Kissela, B. M., Knutson, K. L., . . . Vitani, S. S; American Heart Association Council on Epidemiology and Prevention Statistics Committee and Stroke Statistics Subcommittee. (2019). Heart disease and stroke statistics: 2019 update a report from the American heart association. *Circulation, 139*(10), E56–E528. https://doi.org/10.1161/cir.0000000000000659

Bergerum, C., Engström, A. K., Thor, J., & Wolmesjö, M. (2020). Patient involvement in quality improvement–a 'tug of war' or a dialogue in a learning process to improve healthcare?. *BMC Health Services Research, 20*, 1–13. https://doi.org/10.1186/s12913-020-05970-4

Berwick, D. M. (2009). What 'patient-centered' should mean: Confessions of an extremist. *Health Affairs, 28*(4), 555–565. https://doi.org/10.1377/hlthaff.28.4.w555

Berwick, D. M., Loehrer, S., & Gunther-Murphy, C. (2017). Breaking the rules for better care. *JAMA, 317*(21), 2161–2162. https://doi.org/10.1001/jama.2017.4703

The Beryl Institute. (2024). *Defining patient and human experience*. https://theberylinstitute.org/defining-patient-experience

Blok, A. C., Alexander, C. C., Tschannen, D., & Milner, K. A. (2022). Quality improvement engagement: Barriers and facilitators. *Nursing Management, 53*(3), 16–24. https://doi.org/10.1097/01.numa.0000821708.46746.6f

Bohl, M. A., & Kaplan, G. S. (2020). Using lean process improvement to enhance safety and value. In R. K. Sethi, A. K. Wright, & M. G. Vitale (Eds.), *Value-based approaches to spine care: Sustainable practices in an era of over-utilization* (pp.79–96). Springer Publishing Company.

Bombard, Y., Baker, G. R., Orlando, E., Fancott, C., Bhatia, P., Casalino, S., Onate, K., Denis, J-L., & Pomey, M. P. (2018). Engaging patients to improve quality of care: A systematic review. *Implementation Science, 13*, 1–22. https://doi.org/10.1186/s13012-018-0784-z

Boysen, P. G., II. (2013). Just culture: A foundation for balanced accountability and patient safety. *The Ochsner Journal, 13*(3), 400–406.

Centers for Disease Control and Prevention National Center for Health Statistics. (2017). *Leading causes of death and numbers of deaths, by sex, race, and Hispanic origin: United States, 1980 and 2016.* https://www.cdc.gov/nchs/data/hus/2017/019.pdf

Centers for Medicare and Medicaid Services. (2021, March). Quality assurance guidelines CAHPS® hospital survey (HCAHPS), version 16.0. https://www.cms.gov/files/document/hcahps-qag-v160.pdf#page=211.41

Centers for Medicare and Medicaid Services. (CMS). (2023a). *CMS Measures Inventory.* https://www.cms.gov/medicare/quality/measures/cms-measures-inventory

Centers for Medicare and Medicaid Services. (CMS). (2023b). *Financial report 2023.* https://www.cms.gov/files/document/cms-financial-report-fiscal-year-2023.pdf

Centers for Medicare and Medicaid Services. (CMS). (2023c). *Quality initiatives: General information.* https://www.cms.gov/medicare/quality/initiatives

Centers for Medicare and Medicaid Services. (2024, April 1). *Consumer Assessment of Healthcare Providers & Systems* (CAHPS). https://www.cms.gov/data-research/research/consumer-assessment-healthcare-providers-systems

Chassin, M. R., & Loeb, J. M. (2011). The ongoing quality improvement journey: Next stop, high reliability. *Health Affairs, 30*(4), 559–568. https://doi.org/10.1377/hlthaff.2011.0076

Cochrane, B. S., Hagins, M., Jr., Picciano, G., King, J. A., Marshall, D. A., Nelson, B., & Deao, C. (2017, March). High reliability in healthcare: Creating the culture and mindset for patient safety. In *Healthcare management forum* (Vol. 30, No. 2, pp. 61–68). SAGE Publications.

Cohen, T. N., Kanji, F. F., Zamudio, J., Shouhed, D., Gewertz, B. L., & Sax, H. C. (2024). Why can't we improve turnover time? A systematic review. *World Journal of Surgery, 48*(1), 72–85. https://doi.org/10.1002/wjs.12015

Commission on Accreditation of Healthcare Management Education. (2024). *Quality and safety.* https://cahme.org/accreditation/quality-and-safety

Costello, A., & Huben-Kearney, A. (2023). *Growing as a risk professional.* The American Society for Health Care Risk Management of the American Hospital Association. https://www.md-dc-shrm.org/wp-content/uploads/ASHRM-Chapter-Benefits-White-Paper-2023.pdf

D'Avena, A., Agrawal, S., & Kizer, K. (2020). High-value care every time: Recommendations from the National Quality Task Force. *Health affairs forefront.* https://www.healthaffairs.org/content/forefront/high-value-care-every-time-recommendations-national-quality-task-force

DelliFraine, J. L., Langabeer, J. R., & Nembhard, I. M. (2010). Assessing the evidence of Six Sigma and Lean in the health care industry. *Quality Management in Healthcare, 19*(3), 211–225.

Desveaux, L., & Ivers, N. (2024). Practice or perfect? Coaching for a growth mindset to improve the quality of healthcare. *BMJ Quality & Safety, 33*(4), 1–6. https://doi.org/10.1136/bmjqs-2023-016456.

Donabedian, A. (1966). Evaluating the quality of medical care. *The Milbank Memorial Fund Quarterly, 44*(3), 166–206. https://doi.org/10.2307/3348969

Donaldson, M. S., Corrigan, J. M., & Kohn, L. T. (Eds.). (2000). *To err is human: Building a safer health system.* Institute of Medicine.

Eckelman, M. J., Huang, K., Lagasse, R., Senay, E., Dubrow, R., & Sherman, J. D. (2020). Health care pollution and public health damage in the United States: An update. *Health Affairs, 39*(12), 2071–2079. https://doi.org/10.1377/hlthaff.2020.01247

Eldridge, N., Wang, Y., Metersky, M., Eckenrode, S., Mathew, J., Sonnenfeld, N., Perdue-Puli, J., Hunt, D., Brady, J. P., McGann, P., Grace, E., Rodrick, D., Drye, E., & Krumholz, H. M. (2022). Trends in adverse event rates in hospitalized patients, 2010–2019. *JAMA, 328*(2), 173–183. https://doi.org/10.1001/jama.2022.9600

Emergency Nurses Association. (2024, April 4). *ENA survey: 56 percent of ED nurses assaulted in the past month.* https://www.ena.org/press-room/articles/detail/2024/04/04/ena-survey--56-percent-of-ed-nurses-assaulted-in-the-past-month

Erwin, C. O., Landry, A. Y., Livingston, A. C., & Dias, A. (2019). Effective governance and hospital boards revisited: Reflections on 25 years of research. *Medical Care Research and Review, 76*(2), 131–166. https://doi.org/10.1177/1077558718754898

Fayol, H. (1916). General principles of management. *Classics of Organization Theory, 2*(15), 57–69.

Garman, A. N., Leach, D. C., & Spector, N. (2006). Worldviews in collision: Conflict and collaboration across professional lines. *Journal of Organizational Behavior, 27*(7), 829–849. http://doi.org/10.1002/job.394

Godfrey, M. M., Andersson-Gare, B., Nelson, E. C., Nilsson, M., & Ahlstrom, G. (2014). Coaching interprofessional health care improvement teams: The coachee, the coach and the leader perspectives. *Journal of Nursing Management, 22*(4), 452–464. https://doi.org/10.1111/jonm.12068

Gorzelany, J. (2017). *Death race 2017: Where to find the most dangerous roads in America*. https://www.forbes.com/sites/jimgorzelany/2017/02/16/death-race-2017-where-to-find-the-most-dangerous-roads-in-america/#3bc631be1324

Guo, L., & Hariharan, S. (2012). Patients are not cars and staff are not robots: Impact of differences between manufacturing and clinical operations on process improvement. *Knowledge and Process Management, 19*(2), 53–68.

Hayford, T., & Maeda, J. L. (2017). *Issues and challenges in measuring and improving the quality of health care*. Congressional Budget Office.

Hug, B. L., Witkowski, D. J., Sox, C. M., Keohane, C. A., Seger, D. L., Yoon, C., Matheny, M. E., & Bates, D. W. (2010). Adverse drug event rates in six community hospitals and the potential impact of computerized physician order entry for prevention. *Journal of General Internal Medicine, 25*(1), 31–38. https://doi.org/10.1007/s11606-009-1141-3

Ibrahim, S. A., Reynolds, K. A., Poon, E., & Alam, M. (2022). The evidence base for US joint commission hospital accreditation standards: Cross sectional study. *BMJ, 377*, e063064. https://doi.org/10.1136/bmj-2020-063064

Imai, M. (1986). *Kaizen: The key to Japan's competitive success*. McGraw-Hill.

Imanpour, S., Nwaiwu, O., McMaughan, D. K., DeSalvo, B., & Bashir, A. (2017). Factors associated with antibiotic prescriptions for the viral origin diseases in office-based practices, 2006–2012. *JRSM Open, 8*(8), 2054270417717668. https://doi.org/10.1177%2F2054270417717668

Indeed Editorial Team. (2023, February 16). *9 quality professional certifications to boost your career*. https://www.indeed.com/career-advice/career-development/quality-professional-certifications

Institute for Healthcare Improvement. (2024). *Model for improvement: Forming the team*. https://www.ihi.org/resources/how-to-improve/model-for-improvement-forming-team

Jalilvand, M. A., Raeisi, A. R., & Shaarbafchizadeh, N. (2024). Hospital governance accountability structure: A scoping review. *BMC Health Services Research, 24*(1), 47. https://doi.org/10.1186/s12913-023-10135-0

The Joint Commission. (2024). *Joint commission faqs*. https://www.jointcommission.org/about-us/facts-about-the-joint-commission/joint-commission-faqs

Kaemingk, B. D., Hobbs, C. A., Streeton, A. C., Morgan, K., Schuning, V. S., Melhouse, J. K., & Fang, J. L. (2022). Improving the timeliness and efficiency of discharge from the NICU. *Pediatrics, 149*(5), e2021052759. https://doi.org/10.1542/peds.2021-052759

Khan, S. A., Demidowich, A. P., Tschudy, M. M., Wedler, J., Lamy, W., Akpandak, I., Alexander, L. A., Misra, I., Sidhaye, A., Rotello, L., & Zilbermint, M. (2023). Increasing frequency of hemoglobin A1C measurements in hospitalized patients with diabetes: A quality improvement project using lean six sigma. *Journal of Diabetes Science and Technology*, 19322968231153883. https://doi.org/10.1177/19322968231153883

Knudsen, S. V., Laursen, H. V. B., Johnsen, S. P., Bartels, P. D., Ehlers, L. H., & Mainz, J. (2019). Can quality improvement improve the quality of care? A systematic review of reported effects and methodological rigor in plan-do-study-act projects. *BMC Health Services Research, 19*, 1–10. https://doi.org/10.1186/s12913-019-4482-6

Kolaski, A. Z., & Taylor, J. M. (2019). Critical factors for field staff: The relationship between burnout, coping, and vocational purpose. *Journal of Experiential Education, 42*(4), 398–416. http://doi.org/10.1177/1053825919868817

Kunnen, Y. S., Roemeling, O. P., & Smailhodzic, E. (2023). What are barriers and facilitators in sustaining lean management in healthcare? A qualitative literature review. *BMC Health Services Research, 23*(1), 958. https://doi.org/10.1186%2Fs12913-023-09978-4

Laffel, G., & Blumenthal, D. (1989). The case for using industrial quality management science in health care organizations. *JAMA, 262*(20), 2869–2873. https://doi.org/10.1001/jama.1989.03430200113036

Lancaster, A. K., Thessen, A. E., & Virapongse, A. (2018). A new paradigm for science: Nurturing the ecosystem. *F1000Research, 7*(803). 1–25. https://doi.org/10.12688/f1000research.15078.1

Lee, S. M., & Lee, D. (2022). Developing green healthcare activities in the total quality management framework. *International Journal of Environmental Research and Public Health, 19*(11), 6504. https://doi.org/10.3390/ijerph19116504

Liu, H. C., Zhang, L. J., Ping, Y. J., & Wang, L. (2020). Failure mode and effects analysis for proactive healthcare risk evaluation: A systematic literature review. *Journal of Evaluation in Clinical Practice, 26*(4), 1320–1337. https://doi.org/10.1111/jep.13317

Majed, M., Ayaad, O., AlHasni, N. S., Ibrahim, R., AlHarthy, S. H., Hassan, K. K., Al-Zadjali, R., Al-Awaisi1, H., & Al-Baimani, K. (2024). Enhancing patient safety: Optimizing fall risk management for oncology patients through failure modes and effects analysis. *Asian Pacific Journal of Cancer Prevention, 25*(2), 689–697.

Mantasas, N. (2021). Clinical support services' crucial role in quality improvement. In R. Roberts-Turner & R. K. Shah (Eds.), *Pocket guide to quality improvement in healthcare*. Springer Nature.

Marjoua, Y., & Bozic, K. J. (2012). Brief history of quality movement in US healthcare. *Current Reviews in Musculoskeletal Medicine, 5*(4), 265–273. https://doi.org/10.1007%2Fs12178-012-9137-8

Marshall, T. L., Rinke, M. L., Olson, A. P., & Brady, P. W. (2022). Diagnostic error in pediatrics: A narrative review. *Pediatrics, 149*(Supplement 3), e2020045948D. https://doi.org/10.1542/peds.2020-045948D

Medical Mistakes. (1999). Medical Mistakes: Joint Hearings Before the Subcommittee on Labor, Health and Human Services, and Education, and Related Agencies Committee on Appropriations and the Committee on Health, Education, Labor, and Pensions and the Committee on Veterans' Affairs of the United States Senate, 106th Cong. (1999, December 13). https://www.congress.gov/106/chrg/CHRG-106shrg61732/CHRG-106shrg61732.pdf.

Meese, K. A., Boitet, L. M., Schmidt, J. J., Borkowski, N., & Sweeney, K. L. (2024). Exploring national trends and organizational predictors of violence and mistreatment from patients and visitors. *Journal of Healthcare Management, 69*(1), 29–44. https://doi.org/10.1097/JHM-D-23-00105

Meese, K. A., Colón-López, A., Montgomery, A. P., Boitet, L. M., Rogers, D. A., & Patrician, P. A. (2022). Rules of engagement: The role of mistreatment from patients in the nurse, physician and advanced practice provider experience. *Patient Experience Journal, 9*(2), 36–45. https://doi.org/10.35680/2372-0247.1719

Murray, J., Sorra, J. Gale, B., & Mossburg, S. (2024). *Ensuring Patient and Workforce Safety Culture in Healthcare*. Agency for Healthcare Quality and Research. https://psnet.ahrq.gov/perspective/ensuring-patient-and-workforce-safety-culture-healthcare

National Center for Quality Assurance. (2023, September 21). *About NCQA*. https://www.ncqa.org/about-ncqa

National Nurses United. (2018, December). Johns Hopkins hospital: Reality vs. reputation. https://www.nationalnursesunited.org/sites/default/files/nnu/files/pdf/1118-JHH-Reality-Reputation.pdf

Niv, Y., & Tal, Y. (2024). Risk management and patient safety processes in a Healthcare Organization. In *Patient safety and risk management in medicine: From theory to practice* (pp. 129–174). Springer Nature Switzerland.

Olson, A. P., Graber, M. L., & Singh, H. (2018). Tracking progress in improving diagnosis: A framework for defining undesirable diagnostic events. *Journal of General Internal Medicine, 33*(7), 1187–1191. https://doi.org/10.1007%2Fs11606-018-4304-2

Padilla, T. (2017). Kindness: At the center of patient experience strategies. *Journal of Healthcare Management, 62*(4), 229–233. https://doi.org/10.1097/jhm-d-17-00083

Panagioti, M., Khan, K., Keers, R. N., Abuzour, A., Phipps, D., Kontopantelis, E., Bower, P., Campbell, S., Haneef, R., Avery, A. J., & Ashcroft, D. M. (2019). Prevalence, severity, and nature of preventable patient harm across medical care settings: Systematic review and meta-analysis. *BMJ, 366*, 14185. https://doi.org/10.1136/bmj.l4185

Paterick, Z. R., Patel, N., & Paterick, T. E. (2020). Peer review: Practical aspects and legal/ethical issues faced by the medical staff. *The Journal of Medical Practice Management, 35*(5), 243–246.

Pelletier, L. R., & Beaudin, C. L. (2017). *HQ solutions: Resource for the healthcare quality professional.* Lippincott Williams & Wilkins.

Poku, M. K., Behkami, N. A., & Bates, D. W. (2017). Patient relationship management: What the US healthcare system can learn from other industries. *Journal of General Internal Medicine, 32*(1), 101–104. https://doi.org/10.1007/s11606-016-3836-6

Potthoff, S. J., Mishek, J. H., & Hart, G. W. (2020). *Applied problem-solving in healthcare management.* Springer Publishing, Inc.

Press Ganey. (2024, April 2). *Safety in healthcare 2024.* https://info.pressganey.com/e-books-research/safety-2024

Pruitt, Z. (2024). Health care management. In J. Knickman & B. Elbel (Eds.), *Jonas & Kovner's health care delivery in the United States* (13th ed.). Springer Publishing.

Pruitt, Z., Smith, C. S., & Pérez-Ruberté, E. (2020). *Healthcare quality management: A case study approach.* Springer Publishing Company.

Putnis, N., & Neilson, M. (2022). Environmental sustainability and quality care: Not one without the other. *International Journal for Quality in Health care, 34*(3), mzac066. https://doi.org/10.1093/intqhc/mzac066

Radcliffe, E., Kordowicz, M., Mak, C., Shefer, G., Armstrong, D., White, P., & Ashworth, M. (2020). Lean implementation within healthcare: Imaging as fertile ground. *Journal of Health Organization and Management, 34*(8), 869–884. https://doi.org/10.1108/jhom-02-2020-0050

Rathlev, N. K., Visintainer, P., Schmidt, J., Hettler, J., Albert, V., & Li, H. (2020). Patient characteristics and clinical process predictors of patients leaving without being seen from the emergency department. *Western Journal of Emergency Medicine, 21*(5), 1218–1226. https://doi.org/10.5811%2Fwestjem.2020.6.47084

Rosen, M. A., DiazGranados, D., Dietz, A. S., Benishek, L. E., Thompson, D., Pronovost, P. J., & Weaver, S. J. (2018). Teamwork in healthcare: Key discoveries enabling safer, high-quality care. *American Psychologist, 73*(4), 433–450. https://doi.org/10.1037%2Famp0000298

Rotter, T., Plishka, C., Lawal, A., Harrison, L., Sari, N., Goodridge, D., Flynn, R., Chan, J., Fiander, M., Poksinska, B., Willoughby, K., & Kinsman, L. (2018). What Is lean management in health care? Development of an operational definition for a cochrane systematic review. *Evaluation & the Health Professions, 42*(3), 366–390. https://doi.org/10.1177/0163278718756992

Rubenstein, L., Khodyakov, D., Hempel, S., Danz, M., Salem-Schatz, S., Foy, R., O'Neill, S., Dalal, S., & Shekelle, P. (2014). How can we recognize continuous quality improvement?. *International Journal for Quality in Health care, 26*(1), 6–15. https://doi.org/10.1093%2Fintqhc%2Fmzt085

Sawyer, B., & McDermott, D. (2019). *How does the quality of the U.S. healthcare system compare to other countries?* Retrieved from https://www.healthsystemtracker.org/chart-collection/quality-u-s-healthcare-system-compare-countries/#item-in-hospital-mortality-rate-for-acute-myocardial-infarction-ischemic-stroke-and-hemorrhagic-stroke-2015

Schiff, J. H., & Wagner, S. (2016). Anesthesia related mortality? A national and international overview. *Trends in Anaesthesia and Critical Care, 9,* 43–48. https://doi.org/10.1016/j.tacc.2016.07.001

Schneider, E. C., Shah, A., Doty, M. M., Tikkanen, R. Fields, K., & Williams R. D., II. (2021). *Mirror, mirror 2021: Reflecting poorly.* The Commonwealth Fund. https://www.commonwealthfund.org/publications/fund-reports/2021/aug/mirror-mirror-2021-reflecting-poorly

Shah, A. (2021). Quality improvement in practice—part 1: Creating learning systems. *British Journal of Healthcare Management, 27*(8), 1–8. https://doi.org/10.12968/bjhc.2021.0032

Shortell, S. M., Toussaint, J. S., Halvorson, G. C., Kingsdale, J. M., Scheffler, R. M., Schwartz, A. Y., Wadsworth, P. A., & Wilensky, G. (2023). The Better Care Plan: A blueprint for improving America's healthcare system. *Health Affairs Scholar, 1*(1), qxad007. https://doi.org/10.1093%2Fhaschl%2Fqxad007

Silver, S. A., Harel, Z., McQuillan, R., Weizman, A. V., Thomas, A., Chertow, G. M., Nesrallah, G., Bell, C. M., & Chan, C. T. (2016). How to begin a quality improvement project. *Clinical Journal of the American Society of Nephrology, 11*(5), 893–900. https://doi.org/10.2215/cjn.11491015

Southerland, L. T., Pasadyn, C. L., Alnemer, O., Foy, C., Vaswani, S., Chughtai, S., Young, H. W., & Brownlowe, K. B. (2024). Involuntary sedation of patients in the emergency department for mental health: A retrospective cohort study. *The American Journal of Emergency Medicine, 77*, 53–59. https://doi.org/10.1016/j.ajem.2023.11.059

Stiles, R. A., & Mick, S. S. (1994). Classifying quality initiatives: A conceptual paradigm for literature review and policy analysis. *Journal of Healthcare Management, 39*(3), 309–326.

Sunshine, J. E., Meo, N., Kassebaum, N. J., Collison, M. L., Mokdad, A. H., & Naghavi, M. (2019). Association of adverse effects of medical treatment with mortality in the United States: A secondary analysis of the global burden of diseases, injuries, and risk factors study. *JAMA Network Open, 2*(1), e187041. https://doi.org/10.1001/jamanetworkopen.2018.7041

Tarnutzer, A. A., Lee, S.-H., Robinson, K. A., Wang, Z., Edlow, J. A., & Newman-Toker, D. E. (2017). ED misdiagnosis of cerebrovascular events in the era of modern neuroimaging: A meta-analysis. *Neurology, 88*(15), 1468–1477. https://doi.org/10.1212/wnl.0000000000003814

Thawani, S. (2004). Six sigma: Strategy for organizational excellence. *Total Quality Management & Business Excellence, 15*(5–6), 655–664. http://doi.org/10.1080/14783360410001680143

Thom, B., Sokolowski, S., Abu-Rustum, N. R., Allen-Dicker, J., Caramore, A., Chino, F., Doyle, S., Fitzpatrick, C., Gany, F., Liebhaber, A., Newman, T., Rao, N., Tappen, J., & Aviki, E. M. (2023). Financial toxicity order set: Implementing a simple intervention to better connect patients with resources. *JCO Oncology Practice, 19*(8), 662–668. https://doi.org/10.1200/op.22.00669

Toussaint, J. S., & Berry, L. L. (2013). The promise of Lean in health care. *Mayo Clinic Proceedings, 88*(1), 74–82. https://doi.org/10.1016/j.mayocp.2012.07.025

Tsai, T. C., Jha, A. K., Gawande, A. A., Huckman, R. S., Bloom, N., & Sadun, R. (2015). Hospital board and management practices are strongly related to hospital performance on clinical quality metrics. *Health Affairs, 34*(8), 1304–1311. https://doi.org/10.1377/hlthaff.2014.1282

United Kingdom Civil Aviation Authority. (2013). *Global Fatal Accident Review 2002 to 2011*. https://www.caa.co.uk/publication/download/14559

Vanstone, M., Canfield, C., Evans, C., Leslie, M., Levasseur, M. A., MacNeil, M., Pahwa, M., Panday, J., Rowland, P., Taneja, S., Tripp, L., You, J., & Abelson, J. (2023). Towards conceptualizing patients as partners in health systems: A systematic review and descriptive synthesis. *Health Research Policy and Systems, 21*(1), 12. http://doi.org/10.1186/s12961-022-00954-8

Veazie, S., Peterson, K., Bourne, D., Anderson, J., Damschroder, L., & Gunnar, W. (2022). Implementing high-reliability organization principles into practice: A rapid evidence review. *Journal of Patient Safety, 18*(1), e320–e328. https://doi.org/10.1097/pts.0000000000000768

Wachter, R. M. (2013). Personal accountability in healthcare: Searching for the right balance. *BMJ Quality & Safety, 22*(2), 176–180. https://doi.org/10.1136/bmjqs-2012-001227

Walsh, P. (2019). What is a 'just culture'?. *Journal of Patient Safety and Risk Management, 24*(1), 5–6. https://doi.org/10.1177/2516043519830199

Whittington, J. W., Nolan, K., Lewis, N., & Torres, T. (2015). Pursuing the triple aim: The first 7 years. *The Milbank Quarterly, 93*(2), 263–300. https://doi.org/10.1111/1468-0009.12122

Wilandh, E., Josefsson, M. S., Osowski, C. P., & Sydner, Y. M. (2024). Better Hospital Foodservice–aspects highlighted in research published 2000–2023: A Scoping Review. *Clinical nutrition open science, 54*, 1–40. https://doi.org/10.1016/j.nutos.2024.01.001

Wildi, K., Gimenez, M. R., Twerenbold, R., Reichlin, T., Jaeger, C., Heinzelmann, A., Arnold, C., Nelles, B., Druey, S., Haaf, P., Hillinger, P., Schaerli, N., Kreutzinger, P., Tanglay, Y., Herrmann, T., Weidmann, Z. M., Krivoshei, L., Freese, M., Stelzig, C., Puelacher, C., Rentsch, K., Osswald, S., & Mueller, C. (2015). Misdiagnosis of myocardial infarction related to limitations of the current regulatory approach to define clinical decision values for cardiac troponin. *Circulation, 131*(23), 2032–2040. https://doi.org/10.1161/CIRCULATIONAHA.114.014129

Wirth, T., Peters, C., Nienhaus, A., & Schablon, A. (2021). Interventions for workplace violence prevention in emergency departments: A systematic review. *International Journal of Environmental Research and Public Health, 18*(16), 8459. https://doi.org/10.3390/ijerph18168459

Wolf, J. A., Niederhauser, V., Marshburn, D., & LaVela, S. L. (2021). Reexamining "Defining Patient Experience": The human experience in healthcare. *Patient Experience Journal, 8*(1), 16–29.

Womack, J. P. (2001). *Gemba Walks*. Lean Enterprise Institute, Inc.

Womack, J. P., & Jones, D. T. (1996). *Lean thinking: Banish waste and create wealth in your corporation*. Simon & Schuster.

Woodall, W. H., Adams, B. M., & Benneyan, J. C. (2012). The use of control charts in healthcare. *Statistical Methods in Healthcare*, 251–267.

Zhang, J., IJzerman, M. J., Oberoi, J., Karnchanachari, N., Bergin, R. J., Franchini, F., Druce, P., Wang, X., & Emery, J. D. (2022). Time to diagnosis and treatment of lung cancer: A systematic overview of risk factors, interventions and impact on patient outcomes. *Lung Cancer, 166*, 27–39. https://doi.org/10.1016/j.lungcan.2022.01.015

CHAPTER 13

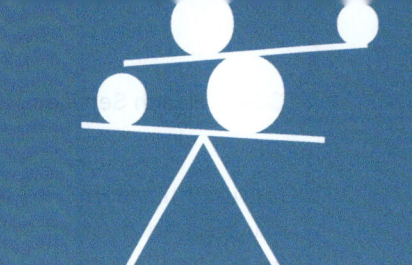

PROJECT MANAGEMENT

Project managers coordinate the temporary efforts of teams under set budgets and tight deadlines.

COMPETENCIES

- Manage projects effectively.
- Influence and motivate others to achieve team goals.
- Provide project oversight and sponsorship.
- Create business cases to gain stakeholder support for new projects.
- Identify and mitigate project risks.
- Prepare comprehensive project plans.
- Facilitate meetings to ensure effective and efficient communications.
- Create and track project budgets and schedules.

CHAPTER OUTLINE

- Project Initiation
- Project Planning
- Project Execution, Monitoring, and Control
- Project Closure

INTRODUCTION

The project management discipline first emerged from large engineering ventures, such as building the Hoover Dam and landing a man on the moon (Seymour & Hussein, 2014). These huge technical undertakings benefited from breaking projects into smaller manageable tasks and ordering them in sequential phases, enabling the development of accurate budgets and schedules. As the professional practice of project management prospered, the tools and practices expanded into other industries, such as technology and building construction. Projects are the temporary endeavors established to solve a specific problem or set of problems before a definite deadline and within a set budget, and project managers are the experts responsible for coordinating teams that deliver products, services, or capabilities on time and within budget (PMI, 2021).

Today, healthcare services managers use the same project management principles as construction and technology to deliver a variety of healthcare projects on time, on budget, and within scope. Projects happen everywhere in health care organizations (HCOs) from clinical care to information technology, to facilities construction, marketing, patient experience, revenue cycle, compliance, and human resources. As a management discipline, project management equips health services managers with a specific set of competencies to manage any group of people in a restricted timeframe. Without the requisite project management competencies, health services managers are doomed to wonder why executives point fingers at them when a given project misses deadlines, the budget swells, and the project gets canceled.

Project managers accept responsibility for project success yet lack the authority to give orders. Successful project managers learn to convince teams to complete high-quality work on schedule and within budget using a combination of interpersonal influence, communication skills, and methods unique to the project management discipline. By adopting a set of tools and processes, project managers can achieve project goals without the need for authoritative interventions from more senior executives. These project management skills help the health services manager succeed with any type of expert on the team, no matter the career level or formal title. Nevertheless, health services managers will encounter problems on projects that will need to be solved under set budgets and tight deadlines. To accomplish these goals, project managers use a standard approach to guide projects through multiple phases, which are organized in this chapter as: (1) project initiation; (2) project planning; (3) project execution, monitoring, and control; and (4) project closure.

PROJECT CONSTRAINTS

Temporary Work Under Tight Deadlines

Project managers who work in healthcare play the same role as other health services managers—plan, organize, staff, direct, and control—except that they specialize in performing temporary work under tight deadlines (Fayol, 1916). Just like all managers, project managers set goals, track progress, divide work tasks, estimate project costs and duration, assemble teams, and communicate with all stakeholders (Drucker, 1954). However, project managers are not concerned with creating routines and standards for ongoing operations. Project managers focus on completing the work and obtaining approval, then shutting down the project and moving on to the next project. Table 13.1 provides examples of healthcare projects and ongoing health services operations.

TABLE 13.1 Examples of Projects and Ongoing Operations

PROJECTS	ONGOING OPERATIONS
Developing clinical protocols for sepsis care	Delivering sepsis services
Implementing RFID technology for hospital pharmacy	Managing pharmacy inventory and supply chain processes
Expanding long-term care facility with a new patient care wing	Maintaining facilities and equipment
Preparing for a planned The Joint Commission accreditation site survey	Sustain The Joint Commission accreditation compliance for possible unannounced survey
Writing a strategic plan with input from physician stakeholders	Engaging physicians in strategy development and performance integration
Installing new software to manage patient registration	Revenue cycle management, including patient registration and health insurance billing
Creating a diversity, equity, and inclusion strategic plan	Recruiting and hiring a diverse workforce in equitable and inclusive ways

RFID, radio frequency identification.

Project Constraints

Limits are placed on every project. The Project Management Institute (PMI, 2021) cites six project limitations or **constraints** that must be carefully managed: time, scope, cost, quality, risk, and resources. Conventionally, project managers focus on controlling three of these constraints: scope, time, and cost. These three constraints are put together in what is called the Triple Constraint Model. When one of the three constraints changes, trade-offs among the other two must be made, as described in Table 13.2 (PMI, 2021). Project managers frame projects in terms of these constraints so that stakeholders can see how their actions impact the project's goals. The ability to successfully deliver the completed project, despite these constraints, enhances the value of the project manager to the team and the organization.

Figure 13.1 illustrates the consequences of prioritizing two constraints over the other. As shown in the figure, a cheap project delivered quickly must be limited in function. For example, project managers at UAB Medicine in Birmingham, Alabama, worked with a team of healthcare professionals to build eleven pop-up COVID-19 vaccination clinics (Klein & Hostetter, 2021). These simple tent structures were built in public locations convenient to high-need populations. Built quickly and cheaply, the clinics could only provide vaccination services and nothing else. Expanding the scope of services, to include COVID-19 testing, would have delayed the delivery of the project and/or increased expenses.

Project managers often deal with more than just these three constraints (scope, time, and cost) alone during the span of a project. The Project Management Institute warns that project managers must also consider quality, risks, and resources (PMI, 2021). Quality is related to scope but remains a different concept. **Scope** is "what" the project is tasked with delivering, and quality is "how good" the project is by comparing the customer's expectations to the actual results (Warner, 2020). For example, a project intended to build a new hospital wing could meet scope requirements (e.g., walls, equipment) but fail to meet The Joint Commission accreditation expectations of quality (e.g., minimums for patient room space). Risks and resources will be discussed later in the chapter.

TABLE 13.2 The Trade-Offs in the Triple Constraint Model

CONSTRAINT	DEFINITION	RELEVANT QUESTION
SCOPE	Collection of tasks that is delivered at the end of the project	We want to add functions to the project (scope), should we add workers, which will be more expensive (cost) or delay the project (time)? A little of both?
TIME	Number of working hours from a certain point to a future deadline	We may miss the deadline for completing the project (time), should we drop certain requirements (scope) or add more workers (cost)?
COSTS	Budgeted amount of money needed to complete a project, including salaries and materials	We need to finish the project sooner than expected (time), should we add workers (cost) or reduce the size of the project (scope)?

FIGURE 13.1 Project management triple constraint Venn diagram.

> **INFORMATIONAL INTERVIEW 13.1**
> *Project Coordinator*
> Access the informational interview online at http://connect.springerpub.com/content/book/978-0-8261-4807-0/chapter/ch00.

PROJECT INITIATION

Project Authorization

A senior manager with formal authority, called the **project sponsor**, formally initiates a project by explaining how the project will solve the specific organizational problem (Westland, 2007). To gain approval to launch the project, the project sponsor presents a formal **business case** that

- clarifies the strategic significance;
- explains how the project will impact the goals of the organization;
- estimates project costs, including labor, materials, and equipment;
- justifies the cost, citing outcomes such as reduced costs, increased revenue, improved patient care, or increased patient experience;
- describes expected benefits;
- identifies any relevant risks; and
- delegates the authority to the project manager for internal project activities.

Once a business case is approved, a **project charter** is written by the project manager which outlines the high-level **deliverables** (products, services, or capabilities) that must be provided upon the completion of a project, the needed resources (e.g., labor, overhead, materials, and equipment), and any potential risk that could derail the success of the project (PMI, 2021). Generally, a charter will outline the initial budget for project planning purposes, but this cost estimate can change when the project scope is completely defined. Table 13.3 illustrates a sample project charter for a fictional project within the facilities planning and construction department called the master facilities plan.

Initial Project Scoping

When a project charter has been approved, the project sponsor—the ultimate decision maker—will delegate authority and responsibility for the project to a project manager. Together, the project sponsor and project manager will host an initial scoping workshop meeting with a group of

TABLE 13.3 Master Facilities Plan Project Charter

PROJECT NAME:	MASTER FACILITIES PLAN	LAST REVISION DATE:	8/18/2026
PROJECT MANAGER:	Steve Doering	Project start date:	9/1/2026
PROJECT SPONSOR:	Olivia Taylor, COO	Expected deadline:	6/30/2027
INITIAL PROJECT BUDGET:	$100,000, including office overhead, staff time, printing and production, and Hawley and Company Architects consultant		
PROJECT PURPOSE AND GOALS:	This project is intended to achieve the following objectives: • Gather resources to inform the planning process. • Conduct a facility needs assessment. • Recommend and describe facilities initiatives necessary to meet strategic and operational needs, including any needed renovations and/or new construction. • Gain approval for facilities initiative recommendations along with detailed clinical conditions and background assumptions as support to operations committee, strategic planning committee, and board of directors.		
DELIVERABLES:	Finalize master facilities plan with maps and graphics, fully vetted and approved through governance process and submitted to the board of directors.		
PHYSICAL RESOURCES:	Project office on corporate floor, including conference room, copier/printer, and materials		
TEAM MEMBERS:	Alicia Day, chief financial officer; Don Zhang, chief information officer; Karen Jensen, chief strategy officer; Sarah Mackenzie, director of facilities management; Edwin Betancourt, director of strategic planning; Jeff Binder, information technology supervisor; Rahul Gupta, CPA, director of finance; Jesse T. Silva-Stone, AIA, NCARB, architect with Hawley and Company Architects; Jean Salvatore, business systems analyst		
PROJECT RISKS:	• A new four-story, 245,000 sq. ft. patient bed tower is being built now, which should be considered in facilities needs assessment. • Changes in certificate-of-need laws could extend the delivery date. • Hospital plans to issue a $90 million bond series through the Public Finance Authority, but final approval has not been made. • Governance committees need to approve, but they only meet every month or every quarter.		

AIA, American Institute of Architects; COO, chief operating officer; CPA, certified public accountant; NCARB, National Council of Architectural Registration Boards.

subject matter experts with specific knowledge or skills who contribute to the project in unique ways (Kendrick, 2012). During this discussion, the team reaches consensus on the project objectives and identifies anything that may have been missed in the project charter (Galbus, 2016). Under the facilitation of the project manager, the initiation workshop seeks to

- confirm that the right people are on the team;
- specify project goals, requirements, and specifications;
- review the budget constraints;
- define the major deliverables;
- explain decision-making processes;
- uncover additional project risks;
- create a communications plan that defines the meeting and status update frequency;
- share project tools and processes for project coordination, such as texting apps or project management websites; and
- agree to measures for project success.

Project Procurement

In some instances, project managers and teams may identify needed products or services that may be purchased from outside sources. Project managers conduct analysis, often called a **buy versus build analysis**, to determine whether the products or services can be created through the in-house team or through outside vendors. If a service is more effective and efficient when purchased from a vendor, then the project manager often works with the procurement or purchasing office to coordinate the purchasing activities for the project. Procurement offices act as professional intermediaries between the project manager and the vendor to coordinate the purchasing processes, such as defining specifications, managing the bidding processes, and engaging in contracts (Miller & Lehoux, 2020).

CAREER BOX 13.1: Early-Career Project Management

For early careerists, project management offers an excellent opportunity to learn how to manage people without formal authority or executive title. Entry-level project management positions include project coordinator, project assistant, or project management associate. These roles are responsible for organizing project materials, coordinating communications among team members, and escalating any observed issues to project managers. While not required, project management certification, such as Google Project Management Professional Certificate or Certified Associate in Project Management (CAPM)® from the PMI, may signal to employers an early careerist's readiness to contribute to projects (Career Employer, 2021).

When contracting services from vendors, health services managers must follow the policies and procedures established by HCO procurement offices. Large competitive contracts, such as building construction or medical equipment purchasing, may require formal bids. HCO procurement offices control the bidding processes to comply with policies and laws related to conflicts of interests and bribery. While the competitive bid process can take longer than direct sourcing of products and services, bidding can result in lower costs and fewer misunderstandings. Competitive bid requirements can sometimes be waived if the contract falls below a certain dollar amount (PMI, 2021).

⚠ KEY IDEA
Vendor selection criteria can also seek to address social goals, such as diversity and equity.

Potential vendors respond to requests for proposals (RFPs) that are evaluated against formal selection criteria. The procurement process will include selection criteria used to evaluate the bidders, often developed in collaboration with the project team. Criteria can include price, past performance, personnel qualifications, insurance capacity, and availability. Vendor selection criteria can also seek to address social goals, such as diversity and equity. For example, a vendor's status, as a minority-owned or women-owned business, can be considered in the evaluation criteria (Wirick, 2009). Project managers and teams are responsible for selecting vendors, evaluating performance, negotiating changes to the contracts, and approving final deliverables.

INFORMATIONAL INTERVIEW 13.2
Program Manager, Informatics
Access the informational interview online at http://connect.springerpub.com/content/book/978-0-8261-4807-0/chapter/ch00.

Once a vendor is chosen from a list of qualified sellers, the project manager and procurement office work with an attorney to create a legal contract that establishes the payment terms and deadlines. Three general types of contracts are used for vendors (Wirick, 2009):

- *Fixed price:* Payment set in advance does not change throughout the project, despite any deviations from the original project time, scope, or quality. Generally, a project manager will negotiate a separate document with the vendor, sometimes called a **service-level agreement** (SLA) or scope of work (SOW), that will establish more detailed terms and conditions for the project operations.
- *Cost reimbursement:* Payment to the vendor is based on their actual costs plus a fee or incentive for meeting or exceeding project objectives.
- *Time and materials:* Payment based on an agreed-upon hourly rate for services on the project multiplied by the number of hours provided plus any costs for supplies and materials.

PROJECT PLANNING

Project Plan

Using the project charter and initial scope, project managers define the requirements of the project in more detail. A **project plan** is a comprehensive document that describes the deliverables in detail (work breakdown), assigns who will complete each deliverable (responsibility matrix), outlines when each deliverable will be started and completed (schedule), decides the sequence of the work (activity sequencing), and estimates how much the project will cost (budget)..

To create the project plan, the project manager first works with the project team to divide deliverables into smaller, more manageable parts, often facilitating multiple problem-solving meetings (Kendrick, 2012). A product of these meetings is the development of a **work breakdown structure** (WBS), which is a chart that illustrates the deliverables and work packages of the project in multiple levels of detail (PMI, 2021). The top level of a WBS states the final deliverable, such as final master facilities plan, as shown in Figure 13.2. The next level states the key deliverables of phases

FIGURE 13.2 Facilities master plan work breakdown structure.

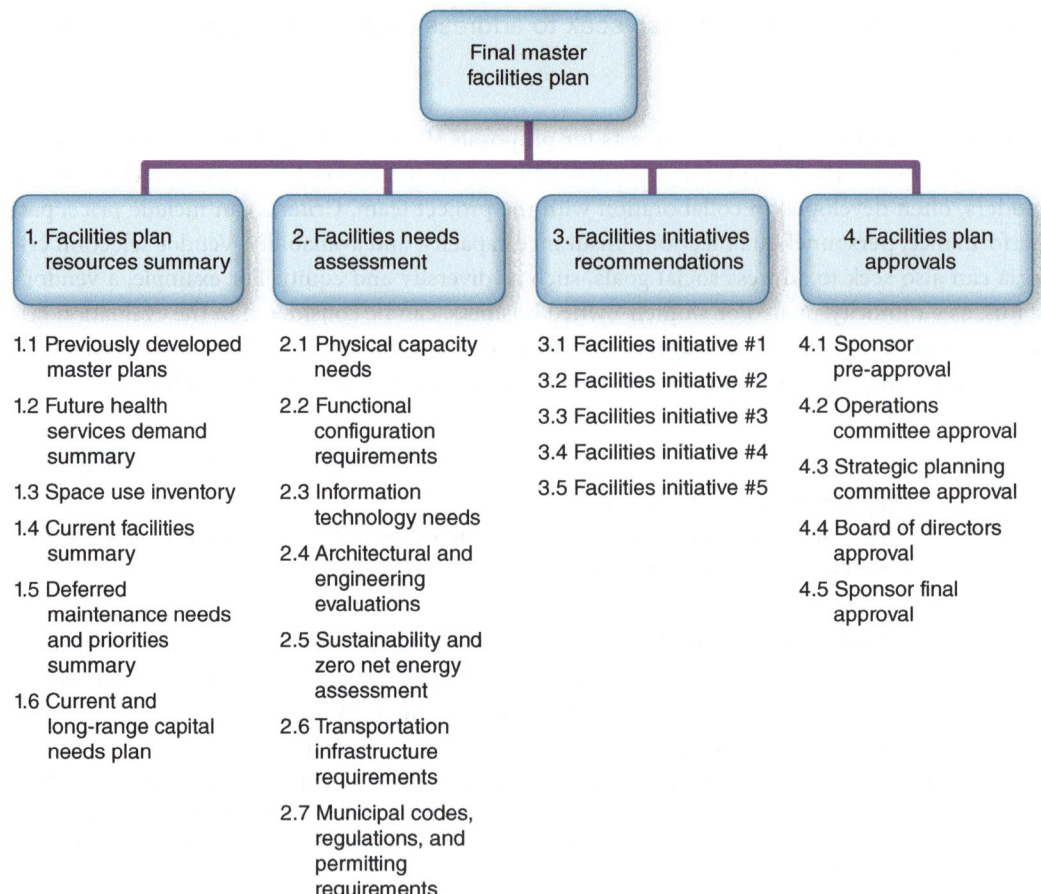

of a project. In the facilities master plan example, the main deliverable is divided into four sub-deliverables, each numbered as follows:

1. facilities plan resource summary
2. facilities needs assessment
3. facilities initiatives recommendations
4. approvals of facilities master plan

The final level of the WBS is the work package. In Figure 13.2, the second deliverable (facilities needs assessment) includes seven different work packages, including physical capacity needs, functional configuration requirements, information technology needs, and so on. When building the WBS, the project manager should focus on specific products that will be delivered rather than actions. The WBS conveys the tangible outcomes of the project—the "what," not the "who" or the "how" (Kendrick, 2012). A WBS can list additional levels of work packages beyond the third level, but generally, three levels are enough detail to effectively manage the project without micromanaging the team.

Responsibility Matrix

Based on the WBS, the project manager collaborates with the project team to assign responsibility for all project deliverables and/or work packages (the "who"). If the team member commits to completing a deliverable or work product, then they accept the responsibility and accountability for that work. To support this effort, the project manager uses a tool called the RACI matrix to document the various roles of a project. Also called a **responsibility matrix**, RACI is an acronym for **R**esponsible, **A**ccountable, **C**onsulted, and **I**nformed.

- *Responsible:* The member of the project team who does the work to create the deliverable. Responsibility for every deliverable should be assigned to at least one person.
- *Accountable:* The person who reviews the work involved in a project. They ensure that the person or team responsible knows the expectations of the project and completes the work on time. Every deliverable should have only one accountable person.
- *Consulted:* Stakeholders who give input and feedback on the work being done in a project because it could affect their current or future work. Project managers get necessary input from these project team members.
- *Informed:* Stakeholders who are given status updates on the work but who are not consulted with the details of the project. Informed people are not on the project team.

Table 13.4 presents a RACI matrix for the "facilities plan resources summary" deliverable described in the master facilities plan example.

In addition to assigning all elements of the work, the RACI matrix prevents confusion about who is responsible for what deliverable or who has authority to give final approval on the completion of a deliverable. While RACI matrices are designed to be used on complex projects that span multiple departments, role confusion can happen even on small projects. An effective project manager should clarify roles and responsibilities for project deliverables and work products irrespective of whether the RACI matrix is implemented or not.

Project Schedule

A well-documented project plan, including the WBS and RACI matrix, enables the project manager and project team to estimate scope, cost, and time with accuracy to avoid any misunderstandings, cost overruns, or missed deadlines. However, estimating the **schedule** often causes project managers the most difficulties—and severe consequences—because project teams often underestimate how long it will take to complete each deliverable or work product (Kendrick, 2012).

CAREER BOX 13.2: Mid-Career Project Management

For mid-careerists, project management experience demonstrates that they possess fundamental skills of the management profession along with the ability to problem-solve when project execution does not go as planned. The high-level skills developed as a project manager—negotiating terms, anticipating issues, resolving conflict, and making sound decisions—transfer to almost any health services manager position, including running clinics or hospital departments. For those who want to advance within the project management discipline, promotion to senior project manager means responsibility for managing larger, more complex projects with bigger budgets and longer timelines (Career Employer, 2021). A director of project management would oversee more junior project managers and manage multiple projects at the same time. Mid-career project managers are responsible for effective project delivery across the organization, often within a department called the project management office (PMO; Gareis, 2000). Mid-careerists who specialize in project management may seek the Project Management Professional (PMP)® certification from the PMI (2017).

TABLE 13.4 RACI Matrix for 1.0 Facilities Plan Resources Summary

TASK/DELIVER-ABLE	LEADERSHIP			PROJECT TEAM						
	CHIEF FINANCIAL OFFICER	CHIEF OPERATING OFFICER (SPONSOR)	CHIEF INFORMATION OFFICER	CHIEF STRATEGY OFFICER	PROJECT MANAGER	DIRECTOR OF FACILI-TIES MAN-AGEMENT	DIRECTOR OF STRATEGIC PLANNING	DIRECTOR OF FINANCE	ARCHITECT	BUSINESS SYSTEMS ANALYST
1.1 Previously developed master plans summary	I	A	I		R	R	C	C	C	
1.2 Future health services demand summary	I	C	I	A	C				C	
1.3 Space use inventory			I		C	A			C	R
1.4 Current facilities summary	I	A	I		C	R			C	
1.5 Deferred maintenance needs and priorities summary	A	C	I		C	R		I	C	
1.6 Current and long-range capital needs plan	A	C	I		C			R	C	

RACI, Responsible, Accountable, Consulted, and Informed.

Using the WBS and RACI matrix, the project manager works with the project team to carefully make a list of the activities or tasks needed to complete each work product (lowest level of the WBS). Activities and tasks are the actions (verbs) that need to happen to complete each deliverable or work product (nouns). Once each of the major activities is defined for a deliverable, then the work is progressively divided into tasks and subtasks. The project manager then collects all these activities, tasks, and subtasks into one document, called an **activity list**. Most activity lists are highly detailed and include all available information regarding the activities and tasks within a project. The list arranges the activities by work product, deliverable, or phase of the project. In addition, effective project managers assign tasks and subtasks to each team member to ensure accountability (PMI, 2021).

After determining all activities and tasks in the activity list, the project manager negotiates with the project team to estimate how much time each project activity or task will take to complete in hours, days, or weeks. This time estimate, which can be described in terms of hours, days, or weeks, is known as the **duration**—the date from when an activity starts to the date when it is completed (PMI, 2021). Activities and tasks with long durations tend to be greatly underestimated, so project managers should encourage project team members to shorten the duration of tasks and subtasks to improve estimation accuracy. Project managers can collect three levels of time estimates for each activity (best case, most likely, and worst case estimate) to improve duration estimation (Wirick, 2009). Duration estimates for tasks and subtasks should be long enough to enable independent work by the project team member but short enough so that the task can be completed in less than two project status update cycles (PMI, 2021). For example, if the project manager updates the status of completion of work products every 2 weeks, then a task or subtask should take less than 4 weeks.

> ⚠ **KEY IDEA**
>
> After determining all activities and tasks in the activity list, the project manager negotiates with the project team to estimate how much time each project activity or task will take to complete in hours, days, or weeks.

Table 13.5 shows an example of an activity list for "future health services demand summary." According to the RACI matrix, the director of strategic planning is responsible for this work project. In collaboration with the project manager, the director of strategic planning would list every action associated with creating the future health services demand summary. Each activity level has an estimated duration assigned such that the total duration of "future health services demand summary" is estimated to take 13 working days to complete from start to finish.

Activity Sequencing

The next step in scheduling a project is to determine the sequence of activities. In many cases, activities can be completed in any order or at the same time (concurrently) by different people. However, when one activity must be completed before another one, the first activity is called a **dependency**. Project managers note which activities must be completed before any of the newly defined activities can begin.

The master facilities plan example contains dependencies. For instance, the activities that create "facilities needs assessment" must be completed before the project team can begin work on "facilities initiatives recommendations." Logically, recommendations cannot be made without first assessing the future needs of the facilities. Therefore, the last completed activity of the "facilities needs assessment" deliverable is a dependency of the first activity in "facilities initiatives recommendations" and should be noted in the project schedule.

TABLE 13.5 Activity List for "Future Health Services Demand Summary"

ACTIVITY OR TASK	RESPONSIBLE PARTY	START DATE	END DATE	DURATION
1.2.1. Summarize service area population trends	Director of strategic planning	30-Sep	1-Oct	2
1.2.2. Summarize top 10 diseases and their growth	Director of strategic planning	2-Oct	2-Oct	1
1.2.3. Summarize technology innovations impacting health services demand	Director of strategic planning	3-Oct	7-Oct	5
1.2.3.1. Research artificial intelligence in health care	Director of strategic planning	3-Oct	3-Oct	
1.2.3.2. Research precision medicine and gene therapy in health care	Director of strategic planning	4-Oct	4-Oct	
1.2.3.3. Research medical equipment innovations in health care	Director of strategic planning	5-Oct	5-Oct	
1.2.3.4. Research predicted pharmaceutical innovations in health care	Director of strategic planning	6-Oct	6-Oct	
1.2.3.5. Research telemedicine innovations in health care	Director of strategic planning	7-Oct	7-Oct	
1.2.4. Summarize trends in health services access barriers and supports	Director of strategic planning	8-Oct	9-Oct	2
1.2.5. Summarize national health expenditure projections by type of service	Director of strategic planning	10-Oct	12-Oct	3

Visualizing Project Timelines

Due to the expectation that the project must be completed by a certain deadline, project managers need to estimate how long the project will take to complete. The total project duration can be determined by analyzing the longest sequence of interdependent activities from the beginning to the end, known as the **critical path**. The project cannot take less time to complete than the sequence of activities that make up the critical path (Moylan, 2002). Project managers can schedule activities that are not on the critical path with slack (or float), which is the amount of time a single activity or task can be delayed without missing the project deadline.

If the project manager appropriately links all interdependent activities using any number of project management software tools, such as Microsoft Project®, they can create a graphical flow of the work activities with related dependencies that illustrates the total duration of the entire project. One such visual representation of the project timeline that simplifies the complexity of the

FIGURE 13.3 PERT chart.

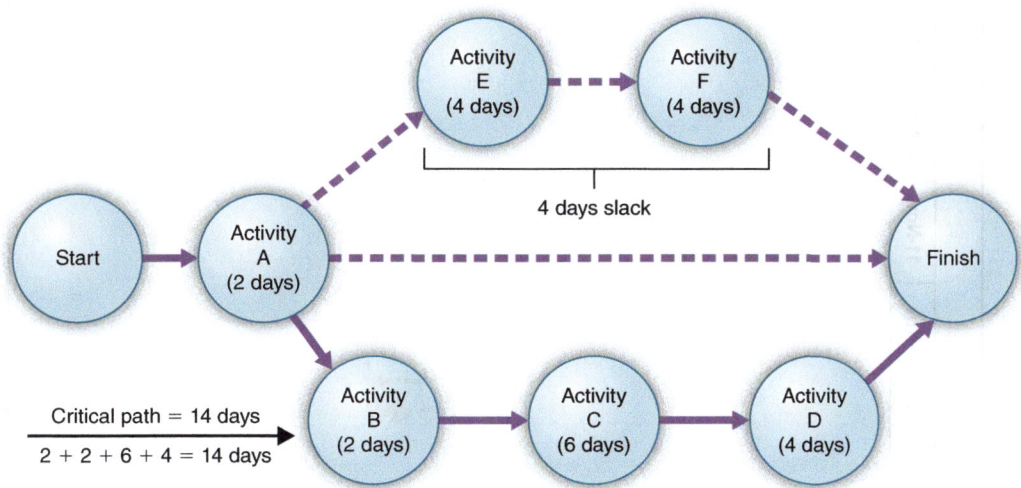

critical path is called the network diagram, sometimes called a Program Evaluation and Review Technique (PERT) chart. Figure 13.3 shows the critical path (the solid line). The critical path example shows that the shortest amount of time this project can take is 14 days (A + B + C + D). The network diagram helps the project manager visualize the critical path and communicate to the project team the importance of completing tasks on time, especially when they are a part of the critical path (Robles, 2018).

One of the most recognizable visual aids for project scheduling is called the **Gantt chart**, named after Henry Gantt, an early 20th-century proponent of scientific management. The Gantt chart is a bar chart with schedules, steps, and deadlines that help project teams visualize project timelines from beginning to end (Robles, 2018). In addition, the Gantt chart shows how the activities are related so that the project manager can communicate the progress against deadlines, especially during project status presentations (PMI, 2021). Gantt charts can be created in Microsoft Project®, Microsoft Excel®, and online project management software.

Figure 13.4 shows an example of the first deliverable of the facilities master plan, "facilities plan resources summary." The Gantt chart includes the following elements:

- *Activity or task:* Each action is listed with an identifier code.
- *Start date:* When the activity or task is estimated to begin.
- *End date:* When the activity or task is estimated to be completed.
- **Duration**: The amount of time each activity or task is estimated to take from start to finish, represented as a bar indicating hours, days, or weeks, depending on the timescale of the project.
- **Milestone**: A diamond shape shows the specific point in time that activities or tasks will be evaluated relative to the initial plan. Lack of progress toward completion becomes a project risk.
- *Dependencies:* Activities or tasks linked with an arrow are interdependent; the bar to the left must be completed before the subsequent activity or task to the right.

Budget Estimation

Project managers also create **budget estimates** in the planning phase. There are many ways to create project management budget estimates, but two of the most common are top-down and

FIGURE 13.4 Gantt chart.

Facilities master plan Gantt chart for facilities plan resources summary deliverable												
Activity or task	**Start**	**End**	**Duration**	**30-Sep**	**7-Oct**	**14-Oct**	**21-Oct**	**28-Oct**	**4-Nov**	**11-Nov**	**18-Nov**	**25-Nov**
1. Facilities plan resources summary												
1.1 Previously developed master plans												
1.1.1 Index previous facility master plans	30-Sep	6-Oct	7									
1.1.2 Summarize previous facility master plans	7-Oct	10-Oct	4									
1.2 Future health services demand summary												
1.2.1. Summarize population trends	14-Oct	15-Oct	2									
1.2.2. Summarize top 10 diseases	15-Oct	18-Oct	4									
1.2.3. Summarize technology innovations	19-Oct	20-Oct	2									
1.2.4. Summarize trends in access barriers	21-Oct	24-Oct	4									
1.2.5. Summarize expenditure projections	25-Oct	26-Oct	2									
Present to project sponsor												
1.3 Space use inventory												
1.3.1. Education space inventory	30-Sep	6-Oct	7									
1.3.2. Administration space inventory	7-Oct	13-Oct	7									
1.3.3. Research space inventory	14-Oct	20-Oct	7									
1.3.4. Outpatient space inventory	21-Oct	27-Oct	7									
1.3.5. Inpatient space inventory	28-Oct	2-Nov	6									
Present to Project Sponsor												
1.4 Current facilities summary												
1.4.1. Summarize current facilities – Education	4-Nov	5-Nov	2									
1.4.2. Summarize current facilities – Research	6-Nov	7-Nov	2									
1.4.3. Summarize current facilities – Outpatient	8-Nov	9-Nov	2									
1.4.4. Summarize current facilities – Inpatient	10-Nov	11-Nov	2									
1.4.5. Summarize current facilities – Admin	12-Nov	13-Nov	2									
Present to project sponsor												
1.5 Deferred maintenance needs and priorities summary												
1.5.1. Deferred maintenance plan	28-Oct	3-Nov	7									
1.5.2. Deferred maintenance summary	4-Nov	5-Nov	2									
1.6 Current and long-range capital needs plan												
1.6.1. Current capital needs plan	5-Nov	17-Nov	13									
1.6.2. Long-range capital needs plan	18-Nov	30-Nov	13									
Present to project sponsor	18-Nov	30-Nov	13									

bottom-up budgeting. The top-down budget is a rough estimate of the total project cost allocated to the various phases or key deliverables. Bottom-up budgeting is a more detailed estimate based on the cost of labor, materials, equipment, and all other resources of each activity.

When calculating the labor costs, project managers should determine the cost associated with the number of hours needed to complete the activity, called effort. Effort is multiplied by the labor cost rate for each person including payroll taxes, social security, medical insurance, paid leave, and benefits. Effort can be measured in hours, days, or weeks. This time estimate of effort can be different from the duration of an activity. While duration is the time between the start date and end date, effort is the actual time it takes to complete the activity (people can work on more than one project in the same period). For example, every project contains inherent delays for which no effort is needed, but the project team may need to wait for it to be completed. Using the example in Figure 13.4, the "gather and index previous facility master plans" work product takes one week to complete. However, this duration includes slack time for the project manager to gather the files from other workers. The labor time required to index the previous master facilities plans might only take one full workday (8 hours).

For activities requiring the efforts of multiple people, the employee labor rates would be multiplied by the total time of effort of the team. For example, the project manager may want to budget all meetings that every project team member would be required to attend, such as the kickoff, the project update reviews, and the closeout. Table 13.6 includes the labor costs for 3 hours of project team meetings.

TABLE 13.6 All-Team Project Meetings Budget Estimate

	HOURLY RATE	TIME OF EFFORT	COST
Olivia Taylor, COO (sponsor)	$165	3	$495
Steve Doering, project manager	$62	3	$186
Alicia Day, chief financial officer	$142	3	$426
Don Zhang, chief information officer	$147	3	$441
Karen Jensen, chief strategy officer	$144	3	$432
Sarah Mackenzie, director of facilities management	$110	3	$330
Edwin Betancourt, director of strategic planning	$123	3	$369
Jeff Binder, information technology supervisor	$45	3	$135
Rahul Gupta, CPA, director of finance	$106	3	$318
Jesse T. Silva-Stone, architect	$75	3	$225
Jean Salvatore, business systems analyst	$49	3	$147
		Subtotal:	$3,504

COO, chief operating officer; CPA, certified public accountant.

PROJECT EXECUTION, MONITORING, AND CONTROL

Project Risk Management

Every project contains potential circumstances that might threaten project success. A **risk** is present when there is uncertainty about whether an event will happen that may negatively affect the project outcomes. Project managers identify, analyze, plan, and control **project risks** throughout the execution phase (PMI, 2021). Any number of risks, as shown in Table 13.7, can result in cost overruns, scope creep, missed deadlines, and/or project cancellation.

Like assigning responsibility for activities, project managers assign ownership of risks to individuals responsible for the associated deliverable or work product (Wirick, 2009). In some cases, project managers assign risks to individual project team members. In other cases, the project sponsor accepts the responsibility for a risk because, after all, sponsors are ultimately accountable for overall project success (Hillson, 2014). Nevertheless, the project manager collaborates with the project team and project sponsor to plan corrective actions for when bad things happen.

TABLE 13.7 Examples of Project Risks

RISK TYPE	RISK EXAMPLES
PROJECT SUPPORT	• Lack of support from executive managers • Lack of project sponsor or authority • Unrealistic expectations of project sponsor • Inadequate budget • Lack of patient or customer involvement
PROJECT SKILL	• Ineffective project management skill • Ineffective communications among project team members • Lack of skill in project team members • Misunderstanding of objectives or requirements • Incorrect schedule estimates • Consistently changing scope (scope creep) • Not managing change properly
PROJECT TEAM	• Changes to membership or availability of the project team • Lack of clearly defined roles and responsibilities • Lack of cooperation/commitment from project team members • Labor shortages • Conflict among project team members • Noncompliance with laws and regulations
ENVIRONMENTAL, EXTERNAL, AND OTHER FACTORS	• Undependable vendors • Unreliable systems or equipment • Delays in government permitting • Information security, privacy breaches, or data loss issues • Acts of nature, such as severe weather conditions • Inflation in prices or unavailability of supplies and materials • Health and safety hazards • Compliance and legal liability issues

Source: Arnuphaptrairong, T. (2011, March). *Top ten lists of software project risks: Evidence from the literature survey*. In Proceedings of the International MultiConference of Engineers and Computer Scientists (Vol. 1, pp. 1–6); Paré, G., Sicotte, C., Jaana, M., & Girouard, D. (2008, January). *Prioritizing clinical information system project risk factors: A delphi study*. In Proceedings of the 41st Annual Hawaii International; Schwalbe, K., & Furlong, D. (2017). Healthcare project management (2nd ed.). Schwalbe Publishing; Shahzad, B., Abdullatif, A. M., Saleem, K., & Jameel, W. (2017). Socio-technical challenges and mitigation guidelines in developing mobile healthcare applications. *Journal of Medical Imaging and Health Informatics*, 7(3), 704–712. https://doi.org/10.1166/jmihi.2017.2050

Change Control

Despite the best efforts of project managers to stick to the plan, projects can change. The initial project scope can expand to include unauthorized tasks or deliverables, a phenomenon called **scope creep**. For example, the master facilities plan charter illustrated in Table 13.3 calls for delivering a facilities needs assessment. The project plan for this example might specifically outline the need for descriptions of relevant municipal codes, building regulations, and necessary permitting requirements. However, if the sponsor or other stakeholders later request that transportation infrastructure permits be approved by the municipal government, it would be a case of scope creep.

> ### △ KEY IDEA
> Despite the best efforts of project managers to stick to the plan, projects can change. The initial project scope can expand to include unauthorized tasks or deliverables, a phenomenon called scope creep.

When unforeseen issues warrant major changes to the approved project plan, effective project managers follow a formal **change control** process. Change control processes enable the project sponsor to make better decisions regarding the trade-offs among the triple constraint model (i.e., scope, time, and cost). While effective managers may insist on producing project deliverables based on the approved project plan, project sponsors may ask for changes to the project scope when they think it will improve the project. Project sponsors hold the formal position of authority, so the change should be evaluated, despite the scope being "frozen" in the approved project plan (Farag, 2021). The project manager analyzes the benefits and the consequences of the change and its impact on the project goals. This analysis allows the project manager to evaluate whether the requested change is justified. Then, the project manager documents the scope change with the reason and the impact to costs, time, or quality and obtains written approval from the project sponsor.

Project Monitoring and Communication

Project managers are responsible for gathering information, such as completed deliverables or missed deadlines, and summarizing the status of the project in reports for the sponsor, project team, and other stakeholders. In the planning phase, a **communication plan** will define the structure and methods by which the project manager will communicate project status and issues. During the execution phase, project managers spend most of their time and effort monitoring and communicating the progress of the projects. For example, summary-level status reports should be sent out regularly (e.g., weekly) to help the sponsor and project team monitor the project progress and react to issues as they arise.

INFORMATIONAL INTERVIEW 13.3
Vice President, Operations
Access the informational interview online at http://connect.springerpub.com/content/book/978-0-8261-4807-0/chapter/ch00.

Communicating project status also helps project managers motivate the team. For example, activities with missed deadlines should be communicated to the project team, sponsors, and other executives (Wirick, 2012). However, the purpose of the status report is to celebrate accomplishments and draw attention to project risks, not shame individuals on the team (Swanson, 2014). Only after sincere attempts have been made to negotiate with team members should a project manager seek assistance from the project sponsor regarding a missed deadline. Senior managers can apply more authoritative pressure to the team members, but such **escalation** of project risks can damage team morale.

> ⚠ **KEY IDEA**
>
> Senior managers can apply more authoritative pressure to the team members, but such **escalation** of project risks can damage team morale.

In addition, regularly scheduled project status meetings enable project managers to ensure collaboration and improve communication (PMI, 2021). While a poorly run meeting can feel like a waste of time, well-run project status meetings can enhance the influence of the project manager and motivate the project team. The following are elements of good project status meetings (Brownlee, 2008; Hansen, 2014; Lencioni, 2007; PMI, 2021):

- *Duration:* Project status meetings should be very short—10 to 25 minutes. Save in-depth discussions for other types of meetings unless the issue is applicable to most team members.
- *Frequency*: Hold project status meetings at consistent frequencies, such as daily or weekly with the project team and monthly with the sponsor or other stakeholders.
- *Format:* Consider requiring the team to stand during project status meetings. These team huddles can ensure that people do not get too comfortable and verge into conversational tangents. For virtual meetings, project managers should insist that team members keep their cameras on to improve focus on other team members' project status updates.
- *Preparation:* Project managers should send the status report or other supporting documents at least 1 day before the project status meeting and insist that project team members review the status report in preparation for the meetings.
- *Agenda:* Project managers should establish a simple standard project status meeting **agenda** that establishes the meeting content and schedule. Typically, project status meetings start with team members presenting short verbal progress updates on their activities, followed by brief discussions about any open issues, risks, or concerns.
- *Updates:* Each team member should be encouraged to give a verbal status presentation on their progress or associated risks for no more than 1 minute, preferably less. Any questions that break the 1-minute time limit for each team member should be moved to the end of the meeting or should be addressed outside the meeting.
- *Visual aids:* To help the project team stay focused, the project manager should prepare a simple visual aid that supports the main topic for discussion. To keep the team focused, the project manager can display snapshots of the Gantt chart, reminders of the critical path, or a simplified activity list.
- *Document meetings:* Following the meeting, the project manager should distribute to all team members a summary of the meeting with new actions or any changes to the project plan.

In *Death by Meeting*, Patrick Lencioni (2007) recommends that managers capture the attention of the team with an engaging hook or theme by focusing on conflict associated with the project. For example, if a team is performing behind schedule of a deliverable, the project manager can engage the team by seeking suggestions for getting back on track. Using the **gap analysis**, a difference between the current status of the project and the planned schedule or budget, can act to focus the team on the message of the meeting.

PROJECT CLOSURE

Project Sign Off

The project sponsor has the final approval on completed deliverables. The project manager presents the sponsor with a summary of the measures of project success (Kendrick, 2012). Potential success measures may include

- actual project duration;
- schedule variance (actual versus estimated);
- actual total costs, including team member effort;
- budget variance (actual versus estimated);
- number of risks encountered; or
- number of scope changes requested and made.

Once final approval is given by the sponsor, the project manager formally closes out the project (Farag, 2021). Project managers will formally release project team members so that they are free to work on other projects or initiatives. If a vendor supplied products or services for the project, the project manager ensures contract closure, which includes reviewing contract terms for satisfactory completion.

At the completion of the project, the project manager conducts a post-project review meeting, sometimes called a postmortem meeting, to review the lessons learned from the project. For example, if there were multiple scope changes, the project team should discuss why these happened and if the requirements could have been included in the original project plan. Also, the project team may have under- or overestimated activities in the original schedule and budget. By documenting these lessons learned, project managers can help the team members improve future project estimates, which in turn enhances the value of the project manager to the organization (Rowe & Sikes, 2006).

> **CAREER BOX 13.3: Late-Career Project Management**
>
> An executive position within the project management discipline can be titled the program manager. This position has responsibility for more long-term (although still temporary), highly complex, interrelated projects. Late-career health services managers with graduate degrees (e.g., MBA or MHA) and extensive experience managing projects in healthcare can also be promoted into executive roles in operations. Instead of managing temporary projects, executive positions, such as Vice President of Operations or Chief Operating Officer, handle the day-to-day functions of the HCO.

Project Transition to Operations

After the sponsor formally approves the completed project deliverables, the project manager transitions the deliverables to ongoing operations of the organization. The project manager transfers knowledge from the project team to the operational teams. In some cases, members of the project team will become a part of the operational staff, but in other cases, new operations will be independent of the project. To prevent future misunderstandings or unexpected events, the project manager should document any outstanding items, activities, risks, or issues. Success of any project also depends on the project manager documenting recommended next steps, updating training manuals, and outlining requirements for ongoing operations (Westland, 2007).

For instance, the Facilities Master Plan example presented in this chapter requires the project team to make a series of recommendations for future facility development based on the facilities plan resources summary and facilities needs assessment. These recommended initiatives should be sufficiently explained so that future teams can effectively launch new facility construction or renovation projects. In addition, the example project plan calls for approval of the facilities master plan by the operations committee, strategic planning committee, and the board of directors, which the project manager should include in the governance committee meeting minutes in the final project documentation.

> △ **KEY IDEA**
>
> **Success of any project also depends on the project manager documenting recommended next steps, updating training manuals, or outlining requirements for ongoing operations.**

Celebrating Successes

Finally, project managers should celebrate accomplishments, such as projects completed on time, at scope, and within budget, and reward professional behaviors, such as effective communication, dedication to the project, and high-quality work. Project managers can express their gratitude to team members in staff meetings or at low-key parties, in an email, or even handwritten thank you notes. These gestures not only solidify relationships between the project manager and project team members but also motivate them to succeed on future projects.

FUTURE DIRECTIONS

Future HCO facility expansions, technology innovations, virtual teams, and tight budgets will likely make project management skills more important than ever. Increased demand for project management skills will mean that all health services managers will need to know how to manage projects. Success will depend on not only the knowledge of project planning, monitoring, and controlling methods but also on strong communication and interpersonal skills. HCOs may not necessarily require specialized project management certifications but will expect that health services managers get projects done on time, on budget, and within scope.

SUMMARY

- Project managers coordinate temporary efforts of a team to accomplish goals that are established by the project sponsor in a project charter and business case.
- Project management is a discipline that specializes in dividing up work, creating teams, negotiating responsibilities and deadlines, tracking progress, facilitating meetings, and solving problems, all while working within budgets and deadlines.
- Often lacking the power to demand that tasks be completed on time; project managers must instead combine exceptional interpersonal skills with discipline-specific tools and processes to accomplish goals. To effectively manage projects and teams, project managers rely on project sponsors, clients, or other stakeholders in positions of authority to approve project plans, scope change requests, and final deliverables.

- Project managers frame projects in terms of the connection between the triple constraint model (scope, time, cost) so that sponsors, team members, and other stakeholders can appreciate the trade-offs associated with making changes to the project plan.
- Requested changes to an approved project plan requires the project manager to analyze potential impacts on scope, schedule, cost, and quality. Major changes to the approved project plan require project managers to follow a change control process designed to prevent scope creep, cost overruns, and missed deadlines.
- Project managers use regular status reports and meetings to communicate project progress and risks. Brief summaries and well-run project status meetings can avoid misunderstandings, improve collaboration, and motivate project teams.
- Once final approval is given by the project sponsor, the project manager formally closes out the project and transitions the deliverables to ongoing operations of the organization.

END-OF-CHAPTER RESOURCES

KEY TERMS*

*For the full list of key terms, please see the online glossary at **http://connect.springerpub.com/content/book/978-0-8261-4807-0.**

activity list
agenda
budget estimates
business case
buy versus build analysis
change control
communication plan
constraint
critical path
deliverables
dependency
duration
escalation

Gantt chart
milestone
project charter
project plan
project sponsor
responsibility matrix
risk
schedule
scope
service-level agreement
subject matter experts
work breakdown structure

LEARNING ACTIVITIES

Professional Development and Reflection

1. When entering a new management or leadership position, people tend to make a series of bad decisions that cost them credibility and potential allies, according to *The First 90 Days* by Micheal D. Watkins. People fail because of their preconceived notions about their new role that makes them rush to act before learning the organizational culture, decision-making processes, and the expectations of their boss. Watkins recommends that people prepare for new positions in advance. Using the tools of project management (e.g., WBS, activity list, Gantt chart, and/or network diagram), plan the first 90 days of a health services management position of interest to you. Base your project plan on Watkins's steps for success, such as define a learning agenda (i.e., learn about organization and meet with people), clarify expectations with your boss, assess the situation, determine how decisions get made, and evaluate and align your team. Or you can devise your own steps

for how to succeed in the first few months of a new job, as long as your project planning includes deliverables (or phase), work products, and activities.
2. Review job websites, such as Indeed, Monster, or LinkedIn, for project coordinator or project manager job listings within the healthcare industry. After reviewing at least three postings, analyze whether the job postings require that job applicants attain advanced project management certifications, such as Google Project Management Professional Certificate, Certified Associate in Project Management (CAPM)®, or Project Management Professional (PMP)®. Or are the certifications just preferred for those types of positions in HCOs? Or are project manager certifications not mentioned at all for healthcare project management jobs? Describe how these kinds of certifications can advance health services management careers.

Discussion Questions

1. Project managers usually lack the authority to demand that project team members complete their work on time and within scope. What are the most important interpersonal skills that can be used to ensure project success?
2. Which are more important to project success during the execution phase—communication skills or technical project management skills, such as Gantt charts and status reports? Why?

RECOMMENDED READING AND MEDIA

Clayton, M. (2019, February 28). *Project management in under 5: What is a gantt chart?* [YouTube]. https://www.youtube.com/watch?v=fB0wsdmV3Sw

Clayton, M. (2017, March 9). *What is a RACI chart? Project management in under 5* [YouTube]. https://www.youtube.com/watch?v=i9J_1N3-ibg

Farag, A. (2021). *Essentials of project management*. Fanshawe College Pressbooks.

Kendrick, T. (2012). *Results without authority: Controlling a project when the team doesn't report to you*. AMACOM.

Lencioni, P. (2007). *Death by meeting: A leadership fable*. Jossey-Bass.

McLachlan, D. (2020, June 11). *The critical path and float—key concepts in project management from the PMBOK* [YouTube]. https://www.youtube.com/watch?v=PIX2FGbLv6A

Watkins, M. D. (2013). *The first 90 days: Proven strategies for getting up to speed faster and smarter*. Harvard Business Review Press.

Witt, J. (2014, June 4). *Project management: What is a work breakdown structure?* [YouTube]. https://www.youtube.com/watch?v=wEWhnodF6ig

Witt, J. (2013, July 22). *What is the project management triple constraint* [YouTube]. https://www.youtube.com/watch?v=wJoipiqjsTc.

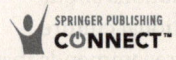

A robust set of instructor resources designed to supplement this text is located at http://connect.springerpub.com/content/book/978-0-8261-4807-0. Qualifying instructors may request access by emailing textbook@springerpub.com.

REFERENCES

Arnuphaptrairong, T. (2011, March). *Top ten lists of software project risks: Evidence from the literature survey*. In Proceedings of the International MultiConference of Engineers and Computer Scientists (Vol. 1, pp. 1–6).

Brownlee, D. (2008). *The secrets to running project status meetings that work!* [Paper presentation]. PMI® Global Congress 2008—North America, Denver, CO, United States of America. Project Management Institute, Newtown Square, PA, United States of America.

Career Employer. (2021, November 26). *Project management career path—the best guide for 2024*. Retrieved January 19, 2023, from https://careeremployer.com/project-management/project-management-career/

Drucker, P. (1954). *The practice of management*. New York: Harper & Row, Publishers, Inc.

Farag, A. (2021). *Essentials of project management*. Fanshawe College Pressbooks.

Fayol, H. (1916). General principles of management. *Classics of Organization Theory, 2*(15), 57–69.

Galbus, A. C. (2016). *Programme management initiation: What to focus on in the first 90 days* [Paper presentation]. PMI® Global Congress 2016 in Barcelona, Spain. Project Management Institute, Newtown Square, PA, United States of America.

Gareis, R. (2000, June 24). *Program management and project portfolio management: New competences of project-oriented organizations* [Conference Paper]. Project Management Institute Annual Seminars & Symposium, Houston, TX. Newtown Square, PA, United States of America.

Hansen, M. (2014, March 31). *The joy of meetings—part 2: The Dreaded status meeting*. Retrieved February 4, 2022, from https://www.credera.com/insights/joy-meetings-part-2-dreaded-status-meeting

Hillson, D. (2014). *Managing overall project risk* [Paper presentation]. PMI® Global Congress 2014—EMEA, Dubai, United Arab Emirates. Project Management Institute, Newtown Square, PA, United States of America.

Kendrick, T. (2012). *Results without authority: Controlling a project when the team doesn't report to you*. AMACOM.

Klein, S., & Hostetter, M. (2021, July 7). *The room where it happens: The role of primary care in the next phase of the COVID-19 vaccination campaign*. The Commonwealth Fund. https://www.commonwealthfund.org/publications/2021/jul/room-where-it-happens

Lencioni, P. (2007). *Death by meeting: A leadership fable*. Jossey-Bass.

Miller, F. A., & Lehoux, P. (2020). The innovation impacts of public procurement offices: The case of healthcare procurement. *Research Policy, 49*(7), 104075. https://doi.org/10.1016/j.respol.2020.104075

Moylan, W. A. (2002). *Planning and scheduling: The yin and yang of managing a project* [Paper presentation]. Project Management Institute Annual Seminars & Symposium, San Antonio, TX. Newtown Square, PA, United States of America.

Paré, G., Sicotte, C., Jaana, M., & Girouard, D. (2008, January). *Prioritizing clinical information system project risk factors: A Delphi study*. In Proceedings of the 41st Annual Hawaii International Conference on System Sciences (HICSS 2008) (pp. 242–242). IEEE.

Project Management Institute. [PMI]. (2021). *A guide to the project management body of knowledge (PMBOK® Guide)* (7th ed.). Project Management Institute.

Robles, V. D. (2018). Visualizing certainty: What the cultural history of the Gantt chart teaches technical and professional communicators about management. *Technical Communication Quarterly, 27*(4), 300–321. https://doi.org/10.1080/10572252.2018.1520025

Rowe, S. F., & Sikes, S. (2006). *Lessons learned: Sharing the knowledge* [Paper presentation]. PMI® Global Congress 2006—EMEA, Madrid, Spain. Project Management Institute, Newtown Square, PA, United States of America.

Seymour, T., & Hussein, S. (2014). The history of project management. *International Journal of Management & Information Systems (IJMIS), 18*(4), 233–240. https://doi.org/10.19030/ijmis.v18i4.8820

Schwalbe, K., & Furlong, D. (2017). *Healthcare project management* (2nd ed.). Schwalbe Publishing.

Shahzad, B., Abdullatif, A. M., Saleem, K., & Jameel, W. (2017). Socio-technical challenges and mitigation guidelines in developing mobile healthcare applications. *Journal of Medical Imaging and Health Informatics, 7*(3), 704–712. https://doi.org/10.1166/jmihi.2017.2050

Swanson, S. A. (2014). Anatomy of an effective status report. *PM Network, 28*(6), 52–61.

Warner, M. H. (2020, February 1). *Scope versus quality*. The Project Management Blueprint. https://www.theprojectmanagementblueprint.com/blog/scope-versus-quality

Westland, J. (2007). *The project management life cycle: A complete step-by-step methodology for initiating planning executing and closing the project*. Kogan Page Publishers.

Wirick, D. (2009). *Public-sector project management: Meeting the challenges and achieving results*. John Wiley & Sons.

CHAPTER 14

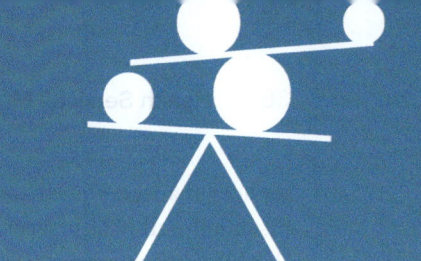

HEALTHCARE FINANCIAL MANAGEMENT

Healthcare financial management entails collecting revenue, controlling costs, reporting financials, planning budgets, and allocating resources to maintain the viability of health care organizations.

COMPETENCIES

- Understand roles and responsibilities of the healthcare finance organization, including financial control systems, third-party contracting, and capital financing.
- Optimize revenues and control expenses in health care organizations.
- Identify and interpret various payment methodologies of third-party payers.
- Manage revenue cycle to increase working capital and improve patient financial services.
- Analyze financial performance using income statements, balance sheets, and cash flow statements.
- Apply cost accounting methods used in health care organizations.
- Appraise organizational performance using financial ratios and metrics.
- Conduct operational and capital budgeting approaches used in financial planning.
- Analyze capital allocation decisions using return-on-investment and discounting methods.

CHAPTER OUTLINE

- Healthcare Finance Organization
- Healthcare Revenue
- Expenses and Costing Methods
- Financial Statements
- Financial Ratios and Metrics
- Budgeting and Planning

INTRODUCTION

Health services managers are responsible for maintaining the financial viability of health care organizations (HCOs) so that physicians, nurses, and other clinicians can care for patients. The health services managers who run financially successful HCOs understand the necessity to generate revenue, collect payments, control unnecessary spending, and squeeze as much usefulness out of buildings and equipment as possible (Nevola, 2016; Oner et al., 2016; Singh & Wheeler, 2012). Some factors are beyond health services managers' control, but excuses are irrelevant when financial realities threaten the viability of the HCO. For struggling HCOs, health services managers need strong financial acumen just to make payroll or to repay bank loans. Essentially, all health services managers need to develop financial competencies to protect the HCO for future generations of patients, clinicians, and communities.

Most health services managers choose to focus on general management roles, not to specialize in healthcare finance (Berman et al., 2013; Erskine et al., 2016). It is the healthcare finance experts who support most of the necessary financial tasks for HCOs, such as budgeting, financial analysis, capital financing, and accounting. Early in health service management careers, financial skills are less important than the ability to communicate effectively and behave professionally (Porter et al., 2016). Mid-career health services managers need to understand how to generate revenues, control costs, allocate resources, track financial performance, and make well-informed business decisions (Berman et al., 2013). As health services managers rise to the senior management ranks, financial skills become especially important to strategic planning, external relations, and financial success (Broom & Hilsenrath, 2015).

This chapter examines the competencies needed to succeed in mid- and early-career health services management positions. As is described, health services managers need to understand how financial experts within HCOs can assist them to meet their performance goals. Moreover, this chapter explains the basics involved with collecting revenues, controlling expenses, analyzing financial performance, and making sound resource allocation decisions. These fundamental competencies must be further developed to succeed in higher level health services management positions.

HEALTHCARE FINANCE ORGANIZATION

Chief Financial Officer

Under the direction of the CFO, the finance department personnel of the HCO are responsible for accounting, financial reporting, investments, revenue cycle, budgeting, resource allocation, financial analysis, and the control of financial processes (Reiter & Song, 2021). Figure 14.1 charts an example of the HCO finance function, including the reporting structure. In addition to overseeing these finance functions, the CFO is responsible for achieving four main goals (Deloitte, 2023; Hegwer & Hut, 2019; Reiter & Song, 2021):

- *Support operations:* Coach health services managers to track financial goals, improve operational performance, and make better fiscal decisions.
- *Create and implement strategy:* Conduct strategic planning, manage mergers and acquisitions, raise money for operations, and implement longer term strategies vital to future performance.
- *Preserve financial resources:* Efficiently manage financial resources, accurately report on the financial position, and ensure proper assessment of risk and compliance with laws and regulations to ensure the long-term financial viability of the HCO.
- *Drive business improvement:* Execute performance improvement initiatives, including cost reduction, supply chain optimization, and payer negotiations.

Controller

The **controller**, also spelled comptroller, is the key financial executive responsible for managing the HCO's accounting operations, payroll, financial reporting, budgeting, and internal controls. Health services **financial accounting** involves recording and summarizing economic events related to the operations, assets, and financing of HCOs (Reiter & Song, 2022). All transactions

FIGURE 14.1 Finance function organizational chart.

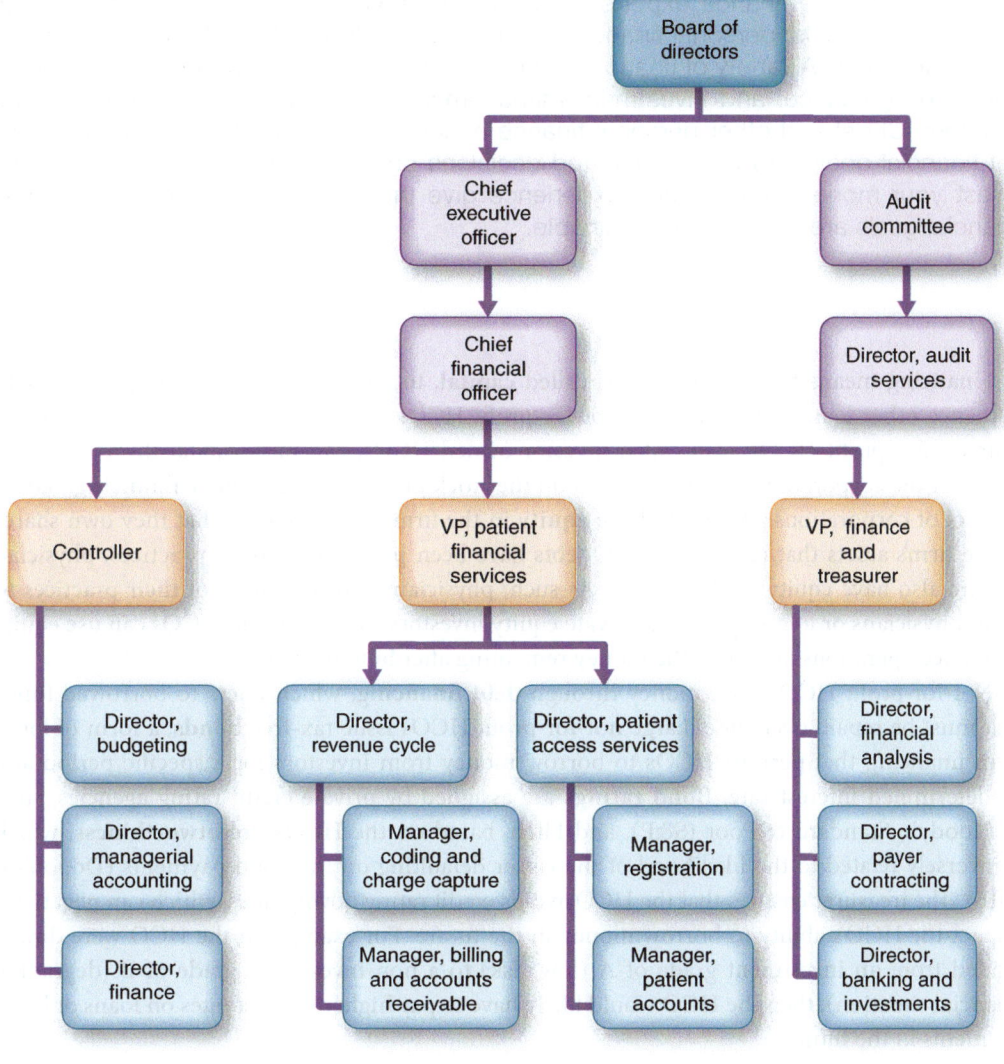

are electronically entered into a **general ledger**, the primary accounting record for all the financial transactions. The controller office is also responsible for budgeting, financial forecasting, cost analyses, and performance reporting that support HCO operations.

Treasurer

Large HCOs employ a senior-level finance executive who runs the treasury, which is the finance function that manages cash flows, investments, and financing of the HCO. Cash management is critical to HCOs for meeting near-term financial obligations, such as payroll, vendor invoices, and debt payments. When HCOs generate surpluses of cash from operations, called **financial reserves**, the treasurer is responsible for investing the money in financial markets. Strong performance in the stock and bond markets protects HCO's money for future use during periods of financial adversity (Kaufman Hall, 2023).

> **CAREER BOX 14.1:** Professional Financial Help
>
> Just as healthcare finance experts assist health services managers to make better decisions for HCOs, personal financial planners can help you to make wise decisions with your money. A variety of financial planning services, such as money management, budgeting guidance, and investment management, are offered by certified financial planners (CFPs) and other personal finance experts. Financial advisors can help you set financial goals and make educated decisions about how to spend and where to invest your money. Training and experience give them financial expertise to ensure financial goals are realistic and attainable.

Financing means borrowing money, called **capital**, to pay for expansion and growth or to refinance other loans. For-profit and not-for-profit HCOs typically raise money from different sources. For-profit HCOs, also called investor-owned HCOs, can raise capital through selling shares of the corporation to investors (i.e., on the stock market), called **equity financing**. Stockholders of corporations are said to have **equity** in the firms, which means that they own shares of the firm's assets that remain after all debts have been paid. For medical practices, physician owners also have equity in their firms. As such, physicians can sell shares of their practices to other physicians or to groups called private equity investors. Not-for-profit HCOs can use equity to finance operations only with the money remaining after bills are paid.

Not-for-profit HCOs raise money through **debt financing**, which refers to borrowed funds that must be repaid over time. Large not-for-profit HCOs issue tax-free **bonds**, a form of long-term financing that permits HCOs to borrow money from investors for a specific period at a predetermined interest rate. **Bond ratings** are assigned by private credit rating agencies, such as Moody's, Standard & Poor (S&P), and Fitch, based on the HCO's **creditworthiness,** which is inversely related to the likelihood of the issuer defaulting on the bond payments (Dopoulos, 2016). The treasurer ensures that the HCO avoids credit rating downgrades, which can negatively impact the HCO's ability to borrow money in the future. For example, if the HCO were downgraded from an investment grade of A (low risk) to a non-investment grade of B (degrading financial situation), then the HCO would likely have to pay higher interest rates on loans or bond payments in the future.

 INFORMATIONAL INTERVIEW 14.1
Financial Analyst
Access the informational interview online at http://connect.springerpub.com/content/book/978-0-8261-4807-0/chapter/ch00.

Board of Directors

The board of directors guides the direction of the HCO and has the collective authority to make the final decisions about financial matters (Erwin et al., 2019). The board reviews financial statements, tracks financial performance, and approves annual budgets. In addition, the board oversees the strategy of the organization to ensure that health services managers act consistently with the mission, vision, and values of the HCO. This involves balancing the financial performance with other important goals, such as medical care quality and community health.

> **△ KEY IDEA**
> Financial controls safeguard the HCO's assets by creating certain checks and balances, such as audit trails and policies related to access to bank accounts.

The board also oversees the HCO's **internal audit function**, ensuring that effective safeguards are in place to protect assets, prevent fraud, and maintain the accuracy of financial reporting. As illustrated in Figure 14.1, the internal auditing department acts as an independent, objective review of the HCO financial operations to identify and categorize risks and to make recommendations for improving finance controls (Reese, 2021). **Financial controls** safeguard the HCO's assets by creating certain checks and balances, such as audit trails and policies related to who can access bank accounts.

HEALTHCARE REVENUE

Seeking Revenue Growth

HCOs generate **revenues** by providing healthcare-related products and services, such as medical diagnostics, treatments, procedures, medications, and surgeries. Most health services managers seek to increase revenue for HCOs through one or more of the following methods (Moon & Shugan, 2020; Pruitt & Pracht, 2013; Rundall et al., 2012; White & Whaley, 2021):

- *Increase patient care **volume***: Add new services, create marketing campaigns to attract patients, improve access to existing services, or improve patient flow.
- *Improve **payer mix***: Attract higher paying patients. Private insurance companies typically pay more for health services than Medicare. Medicaid programs typically pay the lowest rates. Some HCOs create marketing campaigns to attract privately insured patients, which effectively reduces the relative proportion of lower paying government funding sources.
- *Increase **case mix***: Complex and resource-intensive cases typically receive higher payment rates. A higher average case mix increases overall HCO revenue.
- *Improve **service mix***: Build specialized expertise and reputation in providing high-priced premium specialty medical services or make more aggressive treatment choices.

Other revenue sources include fundraising, research grants, educational programs, facility rentals, and investments, all of which can be maximized through sound health services management practices.

Third-Party Payers

The healthcare marketplace is unique in that patients usually do not pay the full amount of the health services bill. Instead, government programs and health insurance companies, also called **third-party payers**, pay for health services on behalf of patients. Almost all of the private health insurers and most of the government programs are operated under a financing mechanism called **managed care** (Hinton & Raphael, 2023; Ochieng et al., 2023). Managed care refers to a group of health insurance activities intended to negotiate lower prices with HCOs, to limit unnecessary health service utilization, and to hold HCOs accountable for performance (Namburi & Tadi, 2023). Table 14.1 describes the basic types of managed care organizations.

Managed care organizations require HCOs to get their permission to deliver services to patients, a process called **utilization review**. In some instances, HCOs need to gain permission before delivering services to patients. To meet this requirement and to qualify for payment,

TABLE 14.1 Managed Care Organization Types

TERM	DEFINITION
HMO	Most restrictive. Members are required to get referrals from primary care physicians to obtain care from specialists. Members must choose HCOs with contracts with HMO to get services paid.
PPO	Moderately restrictive. PPOs contract with HCOs for reduced prices, which are passed on to members. Other HCOs are available, but members must pay higher fees for services.
POS	Least restrictive. Members have to choose a primary care provider but can select any other type of HCO of their choice. Most expensive managed care option.

HCO, health care organization; HMO, health maintenance organization; POS, point of service; PPO, preferred provider organization.

the HCO needs to obtain **prior authorization** from the managed care organization. From the insurance companies' perspective, prior authorizations restrain overuse and unnecessary spending for medical services. **Medical necessity** is a term that describes the determination of whether a specific treatment, procedure, or service is essential for the diagnosis, treatment, or prevention of an illness, injury, or medical condition. HCOs can be denied payment for services delivered and costs incurred if the services are not deemed medically necessary by managed care organizations. Given these circumstances, health services managers are responsible for optimizing payments from third-party payers to ensure the long-term financial viability and success of HCOs.

> ## △ KEY IDEA
>
> **HCOs can be denied payment for services delivered and costs incurred if the services are not deemed medically necessary by managed care organizations.**

Payments are sometimes called **reimbursements**, a term derived from the era when HCOs were paid based on the costs that they incurred (Namburi & Tadi, 2023). Today, the financing of health services is much more complicated than **cost-based reimbursement.** The amounts that HCOs send to payers on their bills for services are called **charges**. The **price** is the total amount an HCO expects to be paid by health insurance companies or government payers for health services. The health insurance company will pay a significantly discounted rate from the charge, which renders the charge amount billed by HCOs meaningless to most consumers. Typically, the only party to pay the full price of the HCO's charge are patients without insurance, also called **self-pay**. Patients without health insurance are often saddled with paying expensive charge amounts that may be unrelated to how much the services cost the HCOs. Unfortunately, uninsured patients do not have as much bargaining power as large insurance companies and are often asked to pay close to the full amount of the charges. Because of this, bills sent to the uninsured patients frequently remain unpaid and become classified as bad debt, also known as **uncompensated care** (Coughlin et al., 2021).

> **CAREER BOX 14.2: Increase Income with a Raise**
>
> Want to increase your income? The best time to ask your boss for a raise is before taking on new responsibilities or after you successfully complete a project (O'Hara, 2015). When asking for a raise, demonstrate to your boss how you add value to the organization with your unique contributions. To determine your worth in the marketplace, gather salary information through your professional network, human resources department, and websites with salary benchmarks. Also, be sure to frame your value in terms of how you can help your boss achieve their goals.

Payments to Health Care Organizations

HCOs are paid by third-party payers based on a variety of schemes and methods. For physicians and other outpatient services, the most common payment scheme is called **fee for service**, in which HCOs are paid a fee for every service provided. For patients with private health insurance, the payments are based on a rate negotiated between the insurance companies and HCOs. Insurance companies negotiate contracts with HCOs and agree to **fee schedules** that outline the payment rates for specific medical procedures. Each of the thousands of services that physicians perform are assigned a unique numerical identifier by the American Medical Association (AMA), called **Current Procedural Terminology (CPT)** codes (AMA, 2020). Medicare calculates fees based on how much the federal government officials think the services cost physicians to perform each CPT code. Under a complex methodology, Medicare generates a **relative value unit (RVU)** for each service based on the time estimate, practice expense, and malpractice expense (Klein et al., 2020). Some commercial insurance companies also use RVUs as a reference when calculating fee schedules (Urwin & Emanuel, 2019).

The fee-for-service method encourages clinicians to deliver more health care services. Thornburg and Meter (2021) call fee-for-service payments the "widget-based compensation methodology" that demotivates physicians. For physicians who are paid for their judgment and advice, a so-called cognitive care, paying for discrete episodes of time undervalues their contributions to patient health outcomes. Compared to physicians who provide procedure-based services, such as surgeries or diagnostics, those who mostly bill for cognitive services, such as many primary care physicians, are paid less. Table 14.2 demonstrates the payment disparity between primary care and specialists for services that take similar amounts of time. The Medicare payment for an RVU of 1.0 was $37.89 per RVU in 2023.

TABLE 14.2 Comparison of Fee-for-Service Payments Among Primary Care and Specialist Physicians

	PRIMARY CARE PHYSICIAN	SPECIALIST PHYSICIAN
SERVICE	History and physical for moderately complex condition	Colonoscopy (physician component)
SERVICE CODE	99204	G0121
TIME ESTIMATE (MINUTES)	45 to 59	30 to 60
RVU	2.60	3.26
TOTAL PAYMENT	$98.51	$123.52

RVU, relative value unit.

Hospitals bill for services separately from physicians. For each inpatient admission, hospitals receive flat fees—at a payment level determined in advance—based on patients' diagnoses. Medicare developed the **prospective payment system** methodology that pays hospitals based on the patients' diagnosis upon admission. The payment methodology uses the *International Classification of Diseases*, 10th Revision (ICD-10) coding system that classifies diagnoses with similar inpatient treatment costs into **diagnosis-related groups (DRGs)**. The DRG-based payment method is attractive to payers because the rate is predetermined upon patient admission, which encourages hospitals to control costs below a fixed amount (Berenson et al., 2016). If the costs associated with the patient stay exceed the DRG payment, then the hospital loses money. As such, the prospective payment system incentivizes careful monitoring of costs by health services managers.

> ⚠ **KEY IDEA**
>
> If the costs associated with the patient stay exceed the DRG payment, then the hospital loses money. As such, the prospective payment system incentivizes careful monitoring of costs by health services managers.

Some payers contract with hospitals to pay based on a **per diem rate,** which is a fixed amount per day. When the insurance company contracts with hospitals, multiple per diems are often negotiated on the basis of service type, such as medical-surgical, obstetrics, intensive care, or heart surgery. Under this payment arrangement, hospitals have no financial incentive to avoid unnecessary days of hospitalization. To prevent runaway costs, payers conduct rigorous utilization reviews of each billed inpatient day. Such reviews can lead payers to deny paying for days in the hospital that are deemed not required to ensure positive patient health outcomes (Berenson et al., 2016).

Unlike payment methodologies that encourage increased volume of care, about 20% of healthcare payments for inpatient care are paid through **advanced payment models** that incentivize quality over quantity, also called **value-based payment models**. A smaller proportion of physician practices have adopted advanced payment models—only 7% of medical revenue among primary care specialties, 6% among surgical specialties, and 15% among nonsurgical specialties (Gliadkovskaya, 2022). This approach incentivizes providers to control costs while maintaining or improving quality of care.

Under more complex value-based contractual arrangements, some HCOs form Accountable Care Organizations (ACOs) to accept responsibility for the total costs of caring for a population of patients. The participating ACOs that lower overall costs may receive financial bonuses from Medicare, if they meet predefined quality targets related to improving equity, care experience, and population health outcomes. For example, HCOs that participate in Medicare's ACO Realizing Equity, Access, and Community Health (REACH) Model accept **capitation payments**, which are fixed payments made on a per-member per-month (PMPM) basis [Centers for Medicare & Medicaid Services (CMS), 2022]. (A member is what insurance companies call their patients.) The HCOs receive predetermined monthly payments regardless of the level of care provided to each individual patient. Under capitation, HCOs are incentivized to control costs. Under advanced payment models, HCOs must meet certain medical care quality targets (Kaufman et al., 2019).

Revenue Cycle Management

Health services managers at all levels are involved in billing for health services, a complex process called the **revenue cycle** (Reiter & Song, 2021). Delays in collecting payments from patients and payers create financial problems for HCOs. Successful health services managers manage the revenue cycle to generate cash that is used to fund daily operations, called **working capital**. Positive working capital indicates that an HCO is financially healthy. Negative working capital usually means that the HCO is not managing the revenue cycle appropriately and can require HCOs to take on short-term debt for temporary working capital needs.

> △ **KEY IDEA**
>
> Effective revenue cycle management ensures accurate and timely bill collection, reduces payment denials from insurance companies, and ultimately improves the financial health of HCOs.

Effective revenue cycle management ensures accurate and timely bill collection, reduces payment denials from insurance companies, and ultimately improves the financial health of HCOs (Singh & Wheeler, 2012). As described in Figure 14.2, the revenue cycle includes multiple steps that can be divided into three main phases: preservice, point of service, and post-service. Effective management in each phase can improve the amount service revenue collected from insurance companies.

FIGURE 14.2 Revenue cycle.

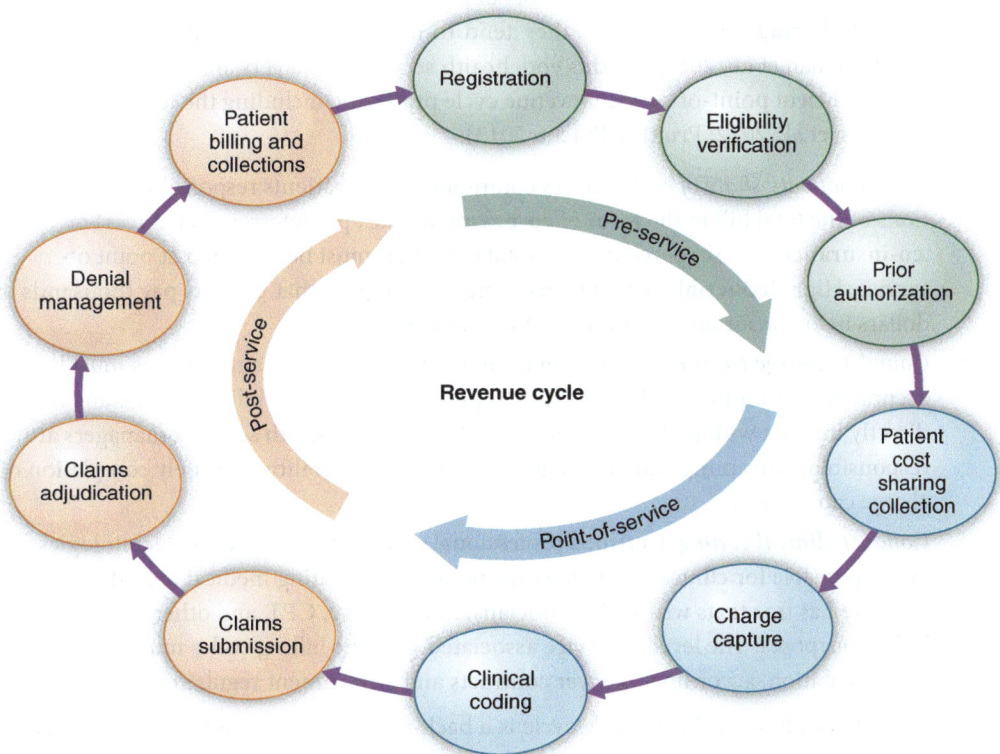

The preservice phase of revenue cycle entails the tasks that occur before a patient receives a service. Nearly half of denials are caused by front-end revenue cycle issues related to patient registration and lack of up-to-date health insurance (Optum, 2023). When patients make appointments, the administrative team establishes patient accounts in the electronic health record (EHR) system, where details such as medical histories and insurance coverages are stored. Prior to the appointment, the steps of the revenue cycle include the following (Chino et al., 2023; Kyle & Song, 2023; Shivan, 2023; Wagner, 2017):

1. *Complete registration:* Gather patient details, including demographic information, insurance coverage, and consent forms prior to the patient visit, if possible, to prevent surprising patients with services for which their insurance company will not cover.
2. *Conduct insurance **eligibility verification**:* For health services to be eligible for payment, patients need to be current with their health insurance membership and the service must be covered by the insurance benefit package. Eligibility verification ensures accurate billing. If not covered by insurance, patients are educated about cost estimates and options for receiving financial help.
3. *Obtain prior authorization:* Health insurance companies require medical reviews for certain procedures, medications, therapies, or supplies to determine if they are eligible for payment.

In the point-of-service phase of the revenue cycle, the health services administrative staff directly interact with patients and their families. Many payers require patients to share financial responsibility for medical care, which can mean they receive large, unexpected bills for services. Many state governments have passed legislation to encourage comparison shopping intended to enhance market competition and reduce prices (Buttorff et al., 2021). **Price transparency** is the term used for HCOs providing pricing information about health services in order to assist the patient in understanding their share of the costs of medical services. When patients fully understand their **cost sharing** responsibilities, they tend to be more satisfied with their health care experiences (Callahan et al., 2018). To this end, health services managers are responsible for creating clear and efficient point-of-service revenue cycle processes, including the following (Cohen et al., 2018; Dong et al., 2022; Pruitt & Pracht, 2013):

4. *Collect patients' share of costs:* Payers commonly make patients responsible for portions of the total bill in the form of **co-payments** (i.e., predetermined flat fees) or **co-insurance** (i.e., set percentage of total bills) that must be collected at point of-service. High **deductible** health plans sometimes require that patients pay thousands of dollars before insurance pays any portion of the bills.
5. *Complete **charge capture**:* Documentation of billable products and services must be accurately input into the EHRs. Charge capture is the responsibility of clinicians who directly interact with patients and provide the services. Health services managers are responsible for training clinicians and ensuring accountability for timely completion of charge capture tasks.
6. *Conduct **clinical coding**:* Certified professional coders and automation technologies are responsible for clinical coding, which involves translating medical records, usually presented as free texts written by clinicians, into ICD-10, CPT, and other codes for billing purposes. The level of service associated with the billing codes must match the documentation, according to payer contracts and government regulations.

The post-service phase of the revenue cycle is a back-office function staffed with various levels of health administrators. The post-service phase of the revenue cycle includes the following (Optum, 2023; Rauscher & Wheeler, 2012):

7. *Submit claims:* Healthcare bills are called **claims**. Claims that are timely, accurate, and free from omissions or errors are called **clean claims**.
8. *Adjudicate claims:* Once submitted, **claims adjudication** is performed by the insurance companies, a process that involves checking for accuracy, medical necessity, and compliance. Claims that contain errors are rejected. Claims that are deemed not medically necessary after the utilization review are denied.
9. *Denial management:* **Denied claims** are sent back to HCOs by health insurance companies with codes describing the reasons for denials. Denial management is the process of identifying resolutions to errors or documentation requests.
10. *Patient billing and collections:* Claims that are paid by the insurance companies are posted to the **patient ledger**, which is the electronic file that stores all history of patient services, charges, payments and adjustments, and remaining balances. When patients still owe money to the HCO after the insurance companies pay the claims, health services managers are responsible for sending bills and collecting payments.

Increases in patient cost sharing responsibilities have increased medical debt, especially in not-for-profit HCOs that serve higher proportions of uninsured and underinsured patients (Khullar et al., 2018). To offset the financial burden assumed by patients, HCOs provide services at no cost or reduced costs, known as **charity care**, also referred to as **financial assistance**. Charity care subsidizes health services for those who are unable to pay for all or a portion of the services, such as uninsured and low-income insured patients (Levinson et al., 2022). The federal government and over half of all states require that not-for-profit hospitals provide some level of charity care as a condition of receiving tax-exempt status. In communities where the financial resources are limited, HCOs provide extensive amounts of free or reduced cost care to patients (Gangopadhyaya et al., 2022; Khullar et al., 2018). For-profit HCOs typically provide a lower proportion of charity care but are required to pay taxes that the government can use to offset uncompensated care (Chletsos & Saiti, 2019).

Philanthropy

Philanthropy is the practice of fundraising from individuals, foundations, and corporations that generates revenue for HCOs whose missions are to care for patient populations who frequently need financial assistance. The amount of money raised through philanthropy is relatively small compared to the overall health system revenues (Association for Healthcare Philanthropy, 2023). However, the costs of fundraising are much smaller than delivering health services, so every dollar received from philanthropy returns about $0.81 in revenue, compared to $0.03 or less for health services (Miller & Sheth, 2023). Therefore, most hospitals and health systems invest in separate philanthropic foundations whose mission is to conduct annual fund campaigns and secure gifts from private philanthropic organizations (Erwin, 2013).

EXPENSES AND COSTING METHODS

Controlling Costs

Health services managers accept responsibility for controlling the costs associated with operating HCOs. The goal of health services managers is to enable clinicians and staff to deliver health services at the most efficient level possible, which includes lowering costs as much as possible while still delivering high-quality medical care. **Expenses** are the costs incurred by an organization to generate revenue. Health services managers seek to control expenses so that they are less than the overall revenues for all HCO services combined. Revenues minus expenses equals **profits**. Not-for-profit HCOs refer to their profits as **retained earnings**, a term that signifies the revenue that remains after expenses are paid and is reinvested back into operations.

> ⚠ **KEY IDEA**
>
> Not-for-profit HCOs refer to their profits as retained earnings, a term that signifies the revenue that remains after expenses are paid and is reinvested back into operations.

The level of expenses associated with each service provided varies widely, depending on the types of health services provided and the size of the HCO (Burgette et al., 2018; Song et al., 2017). Nevertheless, for most HCOs, there are three main drivers of expenses for each patient encounter (Cleverley & Cleverley, 2010; Sutherland & Levesque, 2020):

- *Intensity of services:* Entails quantity and mix of service inputs, such as nursing care, drugs, diagnostic procedures, and hospital length of stay. There is considerable unwarranted variation in the amount of services provided for each patient across HCOs. More care does not necessarily mean better care, but it does cost more.
- *Productivity or efficiency:* Costs incurred for each patient care encounter are related to productivity or efficiency. An example of productivity is the number of hours nurses worked to care for a patient in one day. An example of cost efficiency is cost per laboratory procedure.
- *Prices or salaries:* Increased prices paid for staff or to purchase supplies and drugs make each patient encounter more expensive. Even if the HCO is productive and efficient, if prices and salaries are significantly higher than those paid by its peers, the HCO's overall costs may still be high.

Effective cost control is a widely recognized strategy for creating competitive advantage and may be the most important factor influencing overall HCO financial performance (Cleverley & Cleverley, 2010; Porter, 2008). Some example initiatives that health services managers implement to contain costs in HCOs include the following (Cliff et al., 2021; Kaplan & Haas, 2014; Pure, 2018; Wurth, 2020):

- *Staffing management:* Reduce overtime pay and minimize idle time associated with overstaffing.
- *Supply chain management:* Negotiate lower prices with suppliers.
- *Efficient treatment protocols:* Enable clinicians to create alternative treatment protocols that use resources more judiciously.
- *Energy efficiency:* Implement energy-saving investments, such as solar power, to reduce utility bills.
- *Outsourcing noncore functions:* Hire outside firms to manage non-healthcare functions, such as food service, equipment maintenance, and laundry services.
- *Patient throughput optimization:* Improve patient flow to make better use of resources.
- *Quality improvement initiatives:* Reduce wasteful spending, costly complications, and medical errors.

Controlling costs has become more challenging in healthcare. Between 2019 and 2022, overall hospital expenses increased by 17.5%, primarily due to inflation driving up medical supplies and equipment costs and workforce shortages leading to dramatic increases in salaries [American

Hospital Association (AHA), 2023]. Given that revenues have not kept pace with rising expenses, cost control has become a high priority for health services managers [American College of Healthcare Executives (ACHE), 2023].

Types of Expenses

To effectively manage costs for HCOs, health services managers need to understand the various types of expenses. **Operating expenses** are the costs associated with the day-to-day delivery of health services. Labor is the single largest operating expense category for hospitals and physician practices, although nonlabor supplies can make up a significant proportion of all expenses, depending on the HCO type (Burgette et al., 2018; Song et al., 2017). **Capital expenses** are large, long-term investments, such as buildings, equipment, or technologies. Effective cost management involves careful attention to both operating and capital expenses.

Health services expenses can also be categorized according to whether they are directly attributable to patient care or not. **Direct costs** are connected to health services provided to individuals or communities. These costs can be directly traced to patient care. Examples of direct costs include staffing, medical supplies, diagnostic equipment, and healthcare facilities used in patient care areas. **Indirect costs**, sometimes called **overhead costs**, refer to the expenses that are not directly tied to health services delivery but are necessary for the overall functioning of the HCO. Examples of indirect costs are health services managers in functions that support the HCO operations, such as human resources, information technology, strategic planning and marketing, and finance.

INFORMATIONAL INTERVIEW 14.2
Revenue Cycle Support Manager
Access the informational interview online at http://connect.springerpub.com/content/book/978-0-8261-4807-0/chapter/ch00.

Health services expenses can also be categorized according to whether the costs change depending on the volume of services provided to patients. **Variable costs** in health services delivery are expenses that fluctuate in proportion to the volume of services provided. In other words, the more patients that are treated, the higher the variable costs associated with providing care. Variable costs include medical supplies, medications, and the use of diagnostic equipment. **Fixed costs** in health services delivery are the expenses that remain constant regardless of the volume of health services provided, such as rent or utilities.

CAREER BOX 14.3: Control Expenses With a Budget
Early in your health service management career, your spending will be easier to control than your income. Many early career health services managers struggle with paying day-to-day living expenses and educational debt. Reducing personal spending means being aware of housing expenses, declining more debt, avoiding compulsive purchases, skipping some expensive social events, and planning low-cost vacations. Just like work decisions, wise personal financial decisions can be helped with the use of a budget. To achieve financial stability, health services managers need to create a personal financial budget and stick to it.

TABLE 14.3 Examples of Categories of Expenses Related to Health Services Delivery

	DIRECT	INDIRECT (OVERHEAD)
VARIABLE	• Medical supplies • Labor costs for clinicians involved in patient care • Diagnostic tests and procedures • Pharmaceutical costs • Equipment usage, maintenance, and depreciation costs	• Overtime costs for administrative and support staff. (Base salaries are usually fixed, but overtime costs can vary with increased patient service volume.) • Marketing expenses based on the level of marketing activity for patient care services
FIXED	• Salaries for administrative staff directly involved in supporting patient care activities, such as costs associated with front-office staff • Physical space and utilities specifically designated for patient care	• Salaries and benefits of staff not directly involved in patient care • Building and utility costs that are not directly tied to patient care • General administrative expenses, including office supplies • Technology infrastructure, such as servers and networking equipment

The direct/indirect and variable/fixed categories of expenses are separate concepts that can be combined. For example, variable direct costs, such as medical supplies, are directly used in health services delivery and vary depending on the volume of patient care. Direct fixed expenses are the overhead costs that directly support patient care services, such as the costs of clinical space specifically used for patient care. Indirect fixed costs are the overhead costs indirectly related to patient care that occur irrespective of how many services are provided. Variable indirect costs are expenses that fluctuate with changes in patient volume but are not directly tied to the specific delivery of patient care. Table 14.3 illustrates common health services delivery examples of the combined categories of expenses.

Traditional Costing

To meaningfully lower expenses in HCOs, health services managers need to calculate the true costs of care for each separate health care service (Fang et al., 2021). The full cost of a health service encounter can be calculated as the direct costs plus a predetermined portion of the indirect costs. **Cost accounting** is the practice of estimating and allocating costs to a particular business unit or service line for the purposes of controlling costs, determining profitability, and setting budgets. The operating unit to which expenses are allocated is called a **cost center**. The allocation of direct costs to cost centers is straightforward— assign the full cost of each item to the cost center and divide total costs by the number of services provided for that unit.

To allocate indirect costs (overhead), traditional cost accounting applies a proportion of the total indirect costs to each organizational cost center (Fang et al., 2021). To do this, the traditional cost accounting uses a percentage of a predetermined variable, called a **cost driver**. Total indirect costs are summed up and then multiplied by the cost driver percentage for each cost center. Commonly used cost drivers in health services are the volume of patients seen, quantity of supplies used within the cost center, or factors related to the intensity of expenses associated with providing services, such as Medicare's RVUs.

TABLE 14.4 Traditional Cost Accounting Method Distributing Expenses Into Cost Centers

COST CENTER	PATIENTS	PROPORTION OF COST DRIVER	ALLOCATED INDIRECT COSTS
CLINIC 1	5,000	50%	$150,000
CLINIC 2	4,000	40%	$120,000
CLINIC 3	1,000	10%	$30,000
TOTAL	10,000	100%	$300,000

For example, a multisite physician group with three different clinics might need to allocate $300,000 in indirect costs. If the physician group chooses to use the number of patient visits as the cost driver, then the relative proportion of patients for each clinic would need to be calculated. If the total number of patient visits was 10,000 at the three clinics, with volumes of 5,000, 4,000, and 1,000 patients each, then the proportion of costs allocated to each clinic would be at 50%, 40%, and 10%, respectively. The total indirect costs of $300,000 would be multiplied by each cost driver proportion for each clinic. Table 14.4 illustrates this traditional cost accounting approach.

Traditional cost accounting methods are relatively easy to apply but have been criticized for inaccurate representation of service expenses for each type of service provided (Carroll & Lord, 2016). As such, traditional cost accounting in HCOs limits the ability for health services managers to meaningfully control costs at the service level. In the example above, Clinic 1 might be the most efficient clinic with the highest patient volume per day. But because they care for the most patients, they are charged the highest proportion of the total indirect costs for the physician group. Conversely, Clinic 3 might be chronically unproductive and spend lavishly on overhead, but it assumes the least indirect cost burden of all three clinics. Therefore, the traditional costing method does not directly link overhead costs to productivity or cost control.

Activity-Based Costing

In contrast to traditional cost accounting allocation, **activity-based costing** (ABC) provides a more precise understanding of how indirect costs impact each type of health service delivered to patients (Keel et al., 2017). ABC determines the costs for cost drivers associated with delivering each specific health service, including time, personnel, supplies, and equipment. ABC measures expenses related to patient care and does not account for indirect expenses, including administrative and general overhead costs. Similar to the traditional costing method, indirect costs are allocated to the service based on the proportion of the predetermined cost driver (Fang et al., 2021). In ABC, however, the cost driver is directly related to the cost activities at the service level, not just the department level.

△ KEY IDEA

The ABC method allows health services managers to identify service-level cost reduction opportunities.

The ABC method allows health services managers to identify service-level cost reduction opportunities (Horngren et al., 2015). For example, a health services manager responsible for an orthopedic service line would analyze how surgeons' choice of hip implants relate to the amount of operating room time and patients' average length of stay. If a very expensive hip implant reduces operating room time and average length of stay, then savings in operating room time and average length of stay may be worth the extra medical device expenses.

Time-driven activity-based costing (TDABC) is an extension of ABC frequently used in HCOs. TDABC differs from traditional ABC in that time is used as the only cost driver with the assumption that most health services expenses can be measured in terms of time (Keel et al., 2017). Robert Kaplan and Michael Porter (2011) described a seven-step approach to application of TDABC in health services. In Table 14.5, Kaplan and Porter's TDABC in healthcare approach has been adapted using a pediatric checkup visit for a 4-year-old patient. The personnel costs for this example include compensation and the costs of clinical space, technology, and other direct expenses (Kaplan, 2014). Indirect expenses have not been included. Figure 14.3 illustrates the TDABC Patient Process Map (steps 3 and 4) for a pediatric checkup visit for a 4-year-old patient.

TABLE 14.5 TDABC for a Pediatric Checkup Visit for a 4-Year-Old Patient

STEP	DEFINITION	EXAMPLE
1. Select the medical condition.	Define the beginning and end of the patient care cycle.	Pediatric checkup visit for a 4-year-old patient (CPT: 99383)
2. Define entire patient care value chain.	Identify the full care cycle rather than on individual processes.	Care cycle includes check-in, rooming, clinical visit, vaccination, and checkout.
3. Develop process maps.	Process maps include the steps that patients may follow in their care cycle.	See Figure 14.3.
4. Obtain time estimates for each process step.	Estimate time for patient at each step.	See Figure 14.3.
5. Estimate the direct cost of each care process.	Direct costs include compensation, depreciation or leasing of equipment, supplies, or other operating expenses.	Include personnel compensation and the costs of clinical space, technology, and other direct expenses.
6. Estimate the capacity cost rate of each resource (cost per minute).	Capacity cost rate includes the total cost of resources divided by amount of time available to work on patient care activities in minutes.	Pediatrician = $3.15/min; receptionist = $0.42/min; medical assistant = $0.49/min; patient services = $0.44/min; vaccines = $45.66/min
7. Estimate total costs for cycle of care.	Total cost of patient encounter is calculated by multiplying the capacity cost rates for each resource by the time the patient spent with the resource.	Total costs with vaccines = $574.05; total costs without vaccines = $112.55

CPT, Current Procedural Terminology; TDABC, time-driven activity-based costing.

FIGURE 14.3 TDABC patient process map.

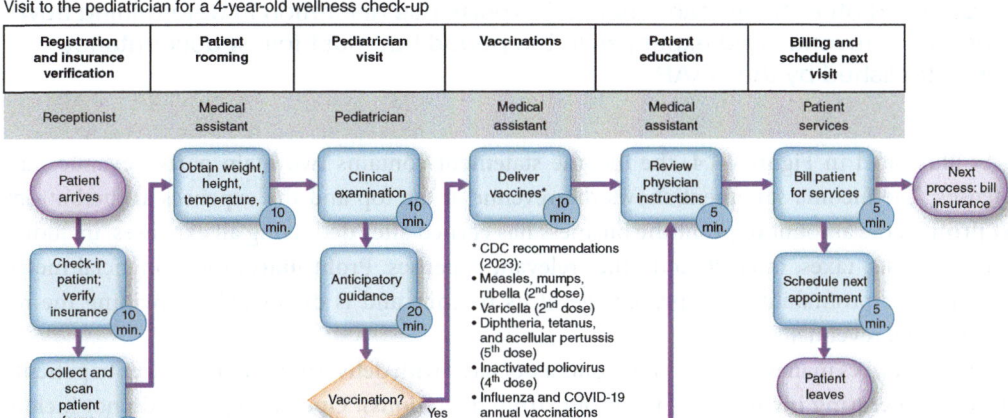

TDABC, time-driven activity-based costing.
Source: Adapted from Centers for Disease Control and Prevention. (2023, November 16). *Child and adolescent immunization schedule by age*. https://www.cdc.gov/vaccines/schedules/hcp/imz/child-adolescent.html; Kaplan, R. S., & Porter, M. E. (2011, September). How to solve the cost crisis in health care. *Harvard Business Review*. https://hbr.org/2011/09/how-to-solve-the-cost-crisis-in-health-care

FINANCIAL STATEMENTS

Importance of Financial Statements

Financial statements are fundamental tools for businesses that reflect concise views of an organization's financial position and performance. The finance organization is responsible for generating the financial statements for the HCO, according to the **generally accepted accounting principles (GAAP)**, which are a set of accounting guidelines used as the default standard by every corporation in the United States. To ensure compliance, internal auditors within the HCO review financial transactions, processes, and documentation to ensure compliance. Independent external auditors, such as accounting firms, are hired by the HCO to provide an objective assessment of the financial statements and submit the audited financial statements to the CEO and board of directors (Hensley-Quinn et al., 2020; Lane et al., 2001; Zare et al., 2022).

Income Statement

The **income statement**, also known as the **profit and loss (P&L) statement**, provides information on revenues and expenses for a specified period. A **fiscal year** is a period used for financial reporting, and unlike the calendar year, can start and end at any point during the year. The CFO and other healthcare financial experts use discretion in determining how to recognize revenue and expenses in the period but must follow accountancy rules established by the GAAP. The **matching principle**, also known as the expense recognition principle, must be followed when preparing the income statement. In essence, the matching principle ensures that the recognition of expenses is tied to the generation of the revenues in that period. The matching principle applies not only to direct costs of services but also to indirect costs and operating expenses. In other words, administrative expenses and other overhead costs must be matched with the revenues generated in the period.

> ⚠ **KEY IDEA**
>
> The CFO and other healthcare financial experts use discretion in determining how to recognize revenue and expenses in the period but must follow accountancy rules established by the GAAP.

As illustrated in Figure 14.4, the income statement contains two main parts: revenues and expenses. The income statement shows the revenue at the top and the expenses at the bottom. **Net profit** is the amount of profit the business has earned after deducting all expenses, including operating costs, taxes, interest, and other relevant expenses. Profit **margin** is a financial metric that expresses profitability as a percentage of its revenue and is calculated by dividing the net profit by total revenue.

Health services managers track the profits associated with delivering health services to patients, called **net operating income** (i.e., net profits from operations). Operating profits do not include investments, unrestricted fundraising donations, and other **nonoperating revenue**. Table 14.6 defines the terms and other income statement terms presented in Figure 14.4 with numbered notations (Levinson et al., 2022; Reiter & Song, 2022).

Because the income statement format lists revenues at the top and the various expenses are deducted sequentially, the net profit at the bottom of the income statement is sometimes referred to as the HCO's bottom line.

FIGURE 14.4 Simplified income statement.

For the fiscal year ended July 31, 2024 (in thousands of dollars)

	2024	2023
(1) **Operating revenues**		
Total patient service revenues (2)	$352,947	$338,829
Contractual allowance (discounts) (3)	$166,734	$160,065
Net patient service revenues (4)	$186,213	$178,764
Other operating revenue (5)	$22,549	$21,647
(6) Total operating revenues	$208,762	$200,412
(7) **Operating expenses**		
Depreciation and amortization (8)	$1,568	$1,602
Interest expense (9)	$156	$151
Other operating expenses (10)	$196,915	$189,038
Total operating expenses (11)	$198,639	$190,790
(12) Net operating income	$10,123	$9,622
(13) **Nonoperating revenue**		
Investment income (14)	$1,498	$1,736
Unrestricted donations (15)	$416	$566
Total nonoperating revenue (16)	$1,924	$2,302
(17) Net income or (loss)	$12,047	$11,924

TABLE 14.6 Income Statement Terms

TERM	DEFINITION
(1) **Operating revenue**	Category of funds that the HCO generates from providing health services
(2) **Total patient service revenues**	Charges billed to patients and third-party payers
(3) Contractual allowance	Difference between the charges for services and the amount paid based on negotiated agreements with third-party payers
(4) **Net patient service revenues**	Revenues collected from patients and third-party payers, after discounts, contractual allowances, and adjustments (2 − 3)
(5) Other operating revenues	Other money generated by the HCO, such as funding for research projects and clinical trials
(6) Total operating revenues	Comprehensive funds derived from providing health services and other core operations of an HCO (4 + 5)
(7) **Operating expenses**	Category of costs that HCO spends related to providing health services
(8) **Depreciation and amortization**	Expenses that reflect the portion of the useful life of the HCO's assets during that particular accounting period
(9) Interest expense	Costs associated with borrowing money, including the interest paid on loans and payments to bondholders
(10) Other operating expenses	Other costs associated with core activities, such as expenses associated with research, education, and uncompensated care (both charity care and bad debt expenses)
(11) Total operating expenses	Comprehensive costs associated with delivering health services and other core operations of an HCO
(12) **Net operating income**	Calculated by subtracting total operating expenses from total operating revenues (6 − 11)
(13) Nonoperating revenue	Category of funds generated from activities that are not directly related to the HCO's core operating functions, such as investment income and unrestricted donations
(14) Investment income	Interest and dividends earned from financial investments such as stocks, bonds, and other securities
(15) Unrestricted donations	Contributions from philanthropic donors, foundations, or government grants that are not tied to specific patient care services
(16) Total nonoperating revenue	Comprehensive funds generated from activities that are not directly related to the HCO's core operating functions (14 + 15)
(17) Net income (or loss)	Total profit or loss of an HCO after all expenses have been deducted from its total revenue; also referred to as retained earnings by not-for-profit HCOs (12 + 16)

HCO, health care organization.

FIGURE 14.5 Simplified balance sheet.

December 31, 2024 (in thousands of dollars)

Assets	2024	2023	Liabilities	2024	2023
Current assets			**Current liabilities**		
Cash and cash equivalents	$536,803	$407,044	Accounts payable	$623,232	$609,021
Short-term investments	$72,009	$74,888	Accrued salaries and benefits	$482,073	$395,637
Supplies inventory	$107,750	$113,421	Short-term debt	$168,200	$158,800
Patient accounts receivable	$1,023,568	$764,948	Other short-term liabilities	$73,742	$79,055
Other current assets	$115,203	$156,168			
Total current assets	$1,855,333	$1,516,469	Total current liabilities	$1,347,247	$1,242,513
Long-term assets			**Long-term liabilities**		
Long-term investments	$1,827,594	$2,058,925	Long-term lease liabilities	$187,592	$233,244
Property and equipment	$3,725,488	$3,619,451	Long-term debt	$2,110,072	$2,135,075
Lease assets	$247,572	$292,588	**Total liabilities**	$3,644,911	$3,610,832
Total assets	$7,655,987	$7,487,433	**Net assets**	$4,011,076	$3,876,601

Balance Sheet

The **balance sheet** is a financial statement that provides a snapshot of what the HCO owns (assets) and what it owes (liabilities) at a specific point in time. **Assets** are economic resources that are expected to provide future benefits, such as cash, property, buildings, and equipment. **Liabilities** are economic obligations to external entities, such as loan payments to banks or paychecks to employees. **Net assets**, also known as fund balance or owner's equity, are what remains after all liabilities have been deducted from the HCO's assets (Reiter & Song, 2022). Figure 14.5 illustrates a simplified balance sheet for an HCO.

Assets and liabilities are categorized as either short term or long term. **Current assets** and **current liabilities** are those financial elements that are expected to be addressed within a short-term period, usually 1 year. **Accounts receivable** (assets) represent the amounts owed to the HCO by patients and third-party payers for health services that have been delivered but not yet paid. The management of accounts receivable is an integral part of managing the revenue cycle. When HCOs collect payments in a timely manner, working capital is increased. **Accounts payable** (liabilities) refers to the outstanding bills that an HCO owes to suppliers, vendors, and other entities for goods and services that have been received but not yet paid. Accounts receivable and accounts payable are two elements of working capital that are strongly linked to operating and total profit margins (Rauscher & Wheeler, 2012).

△ KEY IDEA
Accounts receivable and accounts payable are two elements of working capital that are strongly linked to operating and total profit margins.

Conversely, **long-term assets** (noncurrent assets) and **long-term liabilities** (noncurrent liabilities) are expected to remain longer than 1 year. **Tangible assets** are physical assets that have a definite monetary value, including property, equipment, professional buildings, and vehicles.

These assets are generally used over the long term. **Intangible assets** are nonphysical assets that lack a physical substance but still hold value for an HCO, such as patents, goodwill, brand recognition, and intellectual property.

Asset management involves the strategic planning, acquisition, utilization, and maintenance of tangible and intangible assets within an HCO. For tangible assets, health services managers plan maintenance schedules and plan for upgrades and replacements. As required by the matching principle of accounting, the HCO must match this revenue with the costs of using tangible assets in a manner that reflects the wear and tear over time. **Depreciation** is the systematic allocation of the cost of using tangible assets, such as buildings, machinery, or vehicles, as an expense on the financial statements. Over time, depreciation continues to accrue until the total accumulated amount of depreciation equals the original cost of the asset. Accounting experts within the HCO finance organization will recommend the most appropriate accounting method for depreciation, such as straight line, declining balance, price level, and sum-of-the-years' digits (Reiter & Song, 2022).

Cash Flow Statement

The **cash flow statement** summarizes the total cash receipts and payments as generated by the financial activities of the HCO over a specified period (Reiter & Song, 2022). The cash flow statement represents where money is made and how it is spent. As shown in Figure 14.6, the cash flow statement reports three separate areas: operations, investments, and finance activities.

- *Operating activities:* Cash transactions that result from an HCO's core operations, including receipts from patients and third-party payers
- *Investing activities:* Changes in cash associated with the purchase and sale of long-term capital expenditures and investments
- *Financing activities:* Changes in cash associated with an HCO's debt to fund growth

FIGURE 14.6 Simplified cash flow statement.

Simplified cash flow statement for years ended July 31, 2024 and 2023 (in thousands of dollars)

Cash and cash equivalents, beginning of year	$4,329	$1,492
Operating activities	2024	2023
Adjustments	$3,346	$2,345
Net patient accounts receivable	($4,191)	($3,544)
Net accounts payable	$6,480	$5,385
Net supplies inventories	$546	$389
Pre-paid revenue	$678	$412
Net cash from operating activities	$11,188	$6,479
Investing activities		
Purchases of marketable securities	($9,298)	($4,356)
Purchases of assets (property, equipment)	($7,854)	($5,533)
Proceeds from sales of marketable securities	$12,435	$17,384
Net cash from investing activities	($4,717)	$7,495
Financing activities		
Repayment of loans from banks	($1,585)	($145)
Issuance of bonds	$5,000	–
Net cash from financing activities	$3,415	($145)
Net increase of decrease in cash for period	$9,886	$13,829

Because cash is not subject to managerial discretion, the cash flow statement provides an objective perspective of the HCO's financial performance (Berman et al., 2013). For example, a large investment in a new healthcare facility will be reflected differently on the income statement and the cash flow statement due to the nature of accounting principles and the timing of cash flows. The cost of constructing a new healthcare facility is a capital expenditure and is typically not fully expensed in the period it is incurred. Instead, the cost is depreciated over the useful life of the facility, spread out over several years. Depending on how the new facility was financed, it is possible that the income statement shows a profit, but the cash flow statement reveals a critical shortage of cash needed for day-to-day operations.

FINANCIAL RATIOS AND METRICS

Analyzing and Interpreting Financial Reports

Health services managers use financial statements to analyze the financial position of the HCO. With this information, health services managers can adjust day-to-day operations and use the figures in the financial statements to calculate financial ratios and metrics. Ratios and metrics are examined together for the purposes of the following (Berger, 2014):

- *Benchmarking performance:* Compare the HCO to industry standards and competitors to assess relative strengths and weaknesses.
- *Trending performance*: Identify improvements or deteriorations in financial performance over time.
- *Risk assessment:* Assess financial risks that impact ability to pay bills or borrow money.
- *Operational improvement:* Identify inefficiencies in operations, such as staffing and supply inventories.
- *Strategic planning:* Expand, maintain, or contract operations; negotiate pricing with payers; and manage costs to create advantages over competitors.
- *Stakeholder communication:* Explain financial health and performance to board of directors, bankers, bond rating agencies, regulators, and other stakeholders.

Although there are many useful metrics and ratios from which to choose, the most commonly used categories of financial ratios are profitability, liquidity, capital structure, asset efficiency, and labor productivity (Healthcare Financial Management Association [HFMA], 2020; Kaufman Hall, 2023; Priore, 2021; Turner et al., 2015).

Profitability Ratios

Health services managers use several types of profit metrics and ratios, depending on the operational or financial issue of interest. A **profit margin** is a ratio, usually expressed as a percentage, that divides the difference between revenue and expenses by revenue. For example, an HCO that has $50,000,000 in revenue and $45,000,000 in expenses would have a profit of $5,000,000 and a profit margin of 10% ([$50,000,000 - $45,000,000]/$50,000,000 = 10%). When expenses exceed revenue, the profit margin will be a negative number.

Operating margin measures how much profit an HCO makes on core health services activities. The median operating income margin for hospitals prior to the COVID-19 pandemic was 2.8%. Due to federal government subsidies, the median operating income margin for 2020/2021 was an all-time high of 6.5%, but without federal relief funds, the median operating margin was -1.0% (Gidwani & Damberg, 2023). Commonly used **profitability ratios** are defined in Table 14.7.

Liquidity Ratios

Liquidity is the term that refers to whether assets can be easily converted to cash, such as bank deposits, accounts receivable, and stocks and bonds, to meet short-term financial obligations. **Liquidity ratios** assess whether the HCO has enough cash to pay its bills. Commonly used liquidity ratios and metrics are defined in Table 14.8.

TABLE 14.7 Profitability Ratios and Metrics

TERM	DEFINITION	QUESTIONS ANSWERED
OPERATING MARGIN	Operating revenue minus operating expenses divided by operating revenue; only includes revenues and expenses related to patient care	How much profit is generated for each dollar spent on direct patient care services? Are the profits enough to borrow money to expand operations?
EXCESS MARGIN	Total revenue minus total expenses divided by total revenue; includes operating and nonoperating revenues and expenses (fundraising, government transfers, grants, and investments)	How much profit is generated for each dollar spent on all HCO activities? Are nonoperating revenues offsetting operational losses?
RETURN ON TOTAL ASSETS	Operating profits divided by total assets	How well is HCO using assets to generate a profit?
DEDUCTIBLE RATIO	Percentage discount from listed charges that third-party payers receive	What is the gap between the HCO's charges and the negotiated contract payments?

HCO, health care organization.

TABLE 14.8 Liquidity Ratios and Metrics

TERM	DEFINITION	QUESTIONS ANSWERED
CURRENT RATIO	Current assets divided by current liabilities	How many times the HCO is able to pay its short-term obligations with short-term resources?
DAYS CASH ON HAND	Cash and highly liquid investments divided by average daily cash expenses (total expenses divided by 365)	How many days could the HCO's reserves cover operating expenses if cash flows were suddenly shut off?
DAYS IN ACCOUNTS RECEIVABLE	Total patient accounts receivable divided by the average daily charges for the period being measured (charges divided by the total number of days)	How quickly is the HCO able to collect on patient bills?
AVERAGE PAYMENT PERIOD (DAYS)	Current liabilities divided by average daily cash expenses (charges divided by the total number of days)	How many days does it take to pay current bills?

HCO, health care organization.

Capital Structure Ratios

Capital structure refers to the mix of an HCO's debt and equity used to finance growth (Kaufman Hall, 2023). Capital structure ratios help assess the financial risk of loaning capital or investing in an HCO and reflect the ability to raise money to fund growth initiatives. Table 14.9 defines common capital structure ratios and metrics.

Asset Efficiency Ratios

Asset efficiency ratios measure how well the HCO uses assets to generate revenue and profits. Table 14.10 defines important asset efficiency ratios and metrics.

TABLE 14.9 Capital Structure Ratios and Metrics

TERM	DEFINITION	QUESTIONS ANSWERED
DEBT SERVICE COVERAGE RATIO	Revenue available to pay debt service (principal plus interest) after paying current liabilities divided by debt service (principal plus interest)	Is the HCO able to pay long-term debts, including the principal and interest expenses?
DEBT-TO-CAPITALIZATION RATIO	Long-term debt and capital leases divided by the sum of long-term debt and cash, investments, and other unrestricted current assets	How much debt does the HCO have relative current assets? Can the HCO take on more debt to fund growth?
CAPITAL EXPENSE PERCENTAGE	Total amount spent on long-term debt payments plus depreciation expenses divided by sum of all expenses incurred by the HCO during a specific period times 100	How much does the HCO spend on fixed assets, such as facilities and equipment, relative to all expenses?
CUSHION RATIO	Total debt service (principal and interest payments) minus total cash and cash equivalents	How well are budgets managed? How much cash does the HCO have compared to interest expenses that it has to pay on debt?

CMI, case mix index; FTE, full-time equivalent; HCO, health care organization.

TABLE 14.10 Asset Efficiency Ratios and Metrics

TERM	DEFINITION	QUESTIONS ANSWERED
TOTAL ASSET TURNOVER	Net patient service revenues divided by average total asset expenses for the period	How much revenue is generated per dollar of assets? How efficiently does the HCO use its assets to generate revenue?
INVENTORY TURNOVER RATIO	Total inventory costs for period divided by average on-hand inventory expenses for the period	How much revenue is generated per dollar of inventory? How efficiently does the HCO use inventory to generate revenue?
AVERAGE AGE OF PLANT	Cumulative amount of a fixed asset consumed from the start of its use through a specific date (accumulated depreciation) divided by the portion of a fixed asset consumed in the current period (depreciation expense)	How old are the HCO's fixed assets? How urgent is the short-term need for capital to invest in facilities?

HCO, health care organization.

TABLE 14.11 Labor Costs Ratios and Metrics

TERM	DEFINITION	QUESTIONS ANSWERED
LABOR COST TO REVENUES RATIO	Total labor costs divided by net patient service revenues	Is the HCO staffing and scheduling employees properly? Is the HCO overusing contract labor, such as travel nurses?
LABOR COSTS PER ADJUSTED DISCHARGE	For hospitals, total labor costs divided by the number of inpatient discharges, adjusted by the Medicare CMI	What is the relationship between the labor costs and the volume of patients, adjusted for severity?
TOTAL EXPENSE PER PROVIDER FTE	For medical practices, total direct patient expense divided by the number of full-time equivalent practicing providers	How much direct patient care expense does the HCO incur for every provider employed?

HCO, health care organization.

Labor Cost Ratios and Metrics

Finally, labor costs are the largest category of expense for HCOs (Daly, 2019; Kaufman Hall, 2022). As such, ratios and metrics related to labor expense are critically important for health services managers to track (Berger, 2005). Table 14.11 defines important labor costs ratios and metrics.

BUDGETING AND PLANNING

Budgeting as a Management Competency

Budgeting is the process of planning the allocation of the HCO's resources, coordinating operational units, and controlling the expenses according to that plan for a specified period. For health services managers, budgeting is fundamental competency that relates to the five basic management roles described by Fayol (1916). Budgeting is reflected in Fayol's five functions of the manager, such as the following (Merchant & Van der Stede, 2012):

- *Planning*: Budgets define the expected amount of money that the HCO will need to operate effectively.
- *Organizing*: Managers with authority over an organizational unit's budget are accountable and responsible for making financial decisions.
- *Commanding/leading/directing*: A budget sets the expectations for financial performance and ties financial bonuses to meeting targets.
- *Coordinating*: HCOs need to coordinate spending across functions and service lines to achieve overall goals.
- *Controlling*: Managers track budgets against plans and respond to discrepancies with action.

Operational Budgeting

Although there are many kinds of budgets utilized by health services managers, two major types are used in HCOs—operational and capital budgets. **Operational budgets** predict expenses and revenues based on historical information for a particular department, unit, or service line. Experts in the finance department work with health services managers in their respective areas to budget routine operational items, such as overhead, staffing, supplies, and equipment maintenance. Within operational units, staffing budgets are based on assumptions about how many employees will be needed to meet the future levels of patients at the standards of high-quality patient care, according to applicable law (Han et al., 2021). Staffing budgets also serve to constrain spending by avoiding unnecessary overtime and other staffing expenses that can jeopardize the financial viability of the HCO (Dopoulos, 2016).

> ### △ KEY IDEA
> Experts in the finance department work with health services managers in their respective areas to budget routine operational items, such as overhead, staffing, supplies, and equipment maintenance.

The HCO finance department collaborates with the health services managers in executing budget processes on a standard budget cycle, according to the HCO's policies and procedures (Priore, 2021). Approximately 3 to 4 months before the beginning of the fiscal year, the finance department provides managers with historical data and budgeting templates for their organizational unit. After a period of reviews and revision, budgets are submitted to the finance department by the health services managers. The budget for each level of the organization is rolled up to the corporate level for approval by the board of directors.

Health services managers use a variety of budgeting approaches, depending on policies and procedures set by the HCO finance department, as described in Table 14.12 (Zhang & Bohlen, 2023).

Budget Variance

Health services managers are responsible for staying within the planned budgets for their areas of responsibility. During the fiscal year, the finance department will monitor the operational budget for any unexpected changes. When spending is over or under the target budget, it is called **budget variance**. The HCO finance experts are responsible for giving health services managers reports that track performance and minimize variation. When over budget, health services managers respond by cutting costs, increasing patient care revenues, or both. When health services managers stay under budget, their HCOs generate greater operational profit margins (Slyter et al., 2021).

Capital Budgeting

Capital budgeting plans for multiyear, large-scale investments, including new facilities or expensive equipment, such as robotic surgical systems or PET scanners. Capital funds are allocated annually in accordance with the HCO's capital schedule, which is set during the multiyear strategic and budgeting planning process. In this sense, capital budgeting is a top-down endeavor made by health services management executives and the board of directors. The annual capital budgeting process integrates the strategic and financial plans with the specific investment decisions of the capital allocation process (Sussman, 2017). Through this process, health services managers determine how the HCO's scarce capital resources, including cash and debt capacity, will be budgeted for capital investments based on quality and direction (Sussman, 2017).

TABLE 14.12 Operational Budgeting Approaches

TERM	DEFINITION	NOTES
COMPREHENSIVE BUDGETING	Detailed budget that covers all of the HCO's financial operations and closely aligns strategic objectives	Annual budgeting includes a coordinated calendar and planning cycle that can be time-consuming and expensive.
CONTINUOUS BUDGETS	Budget updated and revised throughout the fiscal year based on actual performance and changes in the business environment, often referred to as rolling budgets	Suitable for HCOs operating in rapidly changing environments. The budgeting period does not end.
FIXED BUDGETS	Budget that assumes patient volumes, revenues, and expenses are constant, regardless of variations in actual activity levels	Actual financial results are compared to the budgeted figures to determine variance.
FLEXIBLE BUDGETS	Budget that models various patient volumes to estimate revenues and expenses under different scenarios.	Useful when patient volumes are difficult to estimate.
INCREMENTAL BUDGETING	Budgeting based on the prior period's budget, with adjustments made for expected changes; also known as baseline budgeting or line-item budgeting	Considered less time-consuming but continues existing expense items without examination of their effectiveness or alignment with organizational goals
ZERO-BASED BUDGETING	Disregards previous budgets and requires managers to justify future expenses	Building the budget from scratch takes a considerable amount of time.

HCO, health care organization.

INFORMATIONAL INTERVIEW 14.3
Senior Vice President, Patient Financial Services
Access the informational interview online at http://connect.springerpub.com/content/book/978-0-8261-4807-0/chapter/ch00.

Capital budgeting can also be viewed as a bottom-up process, in which the medical staff identifies opportunities for investment. In fact, physicians play a uniquely dominant role in almost all aspects of healthcare capital budgeting process (Mukherjee et al., 2016). While health services managers are responsible for deciding where to allocate resources—often for investments related to clinical matters about which they have little expertise—physicians often demand the latest new technologies in large HCOs. However, health services managers may decline to make the requested investments, which can disappoint physicians (Balak et al., 2020). However, HCOs carry the financial risks associated with large investments. As such, effective health services managers make decisions in the best interests of the HCO, regardless of investment requests made by the medical staff.

Analysis of Capital Allocation Options

Health services managers evaluate whether capital investments are worthwhile relative to other investment opportunities (Zhang & Bohlen, 2023). Capital allocation decisions involve determining whether the capital investments make the financial cutoff points set by the HCO and meet nonfinancial objectives, such as organizational mission (Sussman, 2017). To evaluate whether capital investments meet the financial criteria, health services managers also need competency in **managerial accounting**, which is the use of financial mathematics to analyze the various capital allocation options.

First, health services managers determine whether new capital investment opportunities are financially feasible. Two simple metrics that can provide health services managers with quick assessments of the **return on investment**—payback period and break-even analysis. The **payback period** explicitly measures the time required for the initial investment to be recovered. The figure is calculated by dividing the initial investment by the cash inflow. A shorter payback period is better because it indicates a quicker recovery of the initial investment. For example, a $1 million investment that generates $100,000 per year yields a payback period of 10 years.

In health services businesses, the **break-even analysis** simply identifies the number of patient care services that need to be sold to "break even" on the initial investment. Break-even analysis can be used to determine how many services need to be delivered (i.e., volume) to cover the initial investment (e.g., fixed costs). The break-even analysis equation is written as break-even volume equals fixed costs divided by contribution margin. The **contribution margin** is calculated as the price paid for the service minus the variable costs of delivering the service. In other words, break-even analysis reveals the point at which a health service's contribution margin covers the investment (fixed costs) and begins to generate a profit. For example, a $1 million investment in a service line for which an HCO is paid $10,000 and costs $7,500 in direct costs for each service delivered would need to provide 400 service units to pay off the original investment ($1 million divided by $2,500).

> △ **KEY IDEA**
>
> The time value of money is important to consider in long-term capital allocation decisions, especially when comparing investment opportunities that have differing revenues over time.

The payback period or break-even analyses are simple but do not consider the **time value of money**, which is necessary to accurately assess the potential return on an investment. The time value of money is a fundamental concept in finance that recognizes the idea that the value of money changes over time due to factors such as interest, inflation, and the opportunity to earn a return on investment. In essence, a sum of money has a different value today than it will in the future. For example, the value of $952.38 placed in a bank account that earns 5% annual interest would equal $1,000 in 1 year. So, the **present value** of receiving $1,000 1 year from now, with an expected 5% interest rate, is approximately $952.38. Put differently, at 5% interest rate, $952.38 today equals $1,000 a year from now. The time value of money is important to consider in long-term capital allocation decisions, especially when comparing investment opportunities that have differing revenues over time.

The discounted cash flow method considers the time value of money by projecting the value of an investment over its lifespan. Two main approaches to discounted cash flow modeling are **net present value (NPV)** and **internal rate of return (IRR)**. Both are used in capital budgeting to evaluate the financial viability of capital investment opportunities, but they differ in their approaches and what they reveal about the investment. Detailed instructions on their calculations are available through other resources listed in the Recommended Reading and Media section at the end of the chapter.

The **net present value** provides an absolute dollar amount that represents the net gain or loss from the capital investment expressed in the value of today's money. To calculate the NPV, the annual revenue from an initial investment is projected for multiple periods. Then, each annual revenue projection is discounted by the assumed interest rate (i.e., discount rate). For example, $1,000 in annual revenue after the first year at a discount rate of 5% is $952.38. The second year revenue of $1,000 is worth approximately $907.03 in today's money (i.e., present value) at a 5% discount rate over 2 years. Therefore, the NPV of this example equals $1,859.41 ($952.38 plus $907.03). If the initial investment was $1,859.41 or less, then the investment would be considered financially viable.

△ KEY IDEA

When deciding whether or not to invest capital, the IRR needs to exceed the weighted average cost of capital (WACC).

The **internal rate of return** is expressed as a percentage and represents the rate of return on the investment that is needed to exceed the interest expense associated with borrowing the capital. The IRR is a predetermined percentage value set by the healthcare financial experts who understand the overall cost of capital at the HCO. As the executive responsible for the financial function of the HCO, the CFO calculates the minimum return on investment necessary for any investment using the **weighted average cost of capital (WACC)**. The WACC is the average interest rate paid for all capital sources, such as bank loans and bonds issuances. When deciding whether or not to invest capital, the IRR needs to exceed the WACC.

For example, the CFO may determine that the cost of capital in interest payments for an HCO may be 3.5%. An investment of $2,000 that generates $1,000 in revenue after year one and another $1,000 in revenue in year two would have an IRR of approximately 5%. This example would be considered viable since it exceeds the predetermined discount rate of 3.5%. The somewhat complicated IRR calculations can be generated using a financial calculator, online calculators, or Excel templates supplied by healthcare financial experts (Priore, 2021).

The first step of determining capital investments is only considering financial metrics. In health services management, decisions to proceed with capital investments are also dictated by nonfinancial needs (Zhang & Bohlen, 2023). These nonfinancial criteria are essential for a comprehensive evaluation, as they address aspects beyond the immediate financial return. Nonfinancial considerations include the following:

- *Strategy:* Do investments align with the HCO's mission, vision, and values? create long-term competitive advantage?
- *Patient needs:* Do investments improve the experience of patients and their families? enhance health care access?
- *Quality of care:* Do investments enhance the quality of medical care and improve patient outcomes?
- *Operational improvement:* Do investments address facility capacity issues or improve patient flow?
- *Community needs:* Do investments meet community health needs? prevent the future burden of disease in the population?
- *Environmental impact:* Do investments improve energy efficiency or conserve resources?

Such nonfinancial benefits can be included in a **cost-benefit analysis** (CBA) that can be used to more comprehensively quantify the overall impact of a capital investment decision (Wright & Durán, 2020). The CBA approach attempts to capture the financial value of benefits not traditionally included in capital allocation decisions.

FUTURE DIRECTIONS

Fee-for-service payment methodology remains the dominant approach to paying for health services. However, healthcare payers are increasingly turning to value-based contracting that incentivizes HCOs to reduce costs and improve medical care outcomes. This shift to value has the potential to change the structure and function of the healthcare financial organization within HCOs. For example, value-based payments will change how HCOs report revenues on their financial statements. **Deferred revenue**, also known as prepaid revenue, refers to payments that an HCO receives in advance for services that have not yet been delivered and represents a liability on the HCO's balance sheet until the services are provided. Also, when HCOs are paid lump sums for keeping a specified population healthy, the revenue cycle management function drastically changes. Under prepaid payment models, HCOs do not have to chase the payments from third-party payers after care has been delivered.

Value-based contracting will also upend how health services managers deal with expenses for their HCOs. Under value-based contracts, HCOs assume the financial risks associated with the potential for runaway costs of medical care. The HCOs that fail to keep patients healthy or provide too many unnecessary health services will experience financial losses. Therefore, under value-based contracts, health services managers will need to master competencies in costing methodologies and expense management. Moving from transactional to transformative healthcare financing will take time, but when health services managers embrace new payment models, value can be created for patients and payers alike (Kaufman et al., 2019).

SUMMARY

- Healthcare finance experts support functional and service line health services managers to complete most financial tasks, such as budgeting, financial analysis, capital financing, and accounting.
- Health services managers are responsible for facilitating revenue generation through increased patient care volume, more favorable payer mix, or higher patient severity.
- Third-party payers pay HCOs through a variety of methodologies and processes, including fee-for-service and value-based payments. Managed care organizations conduct utilization review processes to restrain overuse and unnecessary spending for medical services.
- Methods of cost accounting, such as ABC, assist health services managers in controlling operating and capital expenses.
- Financial statements, including the income statement, balance sheet, and cash flow statement, provide a comprehensive overview of a company's financial performance over a specific period.
- Financial metrics and ratios are used by health services managers to make intelligent investments and adjust day-to-day operations, such as reducing supply inventories or increasing staffing levels.
- Health services managers are responsible for operational and capital budgeting, which is supported by technical skills, such as variance analysis, return-on-investment analysis, and discounted cash flow method.

END-OF-CHAPTER RESOURCES

KEY TERMS*

*For the full list of key terms, please see the online glossary at **http://connect.springerpub.com/content/book/978-0-8261-4807-0.**

accounts payable
accounts receivable
activity-based costing
asset efficiency ratios
asset management
balance sheet
bond ratings
break-even analysis
budgeting
budget variance
capital
capital budgeting
capital expenses
capital structure
capitation payments
cash flow statement
charges
charge capture
charity care
claims
claims adjudication
clean claims
clinical coding
comprehensive budgeting
continuous budgets
contribution margin
controller
co-insurance
co-payments
cost accounting
cost-benefit analysis
cost center
cost driver
cost sharing
creditworthiness
current assets
current liabilities
Current Procedural Terminology (CPT)
debt financing
deferred revenue
deductible
denied claims
depreciation

depreciation and amortization
diagnosis-related groups (DRGs)
direct costs
eligibility verification
equity
equity financing
expenses
fee for service
fee schedule
financial accounting
financial assistance
financial controls
financial reserves
fiscal year
fixed budgets
fixed costs
flexible budgets
general ledger
generally accepted accounting principles (GAAP)
income statement
incremental budgeting
indirect costs
intangible assets
internal rate of return
internal audit function
International Classification of Diseases, 10th edition (ICD-10)
liabilities
liquidity
liquidity ratios
long-term assets
long-term liabilities
managed care
managerial accounting
matching principle
medical necessity
net assets
net patient service revenue
net present value
net profit
net operating income
nonoperating revenues

operating expenses
operating margin
operating revenues
operational budgets
overhead costs
patient ledger
payer mix
per diem rate
philanthropy
price transparency
prospective payment system
profits
profit and loss statement
profit margin
profitability ratios
relative value unit (RVU)
reimbursements
retained earnings
return on investment
revenues
revenue cycle
self-pay
tangible assets
third-party payers
time-driven activity-based costing
time value of money
total patient service revenues
uncompensated care
utilization review
value-based payment models
variable costs
weighted average cost of capital
working capital
zero based budgeting

LEARNING ACTIVITIES

Professional Development and Reflection

1. When an HCO maintains financial reserves, the organization can survive during periods of financial adversity. Reflect on how personal financial reserves (savings) can preserve career options. Reflect on how living below your means can provide flexibility to take career risks.
2. NPV involves looking at a forecast of cash flows and discounting them for risk. Suppose that one career option provides you with a significant raise next year (to $75,000) but that you will only get a $1,500 raise each year for 10 years. Suppose that another job alternative provides a smaller immediate raise (to $60,000), but you will receive a $5,000 raise each year. Given a 5% discount (inflation) rate, how would you use the discounted cash flow method to decide which job is the better financial offer?

Discussion Questions

1. Which is a higher priority for HCOs? Revenue generation or cost control?
2. Do you think that managed care organizations making medical necessity determinations is a benefit to patients? What role should managed care organizations play in controlling costs and managing utilization of health services?
3. What should the be the responsibility of HCOs to provide charity care? What are the limits to providing uncompensated care, if any?

RECOMMENDED READING AND MEDIA

Fernando, J. (2023, March 30). *Internal Rate of Return (IRR) Rule: Definition and example*. Investopedia. https://www.investopedia.com/terms/i/irr.asp

Finkler, S. A., Jones, C. B., & Kovner, C. T. (2019). *Financial management for nurse managers and executives* (5th ed.). Saunders.

Liu, C. (2021, November). Christine vs. work: How to ask for a raise. *Harvard Business Review*. https://hbr.org/2021/11/christine-vs-work-how-to-ask-for-a-raise

Priore, R. J. (2021). *Improving financial and operations performance: A healthcare leader's guide*. Springer Publishing Company.

Reiter, K., & Song, P. (2022). *Fundamentals of healthcare finance* (4th ed.). Health Administration Press.

Seth, S. (2023, May 29). *Formula to calculate Net Present Value (NPV) in excel*. Investopedia. https://www.investopedia.com/ask/answers/021115/what-formula-calculating-net-present-value-npv-excel.asp

The Finance Storyteller. (2019, July 29). *Net Present Value (NPV) explained* [Video]. YouTube. https://www.youtube.com/watch?v=N-lN5xORIwc

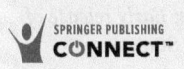

A robust set of instructor resources designed to supplement this text is located at http://connect.springerpub.com/content/book/978-0-8261-4807-0. Qualifying instructors may request access by emailing textbook@springerpub.com.

REFERENCES

American College of Healthcare Executives. (2023). *Survey: Workforce challenges cited by CEOs as top issue confronting hospitals in 2022*. https://www.ache.org/about-ache/news-and-awards/news-releases/survey-workforce-challenges-cited-by-ceos-as-top-issue-confronting-hospitals-in-2022

American Hospital Association. (2023, April). *The financial stability of America's hospitals and health systems is at risk as the costs of caring continue to rise*. https://www.aha.org/costsofcaring

American Medical Association. (2020, September 9). *CPT purpose & mission*. https://www.ama-assn.org/about/cpt-editorial-panel/cpt-purpose-mission

Association for Healthcare Philanthropy. (2023). *Report on giving*. https://www.ahp.org/resources-and-tools/report-on-giving-benchmarking

Balak, N., Tisell, M., & Honeybul, S. (2020). Healthcare economics. In S. Honeybul (Ed.), *Ethics in neurosurgical practice* (pp. 73–84). Cambridge University Press.

Berenson, R. A., Upadhyay D. K., Delbanco S. F., & Murray, R. (2016, April). *Per diem payments to hospitals for inpatient stays*. Urban Institute. https://www.urban.org/sites/default/files/2016/05/03/03_per_diem_payment_to_hospitals_for_inpatient_stays.pdf

Berger, S. (2005). *The power of clinical and financial metrics: Achieving success in your hospital*. Health Administration Press.

Berger, S. (2014). *Fundamentals of health care financial management: A practical guide to fiscal issues and activities*. John Wiley & Sons.

Berman, K., Knight, J., & Case, J. (2013). *Financial intelligence, revised edition: A manager's guide to knowing what the numbers really mean*. Harvard Business Review Press.

Broom, K., & Hilsenrath, P. (2015). ACHE member survey: Perspectives on graduate health management education. *Journal of Health Administration Education, 32*(3), 341–358. https://scholarlycommons.pacific.edu/esob-facarticles/117

Burgette, L. F., Liu, J., Miller, B., Wynn, B. O., Dellva, S., Malsberger, R., Merrell, K., Nguyen, P., Nie, X., Pane, J. D., Qureshi, N., Ruder, T., Zhao, L., & Hussey, P. S. (2018). *Practice expense methodology and data collection research and analysis*. RAND.

Buttorff, C., White, C., Martineau, M., Case, S. R., & Damberg, C. L. (2021). *Increasing price transparency in health care*. Rand Corporation.

Callahan, M., Williams, C., & Wilson, A. E. (2018). *Reinventing revenue cycle management: Delivering next-level patient experiences*. RevSpring Press.

Carroll, N., & Lord, J. C. (2016). The growing importance of cost accounting for hospitals. *Journal of Health Care Finance, 43*(2), 171–185.

Centers for Medicare and Medicaid Services. (2022, March 7). *ACO REACH*. https://www.cms.gov/priorities/innovation/innovation-models/aco-reach

Chino, F., Baez, A., Elkins, I. B., Aviki, E. M., Ghazal, L. V., & Thom, B. (2023). The patient experience of prior authorization for cancer care. *JAMA Network Open, 6*(10), e2338182.

Chletsos, M., & Saiti, A. (2019). For-profit versus not-for-profit hospitals and public hospitals. In *Strategic Management and Economics in Health Care* (pp. 129–149). Springer. https://doi.org/10.1007/978-3-030-35370-4_7

Cleverley, W. O., & Cleverley, J. O. (2010, March). Cost reduction: Identifying the opportunities: With a tough economy forcing hospitals to cut costs, how can executives find areas of the greatest possible savings? *Healthcare Financial Management, 64*(3), 52.

Cliff, B. Q., Avancena, A. L., Hirth, R. A., & Lee, S. Y. D. (2021). The impact of Choosing Wisely interventions on low-value medical services: A systematic review. *The Milbank Quarterly, 99*(4), 1024–1058. https://doi.org/10.1111/1468-0009.12531

Cohen, R. A., Zammitti, E. P., & Martinez, M. E. (2018, May). *Health Insurance coverage: Early release of estimates from the national health interview survey, 2017*. National Center for Health Statistics. https://www.cdc.gov/nchs/data/nhis/earlyrelease/insur201805.pdf

Coughlin, T. A., Samuel-Jakubos, H., & Garfield, R. (2021, April 6). *Sources of payment for uncompensated care for the uninsured*. Kaiser Family Foundation. https://www.kff.org/uninsured/issue-brief/sources-of-payment-for-uncompensated-care-for-the-uninsured/

Daly, R. (2019, October 2). *Hospitals innovate to control labor costs*. Healthcare Financial Management Association. https://www.hfma.org/technology/hospitals-innovate-to-control-labor-costs

Deloitte. (2023). *Four faces of the CFO*. https://www2.deloitte.com/us/en/pages/finance/articles/gx-cfo-role-responsibilities-organization-steward-operator-catalyst-strategist.html

Dong, H., Falis, M., Whiteley, W., Alex, B., Matterson, J., Ji, S., Chen, J., & Wu, H. (2022). Automated clinical coding: What, why, and where we are? *NPJ Digital Medicine, 5*(1), 159. https://doi.org/10.1038/s41746-022-00705-7

Dopoulos, J. (2016). Hospital cost-containment strategies that earn the respect of rating agencies. *Healthcare Financial Management, 70*(1), 32–36.

Erskine, L., Chuang, E., & Finlayson, T. (2016). Great expectations: Factors affecting healthcare management students' choice of graduate degree programs. *Journal of Health Administration Education, 33*(1), 95–120.

Erwin, C. O. (2013). Classifying and comparing fundraising performance for nonprofit hospitals. *Journal of Health and Human Services Administration, 36*(1), 24–60.

Erwin, C. O., Landry, A. Y., Livingston, A. C., & Dias, A. (2019). Effective governance and hospital boards revisited: Reflections on 25 years of research. *Medical Care Research and Review, 76*(2), 131–166. https://doi.org/10.1177/1077558718754898

Fang, C. J., Shaker, J. M., Drew, J. M., Jawa, A., Mattingly, D. A., & Smith, E. L. (2021). The cost of hip and knee revision arthroplasty by diagnosis-related groups: Comparing time-driven activity-based costing and traditional accounting. *The Journal of Arthroplasty, 36*(8), 2674–2679. https://doi.org/10.1016/j.arth.2021.03.041

Fayol, H. (1916). General principles of management. *Classics of organization theory, 2*(15), 57–69.

Gangopadhyaya, A., Blavin, F., Braga, B., & Andre, J. (2022, September 27). *Which hospital financial characteristics are associated with medical debt?* Urban Institute. https://www.urban.org/research/publication/which-hospital-financial-characteristics-are-associated-medical-debt

Gidwani, R., & Damberg, C. L. (2023, July). *Changes in US hospital financial performance during the COVID-19 public health emergency*. JAMA Health Forum, 4(7), e231928. https://doi.org/10.1001/jamahealthforum.2023.1928

Gliadkovskaya, A. (2022, August 26). *Value-based care remains small portion of overall medical revenue, MGMA survey finds*. Fierce Healthcare. https://www.fiercehealthcare.com/providers/value-based-outcomes-and-measures-medical-practices-2022-mgma-report

Han, X., Pittman, P., & Barnow, B. (2021). Alternative approaches to ensuring adequate nurse staffing: The effect of state legislation on hospital nurse staffing. *Medical Care, 59*(10 Suppl 5), S463–S470. https://doi.org/10.1097/MLR.0000000000001614

Healthcare Financial Management Association. (2020, March). *Key hospital financial statistics and ratio medians*. https://www.hfma.org/finance-and-business-strategy/1114

Hegwer, L. R., & Hut, N. (2019, December 16). *The healthcare CFO of the future: How finance leaders are adapting to relentless change*. Healthcare Financial Management Association. https://www.hfma.org/leadership/financial-leadership/the-healthcare-cfo-of-the-future

Hensley-Quinn, M., Butler, J., Kane, N. (2020, March 9). *Snapshot of 12 states' hospital financial transparency laws*. National Academy for State Health Policy. https://nashp.org/snapshot-of-12-states-hospital-financial-transparency-laws

Hinton, E., & Raphael, J. (2023, July 06). *A closer look at the five largest publicly traded companies operating Medicaid managed care plans*. KFF. https://www.kff.org/medicaid/issue-brief/a-closer-look-at-the-five-largest-publicly-traded-companies-operating-medicaid-managed-care-plans

Horngren, C. T., Datar, S. M., Rajan, M. V. (2015). *Cost accounting: A managerial emphasis*. Pearson Education International.

Kaplan, R. S. (2014). Improving value with TDABC. *Healthcare Financial Management, 68*(6), 76–84.

Kaplan, R. S., & Haas, D. A. (2014, November). How not to cut health care costs. *Harvard Business Review*. https://hbr.org/2014/11/how-not-to-cut-health-care-costs

Kaplan, R. S., & Porter, M. E. (2011, September). How to solve the cost crisis in health care. *Harvard Business Review*. https://hbr.org/2011/09/how-to-solve-the-cost-crisis-in-health-care

Kaufman, B. G., Spivack, B. S., Stearns, S. C., Song, P. H., & O'Brien, E. C. (2019). Impact of accountable care organizations on utilization, care, and outcomes: A systematic review. *Medical Care Research and Review, 76*(3), 255–290. https://doi.org/10.1177/1077558717745916

Kaufman Hall. (2022, August 1). *The metrics that matter in today's physician enterprise*. https://www.kaufmanhall.com/insights/article/metrics-matter-todays-physician-enterprise

Kaufman Hall. (2023, April). *The essential role of financial reserves in not-for-profit healthcare*. https://www.aha.org/system/files/media/file/2023/04/Essential-Role-of-Financial-Reserves-in-Not-for-Profit-Healthcare.pdf

Keel, G., Savage, C., Rafiq, M., & Mazzocato, P. (2017). Time-driven activity-based costing in health care: A systematic review of the literature. *Health Policy, 121*(7), 755–763. https://doi.org/10.1016/j.healthpol.2017.04.013

Khullar, D., Song, Z., & Chokshi, D. A. (2018, May 10). *Safety-net health systems at risk: Who bears the burden of uncompensated care?* Health Affairs Forefront. https://www.healthaffairs.org/content/forefront/safety-net-health-systems-risk-bears-burden-uncompensated-care

Klein, L. W., Box, L., Krishnan, S., Kar, S., Ing, F., Cigarroa, J., Mahmud, E., & Committee, G. R. (2020). In defense of the AMA/specialty society RVS update committee (RUC). *Catheterization and Cardiovascular Interventions, 96*(1), 156–157. https://doi.org/10.1002/ccd.28875

Kyle, M. A., & Song, Z. (2023). The consequences and future of prior-authorization reform. *The New England Journal of Medicine, 389*(4), 291–293. https://doi.org/10.1056/NEJMp2304447

Lane, S. G., Longstreth, E., & Nixon, V. (2001). *A community leader's guide to hospital finance: Evaluating how a hospital gets and spends its money*. Access Project.

Levinson, Z., Hulver, S., & Neuman, T. (2022, November 3). *Hospital charity care: How it works and why it matters*. Kaiser Family Foundation. https://www.kff.org/health-costs/issue-brief/hospital-charity-care-how-it-works-and-why-it-matters

Merchant, K. A., & Van der Stede, W. A. (2012). *Management control systems: Performance measurement, evaluation and incentives* (3rd ed.). Pearson Education Limited.

Miller, A., & Sheth, K. (2023, May 31). *3 reasons c-suite leadership at health organizations should invest in philanthropy*. CCS Fundraising. https://www.ccsfundraising.com/insights/roi-philanthropy-health-organizations

Moon, J., & Shugan, S. M. (2020). Nonprofit versus for-profit health care competition: How service mix makes nonprofit hospitals more profitable. *Journal of Marketing Research, 57*(2), 193–210. https://doi.org/10.1177/0022243719901169

Mukherjee, T., Al Rahahleh, N., & Lane, W. (2016). The capital budgeting process of healthcare organizations: A review of surveys. *Journal of Healthcare Management, 61*(1), 58–76. https://doi.org/10.1097/00115514-201601000-00011

Namburi, N., & Tadi, P. (2023, January 30). *Managed care economics*. StatPearls Publishing. https://www.ncbi.nlm.nih.gov/books/NBK556053

Nevola, A. (2016). Revisiting the determinants of hospital profitability in Florida. *Journal of Health Care Finance, 43*(2), 39–60.

Ochieng, N., Biniek, J. F., Freed, M., Damico, A., & Neuman, T. (2023, August 9). *Medicare advantage in 2023: Enrollment update and key trends*. KFF. https://www.kff.org/medicare/issue-brief/medicare-advantage-in-2023-enrollment-update-and-key-trends

O'Hara, C. (2015, March 5). How to ask for a raise. *Harvard Business Review*. https://hbr.org/2015/03/how-to-ask-for-a-raise

Oner, N., Zengul, F. D., Ozaydin, B., Pallotta, R. A., & Weech-Maldonado, R. (2016). Organizational and environmental factors associated with hospital financial performance: A systematic review. *Journal of Health Care Finance, 43*(2), 13–37.

Optum. (2023). *The Optum 2022 revenue cycle denials index*. Change Healthcare. https://info.changehealthcare.com/reduce-denials/denials-index

Porter, J. A., Haberling, K., & Hohman, C. (2016). Employer desired competencies for undergraduate health administration graduates entering the job market. *Journal of Health Administration Education, 33*(3), 355–375.

Porter, M. E. (2008). *Competitive advantage: Creating and sustaining superior performance* (2nd ed.). Free Press.

Priore, R. J. (2021). *Improving financial and operations performance: A healthcare leader's guide*. Springer Publishing Company.

Pruitt, Z., & Pracht, E. (2013). Emergency admissions for non-life-threatening injuries to children. *American Journal of Managed Care, 19*(11), 917–924.

Pure, B. (2018, December 13). *11 cost-cutting ideas for hospitals that you can implement in less than a week*. The Doctors Answer. https://blog.thedoctorsanswer.com/11-cost-cutting-ideas-for-hospitals

Rauscher, S., & Wheeler, J. R. (2012). The importance of working capital management for hospital profitability: Evidence from bond-issuing, not-for-profit US hospitals. *Health Care Management Review, 37*(4), 339–346. https://doi.org/10.1097/HMR.0b013e3182224189

Reese, E. C. (2021). *Why the internal audit function serves as a bulwark against risk for healthcare organizations*. Healthcare Financial Management Association. https://www.hfma.org/accounting-and-financial-reporting/audit-and-internal-controls/why-the-internal-audit-function-serves-as-a-bulwark-against-risk

Reiter, K., & Song, P. (2022). *Fundamentals of healthcare finance* (4th ed.). Health Administration Press.

Reiter, K., & Song, P. (2021). *Gapenski's healthcare finance: An introduction to accounting and financial management* (7th ed.). Health Administration Press.

Rundall, T., Oberlin, S., Salmon, K., Thygesen, B., Salmon, K., & Janus, K. (2012). Success under duress: Policies and practices managers view as keys to profitability in five California hospitals with challenging payer mix. *Journal of Healthcare Management, 57*(2), 94–112. https://doi.org/10.1097/00115514-201203000-00005

Shivan, V. (2023). *Medical revenue cycle management: The comprehensive guide*. Self-published.

Singh, S. R., & Wheeler, J. R. C. (2012). Hospital financial management: What is the link between revenue cycle management, profitability, and not-for-profit hospitals' ability to grow equity? *Journal of Healthcare Management, 57*(5), 325–339. https://doi.org/10.1097/00115514-201209000-00007

Slyter, M., Hernandez, S. R., Hearld, L., Smith, D. G., & Borkowski, N. (2021). Assessing how well hospitals budget operating results by examining the relationship between budget variances and operating margin. *Journal of Health Care Finance, 48*(2), 1–21.

Song, P. H., Reiter, K. L., & Xu, W. Y. (2017). High-tech versus high-touch: Components of hospital costs vary widely. *Journal of Healthcare Management, 62*(3), 186–194. https://doi.org/10.1097/JHM-D-15-00040

Sussman, J. H. (2017). *Strategic allocation and management of capital in healthcare: A guide to decision making* (2nd ed.). Health Administration Press.

Sutherland, K., & Levesque, J. F. (2020). Unwarranted clinical variation in health care: Definitions and proposal of an analytic framework. *Journal of Evaluation in Clinical Practice, 26*(3), 687–696. https://doi.org/10.1111/jep.13181

Thornburg, M., & Meter, R. K. (2021). RIP for the RVU? Transitioning from widget-based production to impactful performance. *Physician Leadership Journal, 8*(3), 58–64.

Turner, J., Broom, K., Elliott, M., & Lee, J. F. (2015). A decomposition of hospital profitability: An application of DuPont analysis to the US market. *Health Services Research and Managerial Epidemiology, 2*, 1–10. https://doi.org/10.1177/2333392815590397

Urwin, J. W., & Emanuel, E. J. (2019). The relative value scale update committee: Time for an update. *JAMA, 322*(12), 1137–1138. https://doi.org/10.1001/jama.2019.14591

Wagner, S. L. (2017). *Fundamentals of medical practice management*. Health Administration Press.

White, C., & Whaley, C. M. (2021). Prices paid to hospitals by private health plans are high relative to Medicare and vary widely: Findings from an employer-led transparency initiative. *Rand Health Quarterly, 9*(2), 5.

Wright, S., & Durán, A. (2020). Decision analysis. In S. Wright & A. Durán (Eds.), *Understanding hospitals in changing health systems* (pp. 193–220). Palgrave Macmillan Cham. https://link.springer.com/chapter/10.1007/978-3-030-28172-4_9

Wurth, M. (2020, January 22). *AHA leader shares how hospitals pave the way to the future*. American Hospital Association. https://www.aha.org/news/healthcareinnovation-thursday-blog/2020-01-22-aha-leader-shares-how-hospitals-pave-way-future

Zare, H., Eisenberg, M. D., & Anderson, G. (2022). Comparing the value of community benefit and Tax-Exemption in non-profit hospitals. *Health Services Research, 57*(2), 270–284. https://doi.org/10.1111/1475-6773.13668

Zhang, R., & Bohlen, J. (2023). *Healthcare business budgeting*. StatPearls Publishing. https://www.ncbi.nlm.nih.gov/books/NBK589707

CHAPTER 15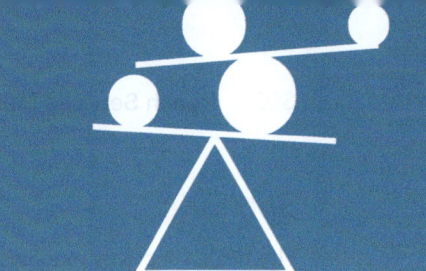

HEALTH SERVICES MANAGEMENT SCENARIOS AND PROJECTS

The following integrated health services management case scenarios and project assignments support the development of health services management competencies.

CASE SCENARIOS AND PROJECTS OUTLINE

1. Conflict on the Interprofessional Team
2. The Diversity, Equity, and Inclusion Initiative at the Healthcare Organization
3. Triple Bottom Line: People, Planet, and Profit
4. The Dark-Side Leader
5. Resisting Private Equity Investors
6. Medical Model Versus Population Health Model
7. Assessing Community Health Needs
8. Design an Accountable Care Organization
9. Home Health Business Plan
10. Performance Review Gone Wrong

CASE SCENARIOS AND PROJECTS

1. CONFLICT ON THE INTERPROFESSIONAL TEAM

Competencies

- Contribute to the interprofessional healthcare team.
- Manage interpersonal conflict through dispute resolution and mediation.
- Role model behaviors beneficial to building a strong organizational culture.
- Adapt interpersonal communication style and content to various management situations.
- Create psychological safety and interpersonal understanding by listening.
- Write credible business communications, including emails and reports.
- Communicate with sensitivity when communicating to diverse audiences.

Introduction

Healthcare teams depend on the contributions of multiple professions. Interprofessional collaboration occurs when individuals from multiple healthcare disciplines work together to care for patients. Unfortunately, interpersonal and task-related conflict can threaten collegial environments and patient care outcomes. While often unrecognized, health services managers play an important role on the interprofessional healthcare team, especially in managing interpersonal conflict.

Scenario

The health services manager for a multispecialty diabetes care clinic, Diabetes Care Plus, wants to maintain a harmonious workplace among the various clinical and nonclinical professions. The health services manager believes that interprofessional collaboration improves patient health outcomes. Based on discussions with the team, the health services manager learned the following troubling opinions (Almost et al., 2016; Brown et al., 2011):

- "I'm overworked. I don't have time to communicate, and neither do my coworkers." (nurse)
- "We are short staffed. This means that I am doing my job and someone else's. I end up doing work that I'm overqualified for." (physician)
- "As the physician, I am solely accountable for patient care." (physician)
- "We all need to be accountable for our jobs. We all have to take responsibility for our assigned actions. Not everyone is owning up to their responsibilities." (nurse)
- "There is a power structure in our clinic. If you disagree with a physician, then it's going to be hard to get them to change." (nurse)
- "I know that some people are afraid to confront others because it makes them uncomfortable." (nurse)
- "Some people don't want to share their concerns, so they just bottle them up. This has been going on so long that some people have formed cliques of disgruntled employees." (patient educator)
- "When I work with people in one clinic department, I have one set of tasks. Then, if I change to a different department, I am expected to do different things. I can never seem to get it right in either place." (medical assistant)
- "I never feel like management is listening to me." (nurse)

Project Assignments

Role of the Health Services Manager

1. Using the case scenario, describe the actions that the health services manager can take to improve interprofessional collaboration at Diabetes Care Plus. State the actions using the management practices of planning, organizing, directing, coordinating, and directing, as discussed in Chapter 1.

Problem-Solving and Evidence-Based Management

2. The team provided good feedback on the various difficulties facing Diabetes Care Plus. Conduct an analysis of the case scenario using problem-solving methods described in Chapter 2. First, start by highlighting or underlining all of the different problems in the scenario. Problems are issues that get in the way of Diabetes Care Plus achieving their organizational objectives. Then, assign each of the identified problems into conceptually similar problem areas. Finally, write a problem statement for each group of problems. The format for simple problem statements is as follows: "How can [the organization] [action verb] given that/in light of [object of problem-solving effort]?" Appendix 1 lists examples of health services management problems.
    a. Based on this feedback, define the problem(s).
    b. Identify potential initiatives or general solutions to the defined problem(s). Support the solutions using an evidence-based management approach.
    c. Define metrics/indicators that measure success. If employee or patient satisfaction is a chosen measure, be sure to be specific (i.e., satisfaction with what?).

Leadership and Change Management

3. Effective health services managers role model collaborative behaviors associated with interprofessional practice. Using the case scenario, write a brief report (less than 500 words) describing the roles that a Diabetes Care Plus Clinic health services manager would play on the interprofessional healthcare team, according to Begun et al. (2011), as discussed in Chapter 1.

Managing Interpersonal Communications

4. Write an agenda, as described in Chapter 3, for a meeting intended to address the issues presented in the case scenario with the clinicians, including nurses, physicians, and others. Be sure to state the meeting topic, meeting purpose, and other written agenda elements presented in Table 3.3.
5. Imagine that a single nurse wrote an email with all of the comments labeled with "nurse" in the case scenario. Write a professional email in response using the elements described in Chapter 3.

References

Almost, J., Wolff, A. C., Stewart-Pyne, A., McCormick, L. G., Strachan, D., & D'Souza, C. (2016). Managing and mitigating conflict in healthcare teams: An integrative review. *Journal of Advanced Nursing, 72*(7), 1490–1505. https://doi.org/10.1111/jan.12903

Begun, J. W., White, K. R., and Mosser, G. (2011). Interprofessional care teams: The role of the healthcare administrator. *Journal of Interprofessional Care, 25*(2), 119–123. https://doi.org/10.3109/13561820.2010.504135

Brown, J., Lewis, L., Ellis, K., Stewart, M., Freeman, T. R., & Kasperski, M. J. (2011). Conflict on interprofessional primary health care teams–can it be resolved? *Journal of Interprofessional Care, 25*(1), 4–10. https://doi.org/10.3109/13561820.2010.497750

2. THE DIVERSITY, EQUITY, AND INCLUSION INITIATIVE AT THE HEALTH CARE ORGANIZATION

Competencies

- Accept professional and social responsibility for diversity, equity, and inclusion.
- Apply evidence-based management skills to health services management challenges.
- Communicate with sensitivity when communicating to diverse audiences.
- Deliver verbal presentations with confidence.
- Motivate individuals and teams to achieve goals.
- Promote and manage processes that create organizational change and innovation.
- Promote diversity, equity, and inclusion for patients, employees, and the community.
- Use governance structures and processes to enhance organizational performance, patient experience, and clinical quality.
- Comply with human resources laws and regulations.
- Apply organizational design concepts to improve performance.
- Define, measure, and monitor indicators of performance.
- Prepare comprehensive project plans

Introduction

Addressing diversity, equity, and inclusion (DEI) are professional imperatives for health services managers, not only because of the ethics related to fairness and justice but also because DEI initiatives can create stronger work cultures, improve decision-making, and create a competitive advantage (American College of Healthcare Executives [ACHE], 2022).

Scenario

You are a forward-thinking CEO of a healthcare organization (HCO) who seeks to improve the diversity of representation, equity of outcomes, and inclusiveness. You also want to improve cross-racial and cross-cultural relationships throughout the HCO. However, previous efforts to enhance DEI were met with confusion, disinterest, and resistance by people in your HCO. So, you decided to ask a variety of coworkers for their thoughts on DEI. Some of the comments you heard when listening to your team mirrored those documented in the DEI scholarship, including the following (Jones & Okun, 2001; Wilkinson, 2021):

- "The efforts we tried in the past were just 'band-aids.' We need meaningful, long-term change to address the racism occurring in this organization."
- "I don't want to participate if we don't have the resources to do DEI right."
- "What are we trying to accomplish? Will these efforts improve our healthcare organization? What are we measuring?"
- "I am frustrated by a lack of progress. Why will this time be different?"
- "Racism and exclusion do not happen here."
- "Why are we only focused on race? What about gender or disability issues?"
- "Any initiative to help one group of people will create division for everyone else."
- "I'm not racist; I'm colorblind. I treat everyone the same."
- "What about other problems, such as our financial performance?"
- "I don't want to be involved because I'm afraid I might say the wrong thing."
- "We should focus on employee performance, not on race, ethnicity, or gender."
- "You don't understand the problem like I do because you have more power than me."
- "When discrimination happens here, our company keeps the complaints private. Why aren't you taking a stand?"

Project Assignments

Role of the Health Services Manager

1. Describe the actions that a health services manager would take to improve health equity in their community and diversity and inclusion in their workplace. State the actions using the management practices of planning, organizing, directing, coordinating, and directing discussed in Chapter 1.

Problem-Solving and Evidence-Based Management

2. The team provided good feedback on the problems associated with creating DEI initiatives at your HCO. Based on this feedback, conduct an analysis of the case scenario using the problem-solving methods described in Chapter 2. First, start by highlighting or underlining all of the different problems in the scenario. Problems are issues that get

in the way of the HCO achieving their organizational objectives. Then, assign each of the identified problems into conceptually similar problem areas. Finally, write a problem statement for each group of problems. The format for simple problem statements is as follows: "How can [the organization] [action verb] given that/in light of [object of problem-solving effort]?" Appendix 1 lists examples of health services management problems.

    a. Define the problem(s).

    b. Identify potential DEI initiatives or general solutions to the defined problem(s). Describe the evidence supporting these initiatives or solutions using an evidence-based management approach.

    c. Measure success with metrics/indicators. If employee satisfaction is a chosen measure, be sure to be specific (i.e., satisfaction with what?).

Managing Interpersonal Communications

3. Write an agenda, as described in Chapter 3, for a meeting intended to address the DEI-related issues presented in the case scenario. Be sure to state the meeting topic, meeting purpose, and other written agenda elements presented in Table 3.3.

4. Write a dramatic-style presentation that anticipates the audience's resistance to DEI programs. Using the story structure described in Table 3.7, explain how sacrifice and hard work will lead to success.

Professionalism and Ethics

5. Identify elements supporting DEI in a written code of ethics from a health services management professional organization, such as the American College of Healthcare Executives, Medical Group Management Association, or healthcare quality professionals. Based on the code of ethics, write a professional DEI statement that could be used to guide your organization's initiative(s).

Leadership and Change Management

6. To improve the diversity of representation, equity of outcomes, and inclusiveness of HCOs, the HCOs need to institute a change management initiative. Choose a change management approach discussed in Chapter 4 and describe the steps needed to create organizational change.

Human Resources Management

7. Develop a position description for new executive management position, called a chief diversity officer, who is responsible for managing diversity, equity, and inclusion activities across the HCO.

Performance Management

8. For the HCO in the scenario, establish at least three (3) performance measures for each of these concepts: diversity, equity, and inclusion.

9. For each defined performance measure, set a target that is challenging but attainable.

Project Management

10. Based on the stated goals and feedback provided in the scenario, create a project plan for one or more healthcare-related DEI initiatives. Define the multiple deliverables or phases of the initiative(s). Then, create a work breakdown structure graphically illustrating at least three (3) levels of deliverables or work products. Use a numbering

system, as described in Chapter 13. Finally, using a table format (e.g., Excel), create a list of activities for each of the work products, including start date, end date, and duration for each. Assign at least one person to each activity (use imagination, if necessary).

References

American College of Healthcare Executives. (2022). *ACHE statement on diversity.* https://www.ache.org/about-ache/our-story/our-commitments/policy-statements/statement-on-diversity

Jones, K., & Okun, T. (2001). White supremacy culture. *Dismantling racism: A workbook for social change.*

Wilkinson, B. (2021) *The diversity gap: Where good intentions meet true cultural change.* HarperCollins Leadership.

3. TRIPLE BOTTOM LINE: PEOPLE, PLANET, AND PROFIT

Competencies

- Maintain or enhance operations of HCOs.
- Write credible business communications, including emails and reports.
- Deliver verbal presentations with confidence.
- Promote and manage processes that create organizational change and innovation.
- Motivate individuals and teams to achieve goals.
- Use governance structures and processes to enhance organizational performance, patient experience, and clinical quality.
- Monitor performance of functional areas of HCOs, including marketing, supply chain, human resources, and clinical quality.
- Apply quality management methodologies and tools to continuous quality improvement initiatives.
- Understand roles and responsibilities of the healthcare finance organization, including financial control systems, third-party contracting, and capital financing.

Introduction

Well-organized community coalitions attempt to influence HCOs to address all types of issues, particularly matters related to the environment (Reed, 2017). Environmental groups are keenly aware that health services delivery systems are responsible for 8.5% of emissions in the United States (Watts et al., 2021). Some hospitals have begun to institute sustainable health services delivery practices that aim to reduce carbon emissions and wastefulness (Greenhill & Khalil, 2023). Social and environmental goals are a part of a concept known as the triple bottom line, which states that businesses should be committed to measuring not only profits but also its social and environmental impact (Senay et al., 2022).

Scenario

At Hopeview General Hospital, board meetings have become a battleground for environmental activism. GreenHeart Community activators, a group of concerned citizens, has asked Dr. Lucila Ontiveros, the Hopeview General Hospital's chief medical officer, to convince the CEO and the board of directors to institute environmentally sustainable health care practices. Dr. Ontiveros is passionate that Hopeview should accept responsibility for their environmental impact and make substantial changes in how they operate. Dr. Ontiveros asked the CEO to adopt green initiatives at the hospital to benefit the environment and improve patient outcomes and reduce costs.

However, Kathryn Kraft, the CEO, questions the financial feasibility of transitioning to environmentally sustainable practices. While she sees the hospital as having a social responsibility, she is caught between the potential long-term benefits advocated by Dr. Ontiveros and Green-Heart Community activators and the immediate financial implications. Nevertheless, Kraft created an agenda item for Dr. Ontiveros to address the board of directors at the next quarterly meeting.

At the board meeting, Dr. Ontiveros passionately argued to the board of directors that an environmentally sustainable hospital would attract socially conscious patients, support the hospital's reputation, and potentially lead to grants and funding opportunities. She pointed to success stories from other HCOs that embraced environmentally friendly practices. However, the chairman of the board, Richard Madison, the pragmatic and financially focused leader, voiced his concerns about the financial burden of Dr. Ontiveros's recommendations. Mr. Madison worried about the upfront costs of implementing sustainable technologies, such as solar panels, energy-efficient equipment, and waste reduction systems. He asked Dr. Ontiveros whether diverting resources to these initiatives would strain the hospital's budget and compromise its ability to provide quality patient care. He asked whether the hospital's funds should instead be directed toward core medical services. The debate intensified during a closed-door board session.

Behind the scenes, whispers circulated among board members, media outlets caught wind of the internal conflict, and public interest grew as citizens rallied both for and against the Hopeview General Hospital's environmental action. As the intrigue reached its climax, a compromise emerged. The board asked Dr. Ontiveros and Ms. Kraft to work with a team of sustainability consultants to develop and present a comprehensive proposal outlining the potential financial, environmental, and reputational benefits of adopting green initiatives.

Project Assignments

Role of the Health Services Manager

1. Write an email from Kathryn Kraft, Hopeview General Hospital's CEO, to Dr. Lucila Ontiveros, the chief medical officer, inviting her to address the board of directors at the next quarterly meeting, as described in the scenario. In the email, refer to Kraft's role, as described by Henry Mintzberg and illustrated in Figure 1.2. of Chapter 1. Because the email will likely be made public, be sure to write the email professionally using the elements described in Chapter 3.

Managing Interpersonal Communications

2. Write a 5-minute pitch that Dr. Ontiveros will deliver to the Hopeview General Hospital board of directors at the scheduled board meeting. The call to action should be a specifically defined investment in environmentally sustainable practices at Hopeview General Hospital. Be sure to address the expected doubts of Richard Madison, chairman of the board, and Kathryn Kraft, the CEO.

3. You are on the team of sustainability consultants asked to develop a comprehensive proposal outlining the potential financial, environmental, and reputational benefits of adopting green initiatives. Write a short report with cited evidence from scholarly

literature that gives a high-level explanation of the pros and cons of hospitals investing in environmentally sustainable practices. The report should include an executive summary, as described in Table 3.8. Be sure to include an attention-grabbing title and write to accomplish objectives.

Leadership and Change Management

4. Using Kotter's 8-Step Change Model, document a plan to manage organizational change at Hopeview General Hospital surgical units. The goal is to encourage surgeons to adopt environmentally sustainable practices in the operating rooms.

Population Health and Community Collaboration

5. Write a brief statement (less than 500 words) for Kathryn Kraft, the CEO, that describes the value to Hopeview General Hospital of forming a partnership with GreenHeart Community activators. Be sure to include elements related to how Hopeview General Hospital can leverage their financial and political influence as an anchor institution that facilitates the community's environmental sustainability.

Professionalism and Ethics

6. Whether or not to invest in environmentally sustainable health care practices can be framed as an ethical dilemma. Write a brief report (less than 500 words) outlining the ethical perspectives, as described in Chapter 5, that may inform Kathryn Kraft's action in this scenario.

Healthcare Governance

7. Write a brief statement (less than 500 words) for Kathryn Kraft, the CEO, that articulates the fiduciary responsibility of the board of directors to commit to an environmentally sustainable hospital. Include the following points:

    a. As CEO, what governance structures and processes can you use to reduce the health system's environmental impact?

    b. Describe the committee's processes, meeting agenda, performance management methods (measures and oversight), and relationship-building approaches that you would use to improve environmental sustainability.

    c. What organizational assets and resources would you allocate to the governance structure and processes to support environmental sustainability?

Performance Management

8. Define at least five performance metrics for Hopeview General Hospital environmental sustainability practices, operationalizing the metrics using the SMART (Specific, Measurable, Assignable, Realistic, and Time bound) goal approach described in Chapter 11.

Healthcare Quality Management

9. The team of sustainability consultants conducted a waste audit of the types and volumes of waste produced by Hopeview General Hospital. It was found that Hopeview General Hospital produced 11 kilograms of medical waste per patient day in the following categories and weights (in kilograms): paper and cardboard (4.18), food waste (2.75), packaging (2.42), infectious waste (0.55), sharps (0.50), genotoxic waste (0.28), chemical waste (0.22), and radioactive waste (0.11). Create a Pareto chart for medical waste per patient day at Hopeview General Hospital, as described in Chapter 12.

Healthcare Financial Management

10. Imagine that the consultants recommended solar panel purchase and installation to offset carbon emissions. Write a capital budgeting request for the solar panels purchase and installation that includes the estimated total expenses and the payback period of the investment. Use the internet to identify solar panel costs, installation costs, commercial per kilowatt costs from the nonsolar sources, and estimated kilowatt-hours generated per kilowatt of peak capacity (kWh/kWp) for a specified location. (Hopeview General Hospital can be assumed to be located anywhere in the United States.)

References

Greenhill, R. G., & Khalil, M. (2023). Sustainable Healthcare depends on good governance practices. *Frontiers of Health Services Management, 39*(3), 5–11. https://doi.org/10.1097/HAP.0000000000000163

Reed, R. (2017, October 20). *Company boards are rife with drama and discontent as directors grapple with social issues.* Chicago Tribune. https://www.chicagotribune.com/business/ct-biz-boardroom-turmoil-robert-reed-1022-story.html

Senay, E., Cort, T., Perkison, W., Laestadius, J. G., & Sherman, J. D. (2022). What can hospitals learn from The Coca-Cola company? Health Care Sustainability Reporting. *NEJM Catalyst Innovations in Care Delivery, 3*(3), CAT-21. https://doi.org/10.1056/CAT.21.0362

Watts, N., Amann, M., Arnell, N., Ayeb-Karlsson, S., Beagley, J., Belesova, K., Boykoff, M., Byass, P., Cai, W., Campbell-Lendrum, D., Capstick, S., Chambers, J., Coleman, S., Dalin, C., Daly, M., Dasandi, N., Dasgupta, S., Davies, M., Di Napoli, C., … Costello, A. (2021). The 2020 report of the Lancet Countdown on health and climate change: Responding to converging crises. *The Lancet, 397*(10269), 129–170. https://doi.org/10.1016/S0140-6736(20)32290-X

4. THE DARK-SIDE LEADER

Competencies

- Role model behaviors beneficial to building a strong organizational culture.
- Develop emotional and social intelligence.
- Acquire and utilize power to influence others or gain commitment for resources.
- Develop a respected professional reputation through executive presence, personal branding, and networking.
- Write credible business communications, including emails and reports.
- Deliver verbal presentations with confidence.
- Apply organizational design concepts to improve performance.

Introduction

Traditionally, patients have been discharged from the hospital into skilled nursing facilities (SNF), where they received health services designed to care for complex medical needs beyond what could be provided in their homes or assisted living facilities. Due to policy developments instituted during the COVID-19 pandemic and technological innovations, a larger share of patients discharged from hospitals are being discharged from the hospital to their homes. This shift represents an opportunity for health systems to expand their services into home-based care.

Scenario

At Harmony Community Hospital, health services managers do not trust the CEO, Lance Wolfe, a leader who prioritizes performance over ethical behaviors. Wolfe's primary goal for his leadership was to get things done. Success is not achieved through cooperation but through political skill. Even though Wolfe's toxic leadership behaviors create stressful work environments and unhappy workers, some ambitious leaders used selfishness, manipulation, and aggression to succeed. Wolfe often ordered two different managers to accomplish the same objective, just to see which person would succeed first.

Marcia MacAfee accepted a position as director of post-acute care, where she was given the responsibility of creating a post-acute care strategy for Harmony. MacAfee was charged with developing and implementing a rehabilitation at home program, in which a multidisciplinary home-based team of post-acute care providers delivered care that was previously delivered in an SNF (Augustine et al., 2020). However, unbeknown to MacAfee, Wolfe privately directed another executive to also manage an initiative—Frank Prince. Relentless in pursuit of success, Prince had been steadily promoted in his 10-year-long career. In his current position as director of business development, Prince was responsible for developing and implementing new business lines for Harmony Community Hospital.

MacAfee was confused by Prince's involvement in the rehabilitation at home program. According to Prince, he was assisting MacAfee and her team with development and implementation. But so far, Prince had done less assisting of MacAfee and more directing of her team. He acted with such supreme self-confidence that MacAfee's team often did just as Prince ordered. MacAfee was blindsided by Prince's ambition, deception, and maneuvering. When MacAfee asked Wolfe about the potential conflict, he told MacAfee to "collaborate as much as possible." This conversation left MacAfee even more concerned, leaving her wondering what her next moves should be.

Project Assignments

Managing Interpersonal Communications

1. Write a professional email, using the elements described in Chapter 3, for Marcia MacAfee to send to her team regarding her authority over the post-acute care initiative. Communicate with confidence, clarity, and credibility to inspire respect and appreciation of her team. Be aware that Frank Prince will likely obtain the email from someone on her team.

Leadership and Change Management

2. As a leader of the post-acute care initiative, Marcia MacAfee needs power, especially more power than Frank Prince, in order to successfully complete the job for which she was hired. Write a brief report to Marcia MacAfee advising her on potential sources of power and the actions she can take to acquire and retain power.
3. Identify self-defense mechanisms that Marcia MacAfee can employ to avoid negative consequences to her career when dealing with organizations led by dark side leaders.
4. Effective health services managers insist on respectfully and directly addressing conflict. Reflecting on conflict management skills, devise a step-by-step plan for Marcia MacAfee to address the conflict with Frank Prince. Use emotional intelligence and political skills.

Organizational Design

5. Create an organizational chart illustrating the authority and responsibilities for the Harmony Community Hospital post-acute care implementation initiative. Illustrate the positions held by Lance Wolfe, Marcia MacAfee, and Frank Prince.

Reference

Augustine, M. R., Davenport, C., Ornstein, K. A., Cuan, M., Saenger, P., Lubetsky, S., Federman, A., DeCherrie, L. V., Leff, B., & Siu, A. L. (2020). Implementation of post-acute rehabilitation at home: A skilled nursing facility-substitutive model. *Journal of the American Geriatrics Society, 68*(7), 1584–1593. https://doi.org/10.1111/jgs.16474

5. RESISTING PRIVATE EQUITY INVESTORS

Competencies

- Solve problems through critical thinking and analysis of the best available evidence.
- Define problems, challenges, or opportunities thoroughly and succinctly.
- Formulate alternative solutions using a variety of credible sources.
- Construct and communicate a shared vision.
- Promote and manage processes that create organizational change and innovation.
- Use governance structures and processes to enhance organizational performance, patient experience, and clinical quality.
- Apply organizational design concepts to improve performance.

Introduction

A private equity firm is a type of investment company that invests in and manages privately owned businesses, including physician practices. These firms raise capital from a variety of investors, such as pension funds, endowments, insurance companies, and wealthy individuals, and pool the money into private equity funds. Private equity funds are generally set up as limited partnerships, with a managing partner making business decisions and limited partners, such as pension funds, endowments, insurance companies, or high-net-worth individuals, contributing capital. The managing partner of the private equity firm runs the medical practice business, and a chief medical officer, who is a physician and a partner in the practice, is responsible for medical decisions. This management structure is referred to as a dyad leadership model.

When private equity investors buy smaller physician practices and consolidate them into larger groups, the practices achieve economies of scale, improve bargaining power with insurers, and streamline administrative functions. Private equity investments allow for growth of physician practices while still remaining independent from hospital control. However, as compared with internal growth initiatives, private equity mergers carry significant risk for physician-owned medical practices. Private equity investment can dilute physician ownership shares in their practices and diminish the influence the physicians have over medical decisions. Moreover, private equity firms may be more interested in generating profits than nonprofit community hospitals (Appelbaum & Batt, 2020).

Scenario

Premier Gastroenterology Associates was started by two young gastroenterologist physicians in 2002. Over time, the Premier grew into a 10-physician practice with three locations in the community. One of the physicians, Dr. Emily Carter, wanted to increase the size of the practice to achieve more bargaining power with commercial insurance companies and suppliers. However, she was resistant to overtures from the local community hospital to purchase their practice, as she and her partner valued independence and the ability to compete with the hospital on certain profitable medical services, such as colonoscopies.

The solution Dr. Carter and her partner preferred was to consolidate with other small- and medium-sized gastroenterology practices. Gastroenterology physician practices have experienced accelerated growth in private equity investment over the last decade (Gilreath et al., 2021). Many gastroenterologist physicians want to take advantage of the economic benefits of large, consolidated practices that can be realized with outside investments from private equity firms. The decision to sell to private equity ownership was controversial, especially among some of the older physicians who practice at Premier Gastroenterology Associates. Private equity firms have a reputation for prioritizing profitability over patient needs. In addition, the management teams in private equity firms often make changes in management practices that affect physicians' autonomy and job satisfaction.

Nevertheless, Dr. Carter and her partner accepted the buyout from the private equity firm that created a large, consolidated gastroenterology practice called Unified Gastroenterology Partners. While this trade-off seemed worth the financial windfall for Dr. Carter and her partner, her fellow physicians were reluctant to change how they practiced under the new organizational structure. They ignored most of the new policies established by the new Unified Gastroenterology Partners medical director who was responsible for creating consistency across all practice locations.

Wanting to create a more collegial environment, she planned an offsite retreat for the physicians from Premier Gastroenterology Associates and the medical director of the new Unified Gastroenterology Partners. Some of the comments from the physicians included the following:

- "I don't think that the physicians in the other practices are as strong clinically as us. They seem to be following the guidelines set by the investors."
- "I'm sorry. I just don't trust nonphysician business leaders. Physicians should be in charge of physician practices."
- "Ever since the merger, I feel constant pressure to maximize profitability. We're being asked to see more patients, perform more procedures, or reduce costs."
- "I think we [physicians formerly employed by Premier Gastroenterology Associates] no longer have the autonomy to make decisions about our own medical practice. Business decisions are made at the corporate level, which really affect how we treat patients."
- "The message from Unified Gastroenterology Partners is to standardize, standardize, standardize. I suppose they want to improve efficiency, but I only see the constraints on my treatment approaches."
- "I lack input into strategic decisions. At Premier Gastroenterology Associates, the practice leaders really listened to our input. Now, I just don't think they listen."
- "I really don't appreciate that they reduced appointment times for some of our services. Now I feel rushed, which is affecting my relationships with patients."

The comments that the physicians provided made Dr. Carter realize that the problems were worse than what she thought. Unfortunately, the merger was already complete. She feared that if she did not figure out how to help the physicians formerly employed by Premier Gastroenterology Associates embrace the change, many of them would look for work elsewhere. Dr. Carter knew that something needed to be done, but she did not know how to go about it. She collected her notes and went to see the new CEO of the Unified Gastroenterology Partners. She hoped that they could develop solutions together.

Project Assignments

Problem-Solving and Evidence-Based Management

1. Based on the approaches described in Chapter 2, conduct an analysis of the case scenario. First, start by highlighting or underlining all of the different problems in the scenario. Problems are issues that get in the way of Unified Gastroenterology Partners achieving their organizational objectives. Then, assign each of the identified problems into conceptually similar problem areas. Finally, write a problem statement for each group of problems. The format for simple problem statements is as follows: "How can [the organization] [action verb] given that/in light of [object of problem-solving effort]?" Appendix 1 lists examples of health services management problems.

2. As described in Chapter 2, for each issue within the problem statement, identify at least two possible solutions. Use scholarly literature or professional whitepapers to brainstorm alternative solutions. For each problem statement, develop a set of decision criteria. Finally, write a research question for each decision criterion. Decision criteria, such as cost-effectiveness or political feasibility, help to select the best solution or solutions.

Leadership and Change Management

3. Using Kotter's 8-Step Change Model, document a plan to manage organizational change at Unified Gastroenterology Partners. Be sure to construct and communicate a shared vision for the HCO.

Healthcare Governance

4. To address the problem(s) identified in the scenario, create a new physician governance committee that will enhance organizational performance, patient experience, and clinical quality. Write a short committee charter (less than 500 words) that defines committee membership, meeting cadence, scope of authority, and parliamentary rules.

5. Assume that Unified Gastroenterology Partners does not have standing committees defined for the new practice. Develop an organizational chart with the standing committees defined. Be sure to include committees that address issues described in the case scenario.

References

Appelbaum, E., & Batt, R. (2020). Private equity buyouts in healthcare: who wins, who loses? *Institute for New Economic Thinking Working Paper Series No. 118*. https://doi.org/10.36687/inetwp118

Gilreath, M., Patel, N. C., Suh, J., & Brill, J. V. (2021). Gastroenterology physician practice management and private equity: Thriving in uncertain times. *Clinical Gastroenterology and Hepatology, 19*(6), 1084–1087. https://doi.org/10.1016/j.cgh.2021.03.015

6. MEDICAL MODEL VERSUS POPULATION HEALTH MODEL

Competencies

- Promote systems thinking in healthcare.
- Balance the concerns of health care access, quality, and cost.
- Write credible business communications, including emails and reports.
- Deliver verbal presentations with confidence.
- Motivate individuals and teams to achieve goals.
- Apply organizational design concepts to improve performance.
- Innovate health services delivery in response to trends in healthcare policy and financing.
- Invest in population health management functions, such as risk-based financing, staff reorganization, and health information technology, to improve quality and reduce costs.
- Define, measure, and monitor indicators of performance.
- Track, analyze, and report quality measures in compliance with national quality initiatives and accreditation standards.

Introduction

The medical model and the population health model represent two different approaches to health services delivery (Johnson et al., 2023). While the medical model excels in diagnosing and treating acute conditions, it often falls short when instituting preventive measures and addressing broader social determinants of health for groups of patients. The population health model, on the other hand, emphasizes prevention and community-based interventions, aiming for long-term health improvement of groups of patients. Population health requires that health care organizations accept financial responsibility for the health of a defined population. The shift away from paying for volume to paying for population health models of care is happening slowly. While the majority of payments to hospitals and doctors are still based on the volume of patients they treat, health insurance companies are moving away from paying hospitals for treatment episodes. For comprehensive healthcare delivery, a combination of both models can lead to better outcomes, ensuring individual patients receive timely and specialized care while also addressing the health needs of communities.

Scenario

Sarah Williams, the vice president of the cardiology service line at St. Jude's General Hospital, wanted to change how the hospital service line practiced medicine. Sarah witnessed how St. Jude's cardiac care team's diligent interventions saved countless lives, consistent with the strengths of the medical model. The cardiology service line

- achieved excellence in diagnosing and treating acute and complex medical conditions;
- featured well-trained, specialized medical professionals with expertise in specific diseases or conditions;
- provided access to specialized care, advanced medical technology, and medical care innovation;
- emphasized personalized treatments based on a patient's specific medical history and condition; and
- offered efficient responses to urgent health issues.

However, she could not ignore St. Jude's glaring deficiencies in preventing heart disease. Patients consistently returned with the same preventable cardiac conditions, and the hospital seemed caught in a cycle of reactive treatment. Sarah noted the following limitations of the medical model:

- focused on individual treatment, often overlooking population-based preventive measures
- can be expensive, with a tendency to overuse medical interventions
- may not address social determinants of health that influence individual well-being

Sarah's epiphany came during a conference where a renowned public health expert spoke about the potential of the population health model. Sarah recognized the urgent need to transition toward more comprehensive care for groups of cardiac patients. Determined to bring about change, Sarah wanted to combine the strengths of both the medical model and the population health model for a more holistic approach.

Sarah understood that population health models are financed differently than the volume-based incentives associated with fee-for-service payments. Sarah knew that St. Jude's General Hospital could contract with insurance companies to be paid predetermined amounts of money regardless of the level of care provided to each individual patient. While St. Jude's General Hospital would risk losing money if the costs of medical care exceed the predetermined payment, the service line could also realize significant profits. Sarah also noted the following strengths of the population health model:

- emphasizes preventive care and health promotion
- addresses the root causes of health issues, including social determinants of health, such as housing, food, education, transportation, and social connectedness
- collaborates with multiple stakeholders for a broader impact

Sarah began by initiating dialogues among her team members, doctors, nurses, and even community representatives about moving beyond medical interventions. She knew that she faced objections from some clinicians who feared that the population health model might compromise the quality of interventional care. Sarah acknowledged the following limitations of the population health model:

- requires sustained efforts and time to achieve measurable results
- may face challenges in funding and resource allocation
- relies on data analysis to identify health trends and tailor interventions, so there is potential for technology-driven decisions to overshadow clinical judgment
- may erode the provider-patient relationship, impacting the quality of communication, trust, and rapport between healthcare professionals and individual patients

However, Sarah was willing to address their concerns. With population health management interventions, such as financial management, organizational design, health information technology, cost control, and operations restructuring, she felt that both the medical model and the population health model could coexist and offer the best of both approaches.

Project Assignments

Managing Interpersonal Communications

1. Write a 5-minute pitch that Sarah Williams can deliver to St. Jude's General Hospital's cardiology service line leadership, including the management director and medical director of cardiac health services, that motivates the creation of a population health model for cardiac care. Be sure to address objections from people who fear that the population health model might compromise the quality of interventional care.

Population Health and Community Collaboration

2. Write a brief statement (less than 500 words) about creating hospital-based health care programs that combine the strengths of both the medical model and the population health model for cardiac care. Identify at least one real-world example of a cardiac care program

that exemplifies a combination of medical and population health models. Use scholarly, such as journal articles, and non-scholarly references, such as news articles, white papers, or company websites. Scholarly sources must be published within the last 5 years.

Performance Management

3. Using the balanced scorecard approach presented in Chapter 11, create at least four strategic perspectives for St. Jude's General Hospital's population health model for cardiac care, as demonstrated in Tables 11.1 to 11.4. For each strategic perspective, devise at least two strategic objectives and the corresponding measures, operationalized definitions, and targets, as described in Table 11.8.

Healthcare Quality Management

4. Define two process measures for the cardiology service line at St. Jude's General Hospital, one for population health model and one for medical care model.

Organizational Design

5. Create an organizational chart for St. Jude's General Hospital cardiology service line that combines various types of services or settings across the continuum of care, such as diagnostics, outpatient specialist care, inpatient care, post-acute rehabilitation, home care, and long-term care. The service line should be an executive health services manager who reports to a more senior executive over multiple service lines.

Reference

Johnson, S., Givens, M., & Gourevitch, M. N. (2023). Population health. In J. R. Knickman & B. Elbel (Eds.), *Jonas and Kovner's health care delivery in the United States* (13th ed., pp. 71–94). Springer Publishing Company.

7. ASSESSING COMMUNITY HEALTH NEEDS

Competencies

- Promote diversity, equity, and inclusion for patients, employees, and the community.
- Assess population health status and respond to changing needs of patient populations.
- Adapt health services operations using public health approaches, such as epidemiology and program planning and evaluation.
- Collaborate with community organizations to improve population health and achieve strategic initiatives.
- Apply evidence-based management skills to health services management challenges.
- Proactively identify current and future problems.
- Define problems, challenges, or opportunities thoroughly and succinctly.
- Write credible business communications, including emails and reports.
- Deliver verbal presentations with confidence.
- Influence organizational strategy and policy through collaborative relationships with the board of directors, medical staff, nurses, and patients.

Introduction

Community health needs assessment (CHNA) reports analyze the health needs of a defined population, the services available to them, and the interventions required to improve community health. Health services managers use the CHNAs to prioritize health needs, set population health goals, and develop programs that address the gaps in community health (Burns et al., 2023). All not-for-profit hospitals and health systems must submit a written CHNAs to the Internal Revenue Service (IRS) every 3 years (Pennel et al., 2016).

Scenario

As the new manager of the Westwood Medical Center, Emma Chung was responsible for coordinating the development of a community health needs assessment—a daunting task that would require her to understand the health concerns of a diverse and growing community. Key community stakeholders were recruited to participate in a focus group by asking a variety of community leaders who they believed would provide valuable information regarding the community. The focus group participants included a variety of community interests, including government leaders, hospital vice president, physician, business owners, local health department leader, director of a nonprofit organization, church leader, school district leader, dietician, social worker, farmer, and a professor of public health. Three different focus group discussions were held, each lasting 60 to 90 minutes.

The focus group interviews included questions about the strengths and weakness of the community; challenges to health and well-being; community resources; and perceptions of HCOs, clinicians, and social care providers. The following comments are from the focus group discussions (Grant et al., 2015; WCRNC, 2019):

- "It's really hard to get an appointment with a specialist. Sometimes, you have to wait for months, and that's if you can afford it."
- "I don't have a car, so getting to the clinic is a real challenge. We need more transportation options."
- "Public transit in the county is not great, so people can't get health care as easily."
- "There are many free screenings offered, but the times often conflict with my work schedule."
- "Health literacy is a big problem. When patients leave their doctors office, they know very little about their condition."
- "I think if we had more community events focused on health and fitness, people would be more motivated to stay active."
- "I think there's a lot of misinformation about health out there. It would be great there were more workshops or classes."
- "Our kids are dealing with so much stress, especially after the pandemic. We need more support in schools for mental health."
- "The cost of medication is so high. Sometimes I have to choose between buying food or getting my insulin."
- "I wish there were more programs to help people with chronic illnesses. It's tough to manage everything on your own."
- "Some doctors don't take certain types of insurance, like Medicaid."
- "I think racism is an issue in health care."
- "It would be great if there were more opportunities for volunteering and getting involved in community health initiatives."
- "Nobody talks about it, but we have a tremendous opioid drug addiction problem."

In addition, a survey was distributed to a variety of community stakeholders asking them to identify the highest priority health problems and barriers. The results of the survey are provided in Table 15.1.

TABLE 15.1 Community-Reported Health Problems and Barriers to Health and Wellness

RANK	PRIORITY HEALTH PROBLEMS	BARRIERS TO HEALTH AND WELLNESS
1	Cardiovascular disease	Costs of health care/insurance/medication
2	Diabetes	Transportation challenges
3	Cancer	Racism in healthcare system
4	Anxiety and depression	Shortage of mental health providers
5	Drug addiction	Scarcity of healthy food options
6	Obesity	Lack of free time to exercise
7	Smoking	Lack of social support for elderly

Project Assignments

Population Health and Community Collaboration

1. Using the elements presented in Chapter 6 and illustrated in Figure 6.1, write a CHNA. For the geographic element of the CHNA, choose any county in the United States as Westwood Medical Center's catchment area. Use the case scenario for the stakeholder input element of the CHNA. Use the data sources cited in Chapter 6, including Healthy People 2030 framework, American Community Survey, U.S. National Center for Health Statistics, and the University of Wisconsin's County Health Rankings model website.

2. Based on the most critical community health problems, identify collaborators that can improve community health for the chosen county. Write a brief proposal (less than 500 words) stating the benefits of community collaboration with Westwood Medical Center. Use evidence from scholarly health services management literature to support the proposal.

Managing Interpersonal Communications

3. Based on the written CHNA report, write and deliver a 15-minute presentation, supplemented with electronic audiovisual media (e.g., PowerPoint). The goal of the presentation is to explain the community health needs to the nonexpert board of directors and health services management executives. See the description of an explanation-style presentation in Table 3.6.

Professionalism and Ethics

4. Health equity seeks to eliminate differences in health outcomes by race, ethnicity, gender, ability status, or neighborhood. Health services managers can actively increase health equity, not only because of the ethics related to fairness and justice but also because of the professional responsibility to reduce health disparities. Within the CHNA report, identify health disparities in the chosen county and make recommendations to eliminate them.

References

Burns, A., Yeager, V. A., Cronin, C. E., & Franz, B. (2023). Community engagement in nonprofit hospital community health needs assessments and implementation plans. *Journal of Public Health Management and Practice, 29*(2), E50–E57. https://doi.org/10.1097/PHH.0000000000001663

Grant, C. G., Ramos, R., Davis, J. L., & Green, B. L. (2015). Community health needs assessment: A pathway to the future and a vision for leaders. *The Health Care Manager, 34*(2), 147–156. https://doi.org/10.1097/HCM.0000000000000057

Pennel, C. L., McLeroy, K. R., Burdine, J. N., Matarrita-Cascante, D., & Wang, J. (2016). Community health needs assessment: potential for population health improvement. *Population Health Management, 19*(3), 178–186. https://doi.org/10.1089/pop.2015.0075

Washington County Regional Medical Center. (2019). *Community health needs assessment*. https://www.wcrmc.com/Community_Health_Needs_Assessment_2020.pdf

8. DESIGN AN ACCOUNTABLE CARE ORGANIZATION

Competencies

- Apply organizational design concepts to improve performance.
- Assess advantages and disadvantages of various organizational designs.
- Build effective collaborations across the continuum of care.
- Understand how organizational structure impacts patient care and experience.
- Examine interdependence, integration, and competition of external organizations.
- Influence organizational strategy and policy through collaborative relationships with the board of directors, medical staff, nurses, and patients.
- Use governance structures and processes to enhance organizational performance, patient experience, and clinical quality.
- Connect organizational goals to individual performance.
- Prepare comprehensive project plans.
- Identify and interpret various payment methodologies of third-party payers.

Introduction

To encourage HCOs to better coordinate care, the Patient Protection and Affordable Care Act of 2010 (ACA) created a new value-based payment arrangement, called the Medicare Shared Savings Program. Participating organizations create formal partnerships between hospitals, physicians, long-term care, and other providers that deliver services across the continuum of care called Accountable Care Organizations (ACOs). Under a distinct contract with Centers for Medicare & Medicaid Services, ACOs accept accountability for overall costs and quality of care of Medicare patients in the area. ACOs are expected to better coordinate care to reduce wasteful spending, such as unnecessary emergency department visits and repeated diagnostic tests (Shortell & Addicott, 2015). The participating ACOs earn bonuses if the ACO decreases costs while achieving certain quality targets (Lewis et al., 2022). Under the Medicare Shared Savings Program, ACOs split any saved dollars with the federal government.

Scenario

The CEO of Sacred Heart Hospital, Juan Carlos Hernández, conducted executive meetings with ferocious efficiency, and this morning was no different. "Good morning, everyone," Juan Carlos began. "I trust you all had a restful weekend. I know it's Monday morning, but I have some news to share from last week's board meeting. The board has approved my recommendation that we apply to participate in the Medicare Shared Savings Program. We have the greenlight to spend the necessary funds to establish an Accountable Care Organization."

Pranita Patel, the CFO, raised an eyebrow. "This will be quite the undertaking, Juan Carlos. Did they agree to the padded budget we developed?"

Juan Carlos nodded and said, "Absolutely. In addition to the legal documentation, we need to hire the right people, implement new technologies, and build population health capabilities in finance and operations. The ACO will require a lot of coordination between departments, and there are risks involved if we don't get these things right."

Dr. Amanda Lee, the chief medical officer, spoke up. "I agree. From a medical perspective, I can see the benefits to patients. But we'd need to ensure we have the right infrastructure to support the kind of care coordination an ACO demands. It involves a lot of data sharing and collaborative decision-making among various providers. Do we have the technological capabilities to make it work?"

Juan Carlos nodded. "Yes, yes. That's where Jake comes in. Jake's team has a plan for handling the IT and data analytics requirements for this."

Jake Turner, the chief technology officer, shrugged. "Yup. We have a plan. We'll also need to create partnerships with the right health care organizations. Do we have partners lined up?"

Juan Carlos replied, "Yes, we have partners lined up, Jake. Our legal team will get the new corporate entity created. You need to make sure technologies allow our partner organizations to collaborate on population health management activities."

Juan Carlos wondered if his team was already doubting themselves or each other, and it troubled him. He paused and held each of his executive's gazes for a beat then spoke. "I know this will take a big effort, but I have confidence in all of you. Let's make this happen." Juan Carlos knew that establishing an ACO would require significant effort, but he was determined to succeed, confident that value-based healthcare was the future of healthcare.

Project Assignments

Managing Interpersonal Communications

1. Write a 5-minute speech for Juan Carlos Hernández that is designed to gain commitment from his team. Use the structure of a pitch-style presentation described in Table 3.7.

Human Resources Management

2. Develop a position description for the top health services management executive of the ACO.

3. Develop a position description for a new position within the ACO, called a performance coordinator, who is responsible for nonclinical coordination activities across the care continuum.

Organizational Design

4. Create an organizational chart for an ACO-specific unit that includes the top executive of the unit and the health services management and clinical team that will report to them. Be sure to include the population health management functions described by Juan Carlos in the case scenario and Chapter 6.

Healthcare Governance

5. Write a brief one-page organizational charter document (less than 500 words) that describes the membership and governance of HCOs belonging to the Sacred Heart Hospital ACO. Define the number of board seats, who would be eligible for membership, and at least five (5) committees. Each of the partner HCO should hold at least one position on the board. Describe how the organizations that partner to form an ACO will improve coordination of patient care.

Performance Management

6. Define at least two organizational performance measures for at least four (4) balanced scorecard perspectives (e.g., financial, patient perspective, learning and growth, and internal business processes).

Healthcare Quality Management

7. Using the flow chart methodology described in Chapter 12, create a swim lane diagram illustrating the coordination of patient care between the following health care settings: inpatient, skilled nursing facility, primary care physician, home care, and therapy.

Project Management

8. Create a project plan for the development of an ACO board of directors from inception to first board meeting. First, create a work breakdown structure (WBS) illustrating the phases of the project, such as bylaws development and meeting logistics.

Healthcare Financial Management

9. Write a brief document (less than 500 words) intended for the Sacred Heart Hospital board of directors that compares and contrasts the traditional health services financing models of inpatient and outpatient services with the value-based financing models associated with Medicare Shared Savings Program. Address issues such as advanced payment models, revenue cycle, capitation, and quality of care benchmarks.

Reference

Lewis, C., Abrams, M. K. Seervai, S., Horstman, C., & Blumenthal, D. (2022, April 28). *The impact of the payment and delivery system reforms of the affordable care act*. The Commonwealth Fund. https://www.commonwealthfund.org/publications/2022/apr/impact-payment-and-delivery-system-reforms-affordable-care-act

9. HOME HEALTH BUSINESS PLAN

Competencies

- Build effective collaborations across the continuum of care.
- Develop business plans that align with organizational strategy.
- Conduct internal and external assessments to determine strategic opportunities.
- Formulate strategic plans to maximize market opportunities.
- Assess strategic alternatives using evidence.
- Allocate resources to improve the long-term viability of the organization.

- Manage hiring processes including recruitment, screening, selection, and onboarding.
- Connect organizational goals to individual performance.
- Write credible business communications, including emails and reports.
- Deliver verbal presentations with confidence.

Introduction

Health systems develop new strategic business units to provide distinct services. Strategic planning at the business level must align with and contribute value to the corporate strategy for new businesses or services to obtain funding from corporate executives. Health services managers develop a written business plan that explains the merits of a particular opportunity and a pitch that persuasively argues for an investment in a new business.

Scenario

Cremont is a growing city that serves as the metropolitan hub for over 2.5 million people in the region. The board of directors and CEO seek to transform Cremont Health System (CHS) into a large integrated delivery system. The strategy is to build or buy many different related businesses that coordinate care across the continuum of care. With this approach, CHS can respond to competition from other health systems in the region.

CHS is considering developing a new home health care business named Cremont Home Health. The demand for home healthcare services is rapidly increasing due to several factors, including an aging population, a rise in chronic diseases, the decreasing payment rates for hospital-based care, and patient preference of convenience and familiarity of home care. In addition, new technologies have enabled hospital-at-home services that feature real-time monitoring of vital signs, regular remote consultations, medication adherence tracking, and remote patient education (Wallis et al., 2024). Hospital-at-home programs provide acute-level medical care to patients in their homes, which can be a viable alternative to inpatient care for certain conditions and treatments. The Cremont regional area home health care market is estimated to gross $5 million in revenue annually.

CHS sees home health as an opportunity to enhance the well-being of patients, especially for elderly individuals with chronic conditions recovering from surgeries or hospitalizations, by providing care in their homes. Cremont Home Health anticipates offering a range of services, including skilled nursing care; rehabilitation therapies; medication management; chronic disease management; palliative and hospice care; personal care assistance; and telehealth solutions that enable remote monitoring, consultations, and medication management. While CHS does not yet have experience in home care, there is an opportunity to develop more specialized care programs following inpatient discharges and to utilize advanced technology for remote patient monitoring and communication. These programs align with the shift toward value-based contracts that require high-quality care at reduced costs.

Three competitors currently operate in the region with similar market shares. These main competitors are ProCerta Home Health Services with 32% market share, Health Plus Home Care with 30% market share, and Caring Touch Home Health with 28% market share. No other health system owns a home healthcare operation, although there are five other small competitors that each have a 2% share of the market. None of these competitors offer strong specialized care and disease management programs. The following analyses were conducted on the three main home health competitors:

- ProCerta Home Health Services has earned a strong brand reputation for quality care. ProCerta offers a comprehensive range of services, including skilled nursing, rehabilitation, and specialized care programs. They currently utilize somewhat limited technologies for remote patient monitoring and telehealth consultations. However, ProCerta also has limited geographic coverage and exclusively covers the city of Cremont. ProCerta charges higher prices to commercial insurance companies compared to some competitors. According to research, they have relatively slower response time in service initiation and frequently change the nurses assigned to patients, which can cause poor care quality and patient satisfaction.
- Health Plus Home Care has extensive experience in the home healthcare industry with strong relationships with insurance providers and a wide coverage network. Health Plus places an emphasis on cultural sensitivity and multilingual staff to cater to diverse populations. However, they do not offer specialized healthcare services, such as pediatric home care for children with special needs and adults with neurodegenerative diseases, nor do they emphasize telehealth solutions. They have relatively low brand awareness outside Cremont.
- Caring Touch Home Health has a robust presence in Cremont and rural areas of the region with a diverse range of services, including skilled nursing, therapy, and nonmedical support. Their focus is on personalized care with individualized treatment plans and proactive engagement with patients' families and caregivers. However, they conduct very limited marketing efforts, resulting in lower market visibility. Most notably, they have inadequate integration of technology for efficient operations and service delivery. They also face challenges with expansion due to their decentralized operations featuring small, somewhat independent district offices.

Additionally, the following facts are relevant to developing and implementing Cremont Home Health:

- There are three health systems in the Cremont regional area: Cremont Health System (four hospitals and a multispecialty physician group), CareBridge Health Services (one hospital in Cremont and eight more in the state), and Eastman Medical Center (one hospital). None of these health systems currently owns a home health operation. Increased competition in home health care could lead to price pressures, reduced market share, and the need for differentiation strategies.
- Labor shortages of skilled healthcare professionals, such as nurses and aides, could limit the ability to provide services, increase labor costs, and affect the quality of care. Recruiting and training skilled healthcare professionals, including RNs, LPNs, and home health aides, will be very important to the home healthcare business. CHS has been more successful than competitors in recruiting and retention because the health system can offer career progression for registered nurses, licensed practical nurses, and home health aides who start in home health settings and progress into higher paid hospital-based positions.
- Inpatient discharges to home will be very important to the success of technology-enabled home care. CHS can act as the primary referral source for patients after they are discharged from the hospital. The CHS electronic health records (EHR) system must be able to assist clinical communications across the continuum of care, and CHS has had success with enhancing EHR in the past.
- There are six commercial health insurance companies in the market, none of which with dominant market power. Medicare is the largest payer type in home health. Shifts in payer mix, such as a decrease in private insurance reimbursements and an increase in lower paying government programs, can impact the financial stability of home health agencies.
- Medicare Certification is required to bill the Medicare program. Medicaid Provider Enrollment is also required to care for Medicaid beneficiaries. Changes in payment rates from Medicare and Medicaid can significantly impact the financial viability of home health agencies.
- The state Agency for Healthcare Regulation (AHR) requires a home health agency license. AHR also requires a nursing registry license to operate as a nursing registry, which allows nurses or certified nursing assistants to provide care. Changes in regulatory frameworks, such as new documentation standards or increased oversight, can increase administrative burdens and compliance costs, potentially impacting profitability.

- Connecting EHRs to remote monitoring technology solutions represents an opportunity to streamline operations and improve patient outcomes. Integrating these technologies into the EHR system requires investment capital.
- CHS has the financial assets to invest in new business ventures. Measures of liquidity (e.g., current ratio) and capital structure (e.g., debt-to-capitalization ratio) are strong.
- CHS has an extensive network of physicians and other healthcare providers who can refer patients to Cremont Home Health. With previous businesses, CHS has experienced success with clinician marketing campaigns, including relationship building by physician relations/marketing manager, to build strong referral networks. Successful marketing tactics include educational workshops and social media campaigns.
- There are a variety of options for creating a management team and staffing clinicians. Other home health businesses in the United States employ an executive director, director of nursing, clinical supervisor, human resources manager, and physician relations/marketing manager. Some larger home health businesses hire operating managers. Some potential clinical staff include home health aides, LPNs, and RNs. CHS does not currently employ executives with home care experience.
- The business requires $100,000 in initial investment to begin operations, including certain technology integration and regulatory approval tasks. The salaries and benefits in Year 1 are expected to be $480,000 per year for staff with another $100,000 in operating expenses, plus variable clinician costs. Annual revenues are estimated to be $300,000 in Year 1 and $1.2 million in Year 5. According to the CHS CFO, the break-even point must be less than 6 years.
- According to CHS executives, the priority performance metrics to track should include market share, profit margin, and proportion of CHS discharges referred to home care.

Project Assignments

Healthcare Strategy and Marketing

1. Act as an analyst for CHS and conduct the following strategic analyses for Cremont Home Health:
    a. Define the strategic direction, including the mission, vision, and values.
    b. Conduct a SWOT (**S**trengths, **W**eaknesses, **O**pportunities, and **T**hreats) analysis for Cremont Home Health and the Cremont regional area.
    c. Identify at least two (2) core competencies that set Cremont Home Health apart from competitors in the marketplace. Be sure that the core competencies are sustainable over a long period of time, valuable to the customer, uncommon among competitors, and difficult to acquire or develop by competitors.
    d. Explain Cremont Home Health's potential competitive advantage, if any.
    e. Conduct a Porter's Five Forces analysis for the Cremont regional area home health market (Porter, 2008). For the overall competitive rivalry of the market, include a Herfindahl–Hirschman Index (HHI) calculation.
    f. Conduct a competitor analysis of the Cremont area home health market.
    g. Describe the strategic and operational support that Cremont Home Health can expect from the CHS corporate headquarters.
2. Write a business plan for Cremont Home Health. Include the following components in the business plan, as described in Chapter 8: executive summary, table of contents, service or business overview, staffing, market analysis, competitor analysis, promotional

tactics, operational logistics, relevant legal and regulatory issues, and performance monitoring. Also include a brief forecast of the financial performance (pro forma) over a 5-year period with a break-even point calculation.

Human Resources Management

3. Develop a position description for the top health services management executive of Cremont Home Health.

Performance Management

4. Using the balanced scorecard approach presented in Chapter 11, create at least four strategic perspectives for Cremont Home Health, as demonstrated in Tables 11.1 to 11.4. For each strategic perspective, devise at least two strategic objectives and the corresponding measures, operationalized definitions, and targets, as described in Table 11.8.

Managing Interpersonal Communications

5. Write a 5-minute pitch to gain approval from the Cremont Health System executives for the Cremont Home Health business plan. See the description of a pitch-style presentation in Chapter 3, Table 3.6.

References

Porter, M. E. (2008). *Competitive advantage: Creating and sustaining superior performance* (2nd ed.). Free Press.

Wallis, J. A., Shepperd, S., Makela, P., Han, J. X., Tripp, E. M., Gearon, E., Disher, G., Buchbinder, R., & O'Connor, D. (2024). Factors influencing the implementation of early discharge hospital at home and admission avoidance hospital at home: A qualitative evidence synthesis. *Cochrane Database of Systematic Reviews, 3*(3), CD014765. https://doi.org/10.1002/14651858.CD014765.pub2

10. PERFORMANCE REVIEW GONE WRONG

Competencies

- Solve problems through critical thinking and analysis of the best available evidence.
- Apply evidence-based management skills to health services management challenges.
- Manage career and professional self-development.
- Comply with human resources laws and regulations.
- Design staff training, development, and engagement programs.
- Create evaluations systems to assess employee performance.

Introduction

A performance evaluation is a formal assessment of an employee's job performance. Most health services managers deliver written and verbal performance evaluations at least once a year, although more frequent conversations are recommended (Murphy, 2020). Fair performance reviews provide specific, measurable, and realistic standards in writing and in advance. When performance ratings are not tied to objective measures related to their position responsibilities, it is called a criterion deficiency. Effective individual performance reviews are based on self-defined goals that are relevant to their job responsibilities (Doheny, 2021).

Scenario

Emily committed herself wholeheartedly to her role at Havenford Clinic, a large multisite primary care physician practice. She worked tirelessly, despite the clinic's challenges, to make sure the patients and clinicians had everything they needed. One morning, Emily received an email notification from the CEO's office, summoning her to an unscheduled performance review. The CEO, Mr. Jerry Reynolds, a stoic figure exuding an aura of authority, sat behind his oak desk at headquarters. Without glancing up, he motioned for Emily to take a seat.

"Emily," he said, his voice carrying a blend of gravity and detachment, "Let's discuss your recent performance. After a thorough review of your recent 360-degree performance evaluation results, I must confess, the feedback was . . . less than satisfactory."

Emily's heart sank. Less than satisfactory? She struggled to understand the feedback. "Is there something specific I need to address?" Emily responded.

Mr. Reynolds, finally raising his eyes, fixed Emily with an intense stare. "Emily, your focus on efficiency and effectiveness has been fine. However, there have been instances of not getting along with other staff members. Frankly, people question your attitude. I've heard from many employees."

Emily believed that her dedication would be enough to earn a glowing review. "Is there documentation on feedback people gave me in the 360-degree review?" Emily asked.

Mr. Reynolds smiled thinly then said, "Emily, your commitment is commendable, but our clinic is like a family, and we cannot afford for our clinic managers to be disagreeable. If you do not show a marked improvement, we may reconsider your place here."

As Emily left the CEO's office that day, her mind swirled with emotions. As Emily left the CEO's office, she recognized that she might be fired. She still had a job at Havenford Clinic today, but it was only a matter of time before she was looking for a new job.

Project Assignments

Problem-Solving and Evidence-Based Management

1. Based on an analysis of the case scenario using problem-solving methods described in Chapter 2, make recommendations to Havenford Clinic to improve performance reviews. First, start by highlighting or underlining all of the different problems in the scenario. Problems are issues that get in the way of Havenford Clinic achieving their organizational objectives. Then, assign each of the identified problems into conceptually similar problem areas. Finally, write a problem statement for each group of problems. The format for simple problem statements is as follows: "How can [the organization] [action verb] given that/in light of [object of problem-solving effort]?" Appendix 1 lists examples of health services management problems.
    a. Define the problem(s).
    b. Identify potential solutions to the defined problem(s). Describe the evidence supporting the solutions using an evidence-based management approach.

Managing Interpersonal Communications

2. Assume Emily has not yet been terminated from her position as clinic manager. Write a professional email, using the elements described in Chapter 3, advising Emily on what she should do next.

3. Assume Emily was terminated from her clinic manager job. Being fired can be a challenging and emotionally charged experience. Write a professional email, using the elements described in Chapter 3, advising Emily on what she should do next.

Human Resources Management

4. Write a brief report (less than 500 words) describing the mistakes that Mr. Reynolds made in this performance review. Was Emily's performance review fair? What processes would you recommend to Mr. Reynolds to make to improve Havenford Clinic's performance reviews? Make recommendations for improvement.

5. Write a synopsis (less than 500 words) for a performance review training program using best practices from management scholarship. Cite at least three (3) journal articles within the last 5 years.

Performance Management

6. Define at least one performance measure for clinic manager at Havenford Clinic for each of the following perspectives:
   a. patient experience
   b. financial
   c. internal business processes
   d. learning and innovation
   e. clinical care

References

Doheny, K. (2021, January 12). *Annual performance review bows out*. SHRM. https://www.shrm.org/resourcesandtools/hr-topics/people-managers/pages/ditching-the-annual-performance-review-.aspx

Murphy, K. R. (2020). Performance evaluation will not die, but it should. *Human Resource Management Journal, 30*(1), 13–31. https://doi.org/10.1111/1748-8583.12259

APPENDIX 1

EXAMPLES OF HEALTH SERVICES MANAGEMENT PROBLEMS

Problems are neither positive nor negative, only a difference between a current situation and a future desired state. In other words, the existence of a problem just means that something needs to change. Problems can be in-the-moment crises, threats to success, improvements in performance, or forward-looking opportunities (Rakich & Krigline, 1996). While no classification of problems exists in health services management literature, the following categories represent common problems faced by health services managers in health care organizations (HCOs): obstacles, challenges, complications, opportunities, issues, concerns, and predicaments.

MANAGEMENT CONTROL AND MONITORING

Management control and monitoring are the processes and systems created by health services managers to ensure that operations are working as intended. These topics are presented in more detail in Chapter 7, "Healthcare Governance"; Chapter 9, "Human Resource Management"; Chapter 11, "Performance Management"; Chapter 12, "Healthcare Quality Management"; and Chapter 14, "Healthcare Financial Management." Table A1.1 lists examples of problem statements related to management control and monitoring.

TABLE A1.1 Problem Statements Related to Management Control and Monitoring

TYPE	EXAMPLE PROBLEM STATEMENT
COST CONTROL	How can supply costs be controlled given that vendor management system encourages unfavorable contracts, physicians demand latest technologies, and a small number of suppliers dominate certain product categories?
EMPLOYEE PERFORMANCE	How can the HCO improve employee performance given ambiguous goal setting, ineffective appraisal processes, and lack of professional accountability?
STAFF SCHEDULING	How can the HCO prevent understaffing and overstaffing of nurses given that future patient volumes are unknown, unions stipulate stringent rules, and nurses prefer predictable working hours?
GOVERNANCE	How can the HCO empower nurses to contribute to decision-making despite that nurses do not have legal authority in the governance structure?

(continued)

TABLE A1.1 Problem Statements Related to Management Control and Monitoring (*continued*)

TYPE	EXAMPLE PROBLEM STATEMENT
ENERGY CONSUMPTION	How can the HCO reduce energy consumption in order to reduce HCO environmental impact and improve financial stability given that HVAC systems are outdated, medical waste management processes are not maximized, and third-party electricity prices are rising rapidly?
BUDGETING	How can the HCO make expense reporting more efficient in light of reconciliation challenges, difficulties generating reports for budgeting, and manual processes that lead to errors?
PROJECT PRIORITIZATION	How can the HCO prioritize technology development project given competing priorities from various business units, undetermined project value, and poorly described business objectives?
QUALITY MEASUREMENT	How can the HCO increase efficiency of quality measurement reporting given that reporting requirements are complex, data exists in multiple data sources, and staff has little expertise in quality measurement?

HCO, health care organization; HVAC, Heating, Ventilation, and Air Conditioning.

GROWTH OPPORTUNITIES

Successful health services managers can proactively identify and create opportunities for growth, sustainability, and profitability. Growth involves implementing initiatives and forging partnerships that drive revenue generation, enhance market share, and improve overall competitive positioning. These topics are presented in more detail in Chapter 8, "Healthcare Strategy and

TABLE A1.2 Problem Statements Related to Growth Opportunities in HCOs

TYPE	EXAMPLE PROBLEM STATEMENT
SERVICE LINE EXPANSION	How can the HCO create new service lines to meet the evolving healthcare needs of the community given that areas of growth potential are unknown, the clinical staffing requirements are unknown, and the revenue and expense projections are unknown?
MERGERS AND ACQUISITIONS	How can the HCOs implement the merger given differing management decision-making approaches, organizational structure duplications, challenges with employee morale related to job security, role changes, cultural change, and employee mistrust?
MARKETING AND ADVERTISING	How can the HCO increase patient referrals by community physicians given that most physicians do not have professional relationships with colleagues or specialists and have concerns regarding the quality of care, patient safety, or the overall patient experience at the HCO?
PARTNERSHIPS AND AFFILIATIONS	How can the HCO align financial goals with the affiliate given the differences in organizational cultures, values, and decision-making approaches?
FACILITY EXPANSION AND RENOVATION	How can the HCO expand the emergency department in light of challenges with significant budget constraints, strict regulations, building codes, safety standards, and concerns about environmental impact?

HCO, health care organization.

Marketing" and Chapter 10, "Organizational Design." Table A1.2 lists examples of problem statements related to growth opportunities in HCOs.

ADAPTATION

Health services managers seek to adapt to adversity within the healthcare organization (HCO) and to threats from the external healthcare environment. While failing to adapt could bring negative consequences to HCOs, health services managers who reframe threats as favorable opportunities for organizational learning are more likely to succeed in addressing such problems creatively (Meyers, 1982). Topics related to adaptation to threats and adversity are presented in more detail in Chapter 6, "Population Health and Community Collaboration"; Chapter 8, "Healthcare Strategy and Marketing"; and Chapter 10, "Organizational Design." Table A1.3 lists examples of problem statements related to adaptation.

RESOURCE ALLOCATION

Resource allocation involves distributing and assigning resources, including money, personnel, equipment, and facilities, to optimize health services delivery and meet the needs of patients. These topics are presented in more detail in Chapter 11, "Performance Management"; Chapter 13, "Project Management"; and Chapter 14, "Healthcare Financial Management." Table A1.4 lists examples of problem statements related to health services resources allocation.

TABLE A1.3 Problem Statements Related to Adaptation

TYPE	EXAMPLE PROBLEM STATEMENT
COMPETITIVE REACTION	What actions should the HCO take to respond to a new competitor in the market, considering that the current services are not differentiated, physician referrals may decrease, and pricing negotiations with payers may evolve?
VALUE-BASED CARE MODELS	How can the HCO build new competencies in value-based care given that care coordination systems are not defined and that analytics capabilities cannot support population health initiatives.
SERVICE MIX	How can the HCO increase service mix to meet the evolving needs of their patient population in light of limited access to capital, unclear patient preferences, and competing interests of the medical staff?
MARKET SHIFTS	How can the HCO make pricing information for medical services and procedures more transparent in response to a more cost-conscious health care consumer given that pricing structures are varied across payers, costs are not adequately allocated across services, and negotiated payment rates are usually confidential?
REGULATORY COMPLIANCE	How can the HCO respond to a new regulation given the lack of staff knowledge and changes in technology requirements?
MERGER, ACQUISITION, AFFILIATION, AND PARTNERSHIPS	How can the HCO restructure the organization following a merger in light of disruptions in decision-making processes and resistance from staff members and clinicians?

HCO, health care organization.

TABLE A1.4 Problem Statements Related to Health Services Resource Allocation

TYPE	EXAMPLE PROBLEM STATEMENT
INVESTMENT DECISIONS	How can the HCO optimize return on investment given that there are two different medical equipment purchase requests from service line leaders?
EMPLOYEE HIRING	How can the HCO optimize support services staffing given resource demands for transportation, environmental services, and dietary services are unknown?
INFORMATION TECHNOLOGY RESOURCES	How can the HCO allocate network resources given regulatory requirements for security and privacy of patient data, increasing volume of data transmission, and outdated technology infrastructure?
BED ALLOCATION AND CAPACITY PLANNING	How can the HCO meet patient demand and optimize bed occupancy given the fluctuating patient admissions, limited physical space, and inadequate physician staffing levels?
SUPPLIES AND EQUIPMENT INVENTORY MANAGEMENT	How can the HCO optimize the disposable supply inventory to meet the needs of various hospital departments given periods of high demand, supply shortages, or unexpected disruptions in the supply chain?

HCO, health care organization.

OPPORTUNITIES FOR IMPROVEMENT

Health services managers employ problem-solving approaches to proactively identify and capitalize on opportunities for improvement. Even when performance is deemed successful, health services managers seek out performance deficiencies and motivate change. These topics are

TABLE A1.5 Problem Statements Related to Opportunities for Improvement

TYPE	EXAMPLE PROBLEM STATEMENT
EMPLOYEE RETENTION	How can the HCO reduce employee dissatisfaction given irregular shift patterns, insufficient support for work-life balance, and disparities in salary structures?
PATIENT EXPERIENCE	How can the HCO improve patient experience scores given the poor communication between clinicians and patients, suboptimal cleanliness of facilities, and excessive noise levels during night?
REVENUE CYCLE	How can the HCO reduce reducing the risk of denied claims due to high proportion of inaccurate health service documentation, such as missing patient information and coding errors?
EQUIPMENT OPTIMIZATION	How can the HCO reduce machine downtime given issues with unexpected breakdowns, operational errors, and replacement part unavailability?
ORGANIZATIONAL CULTURE	How can the HCO improve employee engagement levels despite fear of speaking up; inadequate communication channels for employee feedback; and workplace bullying, incivility, and interpersonal conflicts?

HCO, health care organization.

TABLE A1.6 Problem Statements Related to Emergency Preparedness and Response

TYPE	EXAMPLE PROBLEM STATEMENT
CRITICAL INFRASTRUCTURE DISRUPTIONS	How can the HCO plan to respond to ransomware attacks given that operational contingencies are unknown, legal options are unidentified, and technical remediations are undefined?
NATURAL DISASTERS	How can the HCO ensure that the medical supply chain is functional during a natural disaster given that that medical supply vendors may be unable to deliver key products or services and alternate vendors are unknown?
CHEMICAL AND BIOLOGICAL THREATS	How can the HCO react to chemical spills, hazardous material exposures, or biological threats given that decontamination procedures for both affected individuals and equipment are unknown and the laws and regulations for disposal of hazardous materials and waste are unidentified?
WORKPLACE VIOLENCE	How can the HCO prevent workplace violence in light of understaffing of security personnel, ineffective communication with law enforcement, and limited access controls?
PANDEMICS AND DISEASE OUTBREAKS	How can the HCO acquire personal protective equipment during disease outbreak in light of limited supplies during patient volume surges?
MASS CASUALTY INCIDENTS	How can the HCO respond to a sudden influx of patients with a wide range of injuries and medical needs due to terrorist attacks, transportation accidents, or industrial accidents given that staff lack knowledge of mass casualty triage procedures, patient flow management, and effective communication during high-stress situations?

HCO, health care organization.

presented in more detail in Chapter 11, "Performance Management"; Chapter 12, "Healthcare Quality Management"; and Chapter 14, "Healthcare Financial Management." Table A1.5 lists examples of problem statements related to identifying and capitalizing on opportunities for improvement.

EMERGENCY PREPAREDNESS AND RESPONSE

Health services managers plan for operational continuity during emergencies by anticipating potential disasters and arranging for access to critical resources. Table A1.6 lists examples of problem statements related to emergency preparedness and response.

RELIABLE PATIENT CARE PROCESSES

Broken processes can cause severe patient harm. When medical care endangers patients, health services managers need to marshal resources to address the root causes of the problems. Patient safety and reliable processes are presented in more detail in Chapter 10, "Organizational Design"; Chapter 11, "Performance Management"; and Chapter 12, "Healthcare Quality Management." Table A1.7 lists examples of problem statements related to creating reliable patient care processes.

TABLE A1.7 Problem Statements Related to Creating Reliable Patient Care Processes

TYPE	EXAMPLE PROBLEM STATEMENT
CARE COORDINATION	How can the HCO improve care transitions given challenges in coordinating community-based resources and lack of facility capacity in long-term care?
PATIENT WAIT TIMES	How can the HCO decrease patient wait times given that workflows are not defined, patient scheduling is ineffective, and waste in the patient throughput process exists?
PATIENT SAFETY	How can the HCO prevent falls in assisted living facilities given environmental hazards, including poor lighting, slippery floors, uneven surfaces, cluttered walkways, and inadequate handrails?
PATIENT NO-SHOWS	How can the HCO reduce patient no-shows in light of transportation insecurities, call center wait times, and lack of patient accountability?
PATIENT DISCHARGES	How can the HCO reduce patient discharge delays when there are difficulties in arranging appropriate post-discharge care, delays in coordinating the delivery of durable medical equipment, and challenges related to patient's living situations?
PATIENT READMISSIONS	How can the HCO reduce patient readmissions given delayed or missed follow-up appointments with physician; social isolation; and social factors, such as housing instability, lack of access to healthy food, limited social support, and financial constraints?

HCO, health care organization.

INNOVATION

Healthcare **innovation** refers to the development and implementation of new ideas, technologies, processes, and strategies aimed at improving the delivery, accessibility, affordability, and effectiveness of health services. These topics are presented in more detail in Chapter 4, "Leadership and Change Management"; Chapter 6, "Population Health and Community Collaboration"; Chapter 9, "Human Resource Management"; and Chapter 10, "Organizational Design." Table A1.8 lists examples of problem statements related to innovations in HCOs.

TABLE A1.8 Problem Statements Related to Innovations in HCOs

TYPE	EXAMPLE PROBLEM STATEMENT
ACCESSIBILITY OF CARE	How can the HCO empower patients to monitor their health given the lack of educational resources and difficulties communicating with clinicians?
AFFORDABILITY OF CARE	How can the HCO reduce costs for bundled orthopedic procedures in light of undefined scope of the services, lack of understanding of the costs of services and supplies, and financial risks associated with unexpected complications during the episode of care?
DELIVERY OF CARE	How can the HCO improve care coordination given different service locations, various electronic health record systems, and complex financing schemes that encourage fragmented clinician services?
ENVIRONMENTAL SUSTAINABILITY	How can the HCO reduce carbon emissions given the lack of awareness about sustainable practices among staff and low-efficiency lighting and HVAC systems?
POPULATION HEALTH MANAGEMENT	How can the HCO reduce costs given the inability to predict patient risk levels or develop targeted interventions for high-risk and at-risk patient populations?

HCO, health care organization.

Reference

Rakich, J. S., & Krigline, A. B. (1996). Problem solving in health services organizations. *Hospital Topics*, 74(2), 21–27. https://doi.org/10.1080/00185868.1996.11736053

APPENDIX 2

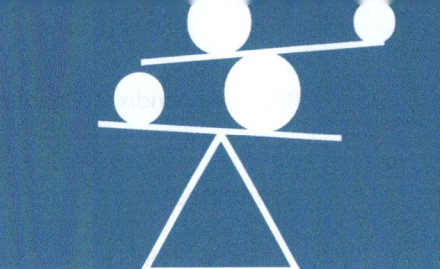

CHAPTER TO CASE SCENARIOS AND PROJECTS CROSSWALK

	CHAPTER	CASE SCENARIO AND PROJECT
1	Role of the Health Services Manager	1. Conflict on the Interprofessional Team; 2. The Diversity, Equity, and Inclusion Initiative at the Health Care Organization; 3. The Triple Bottom Line
2	Problem-Solving and Evidence-Based Management	1. Conflict on the Interprofessional Team; 2. The Diversity, Equity, and Inclusion Initiative at the Health Care Organization; 5. Resisting Private Equity Investors; 10. Performance Review Gone Wrong
3	Managing Interpersonal Communications	1. Conflict on the Interprofessional Team; 2. The Diversity, Equity, and Inclusion Initiative at the Health Care Organization; 3. The Triple Bottom Line; 4. The Dark-Side Leader; 6. Medical Model Versus Population Health Model; 7. Assessing Community Health Needs; 8. Design an Accountable Care Organization; 9. Home Health Business Plan; 10. Performance Review Gone Wrong
4	Leadership and Change Management	1. Conflict on the Interprofessional Team; 2. The Diversity, Equity, and Inclusion Initiative at the Health Care Organization; 3. The Triple Bottom Line; 4. The Dark-Side Leader
5	Professionalism and Ethics	3. The Triple Bottom Line; 7. Assessing Community Health Needs
6	Population Health and Community Collaboration	3. The Triple Bottom Line; 6. Medical Model Versus Population Health Model; 7. Assessing Community Health Needs
7	Healthcare Governance	3. The Triple Bottom Line; 5. Resisting Private Equity Investors; 8. Design an Accountable Care Organization
8	Healthcare Strategy and Marketing	9. Home Health Business Plan
9	Human Resource Management	2. The Diversity, Equity, and Inclusion Initiative at the Health Care Organization; 8. Design an Accountable Care Organization; 9. Home Health Business Plan; 10. Performance Review Gone Wrong
10	Organizational Design	4. The Dark-Side Leader; 5. Resisting Private Equity Investors; 8. Design an Accountable Care Organization

(continued)

(continued)

	CHAPTER	CASE SCENARIO AND PROJECT
11	Performance Management	2. The Diversity, Equity, and Inclusion Initiative at the Health Care Organization; 3. The Triple Bottom Line; 6. Medical Model Versus Population Health Model; 8. Design an Accountable Care Organization; 9. Home Health Business Plan; 10. Performance Review Gone Wrong
12	Healthcare Quality Management	3. The Triple Bottom Line; 6. Medical Model Versus Population Health Model; 8. Design an Accountable Care Organization
13	Project Management	2. The Diversity, Equity, and Inclusion Initiative at the Health Care Organization; 8. Design an Accountable Care Organization
14	Healthcare Financial Management	3. The Triple Bottom Line; 8. Design an Accountable Care Organization

APPENDIX 3

CHAPTER TO THE AMERICAN COLLEGE OF HEALTHCARE EXECUTIVES KNOWLEDGE CROSSWALK

CHAPTER		ACHE KNOWLEDGE
1	Role of the Health Services Manager	Management functions (e.g., planning, organizing, directing, controlling, and evaluating)
		Healthcare and medical terminology
		Healthcare trends
		Levels of healthcare along the continuum of care (e.g., extended care, acute hospital care, ambulatory care, post-acute care)
		Levels of service from a business perspective (e.g., home health, inpatient, outpatient)
		The types of healthcare organizations (e.g., nonprofit, for-profit, federal, public health)
		Ancillary services (e.g., laboratory and imaging services, therapies)
		Support services (e.g., environment of care, plant operations, materials management, hospitality services)
		Potential impacts and consequences of business decision-making on operations, healthcare, human resources, community, and quality of care
2	Problem-Solving and Evidence-Based Management	Evidence-based management practice
		Potential impacts and consequences of financial decision-making on operations, healthcare, human resources, and quality of care
		The potential impact of laws and regulations on operational, financial, quality of care, health resources, and human resources decisions
		Role and function of information technology in business operations (e.g., business intelligence systems)
		Technology trends and clinical applications in a healthcare organization
		Health informatics needed for operational decisions (e.g., data and equipment interoperability standards support)
		Factors that influence selection, acquisition, and maintenance of IT systems (e.g., upgrades and conversions, technology lifecycles)
		Healthcare analytics and clinical informatics applications
3	Managing Interpersonal Communications	Collaborative techniques for engaging and working with clinicians and external stakeholders (e.g., policy makers, payers, community leaders)
		Techniques involved in negotiating contracts or services (e.g., compromise, persuasion) and relevant factors (e.g., utilization review, models)

(continued)

(continued)

CHAPTER		ACHE KNOWLEDGE
4	Leadership and Change Management	Leadership and communication styles and how and in what situations they apply
		Team-building techniques (e.g., communication, use of practical assessment or training tools)
		Change management principles
		Organizational development resources
		Employee motivation and development principles and techniques
5	Professionalism and Ethics	Clinician roles and qualifying criteria (e.g., administrative versus clinical)
		The interrelationships among healthcare access, quality, cost, resource allocation, accountability, and the community
		Diversity, equity, inclusion and justice principles and their influence on team and organizational effectiveness
		Laws relating to confidentiality (e.g., FOIA, release of information)
		Healthcare compliance laws and regulations (e.g., antitrust, conflict of interest, EMTALA, Stark law, No Surprises Act)
		Medicare, Medicaid, and other third-party payment regulations
		Patients' rights laws and regulations (e.g., informed consent, HIPAA, advance directives, involuntary commitments)
		Basic business contracts, such as what constitutes a contractual commitment, and legal and financial implications (e.g., intentional damage to a person or business that causes economic harm)
		Technology policies and regulations (e.g., complying with HIPAA security requirements, complying with HITECH Act, promoting interoperability)
		Professional code of ethical behavior for ACHE
		Patients' rights and responsibilities (e.g., informed consent, withdrawal of care, advance directives)
		Ethics committee's roles, structure, and functions
		Cultural and spiritual diversity of patients and staff as they relate to healthcare needs
		Conflict-of-interest issues and solutions as defined by laws, organizational bylaws, and policies and procedures
		The consequences of unethical actions
		Ethical implications of human-subject research
		Other professional norms and standards of behaviors as defined by professions (e.g., AHA standards/guidelines, physicians' oaths, and other professional pledges)
		Creating an ethical culture in an organization
		ACHE's statement on diversity

(continued)

(continued)

CHAPTER		ACHE KNOWLEDGE
6	Population Health and Community Collaboration	The interdependency of integration within and competition among healthcare sectors including partnerships with academic and social care institutions
		Population health concepts (e.g., patient segmentation, risk-based contracting)
		Social determinants of health (e.g., housing, food insecurity)
		Preventative medicine concepts (e.g., community outreach, wellness initiatives, retail health)
		Emergency preparedness (e.g., contingency planning, emergency response as defined in NIMS)
		The different requirements for nonprofit and for-profit healthcare organizations (e.g., community health needs assessment for nonprofit organizations)
		Utilization review/case management systems
		The impact the socioeconomic environment has on the functions of the organization
		Information systems continuity (e.g., disaster planning, recovery, backup, security, sabotage, natural disasters)
		Public policy matters and legislative and advocacy processes
7	Healthcare Governance	Organizational systems theory and structuring (e.g., span of control, chain of command, interrelationships of organizational units)
		Governance theory (e.g., mission and values, relationships with board of directors, roles of governing board and management)
		Governance structure (e.g., bylaws, articles of incorporation) and operations (e.g., board member selection, education, orientation, and assessment)
		Medical staff structure and its relationship to governing bodies and facility operations (e.g., credentialing, privileging, and disciplinary process)
		The governing board's role (e.g., ultimate accountability, conflict of interest issues, fiduciary responsibility)
8	Healthcare Strategy and Marketing	How to prepare and justify a business model (e.g., make a business case for a new project to gain shareholder support)
		Legal implications for mergers and acquisitions
		The strategic planning process (e.g., scenario planning, forecasting, community needs assessment)
		Business planning processes, including development, implementation, and assessment (e.g., adding new services/ending existing services)
		Marketing principles and tools and how to interpret marketing data (e.g., market analysis, market research, sales, advertising)
		Principles of media relations, advertising, social media, and community relations

(continued)

(continued)

CHAPTER		ACHE KNOWLEDGE
9	Human Resource Management	Collective bargaining (e.g., management's rights during union organizing)
		Human resources laws and regulations (e.g., labor law, wage and hour, FMLA, FLSA, EEOC, ERISA, workers' compensation)
		Recruitment and retention approaches and techniques
		Staffing methodologies and productivity management (e.g., acuity-based staffing, flexible staffing, fixed staffing, capability, capacity, and upskilling)
		Performance management systems (e.g., performance-based evaluation, rewards systems, disciplinary policies and procedures)
		Compensation and benefits practices (e.g., merit-based, provider contracts)
		Employee safety, security, and health issues (e.g., OSHA, workplace violence, employee burnout)
		Conflict resolution and grievance procedures
		Potential impacts and consequences of human resources decision-making on operations, finances, healthcare, and quality of care
		Selection techniques (e.g., commonly available assessments and relative benefits)
		Labor relations practices and strategies
		Job design processes
		Succession planning models
		Mentorship and coaching practices
		Laws and regulations related to collective bargaining
10	Organizational Design	Different staff and functional perspectives in healthcare organizations (e.g., frame of reference, expectations, and responsibilities by discipline and role)
		Patient perspective (e.g., expectations, concerns, healthcare consumerism) and how it differs from the provider perspective
		Different care delivery models and system access points
		Types of healthcare network structures (e.g., clinically integrated network, independent practice association) and their impact on local decision-making
11	Performance Management	Fundamental productivity measures (e.g., hours per patient day, cost per patient day, units of service per labor hour)
		Supply chain systems, structures, and processes (e.g., monitoring the effectiveness of supply chain management and strategic decision-making)
		Employee satisfaction and engagement measurement and improvement techniques
		Inspection and accrediting standards, regulations, and organizations (e.g., OSHA, FDA, NRC, CDC, state and federal accreditation/licensure)
		Benchmarking principles and sources of best practices information (e.g., internal, state, and national standards)

(continued)

(continued)

CHAPTER		ACHE KNOWLEDGE
12	Healthcare Quality Management	The principles and methods of medical staff peer review
		Risk management principles and programs (e.g., insurance, education, safety, injury management, patient complaints, patient and staff security)
		Managerial performance and process improvement tools and techniques (e.g., PDSA cycle, Lean processing, Six Sigma)
		Clinical performance and process improvement tools and techniques (e.g., clinical pathways, evidence-based medicine, population health, pay for performance)
		Quality and performance measurement tools (e.g., patient satisfaction measurements such as HCAHPS, net promoter scores)
		Tools for improving patient safety (e.g., reducing avoidable errors, disclosure of errors)
		How quality impacts operations, staffing, and financing decisions
13	Project Management	Implementation planning (e.g., operational plan, management plan)
14	Healthcare Financial Management	Resource allocation methods (e.g., for addressing conflicts among departments or staff over scarce resources)
		Financial accounting principles needed to analyze and interpret financial reports (e.g., which ratios to look at given your current concerns)
		Operating budget principles (e.g., fixed versus flexible, zero based, variance analysis)
		Asset management (e.g., depreciation schedule)
		Financing, including funding sources, the process of obtaining credit and bond ratings, and issuing bonds
		Philanthropy and foundation work (e.g., as a source of funding for nonprofit organizations or to target for-profit organizations' activities)
		Revenue cycle (e.g., billing, coding, authorizations, collections)
		Capital budgeting principles (e.g., funding sources, long-term implications of capital planning, such as depreciation and value analysis)
		Reimbursement methodologies and their ramifications (e.g., managed care models, national/state programs, value based, fee for service)
		Financial controls (e.g., internal systems for accounts payable, checks and balances, auditing principles)
		Revenue generation (e.g., service line development, new ways to foster revenue, pricing strategies) and implications for payer mix

ACHE, American College of Healthcare Executives; ERISA, Employee Retirement Income Security Act; FDA, Food and Drug Administration; FLSA, Fair Labor Standards Act; FMLA, Family and Medical Leave Act; FOIA, Privacy Act, Freedom of Information Act; HCAHPS, Hospital Consumer Assessment of Healthcare Providers and Systems; HIPAA, Health Insurance Portability and Accountability Act; HITECH, Health Information Technology for Economic and Clinical Health; IT, information technology; NIMS, National Incident Management System; NRC, Nuclear Regulatory Commission; OSHA, Occupational Safety and Health. Administration; PDSA, **P**lan-**D**o-**S**tudy-**A**ct.

Reference

American College of Healthcare Executives. (2023, August 1). *Board of governors exam outline*. https://www.ache.org/fache/the-board-of-governors-exam/board-of-governors-exam-outline

APPENDIX 4

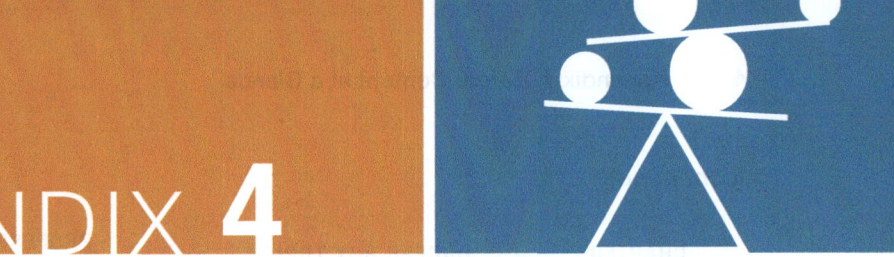

CAREER CONTENT AT A GLANCE

	CHAPTER	CAREER BOX TOPIC	PROFESSIONAL DEVELOPMENT AND REFLECTION TOPIC
1	Role of the Health Services Manager	Early Career Health Services Management; Specialist Versus Generalist Health Services Management; Late-Career Health Services Management	Career options along the continuum of care; conduct an informational interview with a health services manager
2	Problem-Solving and Evidence-Based Management	Cognitive Bias in Career Decision-Making; Analyzing Career Alternatives; Prototyping Career Options	Hypothesis-driven thinking to enhance decision-making; reframing negative career events
3	Managing Interpersonal Communications	Negotiating a Salary; Elevator Pitches; Tell a Story, Land the Job	Executive presence; anxiety associated with public speaking
4	Leadership and Change Management	Envisioning Career Success; Teamwork Promotes Leadership Skills; Ambition or Dissatisfaction	Career impacts of most developed emotional intelligence competencies and three least developed competencies; two versions of your career vision (medium and long term)
5	Professionalism and Ethics	Effort Counts Twice (work ethic); Save Up and Head Out (saving money); Practice Responding to Ethical Dilemmas	Résumé virtues and eulogy virtues; professional relationships: mentor, advisor, career sponsor, political guide, and career coach
6	Population Health and Community Collaboration	Career Assessments; Lifelong Learning; Superconnectors	Career assets; career preferences
7	Healthcare Governance	Managing Upward; Career Board of Directors	Career board members; managing upward
8	Healthcare Strategy and Marketing	Career Core Competencies; Four Ps of Job Searches; Cover Letter as a Press Release	Strengths for career success; organizations matching personal missions, visions, and values
9	Human Resource Management	Negotiating First Positions in Health Services Management; Excelling at Performance Self-Assessments	Performance self-evaluation; write résumé using keywords from the job description

(continued)

(continued)

	CHAPTER	CAREER BOX TOPIC	PROFESSIONAL DEVELOPMENT AND REFLECTION TOPIC
10	Organizational Design	Responsibility and Authority in Entry-Level Jobs; Staff and Line Positions	Level of authority and responsibility desired in the ideal job; staff position or line position?
11	Performance Management	Career Stakeholders; Career Balanced Scorecard; Receiving Performance Evaluations	Career stakeholders; career balanced scorecard
12	Healthcare Quality Management	Specialized Certifications; A Purposeful Career; The Career Ecosystem	Measures of career success; continuous career improvement
13	Project Management	Early-Career Project Management; Mid-Career Project Management; Late-Career Project Management	Planning the first 90 days of a new job; jobs with project management certifications requirements
14	Healthcare Financial Management	Professional Financial Help; Increase Income with a Raise; Control Expenses with a Budget	Savings provide flexibility to take career risks; assessing job opportunities using net present value

INDEX

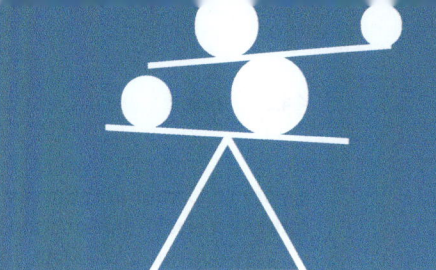

AAAHC. *See* Accreditation Association for Ambulatory Health Care
AAPL. *See* American Association for Physician Leadership
ABC. *See* activity-based costing
abusive behaviors of leaders, organizational checks on, 102–103
ACA. *See* Patient Protection and Affordable Care Act of 2010
academic medical centers, 12
access to care, 44, 124, 148, 203, 314, 315
accountability, 23, 98, 180, 252, 294–295, 304, 343, 345
   definition of, 274
   to stakeholders, 274–277
accountable care organizations (ACOs), 11, 154–155, 156–157, 159–160, 182–183, 264, 366, 415–417
accounts payable, 378
accounts receivable, 378
Accreditation Association for Ambulatory Health Care (AAAHC), 276
accreditors, 179, 186, 276
ACHE. *See* American College of Healthcare Executives
achievement orientation, 98, 273
ACO Realizing Equity, Access, and Community Health (REACH) Model, 366
ACOs. *See* accountable care organizations
acquisitions, 63, 205
active listening, 59
activity lists, 345, 346
activity sequencing, 345
activity-based costing (ABC), 373–375
acuity-based staffing, 235
acute care, 11, 418
ad hoc project teams, 258
ADA. *See* Americans with Disabilities Act
adaptability, 97
adaptability paradox, 97
adaptive strategies, 204
adhocracy, 258
adjusted patient days (APDs), 285
ADKAR® model, 104
administrative functions of human resources, 226
administrative services, 13, 307

advance directive, 134
advanced payment models, 153, 154, 366
advanced practice registered nurses (APRNs), 260
adverse events, 306, 312
advertising, 214
advising (professional development), 125
Aetna, 205
affect heuristic, 33
affiliations, organizational, 265
Age Discrimination in Employment Act of 1967, 234
agency problem, 173
agency theory, 173
agenda (meeting), 67, 68, 352
AHIMA. *See* American Health Information Management Association
AI. *See* artificial intelligence
Alabama Hospital Association, 160–161
algorithms, 46
all-hazards approach, 162–163
alliances, organizational, 265
ALOS. *See* average length of stay
alternative dispute resolution, 62
alternative payment models, 153
alternative solutions (problem-solving), 42–43
   analysis of, 46–47
   analytical plan, 45–46
   data sources, 47–48
   decision criteria, 43–45
   hypothesis-driven thinking, 43
   synthesizing findings, conclusions, and recommendations, 48–49
   transformation of decisions into action, 50
AMA. *See* American Medical Association
ambidextrous leadership, 95
ambition, 98
ambulatory care. *See* outpatient settings
ambulatory surgery centers (ASCs), 13, 208
American Association for Physician Leadership (AAPL), 120
American College of Healthcare Executives (ACHE), 11, 18, 66, 119, 128, 209, 435–439
   Board Certification in Healthcare Management, 120
   Board of Governors exam, 120

American Community Survey, 150
American Health Information Management
    Association (AHIMA), 120, 128
American Hospital Association, 214, 305
American Medical Association (AMA), 210,
    214, 365
American Nurses Credentialing Center, 276
American Organization for Nursing Leadership
    (AONL), 120
Americans with Disabilities Act (ADA), 234
analytical plan (problem-solving), 45–46
analytics, 46
anchor institutions, 161–162
anchor price, 63
anchoring bias, 33
ancillary services, 15, 16
Anti-Kickback Statute, 216
AONL. *See* American Organization for Nursing
    Leadership
APDs. *See* adjusted patient days
appearance, and executive presence, 65
approachability, 60–61, 118
APRNs. *See* advanced practice registered nurses
arbitration, 62, 240
Aristotle, 70, 71
artificial intelligence (AI), 46, 156, 163, 235–236,
    240, 284
ASCs. *See* ambulatory surgery centers
asset efficiency ratios, 382–383
asset management, 379
assets, 378–379
assisted living facilities, 14
audience of presentation, 72
authentic leadership, 93
authority, 101, 252–255
    of board of directors, 172, 173
    dyad model of, 257–258
autocratic leadership style, 94
autonomy, 134, 135, 180, 196, 257, 408
availability bias, 33
average age of plant, 382
average length of stay (ALOS), 290
average payment period, 381
awards, 276

bad debt, 364
balance sheet, 378–379
balanced scorecard, 277–278, 279, 280, 293, 412,
    417, 421
    career, 290
    home healthcare, 286–289
Banner Health, 263

bargaining power of buyers/suppliers, 201
bargaining unit, 240
barriers to entry, 201
BATNA (best alternative to a negotiated
    agreement), 63–64
BCG. *See* Boston Consulting Group Matrix
bed occupancy rate, 285
behavioral interviews, 229
Behavioral Risk Factor Surveillance Survey, 150,
    152
Belmont Report, 135
benchmarking, 277
beneficence, 135
benefits (renumeration), 231–232
best interests standard, 134
best practices, 277
bias. *See* cognitive bias
bidding, 340
big data, 46
Blue Cross Blue Shield of Alabama, 161
board meetings, 184–185, 403
board of directors, 185, 196, 253, 257, 280, 403
    career boards of directors, 177
    and CEO, relationship between, 172–173
    ethical principles of board practice, 178
    overseeing management and clinicians, 176
    and performance management, 274
    recruitment of new board members, 177–178
    representation of external stakeholders, 179
    role in healthcare financial management,
        362–363
    role in healthcare quality management, 305
    setting the strategic direction, 175
    social and environmental measures for
        monitoring, 178
    supporting, 174
bond ratings, 362
bonds, 362
Boston Consulting Group (BCG) Matrix,
    205–206
bottom line. *See* net profit
bottom-up budget, 349
boundary spanning, 7, 160
brainstorming, 43
branding, 214
breach of contract, 131
break-even analysis, 386
budget variance, 384
budget/budgeting, 335, 371
    capital, 384–385
    estimation, 347, 349
    as a management competency, 383
    operational, 383–384, 385

bundled payment, 155
bureaucracy, 255
    machine, 256
    professional, 255–257
burnout, 59
business case, 338
business plans, 207–208, 420–421
business reports, 76–77
business unit strategy, 207–208
business writing, 76
buy *vs.* build analysis, 340
bylaws
    healthcare governance, 184–185
    medical staff, 179, 305

CAHME. *See* Commission on Accreditation of Healthcare Management Education
CAHPS. *See* Consumer Assessment of Healthcare Providers and Systems
Cambridge Health Alliance, 156, 157
capacity, staffing based on, 235
capital, 362
capital allocation, 384, 386–388
capital budgeting, 384–385, 405
capital expenses, 371, 380, 382
capital structure, 382
capital structure ratios, 382
capitation payments, 366
CAPM®. *See* Certified Associate in Project Management
care transitions, 156–157, 265
career assessments, 148
career balanced scorecard, 290
career boards of directors, 177
career coaching, 125
career core competencies, 198
career ecosystem, 317
career ladder, 237
career planning, 123
career purpose, 310
career satisfaction
    and ambition, 98
    and superconnectors, 162
career stakeholders, 275
career success, 67, 96, 122, 290
    and ambition, 98
    barriers faced by women/minorities, 125–126
    of dark leaders, 100
    envisioning, 90
    and organizational awareness, 98
    and political skills, 102
    and work ethic, 122

career vision, 90
Caremark Rx, 205
Carilion Clinic, 104–105
cascading, 281
case consultations, 135
case mix, 201, 363
cash cows (BCG matrix), 205
cash flow statement, 379–380
casuistry, 129
catchment area, 147, 201, 210
cause-and-effect diagram. *See* fishbone diagram
CBA. *See* cost-benefit analysis
Center for Healthcare Leadership model, 18
center of excellence, 263
Centers for Medicare and Medicaid Services (CMS), 11, 159, 182, 183, 186, 215, 264, 275, 276, 308, 415
centralized organizations, 261–262, 265
CEO. *See* chief executive officer
CEO disease, 97
certificate of need, 201
certifications
    of HCOs, 276
    healthcare quality management, 304
    medical practice, 13
    project management, 340, 343
    specialized, 305
Certified Associate in Project Management (CAPM)®, 343
certified financial planners (CFP), 362
Certified Medical Practice Executive (CMPE), 13
Certified Professional in Health Care Risk Management (CPHRM), 305, 306
Certified Professional in Healthcare Quality (CPHQ), 304, 305
Certified Professional in Patient Safety (CPPS), 305
CFO. *See* chief financial officer
CFP. *See* certified financial planners
chain of command, 252, 253
change control, 351
change management, 399, 401, 404, 406, 409, 436, 439
    Kotter's 8 Steps of Change, 104–107
    leadership process, 103–104
charge capture, 368
charges of third-party payers, 364
charismatic leadership, 93
charity care, 369
charters, healthcare governance, 184–185, 417
ChatGPT, 163
check-in meetings, 291

chief executive officer (CEO), 23, 103, 126, 172–173, 174, 176, 253, 274, 317
chief financial officer (CFO), 253, 360, 375, 376, 387
chief medical officer, 179
chief of staff, 179
CHNAs. *See* community health needs assessments
Civil Rights Act of 1964, 234
claims (healthcare bills), 369
claims adjudication (healthcare bills), 369
Cleveland Clinic, 260
clinical coding, 368
clinical decision support systems, 47
clinical education, competency-based education in, 17–18
clinical ethics, 134–135
clinical laboratories, 16
clinical protocols, 251
clinical quality, 279, 283
clinical support services, 307
clinically integrated network, 11
clinicians, 2, 8, 18, 61, 119, 256, 260, 309
   board of directors overseeing, 176
   career ladder, 237
   health promotion by, 159
   marketing to, 216
   moral distress of, 130
   performance of, 274
   productivity, 284–285
   psychological safety of, 59
   role in healthcare governance, 175, 179
      medical practice and other governance structures, 181–183
      medical staff, 179–180
      shared governance councils, 180–181
   role in healthcare quality management, 305
   satisfaction, 44
   standard operating procedures for, 250
   and utilization management, 158
closed system, 7
CMPE. *See* Certified Medical Practice Executive
CMS. *See* Centers for Medicare and Medicaid Services
coaching, 99, 125, 238
codes of ethics, 128, 401
coercive power, 101
cognitive bias, 32–33, 43, 229
   in career decision-making, 34
   that negatively impact problem-solving, 33
co-insurance, 368
collaborative leadership, 92–93
collective bargaining, 240

college internships, 125
Commission on Accreditation of Healthcare Management Education (CAHME), 119, 304
common cause variation, 322
Common Rule, 135
communication adaptability, 58
communication plan (project management), 351
communications. *See* interpersonal communications
communitarianism, 129
community
   contribution to, 123–124
   engagement, 160
   health needs, 44
      assessing, 412–415
   health status, 148–149
   representation, in healthcare governance, 184
   stakeholders, 146–147
community assets, 148
community benefit, 179
community benefit committee, 186
community collaboration, 19, 404, 411–412, 414, 437, 439
   anchor institutions, 161–162
   community engagement, 160
   emergency preparedness and response, 162–163
   health policy advocacy, 160–161
   volunteerism, 163
community health centers, 13
community health needs assessments (CHNAs), 146, 147, 149, 151, 153, 201, 412–413, 414
community hospitals, 12
community standards of care, 158
community volunteerism, 163
compensation, 230–232, 234
compensation committee, 186
compensation philosophy, 231
competency models, 18
competency-based education, 17–18
competitive advantage, 44, 202–203, 241, 370
competitors, 198, 267
compliance department, 234
compliance programs, 132–134
composite score/scoring, 276, 294
comprehensive budgeting, 385
comprehensive outpatient rehabilitation facilities, 14
conclusions (alternative solutions), 49
confidence, and executive presence, 65
confirmation bias, 33
conflict management, 61–62, 99, 406

conflicts of interest, 130, 178, 340
consent agenda, 185
constructive criticism, 97
Consumer Assessment of Healthcare Providers and Systems (CAHPS), 215, 289, 315, 316
consumer governance, 183
context management, 160
contingency leadership, 95
contingency plans, 162
contingent staffing, 235
continuous budget, 385
continuous quality improvement, 317
continuum of care, 10–11, 262–263, 412
contracting, 62–64, 340
contractual allowance, 377
contribution margin, 386
control chart, 322
controller/comptroller, 360–361
convenient care and retail clinics, 13
coordinated divisional structures, 264
coordinating council, 180
coordination of health services, 259
co-payments, 368
core competencies
  career, 198
  of health care organizations, 196–198
corporate social responsibility, 178
corporate strategy, 203–207
cost accounting/costing, 372
  activity-based, 373–375
  traditional, 372–373
cost center, 372
cost control, 369–371
cost driver, 372, 373
cost leadership, 203
cost reimbursement contract, 341
cost sharing, 368
cost-based reimbursement, 364
cost-benefit analysis (CBA), 47, 388
cost-efficient care, 158–159
costs (project constraint), 337
County Health Rankings and Roadmaps program, 149, 150, 152
Cover Alabama, 160
cover letters, 214
COVID-19 pandemic, 97, 104–105, 259, 267, 337, 405
CPHQ. *See* Certified Professional in Healthcare Quality
CPHRM. *See* Certified Professional in Health Care Risk Management
CPPS. *See* Certified Professional in Patient Safety

CPT. *See* Current Procedural Terminology codes
credentials, 119–120, 233
creditworthiness, 362
crisis communications plan, 215
criterion deficiency, 293, 421
critical access hospitals, 12
critical path, 346
critical thinking, 32–34, 43
cultural competence, 132, 133
current assets, 378
current liabilities, 378
Current Procedural Terminology (CPT) codes, 284, 365, 368
current ratio, 381
cushion ratio, 382
CVS, 205
CVS Kidney Care, 205

dark leadership, 99–101, 102–103, 405–407
dashboards, performance, 291, 292
data analytics, 157
data mining, 47
data visualization techniques, 46
data warehouses, 48, 291
days cash on hand, 381
days in accounts receivable, 381
debriefs, 69, 70
debt financing, 362
debt service coverage ratio, 382
debt-to-capitalization ratio, 382
decentralized organizations, 261–262, 265
decision criteria, 43–45, 409
decision-making, 253, 262
  cognitive bias in career decision-making, 34
  and ethical analysis, 129
  heuristic, 32
  in meetings, 68
  shared, 94, 181, 257
Declaration of Helsinki, 135
deductible ratio, 381
deferred revenue, 388
Define, Measure, Analyze, Improve and Control (DMAIC), 322, 323
defined-contribution plan, 232
DEI. *See* diversity, equity, inclusion
delegation, 252–253
delivery (presentation), 71–72
denied claims, 369
deontology, 128
department or profession councils, 181
departmentalization, 252

dependency (activity), 345
depreciation, 379
depreciation and amortization expense, 377
descriptive statistics, 46
design thinking method, 36, 37, 43, 48
diagnosis-related groups (DRGs), 365
dialysis centers, 13
direct costs, 371, 372
director of strategic planning, 345
discharge lounge, 41, 260
disclosure, 126–127
discounted cash flow method, 386–387
discrimination, 132, 234, 238
    definition of, 132
    examples of, 133
    unintentional, 235
disparate impact, 235
disproportionate share hospitals, 12
diversification, 205
diversity, equity, inclusion (DEI), 21–22, 126, 228–229, 238, 242, 278, 279, 399–402
division of labor, 252, 258
divisionalized organizations, 261, 265
DMAIC. *See* Define, Measure, Analyze, Improve and Control
dogs (BCG matrix), 206
Donabedian's healthcare quality measurement, 311
downside risk contracts, 154, 155
dramatic presentation, 73, 74, 401
DRGs. *See* diagnosis-related groups
Drucker, Peter, 3–4
Drucker's 5 steps (problem-solving), 35, 36
duration (activities and tasks), 345
duty of care (board of directors), 178
duty of loyalty (board of directors), 178
duty of obedience (board of directors), 178
dyad model of authority and responsibility, 257–258, 265

economies of scale, 204
education of health services managers, 118–119
EEOC. *See* Equal Employment Opportunity Commission
effectiveness, 282–283
efficiency, 282–283, 285–286, 370
effort (cost), 349
egalitarianism, 129
EHRs. *See* electronic health records
EI. *See* emotional intelligence
Eisenhower Principle, 37
electronic collaboration tools, 78

electronic health records (EHRs), 48, 157, 159, 163, 240, 368, 419, 420
electronic medical records, 203, 211, 291
elevator pitches, 66
eligibility verification, insurance, 368
emails, 78, 406
emergency departments, 13
Emergency Medical Treatment and Labor Act (EMTALA), 133
Emergency Nurses Association, 313
Emergency Operations Plan, 162
emergency preparedness and response, 162–163, 429
emotional intelligence (EI), 96, 406
    relationship management, 99
    self-awareness, 96–97
    self-management, 97–98
emotional self-control, 97
empathy, 37, 72, 98
Employee Retirement Income Security Act of 1974 (ERISA), 234
employee(s). *See also* human resource management
    compliance programs, 132
    engagement, 209, 242
    interpersonal relationships of managers with, 58
    leader's assumptions about, 95
    meeting loads of, 67
    morale of, 93
    performance evaluations, 237, 293–295
    performance self-assessments, 237
    prioritizing, 10
    psychological safety of, 59–61
    relations, 233
    retention, 215, 236
    rewards for, 296
    safety, 239
    satisfaction, 44, 215
    turnover rates, 236
    well-being, 239, 279
EMTALA. *See* Emergency Medical Treatment and Labor Act
end-of-life care, 135
engagement, employee, 209, 242
enlightened self-interest, 125
environmental services, 16, 307
environmental sustainability, 323, 402–405
epidemiologic planning model, 201
epidemiology, 148, 201–202
Equal Employment Opportunity Commission (EEOC), 234, 238
Equal Pay Act of 1963, 234

equity. *See* diversity, equity, inclusion (DEI)
equity (finance), 362
equity theory, 296
ERISA. *See* Employee Retirement Income Security Act of 1974
ethical dilemma(s), 404
   in business of healthcare, 129–131
   clinical ethics, 135
   definition, 129
   practice for responding to, 130
ethical leadership, 93
ethics, 19, 44, 118, 401, 404, 414, 436, 439. *See also* professionalism
   clinical, 134–135
   codes of, 128, 401
   ethical principles of board practice, 178
   future directions, 136
   in marketing, 209–210
   organizational, 131–134
   professional, 127–131
   research, 135–136
ethics committee, 135
ethos (rhetoric), 70, 71
evidence-based management, 398, 400–401, 409, 422, 435, 439. *See also* problem-solving
   challenges, 34
   critical thinking and bias, 32–34
   evidence-based problem-solving, 34
   systematic approaches to problem-solving, 34–36
evidence-based medicine, 34
excess margin, 381
excessive pay, 131
executive committee, 185
executive presence, 64–65, 120
executive sessions, 185
executive summary (business report), 77
expansion strategies, 204–205
expense recognition principle. *See* matching principle
expenses, 369–370, 377, 380, 382
   types of, 371–372
   using budget to control, 371
expert power, 101
explanation presentation, 73, 74
external environmental assessment, 199–202
extrinsic rewards, 296

FACHE® credential (Fellow of the American College of Healthcare Executives), 120
facilitators (meeting), 68
facilities (operations support service), 16

Failure Mode and Effects Analysis (FMEA), 312–313
Fair Labor Standards Act, 234
fall prevention training, 239
False Claims Act, 132
family
   patient and family advisory councils, 183–184
   role in healthcare quality management, 307
Family and Medical Leave Act (FMLA), 234
Fayol, Henri, 2–3, 6, 383
Federal Trade Commission (FTC), 201
Federal-wide Assurance of Compliance, 135
fee schedules, 365
feedback, 7, 58, 61, 97, 106, 107, 173, 183, 291, 293, 294, 398, 400, 401
fee-for-service payment model, 153, 285, 365, 388, 411
fidelity, 124
fiduciary responsibility of board of directors, 178, 404
finance and audit committee, 185
financial accounting, 361
financial analyses, 199
financial assistance. *See* charity care
financial controls, 363
financial management. *See* healthcare financial management
financial ratios and metrics, 199
   analyzing and interpreting financial reports, 380
   asset efficiency ratios, 382–383
   capital structure ratios, 382
   labor cost ratios and metrics, 383
   liquidity ratios, 381
   profitability ratios, 380, 381
financial reserves, 361
financial statements
   balance sheet, 378–379
   cash flow statement, 379–380
   importance of, 375
   income statement, 375–377
findings (alternative solutions), 48–49
fiscal year, 375
fishbone diagram, 39, 40
Five Forces Model, 200–201, 420
five whys analysis, 38
fixed budget, 385
fixed costs, 371, 372
fixed staffing, 235
fixed-price contracts, 341
flat organizational structure, 254–255
flexible budget, 385
flexible spending account, 231

flexible staffing, 235
flowcharts, 319, 417
FMEA. *See* Failure Mode and Effects Analysis
FMLA. *See* Family and Medical Leave Act
food services, 16, 307
forced distribution, 294
forecasting, 47
for-profit health care organizations, 2, 8–9, 176, 179, 205
   charity care in, 369
   financing of, 362
fragmented care, 260–261, 262–263
framing, problem, 40–41
fraud and abuse, 132
freestanding emergency departments, 13
FTC. *See* Federal Trade Commission
functional authority, 253
functional level strategy, 208
functional organizational structure, 252, 265
functional protocols, 250
functional training, 238
fund balance. *See* net assets

GAAP. *See* Generally Accepted Accounting Principles
Gantt chart, 347, 348
gap analysis, 352
Gemba walk, 318
general ledger, 362
Generally Accepted Accounting Principles (GAAP), 375
Geographic Information System (GIS), 147
GIS. *See* Geographic Information System
global capitation, 155
goal setting
   common healthcare goals, 282–286
   defining targets, 286, 287
   definition of, 281
   linking strategic objectives to goals, 281–282
Google Project Management Professional Certificate, 343
governance. *See* healthcare governance
governance committees, 185–186, 305
GPOs. *See* group purchasing organizations
gravitas, 64–65
grievance complaint, 233
group purchasing organizations (GPOs), 63, 266
groupthink, 33

halo effect, 229
hazardous chemicals and bloodborne pathogens training, 239

HCA Healthcare, 262
HCAHPS. *See* Hospital Consumer Assessment of Healthcare Providers and Systems
HCOs. *See* health care organizations
"heads in beds" incentives, 153
health and safety training, 239
health behaviors, 149–151
health care organizations (HCOs), 1, 2. *See also* health services management
   business model of, 207
   consolidation, 10, 186, 216–217
   continuum of care, 10–11
   environmental impacts of, 323
   for-profit, 2, 8–9, 176, 179, 205, 362, 369
   not-for-profit, 2, 8–9, 146, 156, 176, 179, 205, 362, 369, 370
   partnerships/collaborations of, 160, 161
   payments to, 365–366
health disparities, 21, 126, 157, 177, 415
health equity, 21–22, 126, 157, 177, 415
health information exchanges, 48
health information management, 16
health information technology, 157
Health Information Technology for Economic and Clinical Health (HITECH) Act of 2009, 133
Health Insurance Portability and Accountability Act of 1996 (HIPAA), 133, 134, 234
health maintenance organizations (HMOs), 364
health outcomes, definition of, 149
health policy, 201
   advocacy, 160–161
   consumer governance, 183
health promotion, 159
health service demand, calculation of, 201–202
health service utilization, 157
health services management, 1–2, 118
   ancillary services, 15, 16
   balancing margin and mission, 136
   careers, 22–23
   competencies, 17–18, 19
   in the continuum of care, 10–11
   diversity, equity and inclusion, 21–22
   future directions, 24
   inpatient settings, 11–12
   interprofessional team, 18–21
   long-term care (post-acute care) settings, 14–15
   negotiating first positions in, 231
   operations support services, 15, 16–17
   outpatient settings, 12–14
   problems, 32, 425–430
   specialist *versus* generalist, 17
   staff roles/management roles, 17

health services management scenarios/projects, 433–434
  assessing community health needs, 412–415
  dark leadership, 405–407
  DEI initiative, 399–402
  designing an accountable care organization, 415–417
  home health business plan, 417–421
  interprofessional team conflict, 397–399
  medical model *vs.* population health model, 410–412
  performance review, 421–423
  resisting private equity investors, 407–409
  triple bottom line, 402–405
health services managers, 1–2, 118, 304, 435
  analyzing career alternatives, 43
  asking for raise, 365
  early-career, 9, 34, 63, 69, 70, 92, 107, 124, 226–232, 253, 257, 317, 360, 371
  evolution of, 8–9
  impaired, 131
  late-career, 23, 360
  and managers in healthcare businesses, 2
  mid-career, 17, 62, 107, 257, 360
  and physicians, conflict between, 62
  responsibilities of, 9–10
  self-management, 22
health system (integrated delivery network), 10–11
Healthcare Effectiveness Data and Information Set (HEDIS), 275
healthcare financial management, 19, 359–360, 405, 417, 439, 440
  budgeting and planning, 383–388
  cost control, 369–371
  financial ratios and metrics, 380–383
  financial statements, 375–380
  future directions, 388
  healthcare finance organization, 360–363
  personal financial planners, 362
  and population health, 153–155
  revenue, 363–369
  traditional costing, 372–373
  types of expenses, 371–372
Healthcare Financial Management Association (HFMA), 120, 128
healthcare governance, 19, 171–172, 404, 409, 417, 437, 439
  charters and bylaws, 184–185
  committee membership and structures, 185–186
  engagement of medical staff in, 174–175
  future directions, 189
  health system governance structure, 188
  inclusion of nurses and other clinicians in, 175
  managing the boss, 173
  multiorganization governance, 186, 188
  organization governance structure, 185
  policies and procedures, 186, 187
  power sharing, 171
  relationship between board of directors and CEO, 172–173
  role of board of directors in, 175–179
  role of clinicians in, 179–183
  role of patients in, 183–184
  supporting the board of directors, 174
Healthcare Leadership Alliance model, 18, 119
healthcare quality management, 19, 303–304, 404, 412, 417, 439, 440
  access to care, 314, 315
  future directions, 324
  healthcare quality organization, 304–308
  high reliability health care organizations, 322–324
  Lean, 317–320
  methodologies and philosophies, 317
  patient experience, 314–316
  patient safety, 311–313
  quality and safety culture, 308–310
  quality measurement, 311, 426
  Six Sigma, 321–322
  workplace safety, 313–314
healthcare strategy, 195–196, 420–421, 437, 439
  business unit strategy, 207–208
  competitive advantage, 202–203
  corporate strategy, 203–207
  external environmental assessment, 199–202
  functional level strategy, 208
  internal environmental assessment, 196–199
Healthy People 2030
  high priority health behavior measures, 151
  high priority health status measures, 149
HEDIS. *See* Healthcare Effectiveness Data and Information Set
Hennepin Health, 159–160
Herfindahl–Hirschman Index (HHI), 200–201, 420
heuristic decision-making, 32
HFMA. *See* Healthcare Financial Management Association
HHI. *See* Herfindahl–Hirschman Index
HICS. *See* Hospital Incident Command System
high reliability health care organizations, 322–324
Hill-Burton Act, 8
hip replacement, 263
HIPAA. *See* Health Insurance Portability and Accountability Act of 1996

hiring, 253
  negligent, 233
  process, 227–229
hiring managers, 63, 226, 227, 229, 230, 305
HITECH. *See* Health Information Technology for Economic and Clinical Health Act of 2009
HMOs. *See* health maintenance organizations
home healthcare, 14, 286–289, 405–406, 417–421
horizontal expansion, 205
horizontal integration, 204–205
hospice homes, 15
Hospital Compare, 275, 308, 315
Hospital Consumer Assessment of Healthcare Providers and Systems (HCAHPS), 68, 289, 293, 315
Hospital Incident Command System (HICS), 162
hospital outpatient centers, 13
Hospital Readmissions Reduction Program (HRRP), 159, 308
Hospital-Acquired Condition Reduction Program, 308
hostile working environment, 233
HRBPs. *See* human resources business partners
HRIS. *See* human resources information system
HRRP. *See* Hospital Readmissions Reduction Program
huddles, 69, 70
human participants in research, 135
human resource management, 225, 401, 416, 421, 423, 438, 439
  administrative functions, 226
  compensation and benefits, 230–232
  employee relations, 233
  employee safety and well-being, 239
  interviewing, 229–230
  job analysis, 226–227
  job applications, 227
  laws and regulations, 233–235
  onboarding, 232
  organizational culture, 241–242
  performance evaluations, 237
  physician recruitment and retention, 241
  recruitment, 227–229
  selection, 230
  staffing, 235
  strategic, 239–240, 241, 242
  succession planning, 241
  training and organizational development, 237–239
  unions and collective bargaining, 240–241
  workforce planning, 240
  workload forecasting, 235–236
human resources business partners (HRBPs), 232–233, 236, 237
human resources information system (HRIS), 232
hybrid work arrangements, 78
hypothesis-driven thinking, 43

ICD-10. *See* International Classification of Diseases, 10th Revision
ICUs. *See* intensive care units
ideating, 43
IHI. *See* Institute for Healthcare Improvement
imaging and radiology services, 16
implementation intentions, 130
incentives, performance, 295–296
incidence, definition of, 149
inclusion. *See* diversity, equity, inclusion (DEI)
inclusiveness, 60
income statement, 375–377
incremental budgeting, 385
independent practice associations (IPAs), 13
indirect costs, 371, 372, 373, 374
inferential statistics, 47
informational interviews, 124
informed consent, 134, 135
initial project scoping workshop, 339–340
innovation, 36, 44, 97, 430
inpatient readmissions, 37–38, 89–90
inpatient rehabilitation facilities, 12, 15
inpatient settings, 11–12
inspirational leadership, 99
Institute for Healthcare Improvement (IHI), 308
Institute of Medicine (IOM), 146, 303, 312
institutional review boards (IRBs), 135
intangible assets, 379
intangible resources, 198
integrated delivery systems, 186, 196–197, 264
integrity, 126–127
intensive care units (ICUs), 12, 267
interest expense, 377
internal audit function, 363
internal environmental assessment, 196–199
internal marketing, 215–216
internal rate of return, 386–387
Internal Revenue Service (IRS), 146, 179, 413
International Classification of Diseases, 10th Revision (ICD-10), 365, 368
interpersonal communications, 57–58, 399, 401, 403–404, 406, 411, 414, 416, 421, 422–423, 435, 439
  conflict management, 61–62

creating psychological safety, 59–61
future directions, 78
managing interpersonal relationships, 58–59
in meetings, 67–70
negotiation and contracting, 62–64
presentation skills, 70–76
professional reputation, 64–66
written communications, 76–78
interpersonal conflict, 61–62
interpersonal relationships, 58–59, 100
interprofessional team, 18–21
competencies for, 20
conflict, 397–399
interviewing, 229–230
intrinsic rewards, 296
inventory turnover ratio, 382
investment income, 377
investor-owned health care organizations. *See* for-profit health care organizations
IOM. *See* Institute of Medicine
IPAs. *See* independent practice associations
IRBs. *See* institutional review boards
IRS. *See* Internal Revenue Service
Ishikawa diagram. *See* fishbone diagram
issue tree, 40

job analysis, 226–227, 229
job applications, 227
job roles, clarification of, 259–260
job searches, four Ps of, 213
The Johns Hopkins Hospital, 197, 322
The Joint Commission, 186, 233, 239, 276, 308, 322, 323, 337
joint ventures, 264, 265
just culture, 310
justice, 136

Kaiser Permanente, 196–197
kaizen event, 318
kickbacks, 216
knowledge management, 48, 291
knowledge workers, 3
Kotter's 8 Steps of Change, 104, 404, 409
anchoring new approaches in culture, 107
building a guiding coalition, 105
communication of change vision, 106
consolidation of gains and producing more change, 106–107
creating a sense of urgency, 104–105
empowering action, 106
generation of short-term wins, 106

vision and strategy development, 105–106

labor cost to revenues ratio, 383
labor costs
calculation of, 349
ratios and metrics, 383
labor costs per adjusted discharge, 383
labor productivity, 284
laissez-faire leadership style, 94–95
laundry and linens services, 16
law fallacy, 129
law of the instrument, 33
laws/regulations, 44, 176, 419
bylaws, 179, 184–185
ethics, 135
and healthcare strategy, 201
human resources, 233–235
safe harbor, 216
leader-member exchange (LMX), 95
leadership, 87–88, 399, 401, 404, 406, 409, 436, 439. *See also* change management
cost leadership, 203
development programs, 107–108
emotional and social intelligence, 96–99
functions (Northouse), 88
future directions, 107–108
and management, 88
models and theories, 95
and organizational culture, 90–96
power and influence, 99–103
as a process, 103–104
styles, 94–96
training programs, 107
vision setting, 88–90
Lean, 317–320
Lean Six Sigma, 304, 305, 322
legitimate power, 101
Lexington Model, 127
liabilities, 378
licensed independent professionals, 117
life cycle management, 206–207
lifelong learning, 123, 156
line management, 17
line of authority. *See* chain of command
line positions, 257
liquidity, 381
liquidity ratios, 381
LMX. *See* leader-member exchange
logic models, 157–158
logic tree, 39
logos (rhetoric), 70, 71
long-term acute care facilities, 15

long-term assets (noncurrent assets), 378
long-term care settings, 14–15
long-term liabilities (noncurrent liabilities), 378
low-cost strategy, 203

machine bureaucracy, 256
machine learning, 47, 235–236, 240
Magnet Recognition programs, 276
Malcolm Baldrige National Quality Award, 276
maleficence, 135–136
malfeasance, 135
managed care, 363
managed care organizations, 363–364
management, 304
    definitions of, 5–7
    functions
        Drucker, 3–4
        Fayol, 2–3, 383
        Northouse, 88
    and leadership, 88
    problem-solving methods, 35–36
    roles (Mintzberg), 4–5
    and systems theory, 7–8
management by objectives, 4
management letter, 176
management rounds, 61
management services organizations, 13
management-by-walking-around, 118
management-rights clause, 240
managerial accounting, 386
mandatory bargaining issues, 240
market share, 201
marketing, 241, 287, 420–421, 437, 439
    channels, 213
        market segmentation and targeting, 210–212
        marketing mix (four Ps of marketing), 212–213
        trust and ethics in, 209–210
mass casualty emergencies, 251
matching principle, 375
matrix structures, 262
matrixed organizations, 265
Mayo Clinic, 107, 197, 259, 318
McKinsey approach, 36, 40, 43
mediation, 62, 233
Medicaid, 160–161, 275, 363
Medicaid Provider Enrollment, 419
medical errors, 127, 308, 312
Medical Executive Committee, 179
medical futility, 135
Medical Group Management Association (MGMA), 13, 18, 120, 128, 209

medical model, 146, 410–412
medical necessity, 285, 364
medical practices, 12–13, 14, 257
    equity financing of, 362
    governance of, 181–182
    matrix structures in, 262
    and private equity investors, 407–408
medical social work, 16
medical staff
    bylaws, 179, 305
    in healthcare governance, 174–175, 179–180
    organization, 180
medical-surgical hospitals, 12
Medicare, 263, 264, 275, 284–285, 308, 315, 366, 419
Medicare Recovery Audit Program (RAC), 132
Medicare Shared Savings Program (MSSP), 154–155, 264, 308, 415, 417
meeting load, 67
meeting(s), 401
    agenda, 67, 68, 352
    participation in, 67
    planning, coordinating and facilitating, 67–68
    post-project review meeting, 353
    project status, 352
    purpose, 67
    topic, 67
    types of, 68–70
megaproblems, 38–39, 40
mentoring, 99, 125, 238
mergers, 63, 201, 205
Merit-based Incentive Payment System (MIPS), 308
MGMA. *See* Medical Group Management Association
Microsoft Excel, 347
Microsoft Project, 346, 347
middle managers (Mintzberg's organizational framework), 256
Military Health System, 11
Minnesota Method, 35–36, 37, 42
minorities
    barriers to career success faced by, 125–126
    and health disparities, 21
    and pay equity, 231
Mintzberg, Henry, 4–5
MinuteClinic, 205
MIPS. *See* Merit-based Incentive Payment System
mission, 44, 136, 196, 197
modeling of behaviors, 132
monopolistic competition, 201
monopoly, 200

moral distress, 130
moral injury, 130
moral legitimacy, 93
moral-rights approach, 129
morals, 127
MSSP. *See* Medicare Shared Savings Program
multiculturalism, 121
multidimensional appraisal, 294

narcissism, 99
narrative presentation, 73–75
National Association for Healthcare Quality, 305
National Association of Health Services Executives, 66
National Association of Long-Term Care Administrator Boards, 14
National Center for Health Statistics, 150, 152
National Committee for Quality Assurance (NCQA), 275, 308
National Incident Management System (NIMS), 162
National Labor Relations Act, 240
natural language processing, 47
NCQA. *See* National Committee for Quality Assurance
near misses, 310
negligence, 276
negligent hiring, 233
negotiation(s), 62–64, 217, 231, 240
    BATNA (best alternative to a negotiated agreement), 63–64
    deceptive behaviors during, 101
    salary, 63
net assets, 378
net income/loss, 377
net operating income, 376, 377
net patient service revenues, 377
net present value (NPV), 387
net profit, 376
net promoter score (NPS), 290, 315–316
network diagram. *See* Program Evaluation Review Technique (PERT) chart
networking, 66, 124–126, 162
never events, 276
NIMS. *See* National Incident Management System
99214 (CPT code), 284
nominating and governance committee, 186
nonmaleficence, 136
nonoperating revenue, 376, 377
nonverbal communication, 72
Northwell Health Physician Partners, 197

not-for-profit health care organizations, 2, 8–9, 156, 176, 369
    CHNAs of, 146
    financing of, 362
    representation of external stakeholders in, 179
    retained earnings, 370
NPS. *See* net promoter score
NPV. *See* net present value
Nuremberg Code, 135
nurse(s), 256
    in healthcare governance, 175, 180, 181
    patient-to-nurse ratio, 282–283, 322
    performance evaluations for, 293
    staffing, 282–283
    staffing matrix, 236
    standard operating procedures for, 251
    and workplace safety, 313–314
nursing home administrators, 14, 118
nursing homes, 14, 15

Oak Street Health, 205
Occupational Safety and Health Act, 234
Occupational Safety and Health Administration (OSHA), 239
occupational therapy, 16
offsite meetings, 69, 70
oligopoly, 201
onboarding, 232
one-on-one meetings, 69, 70
open system, 7
operating core (Mintzberg's organizational framework), 256
operating expenses, 371, 377
operating margin, 380, 381
operating profit margin, 287
operating revenues, 377
operational budgeting, 383–384, 385
operational efficiency, 285–286
operational plan, 208
operational scorecards, 290–291
operationalization, 282
operations support services, 15, 16–17
organizational awareness, 98
organizational chart, 252, 407, 416
organizational culture, 90, 241–242
    future directions, 242
    incorporation of changes into, 107
    leadership styles, 94–96
    positive leadership theories, 93–94
    quality and safety culture, 308–310, 323
    role modeling, 90–91
    teamwork and collaborative leadership, 91–93

organizational design, 249–250, 407, 412, 416, 438, 440
   alternatives to functional structure, 258–259
   authority and responsibility, 252–255
   centralized and decentralized organizations, 261–262
   clarifying health services roles, 259–260
   clinical protocols, 251
   cooperation among competitors, 267
   coordinated divisional structures, 264
   coordinating health services, 259
   coordinating processes and structures, 260–261
   division of labor, 252
   divisionalized organizations, 261
   dyad model of authority and responsibility, 257–258
   future directions, 267
   organizational affiliations and alliances, 265
   outsourcing to suppliers, 266
   professional bureaucracy, 255–257
   service line structures, 262–264
   staff and line positions, 257
   standard operating procedures, 250–251
   standardized work, 250
organizational development, 237–239
organizational ethics
   compliance programs, 132–134
   creating ethical cultures, 131–132
organizational framework (Mintzberg), 255–256
organizational norms, adapting to, 120–121
OSHA. *See* Occupational Safety and Health Administration
outpatient settings, 12–14, 261
outsourcing to suppliers, 266
overhead costs. *See* indirect costs
owners' equity. *See* net assets

paid parental leave, 232
paid time off (PTO), 232
paired comparative method, 294
palliative care, 15
Pareto chart, 318, 319
parking lot (meeting), 68
parliamentary procedures, 184
participative leadership style, 94
participatory management principles, 58
pathos (rhetoric), 70, 71
Pathway to Excellence programs, 276
patient and family advisory councils (PFACs), 183–184
patient care leadership council, 180
patient care volume, 363

patient discharges, 260, 265, 318–319
   delays in, 40, 41, 43, 49
   labor costs per adjusted discharge, 383
patient experience, 44, 89, 146, 154, 215–216, 289–290, 314–316
patient financial services, 307
patient ledger, 369
patient navigators, 259–260
Patient Protection and Affordable Care Act of 2010 (ACA), 70, 89, 146, 154, 160, 182, 264, 308, 415
patient referrals, 216
patient rights and responsibilities, 134
patient rooming process, process flow for, 320
patient satisfaction, 215, 289, 314
patient services, 16
patient surveys, 211, 291
patient throughput, 290, 314
patient transportation services, 17, 307
patient-centered care, 183
patient-centered governance, 183
patient-centered medical homes (PCMHs), 156
patient-centeredness, 314
patient-to-nurse ratio, 282–283, 322
pay equity, 231
payback period, 386
payer mix, 363, 419
payers, 154, 210, 263, 275, 368, 388
pay-for-performance, 153, 155, 275
payviders, 217
PCMHs. *See* patient-centered medical homes
PDSA. *See* Plan-Do-Study-Act
peer review, 179, 305
per diem rate, 366
perfect competition, 200–201
performance evaluations, 237, 293–294, 421
   delivering, 294–295
   receiving, 295
performance improvement plans (PIPs), 233
performance management, 273–274, 401, 404, 412, 417, 421, 438, 440
   accreditors, 276
   awards and recognitions, 276
   benchmarking, 277
   board of directors, 274
   feedback and learning, 291, 293
   future directions, 296
   healthcare perspectives, 278, 279
   monitoring performance, 290–291
   payers, 275
   performance evaluations, 293–295
   performance incentives, 295–296
   ranking organizations, 276–277

regulators, 275
stakeholder view of performance, 274
strategic performance, 277–278
strategic scoreboard, 277–278
strategic scorecard, 278
performance management cycle, 279
communicating strategic objectives, 281
creating short-term initiatives, 286–290
goal setting, 281–286
setting strategic objectives, 280
performance review, 421–423
performance self-assessments, 237
performance standards, 293
personal branding, 65
personal protective equipment (PPE), 259
person-job fit, 230
person-organization fit, 230
PERT. *See* Program Evaluation Review Technique chart
Peter principle, 237
PFACs. *See* patient and family advisory councils
pharmacies, 16
philanthropy, 124, 369
physical environment, 151
physical therapy, 16
physicians, 35, 260. *See also* medical practices
competencies of, 17–18
dyad model of authority and responsibility, 257–258
and evidence-based medicine, 34
fee-for-service payments among primary care *versus* specialist physicians, 365
and health services managers, conflict between, 62
and interpersonal communications, 58
and marketing, 216
medical practice governance, 181–182
recruitment and retention, 241
role in capital budgeting, 385
role in healthcare governance, 174–175
PIPs. *See* performance improvement plans
pitch presentation, 73, 74, 75, 411, 416, 421
placement (marketing mix), 213
Plan-Do-Study-Act (PDSA), 318–319
PMI. *See* Project Management Institute
PMO. *See* Project Management Office
PMP®. *See* Project Management Professional certification
point of service (POS), 364
point-of-service phase (revenue cycle), 368
political guidance, 125
political skills
elements of, 103

of leaders, 102, 406
population health, 19, 45, 279, 404, 410, 411–412, 414, 437, 439
population health assessment
community assets, 148
community health needs assessment, 146, 147
community stakeholders, 146–147
geographic and demographic characteristics, 147
health behaviors, 149–151
health status, 148–149
physical environment, 151
social and economic factors, 151–152
population health management, 411
cost-efficient care, 158–159
financial management, 153–155
functions, 153
health information technology, 157
health promotion, 159
integrating medical and social care, 159–160
program planning and evaluation, 157–158
value-based health care organizational design, 155–157
population health model, 146, 153, 410–412
portfolio management, 205–206
POS. *See* point of service
position descriptions, 226, 227, 229
positive leadership theories, 93–94, 100
positive outlook, 98
positive reinforcement, 295–296
post-acute care
services, 265, 406
settings, 14–15
post-graduate fellowships, 125
postmortem meeting. *See* post-project review meeting
post-project review meeting, 353
post-service phase (revenue cycle), 368–369
power of leaders
organizational checks on, 102–103
sources of, 101–102
PowerPoint, 76
PPE. *See* personal protective equipment
PPOs. *See* preferred provider organizations
practice and professional development council, 181
pragmatic leadership, 95
pre-authorization, 285
pre-employment screening assessments, 203
preferential treatment, 131
preferred provider organizations (PPOs), 364
pre-paid revenue. *See* deferred revenue

presentation, 414
  and audience, 72
  content, 72–75
  delivery, 71–72
  materials, 76
  software, 76
  structure of a change inspiring presentation compared to a traditional story, 75
  types, goals, and rhetorical devices, 73
  verbal, 70–71
pre-service phase (revenue cycle), 368
press releases, 214, 215
prevalence, definition of, 148–149
price of health services, 203, 364, 370
price transparency, 368
pricing (marketing mix), 213
primary care clinics, 14
prior authorization, 364
private equity funds, 407
private equity investors, 362, 407–410
problem analysis, 37–40
problem definition
  framing and reframing problems, 40–41
  problem analysis, 37–40
  stakeholder analysis, 36–37
problem statement, 40, 41, 398, 401, 409
problems, health services management, 31–32, 425
  adaptation, 427
  emergency preparedness and response, 429
  growth opportunities, 426–427
  innovations, 430
  management control and monitoring, 425–426
  opportunities for improvement, 428–429
  reliable patient care processes, 429–430
  resource allocation, 427, 428
problem-solving, 31–32, 173, 398, 400–401, 409, 422, 435, 439
  alternative solutions, 42–45
    analyzing, 45–50
  decision criteria, 43–45
  defining the problem, 36–41
  evidence-based, 34
  future directions, 50
  hypothesis-driven thinking, 43
  systematic approaches to, 34–36
process improvement, 319
process maps, 319–320
procurement office, 340, 341
product (marketing mix), 212–213
productivity, 284–285, 370
professional bureaucracy, 255–257
professional development, 22–23, 124–125, 237

professional ethics
  ethical analysis and decision-making, 129
  ethical dilemmas in business of healthcare, 129–131
  for health services managers, 127–128
professional legitimacy, 118
professional reputation, 78
  executive presence, 64–65
  networking, 66
  personal branding, 65
professionalism, 19, 118, 401, 404, 414, 436, 439. *See also* ethics
  adapting to organizational norms, 120–121
  building professional connections, 124–126
  contribution to community, 123–124
  credentials, 119–120
  education, 118–119
  elements of, 119
  future directions, 136
  integrity, 126–127
  lifelong learning, 123
  self-management, 123
  trusting relationships, 118
  valuing diversity, equity, and inclusion, 126
  work ethic, 121–122
profit and loss statement. *See* income statement
profit margin, 376, 380
profitability ratios, 380, 381
Program Evaluation Review Technique (PERT) chart, 347
program planning and evaluation, 157–158
progressive discipline systems, 233
project charter, 338–339
project closure
  celebration of successes, 354
  sign off, 353
  transition to operations, 353–354
project initiation
  initial project scoping, 339–340
  project authorization, 338–339
  project procurement, 340–341
project management, 335–336, 401–402, 417, 439, 440
  change control, 351
  early-career, 340
  examples of projects and ongoing operations, 336
  future directions, 354
  late-career, 353
  mid-career, 343
  project closure, 353–354
  project constraints, 337–338
  project initiation, 338–341

project monitoring and communication, 351–352
project planning, 341–349
project risk management, 350
temporary work under tight deadlines, 336
Project Management Institute (PMI), 337, 343
Project Management Office (PMO), 343
Project Management Professional (PMP)® certification, 343
project planning
   activity sequencing, 345
   budget estimation, 347, 349
   project plan, 341–342, 351, 401, 417
   project schedule, 343, 345
   responsibility matrix (RACI matrix), 342–343, 344, 345
   visualizing project timelines, 346–347
project schedule, 343, 345
project sponsor, 338, 339, 350, 351, 353
project status meetings, 352
project timelines, visualizing, 346–347
promise-making, 127
promotion (marketing mix), 213
promotional mix
   branding, advertising, and public relations, 214–215
   internal marketing, 215–216
   marketing to clinicians, 216
prospective payment system, 365
prototyping, 48
proxy, 134
psychological safety, 59–61, 174
PTO. *See* paid time off
public relations, 184, 215

qualified retirement plan, 231
quality and patient safety committee, 185
quality and safety council, 180
quality and safety culture, 323
   empowering self-reliance and responsibility, 309–310
   just culture, 310
   promotion of, 308–309
quality improvement teams, 305–306
quality management. *See* healthcare quality management
quality of care, definition of, 303
question marks (BCG matrix), 205–206

RAC. *See* Medicare Recovery Audit Program
raise, asking for, 365
ranking organizations, 276–277

rating scale method, 294
REACH. *See* ACO Realizing Equity, Access, and Community Health Model
realistic job previews, 230
reasonable accommodations, 226, 234
recommendations (alternative solutions), 49
recruitment, 227–229
   challenges, 228
   of new board members, 177–178
   physician, 241
referent power, 101
reframing, problem, 40–41
regression analysis, 47
regulators, 179, 186, 275, 419–420
rehabilitation therapy team, 16
reimbursements, 364
relationship conflict, 61–62
relationship management, 99
relative value units (RVUs), 284–285, 365
reliability (healthcare quality), 303–304
replacement charts, 241, 242
reports, 73, 76–77, 403–404, 423
representational governance, 182–183
representativeness bias, 33
request for proposal (RFP), 266, 341
research ethics, 135–136
research questions, 44–45
reservation price, 63, 64
reserved powers, 261
resilience, 123
resource allocation, 179, 427, 428
respect for persons, 135
responsibility, 23, 252–255
   dyad model of, 257–258
   empowering, 309–310
   fiduciary responsibility of board of directors, 178, 404
   social, 279, 403
responsibility matrix (RACI matrix), 342–343, 344, 345
résumé screening process, 235
retained earnings, 370, 377
retaliatory discharge, 132, 233
retention, employee, 95, 215, 236, 238, 241
return on total assets, 381
return-on-investment, 386
revenue, healthcare
   payments to health care organizations, 365–366
   philanthropy, 369
   revenue cycle management, 367–369
   seeking growth, 363
   third-party payers, 363–364
reward power, 101

rewards, 99, 100, 124, 290, 296
RFP. *See* request for proposal
risk adjustment, 157, 283
risk management, 306
   professionals, 306
   project, 350
risk stratification, 157
risk-based financing, 154
Robert's Rules of Order, 184
role modeling, 90–91
root cause analysis, 38, 39, 318
rural hospitals, 12, 204
RVUs. *See* relative value units

safe harbor regulations, 216
safe patient handling programs, 239
safety
   culture, 308–310
   employee, 239
   patient, 44, 179, 181, 274, 311–313
   psychological, 59–61, 174
   workplace, 313–314
safety and security (operations support service), 17
safety-net hospitals, 12
salary, 63, 231, 370
salary bands, 231
salespeople, 216
Sarbanes-Oxley Act of 2002, 176
scholarly journals, 48
scientific method, 34–35
scope (project constraint), 337
scope creep, 351
scope of work (SOW), 341
security staff, 307
segmentation, market, 210–212
Select Physical Therapy, 197
selection of candidates (hiring), 230
self-awareness, 96–97
self-dealing, 130
self-evaluation, 123
self-management, 22, 97–98, 123
self-pay, 364
self-protective behaviors of leaders, 100–101
self-serving bias, 33
sentinel events, 276
servant leadership, 93
service differentiation strategy, 202–203
service line organizational structures, 262–264, 265
service mix, 363
service-level agreement (SLA), 341
shared governance, 175

shared governance councils, 180–181
shared vision/values, 89–90
Sherman Anti-Trust Act, 201
short-term disability insurance, 232
short-term strategic initiatives, 286–290
SHRM. *See* strategic human resource management
Signify, 205
situational interviews, 229
situational leadership, 95
Six Sigma, 321–322
skill mix (staffing), 235, 236
skilled nursing facilities, 15
SLA. *See* service-level agreement
SMART goal framework, 281–282, 293, 404
social care partnerships, 159
social determinants of health, 151–152, 159, 163, 410
social health navigators, 159
social learning theory, 91
social media, 215
social responsibility, 178, 279, 403
social risks, 37, 151, 159, 163
solution bias, 33
SOPs. *See* standard operating procedures
SOW. *See* scope of work
span of control, 254
special cause variation, 322
special committees, 185
specialization, 252
specialty hospitals, 12
speech-language pathology, 16
sponsorship, 125
St. Michael's Hospital (Toronto), 107
staff meetings, 69, 70
staff positions, 257
staffing, 235, 242, 282–283
   budgets, 384
   understaffing, 130
staffing matrix, 236
stage-fright, 72
stakeholder analysis, 36–37
stakeholder identification and prioritization theory, 275
stakeholders, 413
   accountability to, 274–277
   career stakeholders, 275
   external, 36, 179, 307–308
   internal, 36
   and population health assessment, 146–147
standard operating procedures (SOPs), 250–251
standardized work, 250
standing committees, 185

Stanford Health Care Cancer Center, 258
STAR technique, 229–230
Stark Laws, 216
stars (BCG matrix), 205
statistical modeling, 47
statistical variation, 321
status meetings, 69, 70
status reports, 351–352
stewardship, 123–124
storytelling, 73, 74
strategic alliance, 205
strategic apex (Mintzberg's organizational framework), 256
strategic business units, 207, 261–262
strategic direction, 175, 196
strategic human resource management (SHRM), 239–240, 241, 242
strategic management process, 208
strategic objectives, 45
   clinical quality, 283
   communicating, 281
   linking to goals, 281–282
   setting, 280
strategic planning committee, 185
strategic scoreboard, 277–278
strategic scorecard, 278
stress management, 123
structured interviews, 229
subject-matter experts, 340
subsidiary boards, 188
succession planning, 125, 241
sunk cost fallacy, 33
superconnectors, 162
supply chain, 17, 266
support staff (Mintzberg's organizational framework), 256
Surgical Safety Checklist, 250
Sutter Health, 106
swim lane diagram, 320, 417
switching costs, 216
SWOT (strengths, weaknesses, opportunities, and threats) analysis, 198, 199, 200, 420
systematic reviews, 48
systems theory, 7–8
systems thinking, 7

tall organizational structure, 254
tangible assets, 378–379
tangible resources, 198
targeting, market, 210–212
targets (goal setting), 286, 287
task conflict, 61

Taylorism, 250
TDABC. *See* time-driven activity-based costing
team leadership, 92
teamwork, 91–93, 99
technostructure (Mintzberg's organizational framework), 256
telehealth, 156, 267
telemedicine, 104–105
Texas Health Resources, 93
ThedaCare, 317
Theory X (leadership), 95
Theory Y (leadership), 95
third-party payers, 203, 209, 213, 363–364
threat of substitution, 201
360-degree feedback, 294
time (project constraint), 337
time and materials contract, 341
time management, 123
time value of money, 386
time-driven activity-based costing (TDABC), 374–375
timeliness of care, 314
Time's Up Healthcare, 107
top-down budget, 349
tortious interference, 131
total asset turnover, 382
total expense per provider full-time equivalent, 383
total nonoperating revenue, 377
total operating expenses, 377
total operating revenues, 377
total patient service revenues, 277
town hall meetings, 69, 70
toxic leadership, 99–101, 102–103, 405–407
traditional costing, 372–373
training, employee, 237–239
transformational leadership, 93
transparency, 126, 182
trauma centers, 12, 251
travel nurses, 235
treasurer, 361–362
Triple Aim framework, 146, 308
triple bottom line, 178, 402–405
triple constraint model, 337–338, 351
trust, 59, 72, 118, 174, 175, 178, 182, 209–210
trustees. *See* board of directors
truthiness, 32
tuition reimbursement, 232
Tuskegee Syphilis Study, 135
two-sided risk contracts, 155

UAB Medicine, 337
uncompensated care, 364

understaffing, 130
unintentional discrimination, 235
unions, 240–241
unity of command, 262
University of Wisconsin, 149
unrelated business income, 131
unrestricted donations, 377
unstructured method (performance evaluation), 294
upcoding, 132
upside risk contracts, 154, 155
URAC. See Utilization Review Accreditation Commission
urgent care clinics, 14
U.S. Agency for Healthcare Research and Quality, 152
U.S. Office of Disease Prevention and Health Promotion, 149
utilitarianism, 129
utilization management, 158
utilization review, 285, 363
Utilization Review Accreditation Commission (URAC), 276

value chain analysis, 198–199
value proposition, 213
value-based health care, 154, 156, 158, 159, 160
　organizational design, 155–157
　payment types, 155
　value equation for, 154
value-based payment models, 89, 263, 275, 366, 388, 415, 417
values, 44, 89, 91, 100, 196, 197
variable costs, 371, 372
vendors
　contract closures, 353
　contracts with, 340, 341
　selection criteria, 341
verbal presentation, 70–72
vertical integration, 204–205, 213
Veterans Health Administration (VHA), 10, 127
VHA. See Veterans Health Administration
videoconferencing applications, 78
violence
　prevention programs, 239
　workplace, 313–314
Virginia Mason Medical Center, 317
virtual meetings, 78
virtual technologies, 267
visibility, 60–61
vision, 74, 105–106, 196, 197

vision setting (leadership)
　career success, 90
　gaining commitment to a shared vision, 89–90
　imagining the future, 89
　management and leadership, 88
　planning future action, 90
volunteerism, 124, 163

WACC. See weighted average cost of capital
Washington Permanente Medical Group, 197
waste (muda), reducing, 318
waste audit, 404
WBS. See work breakdown structure
weighted average cost of capital (WACC), 387
well-being, employee, 239, 279
WellStar Kennestone Regional Medical Center, 260
whistleblowing, 128, 132
WHO. See World Health Organization
wicked problems, 50
women
　barriers to career success faced by, 125–126
　in executive positions, 178
　hiring of, 228–229
　and pay equity, 231
work breakdown structure (WBS), 341–342, 345, 401, 417
work ethic, 121–122
workforce
　planning, 240
　reductions, 131
　shortages, 130, 419
　transformations, 3
workforce analytics, 240
working capital, 367, 378
workload forecasting, 235–236
workplace safety, 313–314
workplace wellness programs, 239
World Health Organization (WHO), 250
written communications
　business reports, 76–77
　business writing style, 76
　emails and collaboration tools, 78
WVU Hospitals and Health Systems, 105

zero based budgeting, 385
zone of possible agreement (ZOPA), 63
Zoom fatigue, 78
ZOPA. See zone of possible agreement